‘Essentials of Cancer Genomic, Computational Approaches and Precision Medicine

Nosheen Masood • Saima Shakil Malik
Editors

'Essentials of Cancer Genomic, Computational Approaches and Precision Medicine

Springer

Editors
Nosheen Masood
Fatima Jinnah Women University
Rawalpindi, Pakistan

Saima Shakil Malik
Fatima Jinnah Women University
Rawalpindi, Pakistan

Armed Forces Institute of Pathology
Rawalpindi, Pakistan

ISBN 978-981-15-1066-3 ISBN 978-981-15-1067-0 (eBook)
https://doi.org/10.1007/978-981-15-1067-0

This Springer imprint is published by the registered company Springer Nature Singapore Pte Ltd.
The registered company address is: 152 Beach Road, #21-01/04 Gateway East, Singapore 189721, Singapore

This book is dedicated to the patients and their families in the past and future, who have both encouraged and will one day benefit from the countless advancements in cancer genomics, and to our own families for their ongoing patience and support for this book.

Foreword

Incidence of cancer in developing countries is rising at much faster pace than improvement in health care facilities. To address this surge, one should devise a holistic approach and contribute in adequate sensitization of all salient stakeholders including clinicians, patients, and researchers. In this book, concise but detailed information related to genetics and epigenetic factors influencing cancer are elaborated. Genetic anomalies related to high-risk penetrance genes are thoroughly discussed in different types of cancers. Effect of DNA repair pathway and key cell signaling pathways in initiation, promotion, and progression of tumorigenesis is also eloquently elaborated.

Metastasis, responsible for the spread of disease to distant organs and also a leading cause of cancer-related death, is also highlighted in the book. Metastasis is a non-randomized process, happening inside human body beginning with loss of cell adhesion from primary site, regulating intravasation, survival in circulation, defying host immunity, extravasation and localization at suitable niche. All plausible genomic and transcriptomic orchestra of cell during these phases is well explained. Biostatistical approaches and precision medicine are the need of the time for correct diagnosis and treatment of cancer, and Dr. Masood outrightly pointed several ongoing and novel potential drugs explicitly to halt this process.

Towards the end, I would like to congratulate Dr. Masood and her coeditor for accomplishing this challenging task of writing scientific book for pathologists, health care professionals, and patients. Simplification of difficult terms without compromising reader interest is extremely pleasant. I highly value the immense efforts of Dr. Masood and Ms Malik to turn this long awaiting book in reality!

COMSATS University
Islamabad, Pakistan

Faraz A. Malik

Preface

This book covers different areas of cancer emphasizing on genomics, proteomics, omics and statistical analysis in the context of precision medicine. The first part highlights cancer genomics, organization and variations in human genome along with various genomic technologies. It sheds light on the importance of genomic technologies in cancer prognosis and treatment. Furthermore, it also covers metabolic changes and their characterization in tumour development. Numerous new techniques and reagents have been introduced into cancer research in the recent past, and these are covered in this book. With overview of basic genomics and processes, groundwork for the next parts of the book is laid.

It is a comprehensive book which is divided into seven parts and each part is composed of chapters on related topics. The first three parts make a very good text for an introductory cancer biology course. It not only covers cancer genomics but also highlights role of genomic instability and cancer metastasis particularly focusing on response of different DNA damage repair pathways, role of mechanotransduction and immunomodulation in cancer metastasis and genomic instability. Description about synthetic genetic strategies and role of nanomedicine in cancer detection and inhibition is an important part of this book. It also highlights the role of transcriptomics, translational genomics and precision medicine in different cancers. The breadth of these chapters provides the information necessary for any researcher to understand how various genomic technologies work for cancer detection, treatment and prevention.

Molecular biology has changed dramatically over the past two decades. Accumulation of data and its interpretation was found to be rate-limiting step in research. Therefore, computational biology has emerged in the past decade as a new subdiscipline of biology. It is great to discuss cancer-related computational approaches and mathematical modelling used to illustrate prognostic and predictive ways towards precision medicine, making this book more unique and comprehensive.

Many new challenges have arisen in the area of oncology clinical trials. New cancer therapies are often based on cytostatic or targeted agents, which pose new challenges in the design and analysis of all phases of trials. Therefore, statistical methods have been evolved to analyse such data in order to get meaningful information. This part is focused on the design and analysis of oncological clinical trials and translational research and is a great edition in this book. Highlighting the importance of pharmacogenomics and proteomics in cancer has become the unique features of this book.

Overall, this book is a single-source collection of up-to-date genomic, proteomic, computational, pharmacogenomics and statistical approaches to research in clinical oncology and precision medicine.

Rawalpindi, Pakistan Nosheen Masood
Rawalpindi, Pakistan Saima Shakil Malik

Acknowledgements

I would like to thank the following reviewers who provided helpful and timely comments on the original proposal for *'Essentials of Cancer Genomic, Computational Approaches and Precision Medicine*, and who gave detailed feedback on chapters from the various iterations that the book went through before evolving into its final form.

Dr. Bibekanand Mallick [Department of Life Science (LS), National Institute of Technology Rourkela, India], Dr. Sajda Ashraf (ICCBS—The International Center for Chemical and Biological Sciences, University of Karachi, Pakistan), Dr. Nadia Zahra (Qarshi University, Lahore, Pakistan), Dr. Shaista Javaid (Institute of Molecular Biology & Biotechnology, University of Lahore New Campus, Lahore, Pakistan), Dr. Abida Yasmeen (Lahore College for Women University, Pakistan), Dr. Rubina Dad (School of Pharmaceutical Science and Technology, Nankai District, Tianjin, China), Sarmad Mehmood (CMH Institute of Medical Sciences Bahawalpur, Pakistan & Atta-ur-Rahman School of Applied Biosciences, National University of Sciences and Technology, Islamabad 44000, Pakistan). Prof. Muhammad Tahir Khadim (Armed Forces Institute of Pathology, Rawalpindi, Pakistan), Sumaira Mubarik (Department of Epidemiology and Biostatistics, School of Health Sciences, Wuhan University, Wuhan 430071, Hubei, People's Republic of China), Muhammad Naeem, Ph.D. (Department of Biological Sciences, National University of Medical Sciences, Rawalpindi, Pakistan), Sophia Shakeel Malik (IT-Services, University of Gujrat, Pakistan), Muhammad Bilal Khan (Sure Bio Diagnostics & Pharmaceuticals, Pakistan) and Dr. Ruqia Mehmood Baig (Department of Zoology, PMAS Arid Agriculture University, Rawalpindi, Pakistan).

Finally, we would like to thank Dr. Bhavik Sawhney (Associate Editor—Biomedicine Springer Nature) for his countless support and guidance in the preparation of this book.

Contents

Part VII

About the Editors

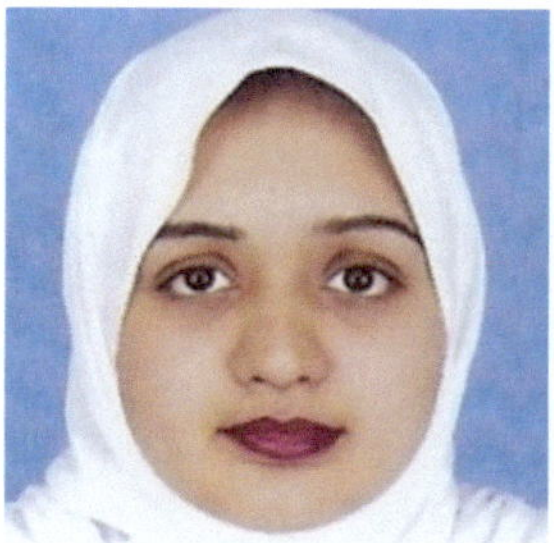

Nosheen Masood is currently working as an Assistant Professor at the Department of Biotechnology, Fatima Jinnah Women University, Rawalpindi, Pakistan. She completed her Ph.D. in Human Molecular Genetics at the Department of Biosciences at COMSATS University, Islamabad, Pakistan. Her main research interests include molecular biology and cancer genetics, with a focus on epidemiological studies, risk assessment, genomic analysis, immunohistochemistry-based diagnostics and protein–protein interactions. She has received various prestigious awards, notably, the Research Productivity Award 2014–2015 from the Pakistan Council of Science and Technology (PCST) category D, and Research Productivity Awards from COMSATS Institute of Information Technology for six consecutive years from 2010 to 2015. She has served as a reviewer for a number of international journals. She has teaching experience in biotechnology, molecular biology, comparative genomics, environmental biology, regulation of gene expression, and molecular evolution.

She has published a number of research articles in respected, peer-reviewed international journals and authored or co-authored various book chapters.

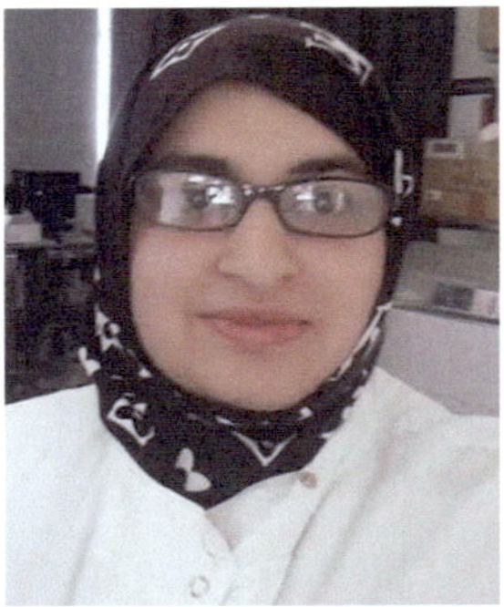

Saima Shakil Malik is currently working as a Scientific Officer at Armed Forces Institute of Pathology, Rawalpindi, Pakistan. She has obtained her Ph.D. from the Department of Biotechnology, Fatima Jinnah Women University, Rawalpindi, Pakistan. Previously, she has worked as a visiting researcher at the School of Cellular and Molecular Medicine at University of Bristol, UK. Her research interests are focused on the cancer genetics and molecular diagnostics. She has teaching experience in biotechnology, molecular biology, and biostatistics. She has numerous publications in internationally reputed journals and authored book chapters.

Part I

Overview of Cancer Genomics, Organization, and Variations in the Human Genome

1

Marriam Yamin, Hadeeqa Gull Raza, and Iffat Fatima

1.1 An Overview of Cancer Genomics

Genomics is an interdisciplinary field covering both structural and functional aspects of whole genomes. Therefore, it is categorized into structural and functional genomics with former characterization of the DNA sequences of haploid genomes while later targeting the entire array of transcripts and encoded proteins from a specific genome. These analyses require the use of high-throughput technologies and complex computational statistics which are continuously updated with recent technological advancements [1]. Being a disease of the genome, cancer research involves an identification of both somatic and germline oncogenic mutations in several tumor suppressor genes. Some of these mutated genes have excellent potential for molecular therapy and disease prognosis [2]. Cancer genomics has evolved with the development of technologies for comprehensive profiling of cancer genomes [3].

1.1.1 Genome Projects and Computational Genomics

Cancer research demands a multidisciplinary approach integrating laboratory experiments, clinical studies, and predictive computational analysis. Bioinformatics

M. Yamin (✉)
Applied Biotechnology and Microbiology, Laboratory of Thermodynamics of Proteins, Department of Biochemistry, State University of Campinas, Sao Paulo, Brazil

H. G. Raza
Applied Biopharmaceutical Biotechnology and Entrepreneurship, Cell Signaling and Cancer Therapeutic Lab, Lahore University of Management Sciences (LUMS), Lahore, Pakistan

I. Fatima
Laboratory of Physiology, Department of Animal Sciences, Quaid-e-Azam University, Islamabad, Pakistan

N. Masood, S. Shakil Malik (eds.), *'Essentials of Cancer Genomic, Computational Approaches and Precision Medicine*,
https://doi.org/10.1007/978-981-15-1067-0_1

has gained huge significance in this field by providing computational tools for collection, storage, distribution, and analyses of genomic data. In this regard, Human Genome Project (HGP) had been logically extended to Cancer Genome Atlas (TCGA) project with the aim of providing a detailed atlas of cancer-related genetic changes. Repositories like Stanford Microarray Database (SMD) and Gene Expression Omnibus (GEO) also exist which mainly facilitate data storage but also offer limited options of data analyses like hierarchical clustering. However, microarray data analysis tools like "Gene Logic's BioExpress® System Oncology Suite" and BioExpress® Oncology Suite are specifically available for cancer research [4]. Recent investigations on different types of cancers including prostate [5], hepatocellular carcinoma [6], and low-grade glioma [7] have demonstrated the association between tumor progression and DNA methylation heterogeneity. Moreover, a link between novel measures of DNA methylation heterogeneity and clinical variables in different types of carcinomas has also been reported recently [8, 9].

1.1.2 Structural Genomics

The term "structural genomics" has been defined in a number of ways which can be converged as "genome characterization via assigning loci to specific chromosomes and physical mapping by using information related to the structural organization of genome provided through both experimental and computational approaches." However, structural genomics is not confined to genome characterization, but it also aims to provide three-dimensional structures of proteins on genomic scale. These objectives are achieved through advanced technologies of sequencing and genomic data analysis.

1.1.3 Characterization of Cancer Genomes

Activation and inactivation of oncogenes and tumor suppressor genes respectively are induced due to nucleotide sequence mutations. Analyses of such alterations in DNA sequence could be performed due to development of sequencing techniques which were first developed in 1975. Initially, somatic mutations in RAS family of genes were discovered followed by determination of tumor suppressor genes. Later on, improvement of sequencing techniques led to discovery of a number of oncogenes which provide potential target for gene therapy [3]. Cancer genomes are characterized by extensively altered copy number and structure of chromosomes as compared to normal genomes. Somatic copy number alterations (SCNAs) in cancer genome which span either a part or full arm of chromosome have been successfully determined owing to the development of comparative genomic hybridization techniques [10]. Although germline DNAs have also been reported from human populations, however, their association with cancer still needs to be investigated [3].

1.1.4 Functional Genomics

Although identification of mutated oncogenes and cancer suppressor genes through sequencing and physical mapping of cancer genomes has abundantly increased genomic data, however, it is unable to completely describe the significance of these mutations during cancer progression [11]. Moreover, many of the oncogenes are not frequently mutated or amplified [12]. Another challenge imposed in cancer research is to analyze functions of genes in specific physiological environment during disease progression. Functional genomics deciphers genes' functions by providing their cellular phenotypes [13].

1.1.5 Challenges in Functional Genomics

Functional genomics can play a significant role in cancer therapeutics by identifying molecular targets of anticancer compounds. It can also be used to screen the genes regulating drug resistance and sensitivity [14]. Practical application of functional genomics in cancer research is a challenging task due to advantages and drawbacks of the technologies used in the process [15]. Therefore, it is necessary to get in-depth knowledge of these techniques or platforms. Measurement of complex phenotypes is made possible in two ways, i.e., either using arrayed or pooled screens. Arrayed screens have the advantage of measuring complex phenotypes of a single population of cells, but their use is costly and labour-intensive, whereas pooled screens are both cost-effective and easy to perform as neither specialized equipment nor many personnel is needed to carry out the analysis. However, they can only measure the cell death, proliferation phenotypes, etc. In conclusion, an optimal functional genomics screen would be the one approaching maximum positive gene hits. To achieve such quality, functional genomics reagents have been continuously improved by researchers [16]. In this regard, recently modified CRISPR algorithms and genomic libraries provide optimal results with higher identification of positive gene hits as compared to previous versions [17].

1.1.6 Genomics' Impact on Cancer Research

Application of genetics and genomics in cancer research was started with the discovery of point mutation in the HRAS gene leading to glycine placement instead of valine at codon 12 [18, 19]. Afterward, mutations were identified in other genes of RAS family including KRAS and NRAS [20, 21]. Proteins encoded by RAS family are involved in signal transduction pathways, thus regulating cell proliferation and survival which make the respective mutated genes the potential target for anticancer therapeutics [22]. Disease management strategies for colon and lung cancer patients are currently focused on testing KRAS mutations before starting epidermal growth factor receptor (EGFR) targeted treatments. This is due to the fact that these mutated genes contribute to resistance against EGFR therapies [23]. Likewise, BRAF mutations are found in malignant melanomas and colorectal, gall bladder, and thyroid cancers. BRAF encodes serine threonine kinase which is the central enzyme in MAPK signaling pathway [24]. In conclusion, advanced sequencing techniques like targeted PCR-based sequencing, etc. have expanded the categories of mutated genes in several types of tumors. Once, genomic data regarding cancer drivers is obtained, further validation through experimental demonstration is needed to understand the mechanism of action and translation of results for clinical practice [3].

1.1.7 Organization of Human Genome

Application of both visual and molecular technologies has enabled the researchers to explore the entire human genome in a folded state. It has been revealed that genomic material spanning approximately 2 meters of length is folded and placed with nucleus having space within micrometer scale. This compactly organized genome is comprised of 46 chromosomes numbered from 1 to 22 somatic pairs based on their size and another pair which determines the sex of the individual. Chromatin is the state in which genomic DNA exists physiologically. Several histone and nonhistone proteins are attached to DNA which is further folded into compact form [25].

1.1.8 Genome in a 3-D Nucleus

Nucleus is a double-membranous organelle which encloses the genome and separates the transcription and translation machineries. Various nuclear substructures are involved in the organization of genome which include nuclear envelop (NE) and nuclear lamina. Several transmembrane proteins populate the inner and outer nuclear membranes of nuclear envelope [26]. These proteins promote the production of nuclear lamina through interaction with lamin proteins. Chromatin remains associated with nuclear lamina through specific domains called lamin-associated domains (LADs) [27].

Similarly, another nuclear substructure regulating genome organization is the nuclear pore complex (NPC). It regulates the transport of several molecules between the nucleus and cytoplasm [28]. These perforations exhibit variation in size, i.e., range from approximately 60 million to 100 million Da [25]. Nucleoli are the structures which play their role in organizing chromatin within nuclear space. These are involved in rRNA synthesis and are found in proximity to rRNA genes at different chromosomes [29]. In addition to aforementioned structures, there exist several other substructures which are associated with chromosome organization within nucleus.

1.1.9 Genes in the Human Genome

Human Genome Project (HGP) has provided valuable information regarding the distribution of genes, sequence homology, and the prevalence of noncoding genes. It has been reported that human genome is comprised of approximately 20,000–25,000 genes [30]. Novel genes have been annotated by using homology analysis and gene prediction tools of bioinformatics. The data generated from these methods is then made available to researchers through various genome browsers [31, 32] This data has revealed that proteome diversity is caused by alternative splicing which exhibits frequency range from 35% to 60% per single gene [33]. Despite the technological advancements, accuracy in prediction of genes, their structures, and alternative splices have not been achieved which inhibits the validation of available genomic data. However, this issue can be resolved by verifying this data through direct experimentation [34].

In addition, a number of noncoding genes have also been reported which produce RNA transcripts with no known function [35]. It is proposed that these noncoding RNAs are involved in regulatory mechanisms such as the regulatory role of antisense transcripts which has been reported for several human genes [36]. MicroRNAs belong to the class of noncoding RNA which were first discovered in animals [37]. More than 800 microRNA genes with unknown function have been found in human genome. Recently, research is underway to discover the biological functions of these genes.

1.1.10 Genes' Distribution

Efforts to determine the distribution of genes within DNA have also revealed some interesting facts. These include the presence of "deserts," i.e., regions devoid of genes usually spanning up to 3Mb [38]. Presence of these regions have not been justified yet, but conserved patterns in the "deserts" have suggested some functions such as the role of enhancers [39]. Likewise, the status of gene clustering which was previously considered due to evolutionary duplication has now been changed to some kind of coordination like same enhancer region or chromatin conformation, etc. [40]. It has been found that 45% of human DNA is comprised of repetitive sequences separated by non-repetitive sequences. Identification of human genes in multiple of four had suggested that whole genome is derived through quadruplicating of a small ancestral genome. However, complete sequencing of human genome has demonstrated the presence of copy number polymorphisms among different individuals [41].

1.1.11 Genetic Variation in the Human Genome

The project named as "The Human Haplotype Map" highlights significant contributions of HGP toward understanding genetics. This project aims at the identification of single-nucleotide polymorphisms (SNPs) in 270 ethnically diverse individuals [42]. These SNPs are categorized as haplotypes which can provide the foundation for mapping of phenotypic and genotypic variations. However, capacity of haplotypes to accurately identify the variations is not found yet [43]. One of the founding principles of HapMAp project was to successfully perform analysis of human genetic disorders. Further development in this project may eventually introduce the novel version of genetic variations in humans. This would ultimately improve the quality of both epidemiological and clinical research and translation of their outcomes into personalized medicine [34].

1.1.12 Genetic Variation and Reference Cancer Genome

Complete profiling of tumor genome is necessary for the respective physician to choose an accurate treatment plan for the patient. Reference for all somatic mutations in all types of cancers has become accessible by discoveries of several mutations including BRAF mutations in melanoma [44], PI3KCA mutations [45] in breast and colon cancers, IDH1 mutations [46] in glioblastoma (GBM), etc. These initial findings have led to the characterization of various types and sub-types of cancers. International Cancer Genome Consortium and (ICGC) and Cancer Genome Atlas (TCGA) are the major contributors to revolutionize the cancer genomics. Although Cancer Genome Atlas is still under development due to certain obstacles in acquisition, generation, and analyses of genomic data, however, it is expected that all oncogenes along with patterns of somatic mutations for all cancer types will soon be compiled [3]. Complete sequencing (high coverage) of cancer genomes would lead to discovery of novel mutations, e.g., those found in neuroblastoma (ALK mutation) [47], prostate cancer (NSLC gene fusion) [48], etc.

1.1.13 Reasoning and Explaining the Cancer Genome

Genomic data available from aforementioned programs have clearly demonstrated that mutations can be functionally categorized into two types which include oncogenic aberrations known as drivers and nonparticipant mutations which are called passengers as they do not exert any oncogenic effect. These two types need to be differentiated for a better understanding of a cancer genome. Bioinformatics plays significant role in this regard by providing computational tools to analyze complex data from cancer genomes. However, to perform such integrated analysis is not an easy task because it demands multidisciplinary approach and background knowledge of mathematics, statistics, bioinformatics, and biology which is not usually feasible for researchers. Additionally, verification through experimentation is also required to distinguish the passengers from driver mutations. Such experiments are performed by experimental biologists who make use of genomic data from cancer genomes. In conclusion, only availability of complex genomic data is not a major accomplishment, but it further needs to be explained so its outcomes could be used directly in clinical practice [3].

1.1.14 Assigning Functions to Genetic Mutations

Experimental proofs are provided in order to verify the significance of a potential mutation in onset, maintenance, and progression of cancer. A single functional assay either in vivo or in vitro cannot verify the cancer-related activity but needs support from multiple functional assay systems which strengthen the claim of the respective gene mutation. In vivo assays have the advantage of being more predictive as compared to in vitro counterparts; however these are mostly laborious and costly. In contrast, in vitro assays can deal with hundreds to thousands of genes at a time within standardized system. However, availability of both reagents and technical expertise are the main obstacles to investigate the cancer-related activities of a candidate gene. Specific model systems are needed to analyze relevance of a mutation with cancer. Such as, EGFRvIII mutations are seen in GBM tumors in the absence of p53 mutations. Therefore, the model system for functional validation of EGFRvIII should be devoid of p53 mutation [49]. Both genetic context and microenvironment need to be considered while investigating the therapeutic targets for progressing tumors. Regarding this aspect of cancer genomics, it is expected that epidemiological and clinical studies for various types of cancer among diverse demographic regions would provide insight into both cellular and genetic contexts of each mutated gene [3].

1.1.15 Translating Cancer Research into Clinical Practice

Human relevance is an essential requirement to evaluate any mutation for its potential as a disease biomarker or target for therapeutics. A criterion for a true human cancer gene is that any mutation deregulates the proteins encoded by it. There is still potential in identifying genes which exhibit alterations in several types of tumors from a significant part of a population until the cancer genomes are not fully saturated. The underlying mechanisms for these alterations include inactivation, deletion, or epigenetic changes which result in gene silencing. Furthermore, large independent cohorts can be screened for prevalence of DNA and protein deregulation in specific types of tumors. In conclusion, integration of genomic, experimental, and epidemiological data will not only relate the mutations in oncogenes with cancer progression but also provide the clues for therapeutic intervention for clinicians [3].

1.2 History of Sequencing

Genome sequencing is, basically, reading an entire genome of an organism or just focusing on sequencing some very specific areas of DNA or RNA. Almost four decades ago, sequencing was introduced to various areas of biological sciences which revolutionized multiple technological advancements, and its applications aim to decrease the cost and time for the biological sample sequencing analysis

[50]. Frederick Sanger, in 1988, introduced sequencing of insulin as biological macromolecule which highlighted the importance of sequencing technique for better understanding of molecules, which opened the doors for several opportunities in medical and biological sciences [51, 52]. Over the past two decades, RNA sequencing brought special consideration to appreciate the genomic state dynamics for both qualitative and quantitative analysis of RNA. Sequencing methods of RNA transcriptome include particularly coding and non-coding regions of RNA transcriptome especially small RNA (sRNA) species, as well as microRNAs, promoter- and terminator-related RNAs [53].

1.2.1 DNA Sequencing

The first DNA sequencing was conducted in the 1960s by Kenneth Murray; he developed a two-dimensional analysis for fractioned oligodeoxyribonucleotides. The earlier limitation was to obtain a sequence of large molecules, and DNA being a large molecule was difficult to sequence by Sanger's method. Therefore, the utilization of single-stranded bacteriophage – ϕX174 – was the only option for the researchers to sequence, as it's size was 5000 nucleotides, which was also quite large for analysis. On the other hand, the absence of degradative enzymes was another obstacle [52].

1.2.2 Principal Mechanism of DNA Sequencing

DNA sequencing is a complex topic. However, once the basics of conventional DNA sequencing, especially Sanger sequencing, are understood, complex processes such as next-generation sequencing can be realized (Fig. 1.1). Molecular biology emphasizes greatly on the importance of Sanger sequencing for being economical and effortless to carry out, in almost any laboratory setup. The main mechanism of sequencing begins with the annealing step in which double-stranded DNA is heated till separation and kept unwind. The insertion of short chemically manufactured DNA sequence known as "primer" facilitates the beginning of the reaction, the sequence of the aforementioned being already known. These primers are corresponding to complementary strand regions, which are attachment sites for DNA polymerase enzyme to carry out DNA synthesis using dNTPs (deoxyribonucleotide triphosphates). The dNTPs are essentially single DNA bases (A, T, C, G) that the polymerase can use for chain elongation by forming a complementary DNA strand. Once the ddNTPs (dideoxyribonucleotide triphosphates) are incorporated in the mixture, which are usually chemically modified sequences, the reaction stops. After the termination of synthesis step, single-strand nucleotide sequence determination is carried out using high-resolution electrophoresis gel equipped with capillary channels. Four color-separated bands are generated by laser excitation of fluorescent-tagged fragments in distinct spectra, which is readable using Sanger's method.

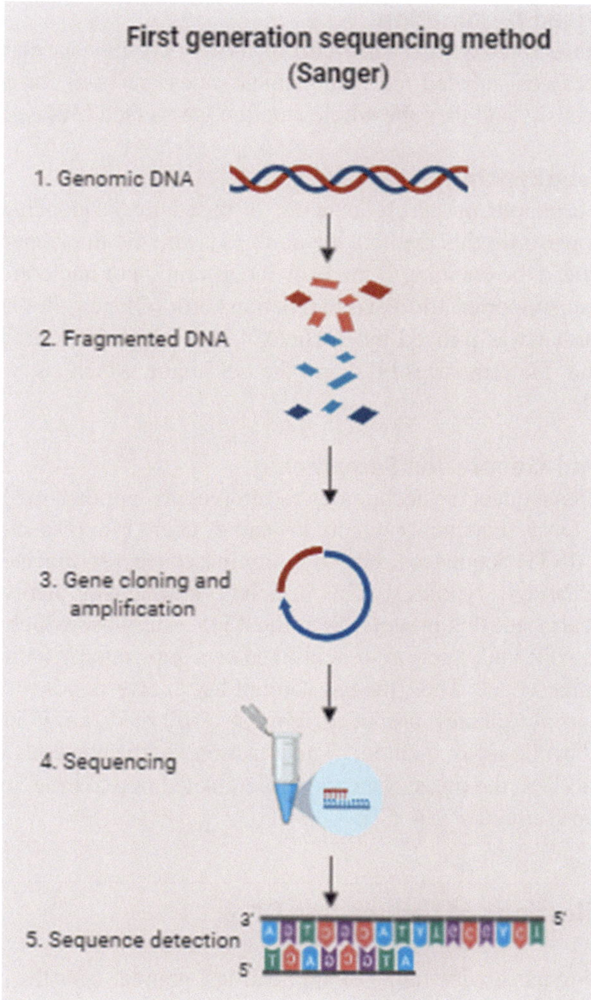

Fig. 1.1 Schematic overview of DNA sequencing (Sanger's method)

There are various software working to distinguish errors in reading of sequences for assigning each base in form of chromatogram peaks [54].

1.2.3 Classification Among DNA Sequencing Technologies

To give more clarity toward global classification of DNA sequencing, it is divided into three main types such as second-generation, massively parallel sequencing of clones, adding value to increase the speed, and decreasing the costs of routine sequencing for the biomedical field [55].

1.2.3.1 Reversed Termination

This method resembles Sanger's method in terms of synthesis manner, but here especially fluorescent-labeled terminator nucleotides are used for chain termination, simultaneously, and then the whole reaction is reversed [56].

1.2.3.2 Pyrosequencing

The working principle of pyrosequencing is based on sequencing-by-synthesis mechanism; however in this method, we don't measure the fluorescence of specific nucleotides instead the counting is made by incorporation of nucleotides. This technology was also supported for discrete reaction form (Qiagen) before a massively parallelized format was utilized by Roche/454. Nowadays both programs support the combination: the sequencer FLX and the GS junior, which carry out low measurements [56].

1.2.3.3 Second-Generation Sequencing

Parallel with the sequencing techniques developments, another methodology was introduced for DNA sequencing which, instead of using Fluorescent-tagged oligonucleotide or dNTP sequences, employs luminescence for the measurement of pyrophosphate bridge synthesis. The principal mechanism involves two main enzymes that carry out this process: first, the ATP sulfurylase which change pyrophosphate into ATP, and, later on, it is utilized as a substrate by luciferase enzyme to produce luminescence. Thus, the emission of light corresponds to the magnitude of multiple pyrophosphates produced, almost $>10^6$ reads/array in the reaction referred to as "cyclic-array method." This reaction is advantageous as it proceeds using natural dNTPs; the measurements are conducted in real time, making it more practical and cost-effective [54, 57].

1.2.4 Applications of Sequencing DNA

DNA sequencing has a wide range of applications, popular over the past few years in an application known as "de novo sequencing," which refers to the complete sequencing of any organism from the beginning. After Human Genome Project (HGP), genome resequencing is another application in which coexisting sequence data is used for comparison of the same species, to determine changes due to environmental stimuli by making gene and physical maps especially. Gene expression analysis is also an important application which is facilitated by. Noninvasive prenatal testing (NIPT) is the most unexpected field of DNA sequencing which has a great impact on human life, that even simple counting of DNA fragment released in maternal circulation by the fetus can be helpful to detect chromosomal abnormalities in pregnancy [50]. Next-generation sequencing (NGS) has also gained promising attention in recent years with respect to its application in many fields such as forensic investigations like in genetic framework, autosomes, mitochondrial, and sex chromosome. Moreover, other applications include construction of DNA database, ancestral studies and phenotypic interpretation, monozygotic twin studies, body fluid and species classification, and forensic animal, plant, and microbiological analyses [58].

1.3 Biomarkers

National Cancer Institute has defined; a biomarker as "a biological molecule found in blood, other body fluids, or tissues that is a sign of a normal or abnormal process, or of a condition or disease." A biomarker can be used to monitor body's response to treatment against specific illness. Therefore, it is also known as a signature molecule or maker. The term "biomarker" is a combination of "biological marker," which denotes a large subclass of clinical signs. National Institutes of Health Biomarkers also described a biomarker as "a characteristic that is objectively measured and evaluated as a hallmark of pathogenic techniques, regular organic approaches, or pharmacologic responses to a healing intervention" in 1998. Joint mission of International Program on Chemical Safety, which was led by World Health Organization (WHO) and coordinated by International Labor Organization and United Nations, has described a biomarker as "any substance, shape, or process that can be measured inside the body or its range and have an impact on or predict the incidence of final results or disease." On the validity of biomarkers in surroundings hazard assessment, according to the WHO report the biomarker's definition includes "nearly any size reflecting an interplay between an organic system and a potential chance, which may be chemical, physical, or organic. The measured reaction can be useful and physiological, biochemical on the cell stage, or molecular interaction." Biomarkers are incredibly newer in medical studies especially laboratory-oriented biomarkers. The bone of contention is to determine the relationship between any given biomarker and applicable medical outcomes [59]. Measurements of metabolites in bloodstream, urine, blood cells, expression of individual genes, and expression of collections of genes can be encompassed within a biomarker. It is from nearly 50 genes out of 5000 genes or greater [60].

1.3.1 Classification

Classification of the biomarkers is based on multiple factors but most importantly on their usage in clinical studies or endpoints, for example, as (a) diagnostic biomarker, (b) prognostic biomarker, (c) pharmacological biomarker, and (d) surrogate biomarker. In this way, the whole class of biomarkers can be divided into four major subclasses: detective, diagnostic, prognostic, and predictive biomarkers [61]. Another classification of biomarkers is based on their utility which includes disorder burden biomarkers and healing efficacy biomarkers. Additionally, they can also be categorized according to their application and can be divided into diagnostic biomarkers, disease-stage biomarkers, disease-analysis biomarkers, and tracking the clinical response to therapy. A comparatively new category of biomarkers is their usage or selection at some point of early drug development, e.g., certain pharmacological reaction, and in dose optimization studies, pharmacodynamic biomarkers are of special interest [62].

1.3.1.1 ROC (Receiver Operating Characteristic) Curve

Relationship between sensitivity and specificity can be represented on a graph, and the curve obtained is cast-off to evaluate the efficiency of a disease or a tumor marker at the various given endpoints. The graph which gives the maximum area under the curve is known as an ideal graph.

1.3.1.2 Screening/Diagnostic Biomarker

Diagnostic markers are used to diagnose or to identify specific disease in a specific individual. Screening biomarkers have high sensitivity/specificity to diagnose a disease, e.g., if Bence Jones protein is present in urine, then it is a diagnostic indicator of multiple myeloma.

1.3.1.3 Prognostic Biomarker

After the disease status is established, prognostic biomarkers are used to predict the progression of the illness. These biomarkers can also be used to predict the disease's recurrence and optimization of clinical therapy. The level of human chorionic gonadotropin and alpha-fetoprotein can be distinguished with survival rates in testicular teratoma.

1.3.1.4 Predictive/Stratification Biomarker

Before starting the treatment, response to a drug can be predicted by stratification marker. It classifies the individuals in responders or nonresponders to a particular treatment. Array-type experiments mainly rise such markers, and it can also help to predict a clinical outcome by predictive biomarker using molecular characteristics of patient's sickness.

1.3.2 Significance/Specification of Biomarkers

Biomarkers have a significant role in:

- Demonstrating the dose-response and progressive relationships between biomarker changes, onset of disease, sternness of disease, and corresponding progression of the disease.
- Identifying the relationship between the extent of biomarker changes and biological outcome; quantitative changes in biomarkers indicate reversibility of the disease.
- Providing passable tissue specificity and ensuring the biomarker not to reflect injury to other organs or stimulation of physiological responses in the target organ not related to disease (Table 1.1).
- Defining biochemical, molecular, genetic, immunological, and physiological responses which link the biomarker to the organ or mechanism of toxicity.

– Providing experimental evidence to connect the biomarker's molecular mechanism response with a biological outcome

1.3.3 Development of Biomarker

Biomarker improvement involves a couple of tactics, linking initial discovery in fundamental studies, validation, and scientific implementation. The closing goal of the procedures is to set up clinically accessible biomarker tests with clinical software, informing scientific decision-making to enhance patient outcomes. However, there are many hurdles evidenced through the low expected compensation (0.1%) of a hit for scientific translation of biomarkers [23].

1.3.4 Identification of Biomarker

Potential biomarkers possibly recognized through more than one procedure. The traditional method was about three factors: candidate biomarker, tumor's biology and tumor's surrounding environment, and metabolism of the pharmaceutical agent. In the recent era of information and latest techniques, biomarkers are regularly being identified by "discovery" method, which includes different strategies, e.g., the high-throughput sequencing, gene expression arrays, and mass spectroscopy, to become aware of individual biomarkers that range among cohorts. The use of these facts generating techniques approach to particular interest should be paid toward layout and statistics evaluation, on the way to limit the risk of figuring out institutions which might be subsequently decided as false positives. The key aspects of improvement in biomarkers to be discussed in detail include cautious examination layout to avoid bias, complete analysis and validation, and accurate reporting of the outcomes [63].

Table 1.1 Specific biomarkers against specific disease condition

Usage	Specificity
For estimation of cancer development risk	Germline mutation_ BRCA1
Screening of the disease	Prostate-specific antigen (PSA)
Diagnosis	Immunohistochemistry for determination of tissue of origin
Determination of course of illness	1. Recurrence score of 21 genes (breast cancer)
To predict the response of therapy	2. KRAS mutation, anti-EGFR antibody
	3. *HER2* expression, anti-Her2 therapy
	4. Estrogen receptor expression
Monitoring the recurrence of a disease	1. Colorectal cancer (CEA mutation)
	2. AFP, LDH, βHCG
Monitoring or progression response in metastatic disease	CEA and CA15-3

1.3.5 Techniques for Biomarker Discovery

Discovery of novel cancer biomarkers is totally renewed with the invention of mass spectrometry, proteomics, DNA arrays, and knowledge of the human genome along with creation of technology. Additionally, modern technologies also offer different approaches to identify new, unpaired cancer biomarkers by using affordable hypotheses and novel analytical techniques. Regardless of intervention of modern techniques, some of the barriers in discovering single, novel cancer biomarkers are still there. Those barriers are related to study design biases, collecting and storing of artifact samples. There are some pieces of evidence that these new techniques often fail to perceive cancer biomarkers and display a bias toward the identification of molecules. However, capacity of technological advances can revolutionize cancer biomarker discovery [64].

1.3.5.1 Profiling of Gene Expression

In the study of gene expression, the genomic microarrays are extensively used. It has witnessed that utility inside gene expression profiling has incredibly increased over past decades. And this increase has helped in subclassification of cancer, vision of cancer pathogenesis, and discovery of huge range of cancer biomarkers for diagnostic purpose.

1.3.5.2 Proteomic Profiling Using Mass Spectrometry

A recent approach which is used to discover cancer biomarkers is proteomic sample profiling. Proteomic approach appears much promising in diagnosing tumor or subclassification of tumor. Mass-spectrometry techniques based on proteomic evaluation and along with the usage of advanced technology, brings higher mass accuracy, detection capability, and shorter biking instances, and allowing extended output and greater-dependable facts. Regardless of accuracy of this method, there are still some limitations. These limitations consist of artifact-related biases (the scientific pattern collection and storage), qualitative nature of mass spectrometers, inability to pick out most cautiously mounted cancer biomarkers and identifying molecules present in serum. Another obstacle concerns feasible bioinformatic artifacts [59]. No product has reached to the medical institution, and also there is no impartial validation research posted despite a considerable time-lapse in the first record of the technology. Serum proteomic profiling for medical use is no longer recommended by experts.

1.3.5.3 Peptidomics

The new focus for discovering the novel cancer biomarkers is peptidomics profiling. In this technique, the low molecular weight serum proteome is used to identify the biomarker. The peptides are being cleaved in coagulation to plasma, including protease inhibition, inflammatory response, or immune modulation. Most of the above-mentioned limitations related to mass spectrometry and protein profiling technologies are also the key points to peptidomics [59].

1.3.6 Biomarker Family

Biomarker family classification is based on "cancer biomarker's own family"; according to this approach, if a member of a protein family is already a biomarker, then other participants of that own family may be the desirable biomarkers (i.e., cancer). Prostate-specific antigen (PSA) is a member of the human tissue protein named kallikrein, and kallikreins are also enzymes which are secreted with trypsin-like/chymotrypsin-like serine proteases. This enzyme (prostate-specific antigen) includes 15 genes which are clustered in tandem on chromosome 19q13.4. Prostate-specific antigens (KLK3, KLK2) are considered clinically critical biomarkers in prostate cancer. Human kallikrein own family participants are also considered in carcinogenesis and utilized for investigation as a biomarker for analysis, e.g., KLK6 is considered as a biomarker for ovarian cancer [65].

As secreted proteins have the very best chance to come into the move, so the candidate serological marker should be a secreted protein. Also, the examination of the tumor-surrounding environment helps in identification of candidate molecules in overlapping researches. There are many evidences regarding the malignancy of the cancerous cells that is dependent on the tumor cells as well as the microenvironment (stroma, endothelial cells, immune and inflammatory cells) around the tumor. The most prominent cancer biomarkers, i.e., CEA, CA125, and HER2, are extensively involved in cancer identification and analysis of membrane-bound proteins in nature and can be released in the blood circulation [66]. The secreted proteins present in tissues or other biological fluids do not suggest that the proteins might be detectable within the sera of most cancers' patients. Serum-based diagnostic tests mostly rely upon the stableness, clearance, and affiliation of targeted protein with other sera proteins and the volume of posttranslational modifications [64].

1.3.7 Other Strategies

There is a wide variety of different techniques present to detect cancer biomarkers. The most important method is based on protein arrays. A tumor-associated antigen is thought as to be a biosensor for developing and progression of cancers because these tumors usually elicit specific immune response in the host system. Furthermore, most hematological cancers arise from the chromosomal translocations and resulting mutations which underlie the solid epithelial tumors. After chromosomal translocation, the gene fusions in most cancers (e.g., prostate) can be diagnosed by gene expression level/set. Another important technique is based on mass-spectrometry imaging of frozen tissue, and it has shown some of its ability to screen candidate biomarkers. There are some significant efforts to unlock the serum proteome using fractionation in order to decrease and simplify the dynamic range of molecules present in sera. Besides proteomic profiling of serum, attempts have been made to decipher the serum proteome. Animal models related to human tumor xenograft experiments are showing strong evidence for cancer-biomarker discovery.

1.3.8 Steps Involved in Evaluating and Reporting Biomarkers

1. The first step involved in the process of evaluation and reporting the biomarkers is preclinical research. A hypothesis is generated for scientific test by comparing the cancerous and non-cancerous cells or specimens to detect most cancers. Different strategies are involved in this process, but most commonly used techniques are gene expression profiling and mass spectrometry. Other approaches can be used to evaluate them.
2. The clinical assay is developed to discriminate the healthy and cancerous specimens to involve in this phase. In this segment, the patients assessed have already set up the disease, but this assay is not used to detect the disease at this stage.
3. The evidences of the biomarker to stumble on preclinical disorder are made and proved by collecting and sorting the samples from healthy individuals, but the improvement of malignancy is monitored at this stage.
4. By using the abovementioned assay and diagnostic approaches, the individuals are screened in this phase; this can help to gauge the stage, nature, and progression of the sickness.
5. A final step of the process and the main objective of this phase is to determine whether the screening has reduced the burden of sickness at a given time in a given population.

1.3.9 Outlook

Biomarkers not only play an important role in the development of drug but also play very critical part in biomedical research enterprise. Understanding the relationship between potential biomarker and clinical consequences is important to modify the existing remedies but will also help to increase the spectrum of therapies for almost all diseases. Biomarkers could best function as authentic replacements for medical relevant endpoints if we absolutely understood the normal physiology of an organic procedure, pathophysiology of that method within disorder state, and consequences of an intervention – pharmacological, tool, or in any other case – on these procedures. Studies that are carried out for evaluation of correlation fulfillment of biomarkers usually need to have minimum retroactive scientific consequences as closing measures. Without continual reassessment of connection between endpoints of surrogate and actual scientific, we again have chance to approve complete instructions regarding medication.

1.4 Microarray Technology

Microarray is a laboratory technique to detect the level of expression of thousands of genes at a time by using microscopic spot of DNA being attached on a solid surface. These DNA spots contain a certain amount of specific DNA sequence which acts as probes to detect the expression of certain genes. These probes are expressed by group of proteins and also called mRNA (messenger RNA) transcripts. The conventional steps of microarray technique involved (1) hybridization of mRNA with DNA template from tissue of origin, (2) multiple samples of DNA assembled for an array, and (3) certain quantity of mRNA on each site of array that indicates the degree of expression different genes, and the range can be run thousand times additionally. All of this information is then amassed which help in generating a profile for the level of expression of profile in a mobile device [67].

1.4.1 Technique Involved in Microarray

In microarray technique known samples are combined with unknown DNA samples using base paring policy. This test uses commonplace assay systems which include microplates or blotting membranes, and the diameter of the spot of a sample is even less than 200 μm, and it includes hundreds of spots on the blotting membrane or microplates. These samples are also known as probes and have known sequences. These samples can be immobilized on a nylon membrane, silicon chip, or on a microscope glass slide. These sample spots can be oligonucleotides, cDNA, or DNA, and complementary binding of an unknown sequence is determined by measuring the level of gene expression or by gene discovery. This test provides enormous information about the real-time genes by using unpaired DNA chip.

1.4.2 Usage of Microarrays

Usage of microarray depends upon the immobilized pattern used and the kind of information drew. The microarray experiments can be divided into three main categories and those are:

1. *Expression microarray*: In this experiment, the cDNA molecule is derived from the known gene's mRNA, and sample is immobilized on an array. Genes present in sample are taken from both diseased and healthy tissues. If the gene is overly expressed in the diseased tissues, then the high-intensity spots are recorded in diseased condition. The expression level of a particular gene in a sample then compared to the gene responsible for the specific disease.
2. *Comparative genomic hybridization*: This technique is used to identify the increase or decrease in chromosomal fragments of sheltering genes involved in a specific disease.
3. *Mutation analysis*: In this technique, the gDNA is used, but genes may vary from each other by single nucleotide polymorphisms (SNPs).

1.4.3 DNA Microarray

DNA microarray involves the hybridization of cDNA to complementary sequences. In this technique, the hybridization of the cDNA is reverse transcribed with a designed complementary DNA probe (known sequence). This probe is mounted on a slide or on an array. So, the DNA microarray basically consists of a library (synthetic nucleic acid probe); these probes are immobilized on a solid surface or matrix. These kinds of microarrays are known as Southern blotting in which the fragments of DNA are attached to the stable matrix or a substrate and are probed by known sequence of specific gene (Fig. 1.2).

In 1995 the primary DNA microarrays were capable of studying lots of sequences constructed by recognizing the known sequences or attaching the synthetic probes on a stable substrate at a specific position. These stable substrates were normally a glass chip (see Fig. 1.2). There are several other ways to produce array, and, in some strategies, a robot is used to print the known-sequenced probes which were mounted to the needles along with chemical matrix. Another technique involved the image-activated interaction and shield to synthesize probes by producing one nucleotide at a time on a surface in multiple hits resulting in multiple probes with unique sequence at a unique place [67].

1.4.4 DNA Microarray Protocol

The basic protocol involved in a DNA microarray is:

1. *Isolation and purification of mRNA*. As gene expression level is compared in the DNA microarray, so experiment sample is compared with the control sample

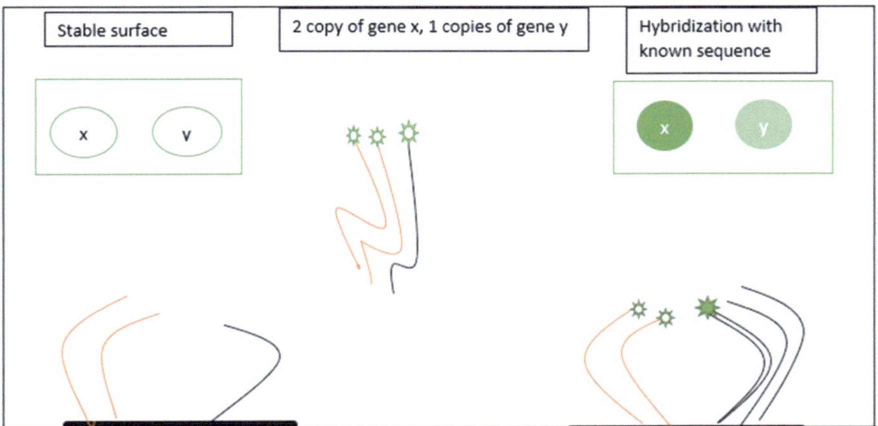

A simplified version of DNA microarray; upper two rectangle boxes are showing two DNA spots x, y on a solid surface before and after hybridization with known sequence. other rectangles at the bottom are showing the side view of the above surface.

Fig. 1.2 DNA microarray technique, before and after hybridization of sample (healthy tissues) expression level of a specific gene in a disease condition vs healthy condition. The mRNA is isolated and purified from the sample of interest.

2. *Reverse transcription and labeling of mRNA*. Firstly, the samples are categorized to detect the transcript by hybridization. The purified sample of mRNA might be in less quantity, so the amplification of the mRNA is recommended. After amplification, the reverse transcription (RT) and complementary DNA (cDNA) are labeled with a fluorescent dye. This dye linked to the DNA nucleotide generates the fluorescent cDNA strand. Both diseased and healthy samples are labeled with different dyes, and they co-hybridize on microarray, equally. In some protocols, the cDNA is not labeled, but in the second step of amplification, the cDNA produced from reverse transcription serves as template and gives rise to cRNA strand.
3. *Hybridization of the labeled target*. Fluorescent-labeled cDNA strands are mounted on a DNA microarray, and these labeled cDNA strands then hybridize with the cDNA probes having known sequence. After hybridization, several washes are required to remove the non-specific bindings onto the surface.
4. *Scanning of the microarray to quantify the signal strength*. Fluorescent labels present on cDNA are excited by using a laser, and a signal is generated from labeled sequences. The strength of the signal after binding the sample with the probe correlates to the stage of expression of different genes in diseased tissues. After detecting the signals, these are quantified to get the virtual picture of DNA microarray. Figure 1.3 is showing the schematic explanation of the DNA microarray procedure.

1.4.5 Applications of DNA Microarray

1.4.5.1 Gene Expression Analysis

Gene expression analysis is the most common use of DNA microarray; expression level of a certain gene can be measured by using this technique. The RNA is extracted and purified from the tissues/cells of interest. This purified RNA can be labeled directly or can be converted to complementary DNA (cDNA) or T7RNA promoter and which transformed into cRNA. There are several methods in place to label the cRNA or cDNA such as biotin labeling. After labeling the cRNA or cDNA, the technique is selected for the amplification of generated signals. The commonly used strategies are incorporation of fluorescently labeled nucleotide or biotin-labeled nucleotide at the synthesis step of cRNA or cDNA. Microarray hybridization takes place on the labeled cRNA or cDNA. The array is washed with several washings, and the signal detection is made by measuring the fluorescence at the given spots. If the samples are labeled with biotin, the array is stained by hybridizing with streptavidin [68]. A laser is used to amplify the fluorescent signals, and the strength of signals is measured by using a scanning confocal microscopy technique. The strength or depth of a signal obtained gives the measurement of the expression stage of a corresponding gene(s).

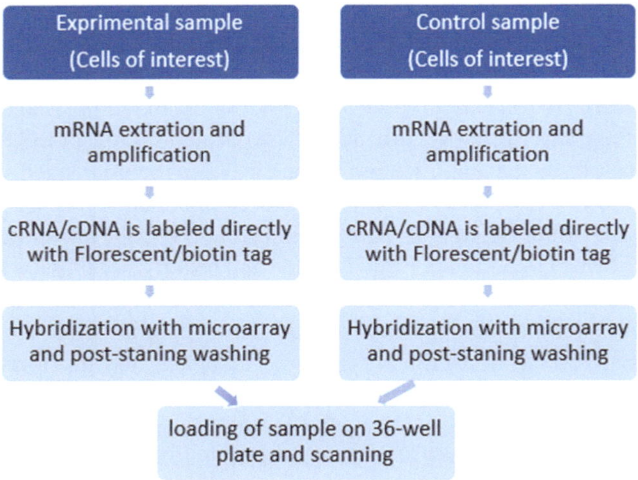

Fig. 1.3 Schematic overview of DNA microarray procedure

1.4.5.2 Transcription Factor Binding Analysis

DNA microarrays can also be used to locate the binding sites of transcription factor/ element along with chromatin immune-precipitation. The transcription factors (TF) of the cell of interest are purified by using affinity method after labeling the transcription factors (TF) with an antibody or a peptide which can docile with the affinity chromatography, i.e., FLAG-, HIS-, myc-, or HA-tag. The DNA released from the transcription factors (TF) after the purification step is subjected to amplification and categorization followed by hybridization to the array. This procedure or method is termed as "ChIP-chip" – chromatin immunoprecipitation on a "chip." The transcription factors (TF) usually bind a bit away from the genes subjected to modify, so the array's layout and the distribution of the length of a fragment are interconnected too [69]. In principle, the array should have the probe which can interrogate the area of DNA too to make sure the transcription factors (TF). In microorganism like yeast, they have small intergenic regions, so the array of the same length can be applied to ChIP-chip. On the other hand, in mammalian system, the intergenic regions are fairly large, and transcription factors (TF) generally bind some kilobase pair (kbp) away from the gene, so the array should be evenly spaced throughout the human or mammalian genome in ChIP-chip [70].

1.4.5.3 Genotyping

In single nucleotide polymorphism (SNP), the microarray is extensively used. There are several approaches to decipher SNP, but the most commonly used technique is allelic discrimination by hybridizing to the Affymetrix. Restriction enzyme is used to fragment the genomic DNA in this technique. After fragmentation, the adaptors are ligated for PCR. Under the specific condition of selective amplification <1 kb in size, the PCR is accomplished. It helps in reducing the genomic complexity for about up to 50×, and the obtained results correspond with the noise of the signal on the array. This SNP array is even capable of detecting >1M human single nucleotide polymorphism (SNP). Moreover, this technique can also be used to detect the copy numbers of a certain gene [59].

1.4.6 Limitations of DNA Microarrays

This technique is very useful in measuring the relative concentrations of DNA or RNA sequences present in a sample, but there are some drawbacks too. Firstly, DNA microarray provides indirect DNA or RNA concentrations, and the signal obtained at a certain point is assumed to be directly proportional to the concentration of specific single molecule present in a sample solution, but this relationship is not always linear. There are very strong chances that the probe may become saturated if the concentration of a specific specie in a solution is high and the equilibrium will not support the high concentrations. Secondly, in mammalian genomes, the designing of the array with multiple related DNA/RNA sequence for a complex mammalian genome is a challenge because the particular sequence may not always bind to a similar probe. There are chances that the sequence which is destined to detect the gene1 can also detect other related genes, and it will create problem in detection of protein family or different splice variants [59].

In addition, the DNA microarray can only detect the sequences which are changed by the array. If the sample solution contains more than one species of DNA or RNA molecule and there is no complementary sequence on the array, these species will not be detected by the array. Additionally, the noncoding RNAs which are not expressed cannot be hybridized on array, and in the variable genome including bacteria, the array is usually designed using information from the reference or model organism. In this way, the array can miss a number of genes present in a specific organism of identical species [71].

1.4.7 Future Outlook of DNA Microarrays

The studies of molecular biology were evolved by the improvement of traditional technologies. It is not possible to research a wide variety of genes by using traditional technique, and DNA microarray is the technology that permits researchers to analyze as well as deal with those problems that have been marked as untraceable. Now expression of many genes can be analyzed in one go speedily and greenway. Scientific community has been empowered to recognize basic factors highlighting boom, improvement of life and to explore genetic causes of irregularities inside functioning of body. DNA microarray has changed unexpectedly the conventional style of sequencing, even for every assay which was performed formerly on microarrays. It is very likely that sequencing methods will absolutely change with the help of DNA microarray in the coming 5–10 years.

This technology has pushed the practical genomics, the subject which particularly looks into the different roles of a certain gene in cellular processes. It also highlights the genome-wide differential RNA expression levels present in the different samples which can help, in particular, in understanding the course of illness, progression of a disease, and response to the therapy. The data being produced in microarray technique can be used in profiling of gene expression, and stages of specific protein expression can also be determined. This technique is equally important in detection of up- and downregulated genes in diseased and healthy conditions, expression styles of the same protein in different environments, detection of the absence and presence of positive stimulus, drug discovery, diagnosing disease, and identification of novel gene.

1.5 Tissue Microarrays

Clinical and biomedical research always demands tissue specimens. So, for that purpose DNA, RNA, and proteins are the main targets in tissues, enriched with the essential information for the improved consideration of disease and its pathological stage toward the development of advanced diagnostic biomarkers. However, the tissues of biopsy collection in biobanks are also small and possessing special value which normally diminishes with the passage of time. Keeping these limitations in mind, with tissue analysis being laborious, expensive, and time-consuming, array-based in situ technologies start to develop in 1977 to get high throughput. Tissue microarray (TMA) technology comprises the use of hundreds to thousands of tissues arranged systematically and thinly sectioned, which can be analyzed molecularly and functionally on a microscopic slide. The examination of multiple replica slides can be done for antibody testing and probing which can facilitate the analysis of pathological state of tissues in a single step, thus detecting many biomarkers in the repeated segment [72, 73].

1.5.1 Applications of Tissue Microarrays Technology

Tissue microarray (TMA) functions in many fields of biomedical and clinical research such as cell line, xenograft tumor, and animal and human tissue-based tissue microarray. It also serves as a diagnostic marker and helps in tumor classification. Interpretation of pathological conditions, screening of pathways and molecular target-dependent treatment decision-making for drug discovery can also facilitate by TMA [74, 75].

1.6 Conclusions

The development of new strategies has always been encouraged for the sake of advancement and betterment of patients' undertreatment. Enhancement in different stages of gene sequencing is revolutionized all over in the past few decades by economizing experimental animal usage, time, and cost, while more innovations are still required in future [57]. The trials with biomarker studies should be allowed with the involvement of the pharmaceuticals industry and governing authorities for the improvement of patients' treatment. On the other hand, the participation of skillful scientists and cooperative work can ease the emergence of biomarker application [76]. Being a neutrally conceptual technique, sequencing can determine the different nucleic acid in the mixture of DNA and RNA, unless the preparation of solution and enzymes are appropriate for the procedure. In contrast with DNA, microarray sequencing does not rely on previously added nucleic acid sequences, which are also related genes. These are the limitation of DNA microarray by virtue of which the reduction in the use of this technique is being observed in comparison with sequencing. The cost of sequencing is also decreasing which is also the reason for the replacement of DNA microarray to sequencing [67]. It is being considered by many researchers that the tissue microarray technique (TMA) is the most tremendous innovation between other histopathology during the past few years. TMA analysis technique influentially works as an important key for opening doors among lab experiments and hospital settings, becoming a helpful tool for researchers and medical students to study diseases. TMA also benefits the study of different proteins and gene expression profile for the extensive range of normal, cancerous, and benign tissues [77]. Cancer genomics can be analyzed inclusively with the assistance of high-throughput implements in the characterization of nucleic acid which would well understand the cellular modifications. Moreover, extensive and intense exertions have recognized a novel site to measure translational potential to cancer genomics.

References

1. Griffiths AJF, Miller JH, Suzuki DT, Lewontin RC, Gelbart WM (2000) An introduction to genetic analysis, 7th edn. W. H. Freeman, New York
2. Garraway LA, Lander ES (2013) Lessons from the cancer genome. Cell 153:17. https://doi.org/10.1016/j.cell.2013.03.002
3. Chin L, Hahn WC, Getz G, Meyerson M (2011) Making sense of cancer genomic data. Genes Dev 25:534
4. Hanauer D, Rhodes D, Sinha-Kumar C, Chinnaiyan A (2007) Bioinformatics approaches in the study of cancer. Curr Mol Med 7:133. https://doi.org/10.2174/156652407779940431
5. Brocks D, Assenov Y, Minner S, Bogatyrova O, Simon R, Koop C, Oakes C, Zucknick M, Lipka DB, Weischenfeldt J, Feuerbach L, Cowper-Sallari R, Lupien M, Brors B, Korbel J, Schlomm T, Tanay A, Sauter G, Gerhäuser C, Plass C (2014) Intratumor DNA methylation heterogeneity reflects clonal evolution in aggressive prostate cancer. Cell Rep 8:798. https://doi.org/10.1016/j.celrep.2014.06.053
6. Lin DC, Mayakonda A, Dinh HQ, Huang P, Lin L, Liu X, Ding LW, Wang J, Berman BP, Song EW, Yin D, Koeffler HP (2017) Genomic and epigenomic heterogeneity of hepatocellular carcinoma. Cancer Res 77:2255. https://doi.org/10.1158/0008-5472.CAN-16-2822
7. Mazor T, Pankov A, Johnson BE, Hong C, Hamilton EG, Bell RJA, Smirnov IV, Reis GF, Phillips JJ, Barnes MJ, Idbaih A, Alentorn A, Kloezeman JJ, Lamfers MLM, Bollen AW, Taylor BS, Molinaro AM, Olshen AB, Chang SM, Song JS, Costello JF (2015) DNA methylation and somatic mutations converge on the cell cycle and define similar evolutionary histories in brain tumors. Cancer Cell 28:307. https://doi.org/10.1016/j.ccell.2015.07.012

8. Landau DA, Clement K, Ziller MJ, Boyle P, Fan J, Gu H, Stevenson K, Sougnez C, Wang L, Li S, Kotliar D, Zhang W, Ghandi M, Garraway L, Fernandes SM, Livak KJ, Gabriel S, Gnirke A, Lander ES, Brown JR, Neuberg D, Kharchenko PV, Hacohen N, Getz G, Meissner A, Wu CJ (2014) Locally disordered methylation forms the basis of intratumor methylome variation in chronic lymphocytic leukemia. Cancer Cell 26:813. https://doi.org/10.1016/j.ccell.2014.10.012
9. Sheffield NC, Pierron G, Klughammer J, Datlinger P, Schönegger A, Schuster M, Hadler J, Surdez D, Guillemot D, Lapouble E, Freneaux P, Champigneulle J, Bouvier R, Walder D, Ambros IM, Hutter C, Sorz E, Amaral AT, De Álava E, Schallmoser K, Strunk D, Rinner B, Liegl-Atzwanger B, Huppertz B, Leithner A, De Pinieux G, Terrier P, Laurence V, Michon J, Ladenstein R, Holter W, Windhager R, Dirksen U, Ambros PF, Delattre O, Kovar H, Bock C, Tomazou EM (2017) DNA methylation heterogeneity defines a disease spectrum in Ewing sarcoma. Nat Med 23:386. https://doi.org/10.1038/nm.4273
10. Hodgson G, Hager JH, Volik S, Hariono S, Wernick M, Moore D, Albertson DG, Pinkel D, Collins C, Hanahan D, Gray JW (2001) Genome scanning with array CGH delineates regional alterations in mouse islet carcinomas. Nat Genet 29:459. https://doi.org/10.1038/ng771
11. Bailey MH, Tokheim C, Porta-Pardo E, Sengupta S, Bertrand D, Weerasinghe A, Colaprico A, Wendl MC, Kim J, Reardon B, Ng PKS, Jeong KJ, Cao S, Wang Z, Gao J, Gao Q, Wang F, Liu EM, Mularoni L, Rubio-Perez C, Nagarajan N, Cortés-Ciriano I, Zhou DC, Liang WW, Hess JM, Yellapantula VD, Tamborero D, Gonzalez-Perez A, Suphavilai C, Ko JY, Khurana E, Park PJ, Van Allen EM, Liang H, Caesar-Johnson SJ, Demchok JA, Felau I, Kasapi M, Ferguson ML, Hutter CM, Sofia HJ, Tarnuzzer R, Yang L, Zenklusen JC, Zhang JJ, Chudamani S, Liu J, Lolla L, Naresh R, Pihl T, Sun Q, Wan Y, Wu Y, Cho J, DeFreitas T, Frazer S, Gehlenborg N, Getz G, Heiman DI, Lawrence MS, Lin P, Meier S, Noble MS, Saksena G, Voet D, Zhang H, Bernard B, Chambwe N, Dhankani V, Knijnenburg T, Kramer R, Leinonen K, Liu Y, Miller M, Reynolds S, Shmulevich I, Thorsson V, Zhang W, Akbani R, Broom BM, Hegde AM, Ju Z, Kanchi RS, Korkut A, Li J, Ling S, Liu W, Lu Y, Mills GB, Ng KS, Rao A, Ryan M, Wang J, Weinstein JN, Zhang J, Abeshouse A, Armenia J, Chakravarty D, Chatila WK, de Bruijn I, Gross BE, Heins ZJ, Kundra R, La K, Ladanyi M, Luna A, Nissan MG, Ochoa A, Phillips SM, Reznik E, Sanchez-Vega F, Sander C, Schultz N, Sheridan R, Sumer SO, Sun Y, Taylor BS, Anur P, Peto M, Spellman P, Benz C, Stuart JM, Wong CK, Yau C, Hayes DN, Parker JS, Wilkerson MD, Ally A, Balasundaram M, Bowlby R, Brooks D, Carlsen R, Chuah E, Dhalla N, Holt R, SJM J, Kasaian K, Lee D, Ma Y, Marra MA, Mayo M, Moore RA, Mungall AJ, Mungall K, Robertson AG, Sadeghi S, Schein JE, Sipahimalani P, Tam A, Thiessen N, Tse K, Wong T, Berger AC, Beroukhim R, Cherniack AD, Cibulskis C, Gabriel SB, Gao GF, Ha G, Meyerson M, Schumacher SE, Shih J, Kucherlapati MH, Kucherlapati RS, Baylin S, Cope L, Danilova L, Bootwalla MS, Lai PH, Maglinte DT, Van Den Berg DJ, Weisenberger DJ, Auman JT, Balu S, Bodenheimer T, Fan C, Hoadley KA, Hoyle AP, Jefferys SR, Jones CD, Meng S, Mieczkowski PA, Mose LE, Perou AH, Perou CM, Roach J, Shi Y, Simons JV, Skelly T, Soloway MG, Tan D, Veluvolu U, Fan H, Hinoue T, Laird PW, Shen H, Zhou W, Bellair M, Chang K, Covington K, Creighton CJ, Dinh H, Doddapaneni HV, Donehower LA, Drummond J, Gibbs RA, Glenn R, Hale W, Han Y, Hu J, Korchina V, Lee S, Lewis L, Li W, Liu X, Morgan M, Morton D, Muzny D, Santibanez J, Sheth M, Shinbrot E, Wang L, Wang M, Wheeler DA, Xi L, Zhao F, Hess J, Appelbaum EL, Bailey M, Cordes MG, Ding L, Fronick CC, Fulton LA, Fulton RS, Kandoth C, Mardis ER, McLellan MD, Miller CA, Schmidt HK, Wilson RK, Crain D, Curley E, Gardner J, Lau K, Mallery D, Morris S, Paulauskis J, Penny R, Shelton C, Shelton T, Sherman M, Thompson E, Yena P, Bowen J, Gastier-Foster JM, Gerken M, Leraas KM, Lichtenberg TM, Ramirez NC, Wise L, Zmuda E, Corcoran N, Costello T, Hovens C, Carvalho AL, de Carvalho AC, Fregnani JH, Longatto-Filho A, Reis RM, Scapulatempo-Neto C, Silveira HCS, Vidal DO, Burnette A, Eschbacher J, Hermes B, Noss A, Singh R, Anderson ML, Castro PD, Ittmann M, Huntsman D, Kohl B, Le X, Thorp R, Andry C, Duffy ER, Lyadov V, Paklina O, Setdikova G, Shabunin A, Tavobilov M, McPherson C, Warnick R, Berkowitz R, Cramer D, Feltmate C, Horowitz N, Kibel A, Muto M, Raut CP, Malykh A, Barnholtz-Sloan JS, Barrett W, Devine K, Fulop J, Ostrom QT, Shimmel K, Wolinsky Y, Sloan AE, De Rose A, Giuliante

F, Goodman M, Karlan BY, Hagedorn CH, Eckman J, Harr J, Myers J, Tucker K, Zach LA, Deyarmin B, Hu H, Kvecher L, Larson C, Mural RJ, Somiari S, Vicha A, Zelinka T, Bennett J, Iacocca M, Rabeno B, Swanson P, Latour M, Lacombe L, Têtu B, Bergeron A, McGraw M, Staugaitis SM, Chabot J, Hibshoosh H, Sepulveda A, Su T, Wang T, Potapova O, Voronina O, Desjardins L, Mariani O, Roman-Roman S, Sastre X, Stern MH, Cheng F, Signoretti S, Berchuck A, Bigner D, Lipp E, Marks J, McCall S, McLendon R, Secord A, Sharp A, Behera M, Brat DJ, Chen A, Delman K, Force S, Khuri F, Magliocca K, Maithel S, Olson JJ, Owonikoko T, Pickens A, Ramalingam S, Shin DM, Sica G, Van Meir EG, Eijckenboom W, Gillis A, Korpershoek E, Looijenga L, Oosterhuis W, Stoop H, van Kessel KE, Zwarthoff EC, Calatozzolo C, Cuppini L, Cuzzubbo S, DiMeco F, Finocchiaro G, Mattei L, Perin A, Pollo B, Chen C, Houck J, Lohavanichbutr P, Hartmann A, Stoehr C, Stoehr R, Taubert H, Wach S, Wullich B, Kycler W, Murawa D, Wiznerowicz M, Chung K, Edenfield WJ, Martin J, Baudin E, Bubley G, Bueno R, De Rienzo A, Richards WG, Kalkanis S, Mikkelsen T, Noushmehr H, Scarpace L, Girard N, Aymerich M, Campo E, Giné E, Guillermo AL, Van Bang N, Hanh PT, Phu BD, Tang Y, Colman H, Evason K, Dottino PR, Martignetti JA, Gabra H, Juhl H, Akeredolu T, Stepa S, Hoon D, Ahn K, Kang KJ, Beuschlein F, Breggia A, Birrer M, Bell D, Borad M, Bryce AH, Castle E, Chandan V, Cheville J, Copland JA, Farnell M, Flotte T, Giama N, Ho T, Kendrick M, Kocher JP, Kopp K, Moser C, Nagorney D, O'Brien D, O'Neill BP, Patel T, Petersen G, Que F, Rivera M, Roberts L, Smallridge R, Smyrk T, Stanton M, Thompson RH, Torbenson M, Yang JD, Zhang L, Brimo F, Ajani JA, AMA G, Behrens C, Bondaruk J, Broaddus R, Czerniak B, Esmaeli B, Fujimoto J, Gershenwald J, Guo C, Lazar AJ, Logothetis C, Meric-Bernstam F, Moran C, Ramondetta L, Rice D, Sood A, Tamboli P, Thompson T, Troncoso P, Tsao A, Wistuba I, Carter C, Haydu L, Hersey P, Jakrot V, Kakavand H, Kefford R, Lee K, Long G, Mann G, Quinn M, Saw R, Scolyer R, Shannon K, Spillane A, Stretch J, Synott M, Thompson J, Wilmott J, Al-Ahmadie H, Chan TA, Ghossein R, Gopalan A, Levine DA, Reuter V, Singer S, Singh B, Tien NV, Broudy T, Mirsaidi C, Nair P, Drwiega P, Miller J, Smith J, Zaren H, Park JW, Hung NP, Kebebew E, Linehan WM, Metwalli AR, Pacak K, Pinto PA, Schiffman M, Schmidt LS, Vocke CD, Wentzensen N, Worrell R, Yang H, Moncrieff M, Goparaju C, Melamed J, Pass H, Botnariuc N, Caraman I, Cernat M, Chemencedji I, Clipca A, Doruc S, Gorincioi G, Mura S, Pirtac M, Stancul I, Tcaciuc D, Albert M, Alexopoulou I, Arnaout A, Bartlett J, Engel J, Gilbert S, Parfitt J, Sekhon H, Thomas G, Rassl DM, Rintoul RC, Bifulco C, Tamakawa R, Urba W, Hayward N, Timmers H, Antenucci A, Facciolo F, Grazi G, Marino M, Merola R, de Krijger R, Gimenez-Roqueplo AP, Piché A, Chevalier S, McKercher G, Birsoy K, Barnett G, Brewer C, Farver C, Naska T, Pennell NA, Raymond D, Schilero C, Smolenski K, Williams F, Morrison C, Borgia JA, Liptay MJ, Pool M, Seder CW, Junker K, Omberg L, Dinkin M, Manikhas G, Alvaro D, Bragazzi MC, Cardinale V, Carpino G, Gaudio E, Chesla D, Cottingham S, Dubina M, Moiseenko F, Dhanasekaran R, Becker KF, Janssen KP, Slotta-Huspenina J, Abdel-Rahman MH, Aziz D, Bell S, Cebulla CM, Davis A, Duell R, Elder JB, Hilty J, Kumar B, Lang J, Lehman NL, Mandt R, Nguyen P, Pilarski R, Rai K, Schoenfield L, Senecal K, Wakely P, Hansen P, Lechan R, Powers J, Tischler A, Grizzle WE, Sexton KC, Kastl A, Henderson J, Porten S, Waldmann J, Fassnacht M, Asa SL, Schadendorf D, Couce M, Graefen M, Huland H, Sauter G, Schlomm T, Simon R, Tennstedt P, Olabode O, Nelson M, Bathe O, Carroll PR, Chan JM, Disaia P, Glenn P, Kelley RK, Landen CN, Phillips J, Prados M, Simko J, Smith-McCune K, VandenBerg S, Roggin K, Fehrenbach A, Kendler A, Sifri S, Steele R, Jimeno A, Carey F, Forgie I, Mannelli M, Carney M, Hernandez B, Campos B, Herold-Mende C, Jungk C, Unterberg A, von Deimling A, Bossler A, Galbraith J, Jacobus L, Knudson M, Knutson T, Ma D, Milhem M, Sigmund R, Godwin AK, Madan R, Rosenthal HG, Adebamowo C, Adebamowo SN, Boussioutas A, Beer D, Giordano T, Mes-Masson AM, Saad F, Bocklage T, Landrum L, Mannel R, Moore K, Moxley K, Postier R, Walker J, Zuna R, Feldman M, Valdivieso F, Dhir R, Luketich J, Pinero EMM, Quintero-Aguilo M, Carlotti CG, Dos Santos JS, Kemp R, Sankarankuty A, Tirapelli D, Catto J, Agnew K, Swisher E, Creaney J, Robinson B, Shelley CS, Godwin EM, Kendall S, Shipman C, Bradford C, Carey T, Haddad A, Moyer J, Peterson L, Prince M, Rozek L, Wolf G, Bowman R, Fong KM, Yang I, Korst R, Rathmell WK, Fantacone-Campbell JL, Hooke JA, Kovatich AJ,

Shriver CD, DiPersio J, Drake B, Govindan R, Heath S, Ley T, Van Tine B, Westervelt P, Rubin MA, Lee JI, Aredes ND, Mariamidze A, Godzik A, Lopez-Bigas N, Stuart J, Wheeler D, Chen K, Karchin R (2018) Comprehensive characterization of cancer driver genes and mutations. Cell 173:371. https://doi.org/10.1016/j.cell.2018.02.060

12. Luo J, Solimini NL, Elledge SJ (2009) Principles of cancer therapy: oncogene and non-oncogene addiction. Cell 136:823
13. Shalem O, Sanjana NE, Zhang F (2015) High-throughput functional genomics using CRISPR-Cas9. Nat Rev Genet 16:299. https://doi.org/10.1038/nrg3899
14. Gerhards NM, Rottenberg S (2018) New tools for old drugs: functional genetic screens to optimize current chemotherapy. Drug Resist Updat 36:30. https://doi.org/10.1016/j.drup.2018.01.001
15. Doench JG (2018) Am I ready for CRISPR? A user's guide to genetic screens. Nat Rev Genet 19:67
16. Hart T, Brown KR, Sircoulomb F, Rottapel R, Moffat J (2014) Measuring error rates in genomic perturbation screens: gold standards for human functional genomics. Mol Syst Biol 10:733. https://doi.org/10.15252/msb.20145216
17. Doench JG, Fusi N, Sullender M, Hegde M, Vaimberg EW, Donovan KF, Smith I, Tothova Z, Wilen C, Orchard R, Virgin HW, Listgarten J, Root DE (2016) Optimized sgRNA design to maximize activity and minimize off-target effects of CRISPR-Cas9. Nat Biotechnol 34:184. https://doi.org/10.1038/nbt.3437
18. Reddy EP, Reynolds RK, Santos E, Barbacid M (1982) A point mutation is responsible for the acquisition of transforming properties by the T24 human bladder carcinoma oncogene. Nature 300:149. https://doi.org/10.1038/300149a0
19. Tabin CJ, Bradley SM, Bargmann CI, Weinberg RA, Papageorge AG, Scolnick EM, Dhar R, Lowy DR, Chang EH (1982) Mechanism of activation of a human oncogene. Nature 300:143. https://doi.org/10.1038/300143a0
20. Capon DJ, Seeburg PH, McGrath JP, Hayflick JS, Edman U, Levinson AD, Goeddel DV (1983) Activation of Ki-ras2 gene in human colon and lung carcinomas by two different point mutations. Nature 304:507. https://doi.org/10.1038/304507a0
21. Shimizu K, Goldfarb M, Suard Y, Perucho M, Li Y, Kamata T, Feramisco J, Stavnezer E, Fogh J, Wigler MH (1983) Three human transforming genes are related to the viral ras oncogenes. Proc Natl Acad Sci 80:2112. https://doi.org/10.1073/pnas.80.8.2112
22. Downward J (2003) Targeting RAS signalling pathways in cancer therapy. Nat Rev Cancer 3:11
23. Allegra CJ, Jessup JM, Somerfield MR, Hamilton SR, Hammond EH, Hayes DF, McAllister PK, Morton RF, Schilsky RL (2009) American society of clinical oncology provisional clinical opinion: testing for KRAS gene mutations in patients with metastatic colorectal carcinoma to predict response to anti-epidermal growth factor receptor monoclonal antibody therapy. J Clin Oncol 27:2091
24. Flaherty KT, Puzanov I, Kim KB, Ribas A, McArthur GA, Sosman JA, O'Dwyer PJ, Lee RJ, Grippo JF, Nolop K, Chapman PB (2010) Inhibition of mutated, activated BRAF in metastatic melanoma. N Engl J Med 363:809. https://doi.org/10.1056/NEJMoa1002011
25. Fraser J, Williamson I, Bickmore WA, Dostie J (2015) An overview of genome organization and how we got there: from FISH to Hi-C. Microbiol Mol Biol Rev 79:347. https://doi.org/10.1128/mmbr.00006-15
26. Amendola M, Van Steensel B (2014) Mechanisms and dynamics of nuclear lamina-genome interactions. Curr Opin Cell Biol 28:61
27. Zuleger N, Robson MI, Schirmer EC (2011) The nuclear envelope as a chromatin organizer. Nucleus 2:339
28. Ptak C, Aitchison JD, Wozniak RW (2014) The multifunctional nuclear pore complex: a platform for controlling gene expression. Curr Opin Cell Biol 28:46
29. Németh A, Conesa A, Santoyo-Lopez J, Medina I, Montaner D, Péterfia B, Solovei I, Cremer T, Dopazo J, Längst G (2010) Initial genomics of the human nucleolus. PLoS Genet 6:e1000889. https://doi.org/10.1371/journal.pgen.1000889

30. International Cancer Genome Consortium, Hudson TJ, Anderson W, Artez A, Barker AD, Bell C, Bernabé RR, Bhan MK, Calvo F, Eerola I, Gerhard DS, Guttmacher A, Guyer M, Hemsley FM, Jennings JL, Kerr D, Klatt P, Kolar P, Kusada J, Lane DP, Laplace F, Youyong L, Nettekoven G, Ozenberger B, Peterson J, Rao TS, Remacle J, Schafer AJ, Shibata T, Stratton MR, Vockley JG, Watanabe K, Yang H, Yuen MMF, Knoppers BM, Bobrow M, Cambon-Thomsen A, Dressler LG, Dyke SOM, Joly Y, Kato K, Kennedy KL, Nicolás P, Parker MJ, Rial-Sebbag E, Romeo-Casabona CM, Shaw KM, Wallace S, Wiesner GL, Zeps N, Lichter P, Biankin AV, Chabannon C, Chin L, Clément B, de Alava E, Degos F, Ferguson ML, Geary P, Hayes DN, Hudson TJ, Johns AL, Kasprzyk A, Nakagawa H, Penny R, Piris MA, Sarin R, Scarpa A, Shibata T, van de Vijver M, Futreal PA, Aburatani H, Bayés M, Botwell DDL, Campbell PJ, Estivill X, Gerhard DS, Grimmond SM, Gut I, Hirst M, López-Otín C, Majumder P, Marra M, McPherson JD, Nakagawa H, Ning Z, Puente XS, Ruan Y, Shibata T, Stratton MR, Stunnenberg HG, Swerdlow H, Velculescu VE, Wilson RK, Xue HH, Yang L, Spellman PT, Bader GD, Boutros PC, Campbell PJ, Flicek P, Getz G, Guigó R, Guo G, Haussler D, Heath S, Hubbard TJ, Jiang T, Jones SM, Li Q, López-Bigas N, Luo R, Muthuswamy L, Ouellette BFF, Pearson JV, Puente XS, Quesada V, Raphael BJ, Sander C, Shibata T, Speed TP, Stein LD, Stuart JM, Teague JW, Totoki Y, Tsunoda T, Valencia A, Wheeler DA, Wu H, Zhao S, Zhou G, Stein LD, Guigó R, Hubbard TJ, Joly Y, Jones SM, Kasprzyk A, Lathrop M, López-Bigas N, Ouellette BFF, Spellman PT, Teague JW, Thomas G, Valencia A, Yoshida T, Kennedy KL, Axton M, Dyke SOM, Futreal PA, Gerhard DS, Gunter C, Guyer M, Hudson TJ, McPherson JD, Miller LJ, Ozenberger B, Shaw KM, Kasprzyk A, Stein LD, Zhang J, Haider SA, Wang J, Yung CK, Cros A, Cross A, Liang Y, Gnaneshan S, Guberman J, Hsu J, Bobrow M, Chalmers DRC, Hasel KW, Joly Y, Kaan TSH, Kennedy KL, Knoppers BM, Lowrance WW, Masui T, Nicolás P, Rial-Sebbag E, Rodriguez LL, Vergely C, Yoshida T, Grimmond SM, Biankin AV, Bowtell DDL, Cloonan N, deFazio A, Eshleman JR, Etemadmoghadam D, Gardiner BB, Gardiner BA, Kench JG, Scarpa A, Sutherland RL, Tempero MA, Waddell NJ, Wilson PJ, McPherson JD, Gallinger S, Tsao M-S, Shaw PA, Petersen GM, Mukhopadhyay D, Chin L, DePinho RA, Thayer S, Muthuswamy L, Shazand K, Beck T, Sam M, Timms L, Ballin V, Lu Y, Ji J, Zhang X, Chen F, Hu X, Zhou G, Yang Q, Tian G, Zhang L, Xing X, Li X, Zhu Z, Yu Y, Yu J, Yang H, Lathrop M, Tost J, Brennan P, Holcatova I, Zaridze D, Brazma A, Egevard L, Prokhortchouk E, Banks RE, Uhlén M, Cambon-Thomsen A, Viksna J, Ponten F, Skryabin K, Stratton MR, Futreal PA, Birney E, Borg A, Børresen-Dale A-L, Caldas C, Foekens JA, Martin S, Reis-Filho JS, Richardson AL, Sotiriou C, Stunnenberg HG, Thoms G, van de Vijver M, van't Veer L, Calvo F, Birnbaum D, Blanche H, Boucher P, Boyault S, Chabannon C, Gut I, Masson-Jacquemier JD, Lathrop M, Pauporté I, Pivot X, Vincent-Salomon A, Tabone E, Theillet C, Thomas G, Tost J, Treilleux I, Calvo F, Bioulac-Sage P, Clément B, Decaens T, Degos F, Franco D, Gut I, Gut M, Heath S, Lathrop M, Samuel D, Thomas G, Zucman-Rossi J, Lichter P, Eils R, Brors B, Korbel JO, Korshunov A, Landgraf P, Lehrach H, Pfister S, Radlwimmer B, Reifenberger G, Taylor MD, von Kalle C, Majumder PP, Sarin R, Rao TS, Bhan MK, Scarpa A, Pederzoli P, Lawlor RA, Delledonne M, Bardelli A, Biankin AV, Grimmond SM, Gress T, Klimstra D, Zamboni G, Shibata T, Nakamura Y, Nakagawa H, Kusada J, Tsunoda T, Miyano S, Aburatani H, Kato K, Fujimoto A, Yoshida T, Campo E, López-Otín C, Estivill X, Guigó R, de Sanjosé S, Piris MA, Montserrat E, González-Díaz M, Puente XS, Jares P, Valencia A, Himmelbauer H, Himmelbaue H, Quesada V, Bea S, Stratton MR, Futreal PA, Campbell PJ, Vincent-Salomon A, Richardson AL, Reis-Filho JS, van de Vijver M, Thomas G, Masson-Jacquemier JD, Aparicio S, Borg A, Børresen-Dale A-L, Caldas C, Foekens JA, Stunnenberg HG, van't Veer L, Easton DF, Spellman PT, Martin S, Barker AD, Chin L, Collins FS, Compton CC, Ferguson ML, Gerhard DS, Getz G, Gunter C, Guttmacher A, Guyer M, Hayes DN, Lander ES, Ozenberger B, Penny R, Peterson J, Sander C, Shaw KM, Speed TP, Spellman PT, Vockley JG, Wheeler DA, Wilson RK, Hudson TJ, Chin L, Knoppers BM, Lander ES, Lichter P, Stein LD, Stratton MR, Anderson W, Barker AD, Bell C, Bobrow M, Burke W, Collins FS, Compton CC, DePinho RA, Easton DF, Futreal PA, Gerhard DS, Green AR, Guyer M, Hamilton SR, Hubbard TJ, Kallioniemi OP, Kennedy KL, Ley TJ, Liu ET, Lu Y, Majumder P, Marra M, Ozenberger B, Peterson J, Schafer AJ, Spellman PT,

Stunnenberg HG, Wainwright BJ, Wilson RK, Yang H (2010) International network of cancer genome projects. Nature 464:993. https://doi.org/10.1038/nature08987
31. Birney E, Andrews TD, Bevan P, Caccamo M, Chen Y, Clarke L, Coates G, Cuff J, Curwen V, Cutts T, Down T, Eyras E, Fernandez-Suarez XM, Gane P, Gibbins B, Gilbert J, Hammond M, Hotz HR, Iyer V, Jekosch K, Kahari A, Kasprzyk A, Keefe D, Keenan S, Lehvaslaiho H, McVicker G, Melsopp C, Meidl P, Mongin E, Pettett R, Potter S, Proctor G, Rae M, Searle S, Slater G, Smedley D, Smith J, Spooner W, Stabenau A, Stalker J, Storey R, Ureta-Vidal A, Woodwark KC, Cameron G, Durbin R, Cox A, Hubbard T, Clamp M (2004) An overview of Ensembl. Genome Res 14:925
32. Karolchik D, Baertsch R, Diekhans M, Furey TS, Hinrichs A, Lu YT, Roskin KM, Schwartz M, Sugnet CW, Thomas DJ, Weber RJ, Haussler D, Kent WJ, University of California Santa Cruz (2003) The UCSC genome browser database. Nucleic Acids Res 31:51
33. Johnson JM, Castle J, Garrett-Engele P, Kan Z, Loerch PM, Armour CD, Santos R, Schadt EE, Stoughton R, Shoemaker DD (2003) Genome-wide survey of human alternative pre-mRNA splicing with exon junction microarrays. Science 302:2141. https://doi.org/10.1126/science.1090100
34. Little PFR (2005) Structure and function of the human genome. Genome Res 15:1759
35. Cheng J, Kapranov P, Drenkow J, Dike S, Brubaker S, Patel S, Long J, Stern D, Tammana H, Helt G, Sementchenko V, Piccolboni A, Bekiranov S, Bailey DK, Ganesh M, Ghosh S, Bell I, Gerhard DS, Gingeras TR (2005) Transcriptional maps of 10 human chromosomes at 5-nucleotide resolution. Science 308:1149. https://doi.org/10.1126/science.1108625
36. O'Neill MJ (2005) The influence of non-coding RNAs on allele-specific gene expression in mammals. Hum Mol Genet 14:R113
37. Lagos-Quintana M, Rauhut R, Lendeckel W, Tuschl T (2001) Identification of novel genes coding for small expressed RNAs. Science 294:853. https://doi.org/10.1126/science.1064921
38. Craig Venter J, Adams MD, Myers EW, Li PW, Mural RJ, Sutton GG, Smith HO, Yandell M, Evans CA, Holt RA, Gocayne JD, Amanatides P, Ballew RM, Huson DH, Wortman JR, Zhang Q, Kodira CD, Zheng XH, Chen L, Skupski M, Subramanian G, Thomas PD, Zhang J, Gabor Miklos GL, Nelson C, Broder S, Clark AG, Nadeau J, McKusick VA, Zinder N, Levine AJ, Roberts RJ, Simon M, Slayman C, Hunkapiller M, Bolanos R, Delcher A, Dew I, Fasulo D, Flanigan M, Florea L, Halpern A, Hannenhalli S, Kravitz S, Levy S, Mobarry C, Reinert K, Remington K, Abu-Threideh J, Beasley E, Biddick K, Bonazzi V, Brandon R, Cargill M, Chandramouliswaran I, Charlab R, Chaturvedi K, Deng Z, di Francesco V, Dunn P, Eilbeck K, Evangelista C, Gabrielian AE, Gan W, Ge W, Gong F, Gu Z, Guan P, Heiman TJ, Higgins ME, Ji RR, Ke Z, Ketchum KA, Lai Z, Lei Y, Li Z, Li J, Liang Y, Lin X, Lu F, Merkulov GV, Milshina N, Moore HM, Naik AK, Narayan VA, Neelam B, Nusskern D, Rusch DB, Salzberg S, Shao W, Shue B, Sun J, Yuan Wang Z, Wang A, Wang X, Wang J, Wei MH, Wides R, Xiao C, Yan C, Yao A, Ye J, Zhan M, Zhang W, Zhang H, Zhao Q, Zheng L, Zhong F, Zhong W, Zhu SC, Zhao S, Gilbert D, Baumhueter S, Spier G, Carter C, Cravchik A, Woodage T, Ali F, An H, Awe A, Baldwin D, Baden H, Barnstead M, Barrow I, Beeson K, Busam D, Carver A, Center A, Lai Cheng M, Curry L, Danaher S, Davenport L, Desilets R, Dietz S, Dodson K, Doup L, Ferriera S, Garg N, Gluecksmann A, Hart B, Haynes J, Haynes C, Heiner C, Hladun S, Hostin D, Houck J, Howland T, Ibegwam C, Johnson J, Kalush F, Kline L, Koduru S, Love A, Mann F, May D, McCawley S, McIntosh T, McMullen I, Moy M, Moy L, Murphy B, Nelson K, Pfannkoch C, Pratts E, Puri V, Qureshi H, Reardon M, Rodriguez R, Rogers YH, Romblad D, Ruhfel B, Scott R, Sitter C, Smallwood M, Stewart E, Strong R, Suh E, Thomas R, Ni Tint N, Tse S, Vech C, Wang G, Wetter J, Williams S, Williams M, Windsor S, Winn-Deen E, Wolfe K, Zaveri J, Zaveri K, Abril JF, Guigo R, Campbell MJ, Sjolander KV, Karlak B, Kejariwal A, Mi H, Lazareva B, Hatton T, Narechania A, Diemer K, Muruganujan A, Guo N, Sato S, Bafna V, Istrail S, Lippert R, Schwartz R, Walenz B, Yooseph S, Allen D, Basu A, Baxendale J, Blick L, Caminha M, Carnes-Stine J, Caulk P, Chiang YH, Coyne M, Dahlke C, Deslattes Mays A, Dombroski M, Donnelly M, Ely D, Esparham S, Fosler C, Gire H, Glanowski S, Glasser K, Glodek A, Gorokhov M, Graham K, Gropman B, Harris M, Heil J, Henderson S, Hoover J, Jennings D, Jordan C, Jordan J, Kasha J, Kagan L, Kraft C, Levitsky A, Lewis M, Liu X,

Lopez J, Ma D, Majoros W, McDaniel J, Murphy S, Newman M, Nguyen T, Nguyen N, Nodell M, Pan S, Peck J, Peterson M, Rowe W, Sanders R, Scott J, Simpson M, Smith T, Sprague A, Stockwell T, Turner R, Venter E, Wang M, Wen M, Wu D, Wu M, Xia A, Zandieh A, Zhu X (2001) The sequence of the human genome. Science 291:1304. https://doi.org/10.1126/science.1058040

39. De La Calle-Mustienes E, Feijóo CG, Manzanares M, Tena JJ, Rodríguez-Seguel E, Letizia A, Allende ML, Gómez-Skarmeta JL (2005) A functional survey of the enhancer activity of conserved non-coding sequences from vertebrate Iroquois cluster gene deserts. Genome Res 15:1061. https://doi.org/10.1101/gr.4004805
40. Caron H, Van Schaik B, Van der Mee M, Baas F, Riggins G, Van Sluis P, Hermus MC, Van Asperen R, Boon K, Voûte PA, Heisterkamp S, Van Kampen A, Versteeg R (2001) The human transcriptome map: clustering of highly expressed genes in chromosomal domains. Science 291:1289. https://doi.org/10.1126/science.1056794
41. Tuzun E, Sharp AJ, Bailey JA, Kaul R, Morrison VA, Pertz LM, Haugen E, Hayden H, Albertson D, Pinkel D, Olson MV, Eichler EE (2005) Fine-scale structural variation of the human genome. Nat Genet 37:727. https://doi.org/10.1038/ng1562
42. Maher MC, Uricchio LH, Torgerson DG, Hernandez RD (2012) Population genetics of rare variants and complex diseases. Hum Hered 74:118–128. https://doi.org/10.1159/000346826
43. Sawyer SL, Mukherjee N, Pakstis AJ, Feuk L, Kidd JR, Brookes AJ, Kidd KK (2005) Linkage disequilibrium patterns vary substantially among populations. Eur J Hum Genet 13:677. https://doi.org/10.1038/sj.ejhg.5201368
44. Davies H, Bignell GR et al (2002) 6-Mutations of the BRAF gene in human cancer. Nature 417:949. https://doi.org/10.1038/nature00766
45. Samuels Y, Wang Z, Bardelli A, Silliman N, Ptak J, Szabo S, Yan H, Gazdar A, Powell SM, Riggins GJ, Willson JKV, Markowitz S, Kinzler KW, Vogelstein B, Velculescu VE (2004) High frequency of mutations of the PIK3CA gene in human cancers. Science 304:554. https://doi.org/10.1126/science.1096502
46. Parsons DW, Jones S, Zhang X, Lin JCH, Leary RJ, Angenendt P, Mankoo P, Carter H, Siu IM, Gallia GL, Olivi A, McLendon R, Rasheed BA, Keir S, Nikolskaya T, Nikolsky Y, Busam DA, Tekleab H, Diaz LA, Hartigan J, Smith DR, Strausberg RL, Marie SKN, Shinjo SMO, Yan H, Riggins GJ, Bigner DD, Karchin R, Papadopoulos N, Parmigiani G, Vogelstein B, Velculescu VE, Kinzler KW (2008) An integrated genomic analysis of human glioblastoma multiforme. Science 321:1807. https://doi.org/10.1126/science.1164382
47. Chen Y, Takita J, Choi YL, Kato M, Ohira M, Sanada M, Wang L, Soda M, Kikuchi A, Igarashi T, Nakagawara A, Hayashi Y, Mano H, Ogawa S (2008) Oncogenic mutations of ALK kinase in neuroblastoma. Nature 455:971. https://doi.org/10.1038/nature07399
48. Soda M, Choi YL, Enomoto M, Takada S, Yamashita Y, Ishikawa S, Fujiwara SI, Watanabe H, Kurashina K, Hatanaka H, Bando M, Ohno S, Ishikawa Y, Aburatani H, Niki T, Sohara Y, Sugiyama Y, Mano H (2007) Identification of the transforming EML4-ALK fusion gene in non-small-cell lung cancer. Nature 448:561. https://doi.org/10.1038/nature05945
49. Verhaak RGW, Hoadley KA, Purdom E, Wang V, Qi Y, Wilkerson MD, Miller CR, Ding L, Golub T, Mesirov JP, Alexe G, Lawrence M, O'Kelly M, Tamayo P, Weir BA, Gabriel S, Winckler W, Gupta S, Jakkula L, Feiler HS, Hodgson JG, James CD, Sarkaria JN, Brennan C, Kahn A, Spellman PT, Wilson RK, Speed TP, Gray JW, Meyerson M, Getz G, Perou CM, Hayes DN, Cancer Genome Atlas Research Network (2010) Integrated genomic analysis identifies clinically relevant subtypes of glioblastoma characterized by abnormalities in PDGFRA, IDH1, EGFR, and NF1. Cancer Cell 17:98. https://doi.org/10.1016/j.ccr.2009.12.020
50. Shendure J, Balasubramanian S, Church GM, Gilbert W, Rogers J, Schloss JA, Waterston RH (2017) DNA sequencing at 40: past, present and future. Nature 550:345–353. https://doi.org/10.1038/nature24286
51. Munshi A (2012) DNA sequencing-methods and applications. InTech, Rijeka
52. Sanger F (1988) Sequences, sequences, and sequences. Annu Rev Biochem 57:1–28
53. Ozsolak F, Milos PM (2011) RNA sequencing: advances, challenges and opportunities. Nat Rev Genet 12:87–98. https://doi.org/10.1038/nrg2934

54. Shendure J, Ji H (2008) Next-generation DNA sequencing. Nat Biotechnol 26:1135–1145. https://doi.org/10.1038/nbt1486
55. Pettersson E, Lundeberg J, Ahmadian A (2009) Generations of sequencing technologies. Genomics 93:105–111. https://doi.org/10.1016/j.ygeno.2008.10.003
56. Moorthie S, Mattocks CJ, Wright CF (2011) Review of massively parallel DNA sequencing technologies. HUGO J 5:1–12. https://doi.org/10.1007/s11568-011-9156-3
57. Heather JM, Chain B (2016) The sequence of sequencers: the history of sequencing DNA. Genomics 107:1–8. https://doi.org/10.1016/j.ygeno.2015.11.003
58. Yaran Y, Xie B, Yan J (2014) Application of next-generation sequencing technology in forensic science. Genomics Proteomics Bioinformatics 12:190–197. https://doi.org/10.13618/j.issn.1001-5728.2017.01.011
59. Aaronson JS, Eckman B, Blevins RA, Borkowski JA, Myerson J, Imran S, Elliston KO (1996) Toward the development of a gene index to the human genome: an assessment of the nature of high-throughput EST sequence data. Genome Res 6:829–845. https://doi.org/10.1101/gr.6.9.829
60. United Nations Environment Programme, International Labour Organisation, World Health Organization, International Program on Chemical Safety (2001) Biomarkers in risk assessment: validity and validation. World Health Organization, Geneva
61. Shaw A, Bradley MD, Elyan S, Kurian KM (2015) Tumour biomarkers: diagnostic, prognostic, and predictive. BMJ 351:h3449. https://doi.org/10.1136/bmj.h3449
62. Frank R, Hargreaves R (2003) Clinical biomarkers in drug discovery and development. Nat Rev Drug Discov 2:566–580. https://doi.org/10.1038/nrd1130
63. Kiviat NB, Critchlow CW (2002) Novel approaches to identification of biomarkers for detection of early stage cancer. Dis Markers 18:73–81. https://doi.org/10.1155/2002/589075
64. Freidlin B, McShane LM, Korn EL (2010) Randomized clinical trials with biomarkers: design issues. J Natl Cancer Inst 102:152–160. https://doi.org/10.1093/jnci/djp477
65. Paliouras M, Borgono C, Diamandis EP (2007) Human tissue kallikreins: the cancer biomarker family. Cancer Lett 249:61–79. https://doi.org/10.1016/j.canlet.2006.12.018
66. Ariztia EV, Lee CJ, Gogoi R, Fishman DA (2006) The tumor microenvironment: key to early detection. Crit Rev Clin Lab Sci 43:393–425. https://doi.org/10.1080/10408360600778836
67. Bumgarner R (2013) Overview of DNA microarrays: types, applications, and their future. Curr Protoc Mol Biol 101:22.1.1–22.1.11. https://doi.org/10.1002/0471142727.mb2201s101
68. Chee M, Yang R, Hubbell E, Berno A, Huang XC, Stern D, Winkler J, Lockhart DJ, Morris MS, Fodor SP (1996) Accessing genetic information with high-density DNA arrays. Science 274:610–614
69. Andrilenas KK, Penvose A, Siggers T (2015) Using protein-binding microarrays to study transcription factor specificity: homologs, isoforms and complexes. Brief Funct Genomics 14:17–29. https://doi.org/10.1093/bfgp/elu046
70. Castle J, Garrett-Engele P, Armour CD, Duenwald SJ, Loerch PM, Meyer MR, Schadt EE, Stoughton R, Parrish ML, Shoemaker DD, Johnson JM (2003) Optimization of oligonucleotide arrays and RNA amplification protocols for analysis of transcript structure and alternative splicing. Genome Biol 4:R66. https://doi.org/10.1186/gb-2003-4-10-r66
71. Russo G, Zegar C, Giordano A (2003) Advantages and limitations of microarray technology in human cancer. Oncogene 22:6497–6507. https://doi.org/10.1038/sj.onc.1206865
72. Bubendorf L, Nocito A, Moch H, Sauter G (2001) Tissue microarray (TMA) technology: miniaturized pathology archives for high-throughput in situ studies. J Pathol 195:72–79. https://doi.org/10.1002/path.893
73. Kallioniemi OP, Kononen J, Sauter G (2012) Introducing tissue microarrays to molecular pathology. Clin Chem 58:1717–1718. https://doi.org/10.1373/clinchem.2012.188748
74. Braunschweig T, Chung JY, Hewitt SM (2005) Tissue microarrays: bridging the gap between research and the clinic. Expert Rev Proteomics 2:325–336. https://doi.org/10.1586/14789450.2.3.325

75. Sauter G, Simon R, Hillan K (2003) Tissue microarrays in drug discovery. Nat Rev Drug Discov 2:962–972. https://doi.org/10.1038/nrd1254
76. Frank R, Hargreaves R, Pike T, Point W (2003) Clinical biomarkers in drug discovery and development. Nat Rev Drug Discov 2:566–580. https://doi.org/10.1038/nrd1130
77. Vokuda RS, Verma SK, Srinivas BH (2018) Tissue microarray technology—a brief review. Natl J Lab Med 7:1–4. https://doi.org/10.7860/NJLM/2018/31639:2271

Metabolic Changes and Their Characterization

2

Noor-ul Ain and Hira Gull

2.1 Metabolic Homeostasis

The term *homeostasis* is described as the sustenance of constant internal environment in the body, irrespective of any fluctuations in external environmental factors or physiological functions. While narrowing down to "metabolic homeostasis," it refers to the maintenance of constant levels of potential energy metabolites mainly creatine phosphate (CrP), adenosine triphosphate (ATP), and others, without getting affected by changes in workload and associated metabolic flux. As the cellular metabolites remain at a steady level, the workload changes will not impact upon cellular processes reliant upon those metabolites [1]. The pathway that is primarily involved in maintenance of metabolic homeostasis in eukaryotic species is oxidative phosphorylation, acting as the controlling element for cellular metabolism and differentiation. The level of ATP that is generated via series of electron transfer steps remains constant as long as the surrounding conditions are devoid of any unfavorable physiological conditions [2]. It must be noted that levels of ATP and ADP are directly correlated to each other at any time in the cell. Under stress condition when cells are necessitated with increased ATP consumption, there is simultaneous rise in the ADP level [3]. This suggests that various mechanisms exist in eukaryotic cells to keep the difference in the levels of ATP and ADP to a minimum in order to achieve an ongoing steady-state. The rates of ATP synthesis and utilization are balanced by means of feedback regulation mechanisms in vivo.

Various factors including mutated genes or pathological influence can lead to disruption of metabolic homeostasis which consequently results in various kinds of metabolic disorders, the most notable among which are Type I, Type II, and maturity-onset diabetes of the young (MODY) [4]. Researches have introduced

N.-u. Ain (✉) · H. Gull
Microbiology and Biotechnology Research Lab, Department of Biotechnology, Fatima Jinnah Women University, Rawalpindi, Pakistan

N. Masood, S. Shakil Malik (eds.), *'Essentials of Cancer Genomic, Computational Approaches and Precision Medicine*,
https://doi.org/10.1007/978-981-15-1067-0_2

number of regulators involved in the maintenance of metabolic homeostasis. Though adipocytes have gained negative reputation with rapid increase in obesity since the last few decades, these fat cells have been investigated as the critical mediators of cell's metabolism. Besides storing triglycerides, adipocytes are involved in the induction of lipolysis by responding to hormonal signals [5]. Immune cells in adipocytes act as the major regulators and maintainers of metabolic homeostasis. Hence, any alterations in their composition or functionality can result in metabolic dysfunction.

Adipocyte specific hormones, typically termed as adipokines influence various body organs and keep metabolism in a steady-state. Multiple adipocyte-secreted hormones that have antihyperglycemic effect in the body include leptin, visfatin, omentin and adiponectin, retinol-binding protein 4 (RBP4), fibroblast grown factor 21 (FGF21), and others [6]. Among various adipocyte secretions, three important mediators with significant impact upon metabolic homeostasis are believed to be leptin, adiponectin, and fatty acids (Fig. 2.1).

Adiponectin usually occur in any of the three structures, i.e., trimer, hexamer, or a multimer having 12–18 subunits. Adiponectin has been recognized as a significant anti-inflammatory and insulin-sensitizing agent [7]. The decreased level of adiponectin in obese conditions results in subsequent decline in anti-inflammatory sensors, thereby instigating soreness of white adipose tissues (WAT) [8]. Enhancement of insulin sensitivity and protection against ectopic lipid accumulation are two of

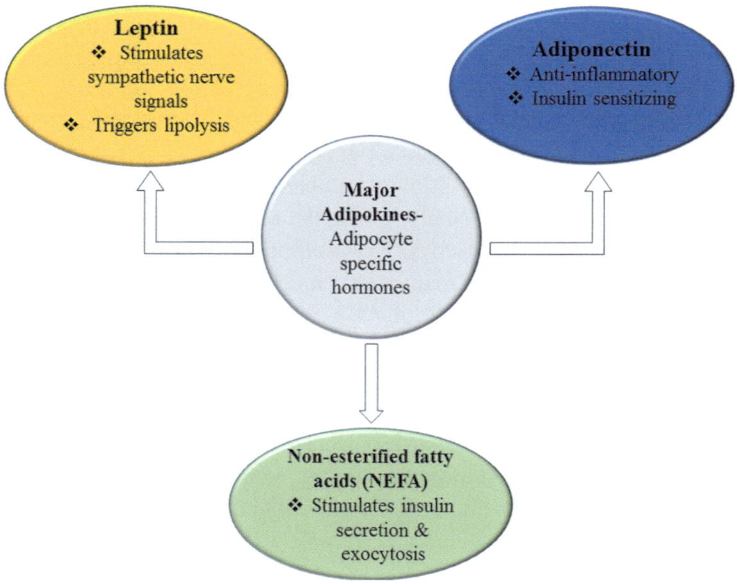

Fig. 2.1 Adipocyte secretions serving as important mediators of metabolic homeostasis. Primary metabolic functions attributed to prominent adipokines are lipolysis (mediated by leptin), protection against lipid accumulation and insulin sensitivity (mediated by adiponectin), and stimulation of insulin secretion (mediated by NEFA)

the most notable attributes of adiponectin [9, 10]. Stern and coworkers suggest that adiponectin decreases hepatic lipogenesis while increasing beta-oxidation by the action of sensory enzyme, AMP protein kinase [11].

Besides adiponectin, another adipokine with profound role in maintaining metabolic homeostasis is leptin whose secretion is modulated by various factors alongside fat deposit. Leptin exerts its influence upon adipose tissue via peripheral nervous system by stimulating sympathetic nerve signals that trigger lipolysis [12] and hence does not depend entirely upon autocrine signaling system as observed in the case of adiponectin. Meanwhile, adipocyte-secreted fatty acids commonly termed as non-esterified fatty acids (NEFA), have long been recognized as a major regulator of energy metabolism by performing dual function, i.e., by inducing as well as reducing insulin secretion in opposing situations [13]. NEFA was recognized as a stimulator of insulin secretion from beta cells by activating GPR40, i.e., G-protein-coupled receptor. This results in increased Ca^{2+} levels in cytosol, consequently paving way toward insulin exocytosis [14].

Besides these hormonal influences upon metabolic regulation, our body has a well-developed and efficient oxygen-sensing mechanism which plays a critical role in modulating metabolic homeostasis [15]. Hypoxia (deficiency of oxygen in tissues) that is mediated by hypoxia-inducible factor (HIF) acts as a stimulant for enhanced expression of leptin-encoding gene. As a result, produced leptin reaches blood-brain barrier, activates its specific receptors in the hypothalamus, and generates signals to stimulate reduced food intake and increased metabolic rate [16].

It is important to note that unbalanced diet and nutrient overloading can lead to irreversible adverse effects upon body's otherwise properly regulated metabolic homeostasis. Metabolic equilibrium is disrupted as a result of excess nutrients in the body causing irreversible damages to organelles [17, 18] or downregulation of AMP-protein kinase [19]. All of these undesirable changes pave way for metabolic disorders. As mitochondria is subjected to excess nutrients, it suffers from a stressed condition where mitochondrial potential to generate NAD^+ and FAD^+ from NADH and $FADH_2$ is significantly impaired [20]. Moreover, nutrient overloading can alter ATP production rate with altered mitochondrial electrical potential and proton gradient [21]. Besides these, there are several other mitochondrial disruptions which lead to reprogramming of bioenergetics pathways thereby inducing metabolic complications [22]. Other than mitochondria, endoplasmic reticulum (ER) has also been reported to be affected by increased lipid and glucose levels that gives rise to ER stress in pancreatic β-cells and reduces insulin expression in those cells, finally resulting in apoptosis [23].

Studies have suggested that metabolic homeostasis is modulated in different manner in opposite genders. It has been observed that females exhibit more specialized mechanism for glucose homeostasis compared to men, mainly because of the involvement of estrogen hormone. Presence of estrogen hormone allows females to utilize lipids as an energy source with lesser glucose utilization [24]. Further, two most important adipokines involved in metabolic regulation, i.e., adiponectin and leptin, have been found in higher concentration in female blood stream compared to men [25]. This suggests that in addition to other factors, sex-specific differences need to be considered while analyzing metabolic regulations, functions, and complications in order to introduce better therapeutic options for metabolic dysfunction or disruption of metabolic homeostasis [26].

2.2 Glycolysis and Warburg Effect

Mammalian cells acquire energy by means of two metabolic pathways, i.e., anaerobic glycolysis and aerobic respiration. Glycolysis or anaerobic fermentation is the multistep pathway occurring in cytosol in which glucose is converted into pyruvate which is then ultimately reduced to lactate. One glucose molecule yields two ATP molecules as a result of glycolysis. Meanwhile, aerobic respiration involves various other complicated energy-yielding mechanisms involving Krebs cycle, oxidative phosphorylation, and others. Although aerobic respiration yields comparatively greater energy, it can occur only in the oxygen-sufficient environment, while lactate fermentation is independent of oxygen supply [27]. Thus, the type of energy-generating cycle adopted by a cell at a particular time depends upon the level of oxygen in the surrounding.

A breakthrough discovery was made in 1922 by Otto Warburg regarding tumor cell metabolism where he proposed that cancer cells have a distinct metabolic pattern in which they prefer lactic fermentation over respiration even in the presence of oxygen. This phenomenon is termed as aerobic glycolysis or Warburg effect [28]. Normal cells generally prefer oxidative phosphorylation in aerobic conditions and glycolysis in oxygen-deficient surrounding. Mitochondrial oxidative phosphorylation results in greater adenosine 5′-triphosphate (ATP) production compared to glycolysis due to which former is preferred over the latter in mammals under aerobic conditions, commonly known as *Pasteur effect*. However, malignant cells execute glucose fermentation into lactate in the presence of oxygen in order to accompany oxidative phosphorylation in meeting energy requirements of uncontrolled cell proliferation [29].

This unique behavior of cancerous cells may arise due to genetic mutations that alter receptor-initiated signaling pathways thereby resulting in increased nutrient uptake so as to fulfill energy demands of rapid cell growth and proliferation [28]. The exact purpose of Warburg effect is debatable as of today because it is believed that the energy demands of malignant cells can be sufficiently fulfilled by ATP generated by oxidative phosphorylation alone, not requiring co-occurrence of glycolysis. Even so, recent studies have concluded that Warburg effect has always been a prerequisite for tumor growth [30] and both mitochondrial metabolism and glycolysis need to be targeted in order to control malignant carcinoma [31]. Following Warburg's hypothesis, Herbert Crabtree analyzed the heterogeneity of glycolysis in various cancer types. He then suggested that there exists great deal of variations in aerobic glycolysis or fermentation undergoing in cancer cells that may be attributed to the genetic and environmental factors [32].

One strong proposal regarding the occurrence of Warburg effect and generation of tumor is the impairment of mitochondria which results in decreased respiratory rate and enhanced reactive oxygen species (ROS) generation [33]. Oxygen in such mutated mitochondria is converted into superoxide O^{2-} (ROS) and hydrogen peroxide (H_2O_2), instead of being reduced to water [34]. These alterations favor aerobic glycolysis over normal metabolism. The underlying reason is the induction of intracellular alkalization by superoxide [35] and stimulation of glycolysis-promoting enzyme, namely, PFK-1 [36]. Also, hypoxia-inducible factor (HIF-1) seemingly plays a crucial role in shifting the trend from oxidative phosphorylation to Warburg effect because HIF-1 has been justified both as activator of aerobic glycolysis and suppressor of oxidative phosphorylation [37]. HIF-1 plays a significant role in transcribing genes that translate such proteins that promote cancer development, metastasis, resistance to apoptosis, and angiogenesis [38]. Meanwhile, nutrient deprivation has also been suggested as an inducer of Warburg effect in order to support cells under starvation conditions. Nutrient-limiting conditions encourage cancer cells to utilize glycolysis to meet energy demands. This switching toward anaerobic glycolysis is facilitated by activation of pyruvate dehydrogenase kinase (PDK) by combined activity of reactive oxygen species (ROS) and AMP-activated protein kinase (AMPK) [39].

Researchers have long sought the exact function of Warburg effect; however, even after a long period since its proposal, the exact reason as to why tumor cells switch from highly efficient mitochondrial metabolism to less efficient anaerobic glycolysis is still doubtful. Liberti and Locasale [40] hypothesized several functions with regard to Warburg effect. These include rapid ATP generation, promoting flux in biosynthetic pathways, establishment of tumor microenvironment, and signal transduction via ROS generation and chromatin mediation [40]. Although these hypotheses are quite compelling, certain questions arise along with each proposed function which reveals that there is still a lot more to go in comprehending the exact function of Warburg effect in tumor growth and proliferation.

As Warburg effect is being investigated more deeply, scientists are of the opinion that this would lead to major advancements in cancer therapy and treatment by focusing more on the metabolic changes in metastatic tissues. In a recent study, Faubert and coworkers proposed that AMPK has the potential to act as tumor suppressor by modulating biosynthetic pathways that minimizes the proliferation of cancer cells [41]. In normal cells, AMPK works to hinder cell growth in nutrient-limiting conditions. Similarly in cancerous cells, the suppression of AMPK during carcinogenesis makes tumor cells sensitive to hypoxic and nutrient-deficient environment, ultimately pushing them toward apoptosis [42]. Loss of AMPK has been observed to increase HIF-1α levels in the absence of hypoxia, that is required for increased glycolysis and biosynthesis observed in AMPK-deficient cells. Thus, AMPK is designated as the negative regulator of Warburg effect [41].

The distinct features of aerobic glycolysis are being studied with gradual understanding of the underlying phenomena. This advancement in knowledge is paving way toward finding more effective novel cancer therapies. Bonuccelli et al. identified a novel prognostic biomarker of human breast cancer. In their study, they identified the deficiency of stromal caveolin-1 in cancerous fibroblasts. This loss of Cav-1 favors growth of cancer cells by upregulating the expression of glycolytic enzymes.

The phenomenon, referred as "reverse Warburg effect," enables the utilization of glycolytic inhibitors in order to treat breast cancer patients diagnosed on the basis of deficient stromal Cav-1 expressions [43]. Moreover, metabolic modulation occurring in cancer cells results in their preference for glycolysis over mitochondrial oxidation. Since glucose oxidation is minimized in such cells with exceeding glycolysis rate, researchers are of the opinion that any approach used for forced activation of oxidative phosphorylation would result in decreased lactate production thereby suppressing metastasis [44]. Thus, new agents recognized as pro-oxidative and anti-aerobic glycolysis features can prove helpful in effective treatment of cancer.

2.3 Mechanisms Responsible for Metabolic Changes

As observed in the case of Warburg effect occurring in metastatic cells, it is quite obvious that the metabolic pathways and functioning of normal cells and cancer cells constitute significant differences. There has been vast research ongoing in recent years in order to elucidate the mechanisms that govern such metabolic alterations. Researches are focused largely upon mitochondria, redox regulations, and bioenergetics since these are associated with most of the metabolic modifications [45]. Mitochondria is the key organelle, changes in which lead to alterations in gene expression profiles, subsequently leading toward cancer onset.

Key metabolic substrates that serve as major energy source for cancer cells include glucose and glutamine. Cancer cells rearrange their metabolic pathways so as to generate excess amount of energy (ATP) to support cancer cells. Conversion of glucose to lactate instead of Acetyl-CoA as observed in the case of aerobic glycolysis is one of the principle metabolic changes occurring in metastatic cells. During glycolysis, either glucose is metabolized to lactate by the action of lactate dehydrogenase A (LDHA) or it may be converted into acetyl-CoA by pyruvate dehydrogenase (PDH), both of which are responsible for generating required ATP [46]. As the tumor onset occurs, hypoxic environment and several oncogenes such as *Ras*, *Src*, and HER2 act to stabilize hypoxia-inducible transcription factor (*HIF-1α*), which works to upregulate pyruvate dehydrogenase kinase 1 (PDK-1) enzyme. PDK-1 inactivates PDH and thereby prevents its role in acetyl-CoA synthesis. Meanwhile, LDHA is upregulated by *HIF-1α* and oncogene *c-Myc* [47], resulting in lactate production accompanied with simultaneous generation of NAD^+ from NADH. Several other genes upregulated by *c-Myc* include hexokinase 2 (HK2), glucose transporter (GLUT1), phosphofructokinase (PFKM), and enolase 1 [48] which collectively contribute to Warburg effect in cancer cells. These metabolic transformations ensure that tumor cells are provided with sufficient ATP even when mitochondrial oxidative phosphorylation becomes insufficient to meet the cell's increased biosynthetic requirements [49].

Glutamine, as already mentioned, is another critical cancer metabolism-regulating substrate [50]. This nonessential amino acid is abundant in blood and acts as a rich energy source through anabolism under normal oxygen levels. Glutamine serves to provide ATP by oxidation via tricarboxylic acid cycle (TCA) and also provide anabolic building blocks during cell growth by synthesis of amino acid, fatty acid, and nucleotide. However, as tumor cells outgrow their blood supply, oxygen tension or hypoxia is induced in the cell. As a result of hypoxic conditions, prominent changes take place in glutamine metabolism in cancer cells. As there is decreased pyruvate oxidation and mitochondrial respiration rate, tumor cells shift their dependence upon other nutrients like glutamine for growth and viability [51]. Glutaminolysis, the catabolism of glutamine, serves as one of the indispensable processes in cancer proliferation. In TCA cycle, as glutamine is converted to α-ketoglutarate, it serves as the major source of oxaloacetate, malate, and NADH. All of these are involved in fatty acid synthesis in tumor cells [52]. High dependence of tumor cells upon glutamine leads to boosted glutamine catabolism by means of reprogrammed mitochondrial metabolism. It has been observed that tumor-related changes in glutamine metabolism are mainly regulated by c-Myc expression. With overexpression of c-Myc, hypoxic cells are able to oxidize glutamine with simultaneous conversion of glucose to lactate. Overexpressed c-Myc can even induce glutamine catabolism in TCA cycle even in the absence of glucose [53]. The underlying reason behind the upregulation of glutamine catabolism is the transcriptional repression of two miRNAs, i.e., miR23a and miR23b, that results in increased expression of mitochondrial glutaminase (GLS), their target protein involved in glutamine catabolism. This leads to subsequent upregulation of glutamine conversion to glutamate, finally resulting in higher production of glutathione. Glutathione functions as an efficient oxygen scavenger by controlling reactive oxygen species in mitochondria and, in this way, protects the cell from apoptosis [54, 55]. Also in case of dysfunctional mitochondria where pyruvate is not oxidized to acetyl-CoA, α-ketoglutarate synthesized by glutamine is transformed into citrate via reductive carboxylation by the action of isocitrate dehydrogenase-2 (IDH-2) enzyme. This reductive carboxylation pathway serves as an alternate path for lipid synthesis [56].

As metastatic cells proliferate uncontrollably, certain regions of the tumor become deficient of the required oxygen supply, giving rise to the condition of hypoxia. As the tumor becomes aggressive, hypoxic condition results in the generation of signals [57] which are actually employed by tumor cells as a metabolic adaptation to prevent apoptosis [58]. An important transducer of hypoxia cells is the hypoxia-inducible transcription factor 1a (HIF1a). This transcription factor drives expression of different enzymes [GLUTs, hexokinase 2 (HK2), phosphofructokinase 1 (PFK1) and lactate dehydrogenase A (LDHA)] and also works to inhibit the expression of pyruvate dehydrogenase kinase 1 that is involved in minimizing the rate of oxidative phosphorylation by reducing pyruvate flux in TCA cycle [46].

In addition to aforementioned modifications, metastatic cells also have altered lipid metabolism. Fatty acids are required in abundance in order to provide the rapidly growing cancer cells with required building blocks for synthesis of metabolites, new membranes, and energy generation via oxidation of fatty acid oxidation. Under this context, fatty acid metabolism is believed to play a crucial role in metastasis, as observed in recent findings. It has been suggested by Pascual et al. that fatty acids in metastasis-initiating cells (MICs) are responsible for their rapid proliferation during metastasis. There is found increased expression of CD36 fatty acid receptor in MICs, i.e., in the models of human oral squamous cell carcinoma (OSCC) [59]. Although epithelial to mesenchymal transition which gives rise to metastatic transformation of cells is not directly associated with CD36 expression, Nath and coworkers observed the occurrence of EMT in liver cells followed by fatty acid uptake by CD36 and FA-binding proteins 1 and 4 (FABP1 and FABP4) [60]. A strong correlation between dietary lipids and cancer proliferation was observed as blockage of enzyme monoacylglycerol lipase (MAGL) that produces free fatty acids was found to be directly involved in the impairment of ovarian cancer growth and migration capacity [61]. Though the strong correlation between fatty acid metabolism and malignant tumors has been established through various studies, there is still required in-depth study of the exact mechanism which could further elaborate the link between these two occurrences.

2.4 Metabolic Reprogramming of Cancer Cells

2.4.1 Altered Metabolic Enzymes

It has now been well acknowledged that cancer cells possess specific altered metabolic activities which induce their metastatic nature. Cancer-related deaths usually occur when the human body is unable to defend itself against the induced changes in normal metabolic pathways. Several transitioning programs including various altered enzymes and growth factors work collectively toward cancer progression (Fig. 2.2) as maximized supply of proteins, lipids, nucleotides, and other cellular components is required for rapid doubling of cell biomass so that it could divide into two daughter cells in minimum time.

Studies aimed toward investigation of underlying mechanisms in cancer proliferation reveal that isoforms of certain glycolytic enzymes serve as key modulators of glucose metabolism in metastatic cells [29]. Hexokinase (HK) is undeniably one of the most basic enzymes involved in glycolytic pathway as it catalyzes the conversion of glucose to glucose-6-phosphate (G-6-P) in TCA cycle. This reaction facilitates the entrapment of glucose inside the cell for it to be utilized either as an energy source or for other biosynthetic reactions. As the fact was validated that increased glucose entrapment in the cell is facilitated by hexokinase, researchers concluded that hexokinase is particularly involved in boosting up glycolysis in malignant tumors [62].

Later on, another interesting discovery revealed that one of the isoforms of hexokinase, i.e., HK-2, localized on outer mitochondrial membrane protein, is overexpressed in cancer cancers. The strategic positioning of HK-2 allows it to gain access to mitochondrial ATP and also protects it against feedback inhibition control [63]. Several reasons have been proposed as to why HK-2 is preferentially overexpressed by cancer cells instead of other hexokinases. The most convincing explanation is that only HK-2 has the ability to bind to mitochondria's VDAC protein due to exclusive nature of its N-terminal hydrophobic domain which enhances

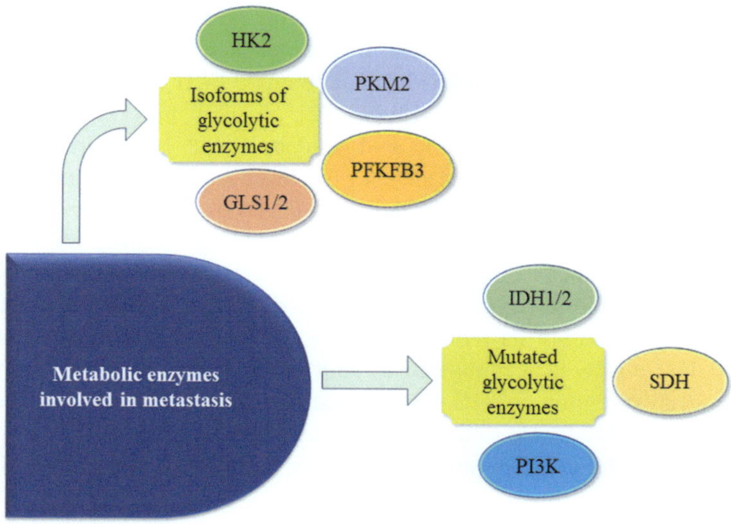

Fig. 2.2 General metabolic enzymes associated with glucose metabolism of metastatic cells. Isoforms of metabolic enzymes which regulate glycolysis in normal cells are overexpressed in tumor cells for maximum glycolytic efficacy. Certain glycolytic enzymes undergo missense mutations that maximizes their ability to favor malignant environment

its ATP-binding affinity [64] and also protects it from its own product (G-6-P) [65]. With better substrate affinity, reduced product inhibition, and increased catalytic efficiency, HK-2 is thus selectively overexpressed by malignant cells for maximum glycolytic efficiency. Other notable enzymes that exist as unique isoforms in cancer cells include pyruvate kinase M 2 (PKM2), phosphofructokinase 2 FB3 (PFKFB3), and glutaminase 1 and 2 (GLS1, GLS2). Besides such enzymes whose unique isoforms exist in overexpressed state in malignant tumors and control their growth and proliferation, cancer metabolism also appears to be predominantly regulated by mutated forms of certain enzymes. Isocitrate dehydrogenase is one prominent enzyme which undergoes point mutation in both of its forms IDH1 and 2. In normal cell, IDH1/2 work to generate α-ketoglutarate (αKG) from isocitrate while producing an essential reducing factor that is responsible for defending the cell against oxidative damage [66].

Somatic mutation in IDH enzymes leads to the conversion of alpha-ketoglutarate to an oncometabolite, D-2-hydroxyglutarate (2-HG), the excess accumulation of which favors tumorigenesis [52] The link between IDH mutations and 2-HG is quite strong as no tumor with IDH mutants has been found devoid of 2-HG. However, the exact mechanism behind IDH mutations and 2-HG accumulation is still under investigation. Several studies have reported the identification of IDH as mutation hot spot in cancers including myelodysplastic syndromes (MDS), acute myeloid leukemia (AML), myeloproliferative neoplasms (MPN), and cholangiocarcinoma [67–69]. In 2008, a study undertaken by Parsons and colleagues served as the basis for understanding exact mutation that existed in IDH1/2. In an effort to recognize the probable treatment for glioblastoma multiforme (GBM), they identified recurring missense mutation at arginine 132 in five out of six secondary GBMs [70]. Meanwhile, several other secondary GBMs and grade II/III gliomas were found to possess mutation at codon 172 of IDH2 [71, 72].

These mutations arising in amino acid residues of IDH1/2 result in decreased binding affinity of enzyme's active sites for isocitrate while, at the same, increased affinity for NADPH that nullifies the oxidative decarboxylation activity possessed by normal enzymes [48]. As the mutant IDH1/2 catalyze the conversion of 2-oxoglutarate (produced initially by oxalosuccinate decarboxylation by native IDH1/2) to 2HG, the mutant enzymes lack the catalytic activity to carboxylate 2OG, thus favoring only its reduction. Given this altered enzymatic activity of mutant IDH1/2, 2HG is accumulated in bulk concentration in malignant tumors [73]. The overexpression of 2HG has been validated as the inducer of histone and DNA hypermethylation by acting as inhibitor of αKG-dependent dioxygenase. Consequently, cellular differentiation is hindered, and tumorigenesis is favored [74, 75].

Another important mitochondrial enzyme with an established role as tumor repressor is succinate dehydrogenase, as observed through various studies involving paragangliomas, renal cell carcinoma, and gastrointestinal stromal tumors [76–78]. While somatic mutations are responsible for altered IDH1/2 enzymes, germline mutations are associated with SDH. SDH comprises of four subunits, viz., SDHA, SDHB, SDHC, and SDHD [79]. SDH is the major enzyme that catalyzes the conversion of succinate to fumarate in TCA cycle. In response to the mutations arising in SDH-encoding genes, a "tumor microenvironment" develops in the cell that favors the survival of cancer cells. Dysfunctional succinate dehydrogenase (SDH) is a prominent inducer of malignancy as it results in the excessive accumulation of succinate inside the cell. Succinate acts as an inhibitor of 2-oxoglutarate (2-OG)-dependent HIF prolyl-hydroxylases [80]. Resultantly, hypoxia-inducible factors (HIFs) are stabilized and activated, favoring angiogenesis and ultimately paving way toward metastasis.

One noteworthy fact regarding SDH mutations is that different subunit mutations give rise to distinct tumors. Mediastinal paragangliomas (PGLs) have been found linked with SDHD gene mutation [81] while SDHB and SDHC gene mutations were observed to be associated with sporadic head and neck paraganglioma [82]. Likewise, SDHB domain alteration showed implication in renal cell carcinoma and papillary thyroid cancer [83, 84].

Another enzyme-related germline gene mutation that is found directly correlated with oncogenic transformations is that of phosphatidylinositol 3-kinase (PI3-kinase). PIK3CA, gene encoding catalytic subunit p110α of PI3-kinase, has been found overexpressed in ovarian cancer [85]. Meanwhile, mutations have been reported in PIK3CA gene in several types of cancers.

PIK3CA undergoes missense mutations in exons 9 and 20 of coding sequence. The two residues E542 and E545 located in exon 9 of p110α are most frequently altered, usually testified with lysine substitution [86]. Another residue H1047 positioned in exon 20 is normally substituted with arginine residue in various cancers.

Mutations found in P13 kinase exhibited increased lipid kinase potential in contrast to the non-mutated enzyme [87]. The ability of three abovementioned mutations to induce malignancy was again validated by Kang et al. by analyzing the potential of mutated P13-kinase in transforming cultures of chicken embryo fibroblasts [88]. Other than few of the aforementioned examples of altered metabolic enzymes that mediate the onset of metastasis, researchers are continuously investigating other factors and underlying mechanisms with an aim to find therapeutic solutions for various types of cancers.

2.4.2 Cancer Stem Cells

Cancer stem cells have long been a matter of great interest from diagnostic and therapeutic view point given their exclusive characteristics. Nguyen et al. [89] defined cancer stem cells (CSCs) as cells which possess malignant clonal population that are able to proliferate cancer in a way that their eradication can lead toward the cure. This implies that CSCs have a separate distinction which is not found in all malignant cells. CSCs have the ability to generate all forms of malignant cells including those with and without cell-propagating ability. The type of cell generated by CSCs depends upon the intracellular molecular response network that depends upon the parent tissue from which CSCs are originated [89].

The concept of cancer stem cells dates back to the nineteenth century AD when a link between cancer cells and embryonic tissue was identified for the first time in history. As a result "embryonic rest theory" was postulated that was based upon the hypothesis that the causative agent of cancer is the type of cells much similar in nature to early embryo. Teratocarcinomas were then identified in 1941 as malignant structures which constituted many types of differentiated cells. This suggested the origin of malignant structures from tumorigenic "stem cells" [90]. Human CSCs were first recognized in adult acute myeloid leukemia (AML) as $CD34^{+}/CD38^{-}$ cell subpopulation following transplantation into severe combined immunodeficient (SCID) mice. Leukemia-initiating cells were found capable of instigating AML even though they were not mature enough as colony forming cells [91].

One of the prominent features of CSCs that acts as a hindrance toward anticancer therapies is their heterogeneous nature which allows them to acquire distinct gene expressions [92], making them more resistant toward treatment strategies. Some of the distinguishable features of CSCs which mark their exclusive nature include metabolic reprogramming [93], their ability to survive in nutrient-limited environment [94] and also their capacity of drug efflux via ABC transporters, i.e., ATP-binding cassette transporter [95].

CSCs with heterogeneous functional and phenotypic characteristics have been identified in various types of tumors including ovarian, breast, and squamous cell carcinomas [96–98].

Such heterogeneity that leads to prominent differences among cancerous cells can be influenced by various factors such as genetic [99] or epigenetic changes [100] as well as differences in tumor located in distinct regions [101]. An interesting phenomenon that has been studied regarding CSCs is that in the case of certain tumors, cancerous stem cells have the ability to differentiate into non-cancerous cancer cells [102, 103].

According to the CSC theory, tumor growth is initiated by limited numbers of tumor stem cells that are located in the niche of cancerous region. This might be the probable reason as to why certain tumors recur even after successful implementation of initial chemotherapy/radiation therapy sessions. Pancreatic CSCs, i.e., $CD44^+/CD24^+/ESA^+$, were also identified by confirming their potential to induce tumor formation in orthotopic pancreatic tail injection model [104]. Several other researches have been performed for identification of CSCs in commonly occurring cancer types [105–107]. Given the chief role of CSCs in cancer sustenance, most of the cancer treatment strategies at present are focused upon identification and extermination of CSCs, the actual cell population involved in long-term sustenance of cancer [108].

Plasticity is another prominent aspect which allows both CSCs and non-CSCs to undergo phenotypic transitions as a result of suitable stimulus. As three types of cell subpopulations were retrieved from breast cancer cell lines, it was clearly observed that these subpopulations were able to generate two phenotypes that were fully functional as stem-cell like cell-population and inherited the ability to generate tumors upon xenotransplantation. Meanwhile, the tumorigenic potential of cells was directly influenced by the environmental stimuli such that when three subpopulations were subjected to certain environment fluctuation, all tumor cells acquired the ability to generate tumors [109]. This plasticity is another significant feature of cancer stem cells that provides resistance against cancer therapeutic treatments.

While studies were conducted in order to distinguish CSCs from non-CSCs population by means of their metabolic preferences, no universal patterns have been observed among two cell types. Both types use glycolysis or oxidative phosphorylation according to their own preferences. Plasticity as a response to environmental fluctuations was again found to be prominent in the case of CSCs' metabolic patterns in existing literature [110]. Glioma CSCs were observed to prefer oxidative phosphorylation to meet their energy demands but possess the potential to switch to glycolysis in conditions unfavorable for oxidative metabolism [111]. This metabolic adaptation of cancer cells mediated by HIF-1α protein is the "Warburg effect" as already discussed in the previous section.

In addition to glucose metabolism, there exist certain reports where tumor cells acquire energy via fatty acids. This process is mediated by fatty acid receptor "CD36" located in a subset of CSC population [112]. Likewise, $CD36^+$ leukemic stem cells oxidize fatty acids from gonadal adipose tissue that acts as a niche for chemotherapeutic resistance [113]. Hence, specific energy requirements of CSCs during cancer growth indicates an opportunity to cure cancer at later stages.

Cell plasticity by means of epithelial-mesenchymal transition (EMT) is also found linked to metabolic adaptation of CSCs. Pancreatic tumor cells that were deficient of EMT transcription factor ZEB1 were found incapable of EMT; as a result of which, they were unable to switch toward glycolytic metabolism even when oxidative phosphorylation was inhibited [114]. This concludes that glucose- and oxygen-sufficient environment favors glycolysis, suggesting considerable impact of microenvironment upon the CSCs' preferences.

To date, most of the cancer treatment strategies are solely aimed at reducing and localizing malignant tumors, whereas the agents that could target CSCs could prove equally or even more beneficial than the existing strategies. Further research in this dimension by identification of CSCs can pave way toward improved diagnostic and therapeutic procedures. The results by anti-CSC agents would be gradually observable once the tumor growth halts and a benign mass is left behind. The clinical evidence for this approach is quite obvious in the case of teratocarcinomic patients where CSCs were deleted by chemotherapy such that only mature, differentiated cells were left behind. The results revealed that patients with only mature teratomas were completely cured after the elimination of CSC population [115]. Thus, improved CSC identification techniques are much needed at the moment for further progress in this dimension.

2.4.3 Metabolic Related Role of Tumor Suppressor and Oncogenes

Tumor suppressor genes, also referred as anti-oncogenes, have been validated as critical metabolic regulators which suppress tumor growth and proliferation under conditions of limited nutrient availability. Cancer-inducing metabolic reprogramming of cells is considered as the primary task of activated oncogenes and inactivated tumor suppressors, as demonstrated through various researches [116, 117]. In other words, we can say that metabolic shift in cancer cells is directly influenced by tumor suppressor genes. Some of the highly active tumor suppressors have been illustrated in Fig. 2.3.

Phosphatidylinositol 3-kinase (PI3K) is a lipid kinase that acts as a major metabolism regulator in both wild-type and mutated cells by regulating concentration of phosphorylated phosphatidylinositol (PIP3) in plasma membrane. In healthy cells, activation of PI3K is controlled by way of PIP3 de-phosphorylation which is performed by the action of critical tumor suppressor, i.e., phosphatase and tensin homologue or PTEN. In the case of mutated cells, this pathway is deregulated by various means such as loss of PTEN [118] or activation of PI3K [119].

The key function associated with PTEN includes modulation of cell proliferation and metabolism; thus it acts as a strong tumor inhibitor [120]. As its level decreases in the cell or PTEN gene expression is altered by some way or other, the cell becomes susceptible to cancer [121]. On the contrary, elevated level of PTEN can reverse the metabolic reprogramming of cancer cells, thereby shifting the trend from glycolysis to oxidative phosphorylation [122]. Mutated PI3K signaling can directly favor tumor induction among humans [123]. If protein translation is deregulated due to certain mutation, it would favor tumorigenesis due to lack of certain essential component. mTOR is a member of P13K family that acts as the central unit in TOR complex 1 and 2, namely, TORC1 and TORC2. The major role of mTOR is to initiate translation by controlling the activity of transcription inhibitors.

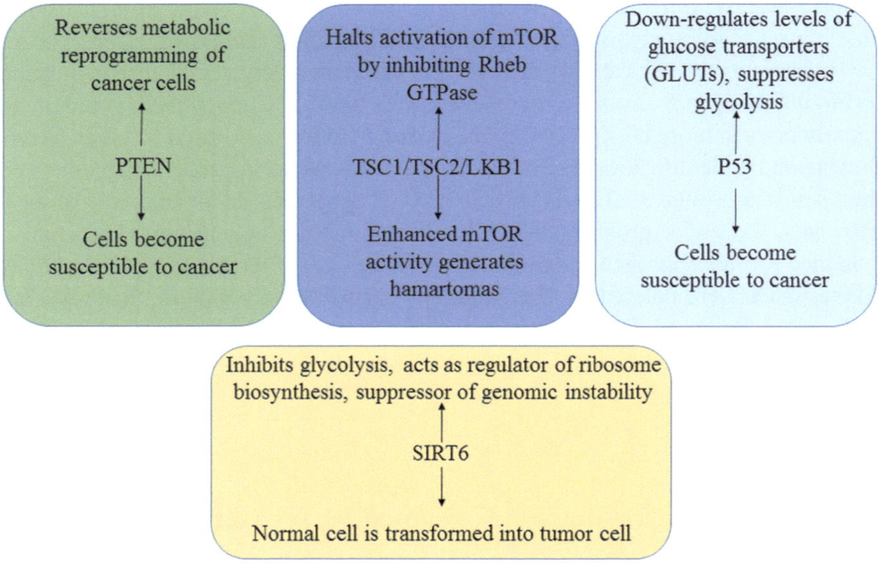

Fig. 2.3 Effect of up- and down regulation of crucial tumor suppressors in cellular metabolism. Decreased expressions of tumor suppressor genes favor metabolic reprogramming of tumor cells whereas their enhanced expressions contribute to suppression of cancer-associated modifications

The activity of TOR complex is kept in check by tumor suppressors, TSC1/TSC2 and LKB1. These tumor suppressors halt activation of mTOR by inhibition of the GTPase Rheb. Mutations among tumor suppressor genes lead to enhanced mTOR activity, resulting in hamartomas [124, 125].

Another critical tumor suppressor gene p53, a transcription factor, is involved in numerous cellular responses such as apoptosis, metabolic regulation, cellular aging, and other physiological functions. P53 controls intracellular metabolism by modulating gene expressions while acting as key element of metabolic regulatory mechanisms. As suggested in various studies, more than 50% of human cancers constitute mutated p53 gene [126, 127], which signifies the role of p53 gene in tumor suppression.

p53 in its original state deregulates glycolysis negatively via transcriptional repression of two glucose transporters *GLUT1* and *GLUT4*, along with transactivation of glycolytic inhibitors, namely, *RRAD* and *TIGAR* [128–130]. In addition to these, p53 also works to inhibit glucose-6-phosphate dehydrogenase, resulting in suppression of glucose metabolism [131]. Thus in the case of non-mutated cells, p53 regulates the metabolic pathways in a cell. Various mechanisms by which p53 is regulated to perform its role in tumor suppression include ubiquitination and degradation by E3 ubiquitin ligases like MDM2 [132, 133]. P53 regulates glucose metabolism by repressing transcription of glucose transporters (GLUTs), reducing glucose uptake [129]. Besides downregulating levels of GLUTs, P53 also prevents translocation of GLUTs to plasma membrane by activating transcription of RRAD which in turn binds p65 of NF-κB thus inhibiting its activity and suppressing GLUT translocation [130]. Downregulation of hexokinase 2 and protein levels and phosphoglycerate mutase 1 protein levels is induced by p53 that also result in glycolysis suppression [134]. Moreover, p53 transcriptionally prompts TIGAR (TP53-induced glycolysis regulatory phosphatase) to lower intracellular levels of fructose-2, 6-bisphosphate, stimulates glycolysis, and consequently suppresses glycolysis [128]. All these glycolysis-suppressing activities performed by p53 work in unison in preventing tumor growth and proliferation.

Sirtuin 6 or SIRT6 is another tumor suppressor gene that mediates aerobic glycolysis in cancer cells. Deletion of SIRT6 from the cell results in transformation of normal cell to tumor cell. SIRT6 is a chromatin-bound factor that was originally known as a suppressor of genomic instability by means of stimulating base excision DNA repair (BER) [135]. Various studies have established the role of SIRT6 as DNA repair factor as it has been found associated with DNA double-strand break (DSB) repair by regulating activity of three relevant proteins, i.e., C-terminal-binding protein (CtBP), interacting protein (CtIP) [136], and poly-ADP-ribose polymerase 1 (PARP1) [137].

SIRT6 is actively involved in defending cells against metastasis by inhibiting glycolysis that is the prerequisite for tumor formation. Moreover, SIRT6 has also been found to act as regulator of ribosome biosynthesis. Given the two crucial roles of SIRT6, it acts as an essential factor in metabolic reprogramming of cancer cells [138].

Alongside tumor suppressors, other major regulators of cancer metabolic pathways are the oncogenes, most prominent among which are c-Myc, H-ras, Src, and Akt [139, 140]. Most importantly, proto-oncogene c-Myc is the chief regulator of biosynthetic activities and metabolic pathways essential for cancer proliferation [141].

Myc gene favors the production of glutamate by stimulating the transcription of glutaminase-1, the first enzyme involved in glutaminolysis [142]. Also, Myc transcribes ribosomal RNA genes and the ribosomal protein genes which resultantly boosts protein synthesis rate and cell mass. The transcriptional repression of miR-23a and miR-23b (miRNAs targeting glutaminase 1) results in enhanced levels of the glutaminase 1 and in turn upregulates glutamine catabolism [143].

Myc usually regulates cancer cell metabolism in two ways. On the one hand, it generates exceptionally large amount of ammonia during c-Myc-dependent glutaminolysis that paves way toward cell senescence [144], while on the other hand, c-Myc-dependent glutaminolysis delivers extended supply of NADPH to cells to support anabolic synthesis [70].

Besides Myc, other oncogenes involved in stimulation of glycolysis and glutaminolysis include nuclear factor kB (NF-κB), Akt, and tyrosine kinase receptors. Increased AKT and mTOR activities lead to higher HIF activity. Both the myc and HIF-1 transcription factors increase the rate of transcription of some of the GLUT transporters and hexokinase 2, enhancing both glucose uptake and its retention in the cell [145].

Autophagy is one of the most commonly used mechanisms utilized by cells in order to suppress tumors. In the similar manner as metabolic transformation, oncogene and tumor suppressor pathways influence autophagy in opposing ways. Prominent oncogenes such as Akt, mTOR, and Bcl2 act as inhibitors of autophagy whereas tumor suppressors like PTEN, LKB1, and HIF1α stimulate autophagy [146]. p53 works in a unique manner as it promotes autophagy in stressed conditions by controlling transcription of autophagy regulators, e.g., DRAM [147], while on the contrary, p53 deregulates autophagy when located in cytoplasm [148, 149].

2.4.4 Drug Resistance Patterns

The major threat toward the treatment of cancer is the drug resistance acquired by tumor cells which are initially susceptible to chemotherapy. This drug resistance is basically the outcome of various epigenetic events that influence the heterogeneity in gene expression patterns which continuously evolve to provide defense against selected drug treatment (Fig. 2.4)

Chemotherapeutic drug resistance of tumor cells is generally divided into two types: intrinsic and acquired resistance. Intrinsic resistance refers to the inherent resistance potential of cell before receiving chemotherapy, and such resistance-mediating factors normally preexist in tumor cells and make the therapy unsuccessful. On the

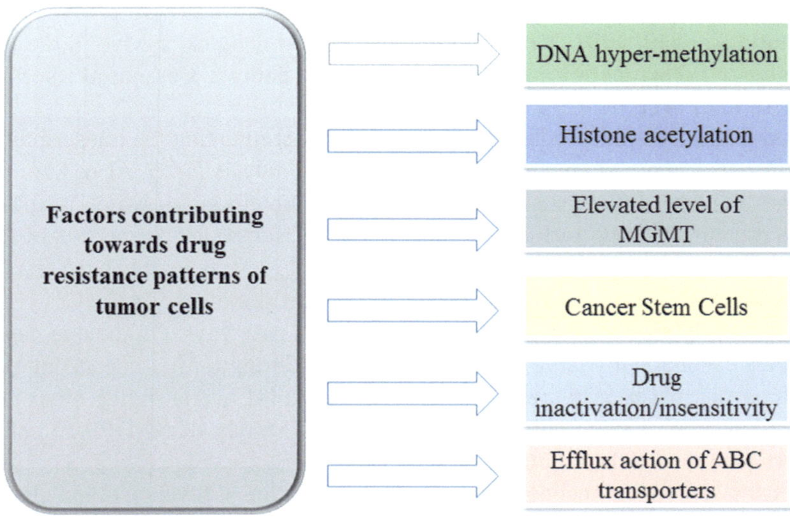

Fig. 2.4 Different mechanisms and elements that impart drug resistance to metastatic cells. Epigenetic occurrences like hypermethylation of tumor suppressor genes (anti-oncogenes) and hypomethylation of oncogenes confer drug resistance to cancer cells. CSCs possess intrinsic resistance against drugs due to their heterogeneity and plasticity. Certain cellular mechanisms including drug inactivation and efflux action of ATP-binding cassette transporters also contribute to drug resistance of tumor cells

other hand, acquired drug resistance develops among the treated tumors which were initially sensitive but later develop resistance as a result of genetic mutations or through other adaptive responses, e.g., overexpression of the therapeutic target or activation of substitute compensatory signaling pathways [150].

Epigenetic occurrences such as gene promoter DNA hypermethylation, which correlate to the alterations in gene expressions, have been observed as prominent causative agents of acquired chemotherapeutic drug resistance by cancer cells [130, 151]. The two striking epigenetic events that confer drug resistance to cancer cells include DNA methylation and histone acetylation/methylation. In DNA methylation, methyl groups are linked to cytosine within regions of CpG islands, position at CG-dinucleotide sequences. Meanwhile, histone acetylation and deacetylation results in loosening and tightening of chromatin structure, respectively. These are the mechanisms that regulate gene expression in normal cells but are deregulated in mutated cancer cells. Hypermethylation-associated silencing of tumor suppressor genes along with hypomethylated activation of oncogenes are some of the epigenetic events that alter gene expressions conferring drug resistance to cancer cells [152].

DNA repair enzyme O^6-methylguanine-DNA methyltransferase (MGMT) plays a substantial role in cancer treatment strategies. MGMT is associated with repair of DNA lesion O^6-methylguanine (generated by the action of alkylating drugs) and converts it back to guanine thus protecting the cell from apoptosis. Thus, increased levels of MGMT in tumor cells impart resistance to chemotherapeutic treatments, and further research to control this drug damage response (DDR) mechanism is required to make mutated cells vulnerable to drugs [153].

Recently, insensitivity of cancer cells toward treatment in certain settings has been credited to the cancer stem cells which possess intrinsic defense in response to various therapeutic approaches [154]. Cancer stem cells (CSCs) are comparatively much more resistant to chemotherapy compared to non-CSCs in such a manner that they also make non-CSCs insensitive to treatment due to their persisting behavior [155]. It has been observed through genetic analysis of hematological tumors that subclones that are minute before therapy become dominant after treatment [156, 157]. This is again attributed to the genetic alterations that become the cause of drug resistance.

Another mode of action by means of which cancer cells defend themselves against therapeutic drugs is through drug inactivation. This has been observed in the case of a nucleoside drug "cytarabine (AraC)" used for the treatment of acute myelogenous leukemia. This drug is activated after conversion into to AraC-triphosphate following several phosphorylations [158]. As the phosphorylation pathway of AraC is deregulated or mutated, AraC fails to activate and, thus, drug becomes inactive.

Changes directed toward apoptosis-related proteins like tumor suppressor p53 can also impart drug resistance. p53 is normally involved in apoptosis of cancer cells as a result of chemotherapy; however if the p53 gene is deleted, mutated, or silenced by some means, it fails to carry out its apoptotic role and becomes nonfunctional [159].

Inactivation of P53 regulators like caspase-9 and cofactor "apoptotic protease activating factor 1 (Apaf-1)" can also result in drug insensitivity [160].

Besides drug inactivation mechanisms, drug resistance is also governed by changes in signal transduction processes, regulating drug activation. A monoclonal antibody trastuzumab (Herceptin) is used for effective treatment of HER2-positive breast cancer tumors. However, drug resistance was observed among patients who were initially sensitive to trastuzumab. Resistance mechanisms believed to be associated with drug insensitivity are inhibition of cell cycle co-expression of growth factor receptors, loss of activity of tumor suppressor PTEN, as well as activation of PI3K/Akt pathway [161, 162].

Another mechanism involved in contributing toward drug resistance in cancer cells is efflux action of ATP-binding cassette (ABC) transporters. Three main transporters that are usually involved in drug-resistant cancers are multidrug resistance protein 1 (MDR1), multidrug resistance-associated protein 1 (MRP1), and breast cancer resistance protein (BCRP). These transporters have wide-ranging substrate specificity and possess the potential to efflux numerous xenobiotic compounds, namely, epipodophyllotoxins, anthracyclines, kinase inhibitors, vinca alkaloids, and taxanes from the cells [163]. Playing their role effectively, these transporters defend cancer cells against chemotherapies.

Octamer 4 encoded by Pou5f1 gene is considered an important protein that imparts chemoresistance to cancer cells. Studies have demonstrated that drug-resistant cells undergo gene demethylation leading toward enhanced expression of Oct4. Overexpression of Oct4 favored drug resistance, while deletion of Oct4 decreased drug resistance of liver cells. As Oct4 is overexpressed, TCL1 expression is enhanced correspondingly, followed by Akt activation [164]. Consequently, cancer cells become equipped with anti-apoptotic potential.

Furthermore, drug insensitivity of cancer cells may also arise as the result of signaling processes of differentiation that are indispensable for *epithelial-to-mesenchymal transition* (EMT). The differentiation process that occurs during EMT gives rise to metastatic cancer cells with diversified cellular morphology [165]. In EMT, cell adhesion molecules residing on stromal cells and extracellular matrix proteins bind to the cell adhesion molecules located on cancer cells. Stromal cells and cancer cells also release factors which mediate EMT. As EMT favors the formation of increased number of metastatic cancer cells, it also produces signals for increased cell survival which imparts drug resistance attribute to tumor cells [152].

Thus, various genetic alterations either individually or collectively work to provide cancer cells with defense mechanism against therapeutic drug treatments. There is a need for better understanding of resistance mechanisms at molecular level through clinical assessment of rational drug combinations among selected group of patients so as to generate such therapies which could ward off resilient modes of anticancer drugs.

2.4.5 Therapeutic Approaches Targeting Cancer Cell Metabolism

Cancer cells reprogram their anabolic and catabolic metabolism for energy production in order to initiate and progress their cellular activities even when the nutrients are limited in the environment. Three types of pathways are involved in redirecting energy in high-proliferating and malignant cells. These are c-Jun N-terminal kinases (JNKs), mitogen-activated protein kinase (MAPKs), and extracellular signal-regulated kinase (ERKs) pathways [166]. Metabolic reprogramming is the property of cancerous cells in which the cells alter their metabolism in order to support the elevated energy demands due to rapid proliferation and continuous growth.

Inhibitory glycolysis is a main therapeutic strategy for cancerous cells that are extremely glucose dependent [167]. For those tumorous cells that depend on glutamine for the division and surveillance of cell, inhibition of glutamine in metabolism is the most logical strategy. Different agents are used in metabolic treatment of cells that can actively bind different metabolic pathways within cells. To target cancer metabolism, different therapeutic strategies are used in which active agents are employed for treatment. Treatment strategies are mentioned as follows:

1. Inhibition of glycolysis
2. Interfering glutamine metabolism
3. Targeting energy regulators and sensors

2.4.5.1 Inhibition of Glycolytic Pathway (IGP)

It has been seen that level of hexokinase 2 (HKII) is elevated in tumor cells. It is the main compound in glycolytic pathway of oncogenic cells that using 2-deoxyglucose (non-metabolically active glucose analog) directly inhibits the hexokinase activity and suppresses the tumor cells [168]. In human neck and head cancer, cytotoxicity of cells is increased by combining cisplatin with 2-deoxyglucose and 3-bromopyruvate. It is another inhibitor of hexokinase that has the ability to inhibit the glycolysis pathway in tumor cells. This leads to the starvation and ultimately results in the apoptosis of cancer cells [169]. Moreover, derivative of indazole-3-carboxylic acid, called lonidamine, has the potency to inhibit the growth of cancer cell by inhibiting HK, reducing oxygen, depleting ATPs, and reducing lactate production in the cell. This compound possesses the ability to treat highly glycolytic cancer types (HGC) [170].

Active glycolysis in cancer cells is repressed by inhibiting the activity of glucose transporters. In hypoxic conditions, phloretin, an inhibitor of glucose transporter can cause apoptosis, and it overcomes the property of drug resistance [171]. In glycolysis, one of the regulatory enzyme is phosphofructokinase (PFK), thus making it the main target for antitumorous drugs [172]. Small molecule that is inhibitor of phosphofructokinase (PFK) is PFKFB3-3(3-pyridinyl)-1-(4-pyridinyl)-2-propen-1-one (3PO). In adenocarcinoma and in human malignant hematopoietic cell lines, this molecule has shown the capacity to reduce glucose uptake and suppress tumor cell formation [173].

2.4.5.2 Inhibition of Glutamine Metabolism (IGM)

Cancer cells depend on exogenously produced glutamine to maintain their regular cellular functions and for survival during starvation situations, and this phenomenon is referred as glutamine addiction (GA) [174]. For inhibition of glutamine metabolism, glutamine analogues show potential as antitumor or anticancerous activity. Some examples of glutamine analogues are azaserine, L-DON (6-dizo-5-oxo-L-norleucine), and acivicin [175].

Different types of agents are used that play an important role in lowering the concentration of glutamine in the blood and directly lead to the inhibition of glucose metabolism (IGM). For this purpose, phenylbutyrate and L-asparaginase have shown strong potential [176]. In the treatment of PALL (pediatric acute lymphoblastic leukemia) an enzyme, L-asparaginase, is used. This enzyme produces aspartic acid by hydrolyzing asparaginase. Glutamic acid and ammonia are produced on the hydrolysis of glutamate by L-asparaginase, and in this way it reduces the glutamate concentration in the blood stream.

Biphenyl and Ammonaps also named as phenylbutyrate are agents which have the potential to treat hyperammonemia. After metabolizing inside the human body, these agents are converted into phenyl acetate. After conversion, phenyl acetate binds with glutamine to form a compound known as phenylacetylglutamine that is excreted out by the kidneys. Glutamine concentration in plasma is depleted by phenylbutyrate and inhibits glutamate metabolism [177].

SLC1A7 and SLC1A5 (ASCT2) are transporters of glutamine in cancer cells. By inhibiting the activity of these transporters, glutamate uptake by the defected cells is directly inhibited [178]. GPNA (IL-γ-glutamyl-*p*-nitroanilide) is an agent that is inhibitor of SLC1A5. It shows the potential to inhibit the mTOR (mammalian target of rapamycin) activation that is dependent on glutamine and also inhibit the uptake of glutamine by the cells [179]. Such kinds of inhibition become the reason of autophagy (self-eating) of cancer cells [180].

For the survival of cancer cells, an energy-metabolizing enzyme also plays an important role. This enzyme, known as glutaminase, produces glutamate and ammonia by hydrolyzing glutamine [181]. Hence, inhibiting the activity of this enzyme will result in the inhibition of glutamate metabolism. Transamination is the main pathway or route through which glutamine enters the tricarboxylic acid cycle (TCA). Hence the inhibitor of transaminase, AOA (aminooxyacetic acid), exhibits the potential as an agent in treatment of cancer cells. This compound exerts cytotoxic effect on all cancer cells that are dependent on glutamine for their survival [182].

2.4.5.3 Targeting Energy Sensors and Regulators (ESAR)

HDAC Inhibitors and AMPK Activators

Cellular energy homeostasis is maintained by the AMPK enzyme (AMP-activated protein kinase) [183]. Under different stress conditions, e.g., glucose deprivation, hypoxia, and oxidative stress, this enzyme is activated. Thus when the body is under stress, AMPK activates and shows the therapeutic potential in treating cancer.

Thiazolidinedione (troglitazone) is a compound that activates AMPK enzyme and shows the anticancerous property [184].

HDAC (histone deacetylase inhibitor) is one of the other therapeutic approaches for treatment of cancer. Suberoylanilide hydroxamic acid (SYHA) inhibitor has potential to induce autophagy, oxidative stress, and apoptosis in chronic myelogenous leukemia (CML) [185].

Inhibition of P13K/AKT/mTOR Axis

In different tumor cells, AKT/P13K and mTOR signaling pathways play a crucial role in proliferation of cancer cells as well as maintaining the normal energy level. These pathways provide a target for treating cancerous cells. For the treatment of prostate cancer, different types of agents have been tested that target the AKT pathways, e.g., perifosine, genistein, and celecoxib are potential target agents [186]. Wortmannin is a P13K inhibitor and possesses the therapeutic potential for cancer treatment [187]. Transcription factor HIF1 is activated by mTOR pathway and enhances glycolysis process in tumor cells. Due to this reason, inhibiting mTOR pathway by different compounds can inactivate the transcription factor and glycolysis. For instance, rapamycin shows antitumor property, but some inhibitors, e.g., temsirolimus (CC1-779) and everolimus (RAD-001), are under clinical trials for cancer treatment [188].

Targeting Other Regulators of Cancer Metabolism

Transcription factor c-Myc is encoded by Myc-oncogene that is useful in cellular metabolic processes in cancer cells. Myc shows the special ability to regulate other genes that are involved in cellular metabolism process, e.g., HK11, GLUT1, LDH-A, PFKM, glutaminase, etc. For sensing the changing environment inside the cell and promotion of glycolysis process by regulating different enzymes, HIF1 protein plays primary role [189]. For treating cancer at different stages, various strategies are used that use agents to target such regulatory molecules and transcription factors (proteins) [190].

2.5 Metabolic Related Diets

2.5.1 Low-Carbohydrate Diet

American diabetes council defines low-carbohydrate diet (LCD) as "the diet that gives less than 130 g/day or 26% of energy from total energy intake (TEI)" [191]. LCD was the best method for treating diabetes before the discovery of insulin [192]. Dietary carbohydrate (DC) are the main reason for the increase in blood glucose level of diabetic patient. It was suggested that reducing the intake of energy from carbohydrates will help in control of glycemia and attaining the standard glycated hemoglobin (GH) that is HbA1c <7.0% or 53 mmol/mol [193]. Kevin and Stephanie elaborated that LCD is very fruitful for weight loss as other diets do [194]. This diet is good for the control of hyperinsulinemia and glycemia but alternatively results in sensitivity for insulin and impairment of insulin secretion stimulated by glucose [195].

LCD lowers the appetite and stimulates the increased level of ketone species in the circulatory system [196]. It results in the high intake of proteins that leads to the feeling of satiety (fullness) and lowers the total energy intake and directly reduces the body fat [197].

Drawback of such kind of LCD is that they can increase the HDL (high-density lipoprotein) cholesterol and lower the TAG (triacylglycerides) in the blood when one is in a state of fasting [198]. Increased level of HDL and decreased level of LDL (low-density lipoprotein) is the main cause of coronary heart diseases. Unlike HDL, LDL is good for maintaining normal body functions. Dietary fats (protein content) are the main reason for increased level of HDL. Risk of cardiovascular diseases increases with the increase in level of HDL in blood. Such kinds of diets play an important role in proper metabolism of lipids in the body [199].

Generally there are two types of very low-carbohydrate diet. One is semi-starvation ketogenic diet (low caloric diet), while the other is eucaloric ketogenic diet. It gives more calorie than the first one because use of fat in this case is for maintaining normal metabolic functions [200].

2.5.2 Ketogenic Diet (KT)

KT (ketogenic diet) is basically a nutritional diet that consists of low level of carbohydrates that are insufficient to meet metabolic demands, i.e., maximum level of proteins and high level of fats [201]. In the case of ketogenic diets, daily carbohydrate meal is replaced by fats. Ketone bodies' synthesis begins with depletion of glycogen stores in the liver. Acetoacetate, acetone, and beta-hydroxybutyrate are the main ketone bodies. Mitochondria metabolize acetoacetate and beta-hydroxybutyrate but not acetone [202, 203].

Earlier, ketogenic diet was used to treat epilepsy, but as the research progresses, different studies have shown the potential of KT in treating different metabolic diseases like diabetes, cancer, and epilepsy as well as in weight reduction [204].

By comparing high-carbohydrate low-fat diet (HCLF) mode that includes doughnut, rice ball, and spaghetti with the low-carbohydrate high-fat (LCHF) mode diet that includes avocado, poultry, and cheese, scientists observed that LCHF provides more benefit than HCLF by means of improving appetite and controlling weight and directly helps in decreasing appetite-related obesity [205].

KD plays an important role in treatment of cancer. Warburg effect is targeted by the KDs in which the oncogenic cells (cancerous cells) instead of utilizing the oxidative pathway for ATP production and consumption are consumed by glycolysis pathway [206]. In CT (cancer therapy), the main purpose of providing LCHF to patients is that it reduces the level of circulating glucose and induction of ketosis in blood. In this way, cancerous cells face starvation because these cells cannot metabolize ketone bodies. As a result, fat bodies are produced when glucose is less in the body and act as energy source inside the body as cells face energy-less environment.

Alternatively normal cells adopt routine metabolic pathway that is necessary for survival of cells by breaking down ketone bodies [207].

Ketogenic diet constitutes neuroprotective properties. Neurons are influenced by the ketone bodies at three different levels:

1. Bioenergetic and metabolic level (BEML)
2. Signaling level (SL)
3. Epigenetic level (EL)

2.5.2.1 Bioenergetic and Metabolic Level (BEML)

Ketone body (KB) serves as efficient and effective energy substrates as compared to glucose. During starvation condition, the brain gets energy from the molecule that results from the metabolism of fat bodies [208]. These bodies act as a molecule that plays an important role in balancing the synthesis of glutamate and gamma-aminobutyric acid (GABA), leading to storage of GABA in the central nervous system and protecting the nerves from inhibitory synaptic transmission (IST) [209].

2.5.2.2 Signaling Level (SL)

For G-protein-linked receptor HCA (hydroxycarboxylic acid), ketone bodies function as a ligand [210]. Microglial cells are inhibited by ketogenic diets that reduce the level of interleukin and promote the neuroprotective phenomenon of the brain [211].

2.5.2.3 Epigenetic Level (EL)

Epigenetic changes are the kind of changes that are associated with genome but not associated with the change in sequence of nucleotides in DNA. These changes may or may not be heritable [212]. Such changes in genome change the level of gene expression and prepare the individual for adjustment in the environment. Histone modification and DNA methylation are prime changes in DNA. Histone acetylase inhibitors are butyrate and beta-hydroxybutyrate. Synthesis of antioxidant enzymes increases with the inhibition of histone acetylase that causes changes in folding of histone [213]. Either by blood-brain barrier (BBB) or by neural plasma membrane (NPM), ketone bodies are transported to the brain where they play effective role in neuroprotection of neurons [214]. Ketogenic diet (KT) is different from ketoacidosis (KA) in a sense that KT promotes neuroprotection by the help of ketone bodies, whereas KA promotes acidification and thus leads to neurotoxicity of nerve cells [215].

2.6 Conclusion

Various metabolic transformations arise as normal cells transform into cancer cells by a series of events. Associated with these metabolic changes are various metabolic genes and enzymes whose mutated expressions alter the metabolic pathways of cancer cells and maximize their growth rates as well as nutritive requirements. A thorough understanding of the underlying mechanisms particularly the "Warburg effect" while identifying ways and means that could restrain or reverse aerobic glycolysis can significantly contribute toward development of novel treatment strategies which could limit the rapidly increasing number of cancer-related deaths.

References

1. Balaban RS (2006) Maintenance of the metabolic homeostasis of the heart. Ann N Y Acad Sci 1080(1):140–153
2. Wilson DF (2017) Oxidative phosphorylation: regulation and role in cellular and tissue metabolism. J Physiol 595(23):7023–7038
3. Chance B, Williams G (1955) Respiratory enzymes in oxidative phosphorylation III. The steady state. J Biol Chem 217(1):409–428
4. Wu J (2017) New ways to maintain or disrupt metabolic homeostasis. J Mol Cell Biol 9(5):351–351. https://doi.org/10.1093/jmcb/mjx049
5. Arner P, Bernard S, Salehpour M, Possnert G, Liebl J, Steier P, Buchholz BA, Eriksson M, Arner E, Hauner H (2011) Dynamics of human adipose lipid turnover in health and metabolic disease. Nature 478(7367):110
6. Allison MB, Myers MG Jr (2014) Connecting leptin signaling to biological function. J Endocrinol 223(1):T25
7. Lumeng CN, Saltiel AR (2011) Inflammatory links between obesity and metabolic disease. J Clin Invest 121(6):2111–2117
8. Ouchi N, Parker JL, Lugus JJ, Walsh K (2011) Adipokines in inflammation and metabolic disease. Nat Rev Immunol 11(2):85
9. Holland WL, Miller RA, Wang ZV, Sun K, Barth BM, Bui HH, Davis KE, Bikman BT, Halberg N, Rutkowski JM (2011) Receptor-mediated activation of ceramidase activity initiates the pleiotropic actions of adiponectin. Nat Med 17(1):55
10. Xu A, Wang Y, Keshaw H, Xu LY, Lam KS, Cooper GJ (2003) The fat-derived hormone adiponectin alleviates alcoholic and nonalcoholic fatty liver diseases in mice. J Clin Invest 112(1):91–100
11. Stern JH, Rutkowski JM, Scherer PE (2016) Adiponectin, leptin, and fatty acids in the maintenance of metabolic homeostasis through adipose tissue crosstalk. Cell Metab 23(5):770–784
12. Zeng W, Pirzgalska RM, Pereira MM, Kubasova N, Barateiro A, Seixas E, Lu Y-H, Kozlova A, Voss H, Martins GG (2015) Sympathetic neuro-adipose connections mediate leptin-driven lipolysis. Cell 163(1):84–94
13. Eldor R, Raz I (2006) Lipotoxicity versus adipotoxicity—the deleterious effects of adipose tissue on beta cells in the pathogenesis of type 2 diabetes. Diabetes Res Clin Pract 74(2):S3–S8
14. Itoh Y, Kawamata Y, Harada M, Kobayashi M, Fujii R, Fukusumi S, Ogi K, Hosoya M, Tanaka Y, Uejima H (2003) Free fatty acids regulate insulin secretion from pancreatic β cells through GPR40. Nature 422(6928):173
15. Palmer BF, Clegg DJ (2014) Oxygen sensing and metabolic homeostasis. Mol Cell Endocrinol 397(1-2):51–58
16. Yingzhong Y, Droma Y, Rili G, Kubo K (2006) Regulation of body weight by leptin, with special reference to hypoxia-induced regulation. Intern Med 45(16):941–946
17. Kaufman RJ, Scheuner D, Schröder M, Shen X, Lee K, Liu CY, Arnold SM (2002) The unfolded protein response in nutrient sensing and differentiation. Nat Rev Mol Cell Biol 3(6):411
18. Liesa M, Shirihai OS (2013) Mitochondrial dynamics in the regulation of nutrient utilization and energy expenditure. Cell Metab 17(4):491–506

19. Hardie DG, Ross FA, Hawley SA (2012) AMPK: a nutrient and energy sensor that maintains energy homeostasis. Nat Rev Mol Cell Biol 13(4):251
20. Kim H-J, Kim JH, Noh S, Hur HJ, Sung MJ, Hwang J-T, Park JH, Yang HJ, Kim M-S, Kwon DY (2010) Metabolomic analysis of livers and serum from high-fat diet induced obese mice. J Proteome Res 10(2):722–731
21. Mollica MP, Iossa S, Liverini G, Soboll S (1998) Steady state changes in mitochondrial electrical potential and proton gradient in perfused liver from rats fed a high fat diet. Mol Cell Biochem 178(1-2):213–217
22. Qiu H, Schlegel V (2018) Impact of nutrient overload on metabolic homeostasis. Nutr Rev 76(9):693–707
23. Laybutt D, Preston A, Åkerfeldt M, Kench J, Busch A, Biankin A, Biden T (2007) Endoplasmic reticulum stress contributes to beta cell apoptosis in type 2 diabetes. Diabetologia 50(4):752–763
24. Widdowson EM (1976) The response of the sexes to nutritional stress. Proc Nutr Soc 35(2):175–180
25. Nishizawa H, Shimomura I, Kishida K, Maeda N, Kuriyama H, Nagaretani H, Matsuda M, Kondo H, Furuyama N, Kihara S (2002) Androgens decrease plasma adiponectin, an insulin-sensitizing adipocyte-derived protein. Diabetes 51(9):2734–2741
26. Mauvais-Jarvis F (2015) Sex differences in metabolic homeostasis, diabetes, and obesity. Biol Sex Differ 6(1):14
27. Nelson DL, Lehninger AL, Cox MM (2008) Lehninger principles of biochemistry. Macmillan, London
28. Warburg O (1925) The metabolism of carcinoma cells. J Cancer Res 9(1):148–163
29. Vander Heiden MG (2011) Targeting cancer metabolism: a therapeutic window opens. Nat Rev Drug Discov 10:671. https://doi.org/10.1038/nrd3504
30. Fantin VR, St-Pierre J, Leder P (2006) Attenuation of LDH-A expression uncovers a link between glycolysis, mitochondrial physiology, and tumor maintenance. Cancer Cell 9(6):425–434
31. Birsoy K, Wang T, Chen WW, Freinkman E, Abu-Remaileh M, Sabatini DM (2015) An essential role of the mitochondrial electron transport chain in cell proliferation is to enable aspartate synthesis. Cell 162(3):540–551
32. Crabtree HG (1929) Observations on the carbohydrate metabolism of tumours. Biochem J 23(3):536
33. Bonora E, Porcelli AM, Gasparre G, Biondi A, Ghelli A, Carelli V, Baracca A, Tallini G, Martinuzzi A, Lenaz G (2006) Defective oxidative phosphorylation in thyroid oncocytic carcinoma is associated with pathogenic mitochondrial DNA mutations affecting complexes I and III. Cancer Res 66(12):6087–6096
34. López-Lázaro M (2008) The warburg effect: why and how do cancer cells activate glycolysis in the presence of oxygen? Anti Cancer Agents Med Chem 8(3):305–312
35. Ikebuchi Y, Masumoto N, Tasaka K, Koike K, Kasahara K, Miyake A, Tanizawa O (1991) Superoxide anion increases intracellular pH, intracellular free calcium, and arachidonate release in human amnion cells. J Biol Chem 266(20):13233–13237
36. Erecińska M, Deas J, Silver I (1995) The effect of pH on glycolysis and phosphofructokinase activity in cultured cells and synaptosomes. J Neurochem 65(6):2765–2772
37. Papandreou I, Cairns RA, Fontana L, Lim AL, Denko NC (2006) HIF-1 mediates adaptation to hypoxia by actively downregulating mitochondrial oxygen consumption. Cell Metab 3(3):187–197
38. Semenza GL (2006) Development of novel therapeutic strategies that target HIF-1. Expert Opin Ther Targets 10(2):267–280
39. Wu C-A, Chao Y, Shiah S-G, Lin W-W (2013) Nutrient deprivation induces the Warburg effect through ROS/AMPK-dependent activation of pyruvate dehydrogenase kinase. Mol Cell Res 1833(5):1147–1156
40. Liberti MV, Locasale JW (2016) The Warburg effect: how does it benefit cancer cells? Trends Biochem Sci 41(3):211–218

41. Faubert B, Boily G, Izreig S, Griss T, Samborska B, Dong Z, Dupuy F, Chambers C, Fuerth BJ, Viollet B (2013) AMPK is a negative regulator of the Warburg effect and suppresses tumor growth in vivo. Cell Metab 17(1):113–124
42. Svensson RU, Shaw RJ (2012) Cancer metabolism: tumour friend or foe. Nature 485(7400):590
43. Bonuccelli G, Whitaker-Menezes D, Castello-Cros R, Pavlides S, Pestell RG, Fatatis A, Witkiewicz AK, Vander Heiden MG, Migneco G, Chiavarina B (2010) The reverse Warburg effect: glycolysis inhibitors prevent the tumor promoting effects of caveolin-1 deficient cancer associated fibroblasts. Cell Cycle 9(10):1960–1971
44. Lu J, Tan M, Cai Q (2015) The Warburg effect in tumor progression: mitochondrial oxidative metabolism as an anti-metastasis mechanism. Cancer Lett 356(2):156–164
45. Hammoudi N, Ahmed KBR, Garcia-Prieto C, Huang P (2011) Metabolic alterations in cancer cells and therapeutic implications. Chin J Cancer 30(8):508
46. Semenza GL (2010) Defining the role of hypoxia-inducible factor 1 in cancer biology and therapeutics. Oncogene 29(5):625
47. Ramanathan A, Wang C, Schreiber SL (2005) Perturbational profiling of a cell-line model of tumorigenesis by using metabolic measurements. Proc Natl Acad Sci 102(17):5992–5997
48. Dang L, White DW, Gross S, Bennett BD, Bittinger MA, Driggers EM, Fantin VR, Jang HG, Jin S, Keenan MC (2009b) Cancer-associated IDH1 mutations produce 2-hydroxyglutarate. Nature 462(7274):739
49. Vander Heiden MG, DeBerardinis RJ (2017) Understanding the intersections between metabolism and cancer biology. Cell 168(4):657–669
50. Altman BJ, Stine ZE, Dang CV (2016) From Krebs to clinic: glutamine metabolism to cancer therapy. Nat Rev Cancer 16(10):619
51. Eales K, Hollinshead K, Tennant D (2016) Hypoxia and metabolic adaptation of cancer cells. Oncogenesis 5(1):e190
52. Dang CV (2010) Rethinking the Warburg effect with Myc micromanaging glutamine metabolism. Cancer Res 70(3):859–862
53. Le A, Lane AN, Hamaker M, Bose S, Gouw A, Barbi J, Tsukamoto T, Rojas CJ, Slusher BS, Zhang H (2012) Glucose-independent glutamine metabolism via TCA cycling for proliferation and survival in B cells. Cell Metab 15(1):110–121
54. Dang CV, Le A, Gao P (2009a) MYC-induced cancer cell energy metabolism and therapeutic opportunities. Clin Cancer Res 15(21):6479–6483. https://doi.org/10.1158/1078-0432.ccr-09-0889
55. Mullen AR, Wheaton WW, Jin ES, Chen P-H, Sullivan LB, Cheng T, Yang Y, Linehan WM, Chandel NS, DeBerardinis RJ (2011) Reductive carboxylation supports growth in tumour cells with defective mitochondria. Nature 481:385. https://doi.org/10.1038/nature10642
56. Mullen AR, Hu Z, Shi X, Jiang L, Boroughs LK, Kovacs Z, Boriack R, Rakheja D, Sullivan LB, Linehan WM, Chandel NS, DeBerardinis RJ (2014) Oxidation of alpha-ketoglutarate is required for reductive carboxylation in cancer cells with mitochondrial defects. Cell Rep 7(5):1679–1690. https://doi.org/10.1016/j.celrep.2014.04.037
57. Rankin EB, Giaccia AJ (2016) Hypoxic control of metastasis. Science 352(6282):175–180. https://doi.org/10.1126/science.aaf4405
58. Benjamin DI, Cravatt BF, Nomura DK (2012) Global profiling strategies for mapping dysregulated metabolic pathways in cancer. Cell Metab 16(5):565–577. https://doi.org/10.1016/j.cmet.2012.09.013
59. Pascual G, Avgustinova A, Mejetta S, Martín M, Castellanos A, Attolini CS-O, Berenguer A, Prats N, Toll A, Hueto JA, Bescós C, Di Croce L, Benitah SA (2016) Targeting metastasis-initiating cells through the fatty acid receptor CD36. Nature 541:41. https://doi.org/10.1038/nature20791
60. Nath A, Li I, Roberts LR, Chan C (2015) Elevated free fatty acid uptake via CD36 promotes epithelial-mesenchymal transition in hepatocellular carcinoma. Sci Rep 5:14752–14752. https://doi.org/10.1038/srep14752

61. Nomura DK, Long JZ, Niessen S, Hoover HS, Ng S-W, Cravatt BF (2010) Monoacylglycerol lipase regulates a fatty acid network that promotes cancer pathogenesis. Cell 140(1):49–61. https://doi.org/10.1016/j.cell.2009.11.027
62. Mathupala SP, Ko YH, Pedersen PL (2009) Hexokinase-2 bound to mitochondria: cancer's stygian link to the "Warburg Effect" and a pivotal target for effective therapy. Semin Cancer Biol 19(1):17–24. https://doi.org/10.1016/j.semcancer.2008.11.006
63. Mathupala SP, Ko YH, Pedersen PL (2006) Hexokinase II: cancer's double-edged sword acting as both facilitator and gatekeeper of malignancy when bound to mitochondria. Oncogene 25(34):4777–4786. https://doi.org/10.1038/sj.onc.1209603
64. Bustamante E, Pedersen PL (1980) Mitochondrial hexokinase of rat hepatoma cells in culture: solubilization and kinetic properties. Biochemistry 19(22):4972–4977. https://doi.org/10.1021/bi00563a006
65. Bustamante E, Morris HP, Pedersen PL (1981) Energy metabolism of tumor cells. Requirement for a form of hexokinase with a propensity for mitochondrial binding. J Biol Chem 256(16):8699–8704
66. Biaglow JE, Miller RA (2005) The thioredoxin reductase/thioredoxin system: novel redox targets for cancer therapy. Cancer Biol Ther 4(1):6–13. https://doi.org/10.4161/cbt.4.1.1434
67. Borger DR, Tanabe KK, Fan KC, Lopez HU, Fantin VR, Straley KS, Schenkein DP, Hezel AF, Ancukiewicz M, Liebman HM, Kwak EL, Clark JW, Ryan DP, Deshpande V, Dias-Santagata D, Ellisen LW, Zhu AX, Iafrate AJ (2012) Frequent mutation of isocitrate dehydrogenase (IDH)1 and IDH2 in cholangiocarcinoma identified through broad-based tumor genotyping. Oncologist 17(1):72–79. https://doi.org/10.1634/theoncologist.2011-0386
68. Kosmider O, Gelsi-Boyer V, Slama L, Dreyfus F, Beyne-Rauzy O, Quesnel B, Hunault-Berger M, Slama B, Vey N, Lacombe C, Solary E, Birnbaum D, Bernard OA, Fontenay M (2010) Mutations of IDH1 and IDH2 genes in early and accelerated phases of myelodysplastic syndromes and MDS/myeloproliferative neoplasms. Leukemia 24(5):1094–1096. https://doi.org/10.1038/leu.2010.52
69. Mardis ER, Ding L, Dooling DJ, Larson DE, McLellan MD, Chen K, Koboldt DC, Fulton RS, Delehaunty KD, McGrath SD, Fulton LA, Locke DP, Magrini VJ, Abbott RM, Vickery TL, Reed JS, Robinson JS, Wylie T, Smith SM, Carmichael L, Eldred JM, Harris CC, Walker J, Peck JB, Du F, Dukes AF, Sanderson GE, Brummett AM, Clark E, McMichael JF, Meyer RJ, Schindler JK, Pohl CS, Wallis JW, Shi X, Lin L, Schmidt H, Tang Y, Haipek C, Wiechert ME, Ivy JV, Kalicki J, Elliott G, Ries RE, Payton JE, Westervelt P, Tomasson MH, Watson MA, Baty J, Heath S, Shannon WD, Nagarajan R, Link DC, Walter MJ, Graubert TA, DiPersio JF, Wilson RK, Ley TJ (2009) Recurring mutations found by sequencing an acute myeloid leukemia genome. N Engl J Med 361(11):1058–1066. https://doi.org/10.1056/NEJMoa0903840
70. Parsons DW, Jones S, Zhang X, Lin JC, Leary RJ, Angenendt P, Mankoo P, Carter H, Siu IM, Gallia GL, Olivi A, McLendon R, Rasheed BA, Keir S, Nikolskaya T, Nikolsky Y, Busam DA, Tekleab H, Diaz LA Jr, Hartigan J, Smith DR, Strausberg RL, Marie SK, Shinjo SM, Yan H, Riggins GJ, Bigner DD, Karchin R, Papadopoulos N, Parmigiani G, Vogelstein B, Velculescu VE, Kinzler KW (2008) An integrated genomic analysis of human glioblastoma multiforme. Science 321(5897):1807–1812. https://doi.org/10.1126/science.1164382
71. Hartmann C, Meyer J, Balss J, Capper D, Mueller W, Christians A, Felsberg J, Wolter M, Mawrin C, Wick W, Weller M, Herold-Mende C, Unterberg A, Jeuken JW, Wesseling P, Reifenberger G, von Deimling A (2009) Type and frequency of IDH1 and IDH2 mutations are related to astrocytic and oligodendroglial differentiation and age: a study of 1,010 diffuse gliomas. Acta Neuropathol 118(4):469–474. https://doi.org/10.1007/s00401-009-0561-9
72. Yan H, Parsons DW, Jin G, McLendon R, Rasheed BA, Yuan W, Kos I, Batinic-Haberle I, Jones S, Riggins GJ, Friedman H, Friedman A, Reardon D, Herndon J, Kinzler KW, Velculescu VE, Vogelstein B, Bigner DD (2009) IDH1 and IDH2 mutations in gliomas. N Engl J Med 360(8):765–773. https://doi.org/10.1056/NEJMoa0808710
73. Losman JA, Kaelin WG Jr (2013) What a difference a hydroxyl makes: mutant IDH, (R)-2-hydroxyglutarate, and cancer. Genes Dev 27(8):836–852. https://doi.org/10.1101/gad.217406.113

74. Chowdhury R, Yeoh KK, Tian YM, Hillringhaus L, Bagg EA, Rose NR, Leung IK, Li XS, Woon EC, Yang M, McDonough MA, King ON, Clifton IJ, Klose RJ, Claridge TD, Ratcliffe PJ, Schofield CJ, Kawamura A (2011) The oncometabolite 2-hydroxyglutarate inhibits histone lysine demethylases. EMBO Rep 12(5):463–469. https://doi.org/10.1038/embor.2011.43
75. Xu W, Yang H, Liu Y, Yang Y, Wang P, Kim SH, Ito S, Yang C, Wang P, Xiao MT, Liu LX, Jiang WQ, Liu J, Zhang JY, Wang B, Frye S, Zhang Y, Xu YH, Lei QY, Guan KL, Zhao SM, Xiong Y (2011) Oncometabolite 2-hydroxyglutarate is a competitive inhibitor of alpha-ketoglutarate-dependent dioxygenases. Cancer Cell 19(1):17–30. https://doi.org/10.1016/j.ccr.2010.12.014
76. Baysal BE, Ferrell RE, Willett-Brozick JE, Lawrence EC, Myssiorek D, Bosch A, van der Mey A, Taschner PE, Rubinstein WS, Myers EN, Richard CW, Cornelisse CJ, Devilee P, Devlin B (2000) Mutations in SDHD, a mitochondrial complex II gene, in hereditary paraganglioma. Science 287(5454):848–851. https://doi.org/10.1126/science.287.5454.848
77. Janeway KA, Kim SY, Lodish M, Nose V, Rustin P, Gaal J, Dahia PL, Liegl B, Ball ER, Raygada M, Lai AH, Kelly L, Hornick JL, O'Sullivan M, de Krijger RR, Dinjens WN, Demetri GD, Antonescu CR, Fletcher JA, Helman L, Stratakis CA (2011) Defects in succinate dehydrogenase in gastrointestinal stromal tumors lacking KIT and PDGFRA mutations. Proc Natl Acad Sci U S A 108(1):314–318. https://doi.org/10.1073/pnas.1009199108
78. Ricketts C, Woodward ER, Killick P, Morris MR, Astuti D, Latif F, Maher ER (2008) Germline SDHB mutations and familial renal cell carcinoma. J Natl Cancer Inst 100(17):1260–1262. https://doi.org/10.1093/jnci/djn254
79. Sun F, Huo X, Zhai Y, Wang A, Xu J, Su D, Bartlam M, Rao Z (2005) Crystal structure of mitochondrial respiratory membrane protein complex II. Cell 121(7):1043–1057. https://doi.org/10.1016/j.cell.2005.05.025
80. Brière J-J, Favier J, Bénit P, Ghouzzi VE, Lorenzato A, Rabier D, Di Renzo MF, Gimenez-Roqueplo A-P, Rustin P (2005) Mitochondrial succinate is instrumental for HIF1α nuclear translocation in SDHA-mutant fibroblasts under normoxic conditions. Hum Mol Genet 14(21):3263–3269. https://doi.org/10.1093/hmg/ddi359
81. Michalowska I, Cwikla J, Prejbisz A, Kwiatek P, Szperl M, Michalski W, Wyrwicz L, Kusmierczyk M, Januszewicz A, Maciejczyk A, Roszczynko M, Peczkowska M (2016) Mediastinal paragangliomas related to SDHx gene mutations. Kardiochir Torakochirurgia Pol 13(3):276–282. https://doi.org/10.5114/kitp.2016.62624
82. Bayley JP, van Minderhout I, Weiss MM, Jansen JC, Oomen PH, Menko FH, Pasini B, Ferrando B, Wong N, Alpert LC, Williams R, Blair E, Devilee P, Taschner PE (2006) Mutation analysis of SDHB and SDHC: novel germline mutations in sporadic head and neck paraganglioma and familial paraganglioma and/or pheochromocytoma. BMC Med Genet 7:1. https://doi.org/10.1186/1471-2350-7-1
83. Kuroda N, Yorita K, Nagasaki M, Harada Y, Ohe C, Jeruc J, Raspollini MR, Michal M, Hes O, Amin MB (2016) Review of succinate dehydrogenase-deficient renal cell carcinoma with focus on clinical and pathobiological aspects. Pol J Pathol 67(1):3–7
84. Vanharanta S, Buchta M, McWhinney SR, Virta SK, Peçzkowska M, Morrison CD, Lehtonen R, Januszewicz A, Järvinen H, Juhola M (2004) Early-onset renal cell carcinoma as a novel extraparaganglial component of SDHB-associated heritable paraganglioma. Am J Hum Genet 74(1):153–159
85. Shayesteh L, Lu Y, Kuo WL, Baldocchi R, Godfrey T, Collins C, Pinkel D, Powell B, Mills GB, Gray JW (1999) PIK3CA is implicated as an oncogene in ovarian cancer. Nat Genet 21(1):99–102. https://doi.org/10.1038/5042
86. Broderick DK, Di C, Parrett TJ, Samuels YR, Cummins JM, McLendon RE, Fults DW, Velculescu VE, Bigner DD, Yan H (2004) Mutations of PIK3CA in anaplastic oligodendrogliomas, high-grade astrocytomas, and medulloblastomas. Cancer Res 64(15):5048–5050. https://doi.org/10.1158/0008-5472.can-04-1170
87. Samuels Y, Wang Z, Bardelli A, Silliman N, Ptak J, Szabo S, Yan H, Gazdar A, Powell SM, Riggins GJ, Willson JK, Markowitz S, Kinzler KW, Vogelstein B, Velculescu VE (2004)

High frequency of mutations of the PIK3CA gene in human cancers. Science 304(5670):554. https://doi.org/10.1126/science.1096502
88. Kang S, Bader AG, Vogt PK (2005) Phosphatidylinositol 3-kinase mutations identified in human cancer are oncogenic. Proc Natl Acad Sci U S A 102(3):802–807. https://doi.org/10.1073/pnas.0408864102
89. Nguyen LV, Vanner R, Dirks P, Eaves CJ (2012) Cancer stem cells: an evolving concept. Nat Rev Cancer 12(2):133–143. https://doi.org/10.1038/nrc3184
90. Jackson EB, Brues AM (1941) Studies on a transplantable embryoma of the mouse. Cancer Res 1(6):494–498
91. Lapidot T, Sirard C, Vormoor J, Murdoch B, Hoang T, Caceres-Cortes J, Minden M, Paterson B, Caligiuri MA, Dick JE (1994) A cell initiating human acute myeloid leukaemia after transplantation into SCID mice. Nature 367(6464):645–648. https://doi.org/10.1038/367645a0
92. Easwaran H, Tsai HC, Baylin SB (2014) Cancer epigenetics: tumor heterogeneity, plasticity of stem-like states, and drug resistance. Mol Cell 54(5):716–727. https://doi.org/10.1016/j.molcel.2014.05.015
93. Wu Z, Wei D, Gao W, Xu Y, Hu Z, Ma Z, Gao C, Zhu X, Li Q (2015) TPO-induced metabolic reprogramming drives liver metastasis of colorectal cancer CD110+ tumor-initiating cells. Cell Stem Cell 17(1):47–59. https://doi.org/10.1016/j.stem.2015.05.016
94. Ishimoto T, Oshima H, Oshima M, Kai K, Torii R, Masuko T, Baba H, Saya H, Nagano O (2010) CD44+ slow-cycling tumor cell expansion is triggered by cooperative actions of Wnt and prostaglandin E2 in gastric tumorigenesis. Cancer Sci 101(3):673–678. https://doi.org/10.1111/j.1349-7006.2009.01430.x
95. Dean M (2009) ABC transporters, drug resistance, and cancer stem cells. J Mammary Gland Biol Neoplasia 14(1):3–9. https://doi.org/10.1007/s10911-009-9109-9
96. Meyer MJ, Fleming JM, Lin AF, Hussnain SA, Ginsburg E, Vonderhaar BK (2010) CD44posCD49fhiCD133/2hi defines xenograft-initiating cells in estrogen receptor-negative breast cancer. Cancer Res 70(11):4624–4633. https://doi.org/10.1158/0008-5472.can-09-3619
97. Schober M, Fuchs E (2011) Tumor-initiating stem cells of squamous cell carcinomas and their control by TGF-beta and integrin/focal adhesion kinase (FAK) signaling. Proc Natl Acad Sci U S A 108(26):10544–10549. https://doi.org/10.1073/pnas.1107807108
98. Stewart JM, Shaw PA, Gedye C, Bernardini MQ, Neel BG, Ailles LE (2011) Phenotypic heterogeneity and instability of human ovarian tumor-initiating cells. Proc Natl Acad Sci U S A 108(16):6468–6473. https://doi.org/10.1073/pnas.1005529108
99. Nowell PC (1986) Mechanisms of tumor progression. Cancer Res 46(5):2203–2207
100. Baylin SB, Jones PA (2011) A decade of exploring the cancer epigenome – biological and translational implications. Nat Rev Cancer 11:726. https://doi.org/10.1038/nrc3130
101. Bissell MJ, Hines WC (2011) Why don't we get more cancer? A proposed role of the microenvironment in restraining cancer progression. Nat Med 17(3):320–329. https://doi.org/10.1038/nm.2328
102. Dick JE (2008) Stem cell concepts renew cancer research. Blood 112(13):4793–4807. https://doi.org/10.1182/blood-2008-08-077941
103. Shackleton M, Quintana E, Fearon ER, Morrison SJ (2009) Heterogeneity in cancer: cancer stem cells versus clonal evolution. Cell 138(5):822–829. https://doi.org/10.1016/j.cell.2009.08.017
104. Li C, Heidt DG, Dalerba P, Burant CF, Zhang L, Adsay V, Wicha M, Clarke MF, Simeone DM (2007) Identification of pancreatic cancer stem cells. Cancer Res 67(3):1030–1037. https://doi.org/10.1158/0008-5472.can-06-2030
105. Bonnet D, Dick JE (1997) Human acute myeloid leukemia is organized as a hierarchy that originates from a primitive hematopoietic cell. Nat Med 3(7):730–737
106. O'Brien CA, Pollett A, Gallinger S, Dick JE (2007) A human colon cancer cell capable of initiating tumour growth in immunodeficient mice. Nature 445(7123):106–110. https://doi.org/10.1038/nature05372

107. Singh SK, Hawkins C, Clarke ID, Squire JA, Bayani J, Hide T, Henkelman RM, Cusimano MD, Dirks PB (2004) Identification of human brain tumour initiating cells. Nature 432(7015):396–401. https://doi.org/10.1038/nature03128
108. Batlle E, Clevers H (2017) Cancer stem cells revisited. Nat Med 23(10):1124–1134. https://doi.org/10.1038/nm.4409
109. Gupta PB, Fillmore CM, Jiang G, Shapira SD, Tao K, Kuperwasser C, Lander ES (2011) Stochastic state transitions give rise to phenotypic equilibrium in populations of cancer cells. Cell 146(4):633–644. https://doi.org/10.1016/j.cell.2011.07.026
110. Peiris-Pagès M, Martinez-Outschoorn UE, Pestell RG, Sotgia F, Lisanti MP (2016) Cancer stem cell metabolism. Breast Cancer Res 18(1):55–55. https://doi.org/10.1186/s13058-016-0712-6
111. Vlashi E, Lagadec C, Vergnes L, Matsutani T, Masui K, Poulou M, Popescu R, Della Donna L, Evers P, Dekmezian C, Reue K, Christofk H, Mischel PS, Pajonk F (2011) Metabolic state of glioma stem cells and nontumorigenic cells. Proc Natl Acad Sci U S A 108(38):16062–16067. https://doi.org/10.1073/pnas.1106704108
112. Pascual G, Avgustinova A, Mejetta S, Martin M, Castellanos A, Attolini CS, Berenguer A, Prats N, Toll A, Hueto JA, Bescos C, Di Croce L, Benitah SA (2017) Targeting metastasis-initiating cells through the fatty acid receptor CD36. Nature 541(7635):41–45. https://doi.org/10.1038/nature20791
113. Ye H, Adane B, Khan N, Sullivan T, Minhajuddin M, Gasparetto M, Stevens B, Pei S, Balys M, Ashton JM, Klemm DJ, Woolthuis CM, Stranahan AW, Park CY, Jordan CT (2016) Leukemic stem cells evade chemotherapy by metabolic adaptation to an adipose tissue niche. Cell Stem Cell 19(1):23–37. https://doi.org/10.1016/j.stem.2016.06.001
114. Krebs AM, Mitschke J, Lasierra Losada M, Schmalhofer O, Boerries M, Busch H, Boettcher M, Mougiakakos D, Reichardt W, Bronsert P, Brunton Valerie G, Pilarsky C, Winkler TH, Brabletz S, Stemmler MP, Brabletz T (2017) The EMT-activator Zeb1 is a key factor for cell plasticity and promotes metastasis in pancreatic cancer. Nat Cell Biol 19:518. https://doi.org/10.1038/ncb3513
115. Clarke MF, Hass AT (2006) Cancer stem cells. In: Reviews in cell biology and molecular medicine. Wiley, Hoboken
116. Dang CV (2012) MYC on the path to cancer. Cell 149(1):22–35. https://doi.org/10.1016/j.cell.2012.03.003
117. Ward PS, Thompson CB (2012) Metabolic reprogramming: a cancer hallmark even warburg did not anticipate. Cancer Cell 21(3):297–308. https://doi.org/10.1016/j.ccr.2012.02.014
118. Cairns P, Okami K, Halachmi S, Halachmi N, Esteller M, Herman JG, Jen J, Isaacs WB, Bova GS, Sidransky D (1997) Frequent inactivation of PTEN/MMAC1 in primary prostate cancer. Cancer Res 57(22):4997–5000
119. Jia S, Liu Z, Zhang S, Liu P, Zhang L, Lee SH, Zhang J, Signoretti S, Loda M, Roberts TM, Zhao JJ (2008) Essential roles of PI(3)K-p110beta in cell growth, metabolism and tumorigenesis. Nature 454(7205):776–779. https://doi.org/10.1038/nature07091
120. Carracedo A, Pandolfi PP (2008) The PTEN-PI3K pathway: of feedbacks and cross-talks. Oncogene 27(41):5527–5541. https://doi.org/10.1038/onc.2008.247
121. Alimonti A, Carracedo A, Clohessy JG, Trotman LC, Nardella C, Egia A, Salmena L, Sampieri K, Haveman WJ, Brogi E, Richardson AL, Zhang J, Pandolfi PP (2010) Subtle variations in Pten dose determine cancer susceptibility. Nat Genet 42(5):454–458. https://doi.org/10.1038/ng.556
122. Garcia-Cao I, Song MS, Hobbs RM, Laurent G, Giorgi C, de Boer VC, Anastasiou D, Ito K, Sasaki AT, Rameh L, Carracedo A, Vander Heiden MG, Cantley LC, Pinton P, Haigis MC, Pandolfi PP (2012) Systemic elevation of PTEN induces a tumor-suppressive metabolic state. Cell 149(1):49–62. https://doi.org/10.1016/j.cell.2012.02.030
123. Shaw RJ, Cantley LC (2006) Ras, PI(3)K and mTOR signalling controls tumour cell growth. Nature 441(7092):424–430. https://doi.org/10.1038/nature04869
124. Corradetti MN, Inoki K, Bardeesy N, DePinho RA, Guan KL (2004) Regulation of the TSC pathway by LKB1: evidence of a molecular link between tuberous sclerosis complex

and Peutz-Jeghers syndrome. Genes Dev 18(13):1533–1538. https://doi.org/10.1101/gad.1199104
125. Inoki K, Zhu T, Guan KL (2003) TSC2 mediates cellular energy response to control cell growth and survival. Cell 115(5):577–590
126. Muller PA, Vousden KH (2013) p53 mutations in cancer. Nat Cell Biol 15(1):2–8. https://doi.org/10.1038/ncb2641
127. Vousden KH, Prives C (2009) Blinded by the light: the growing complexity of p53. Cell 137(3):413–431. https://doi.org/10.1016/j.cell.2009.04.037
128. Bensaad K, Tsuruta A, Selak MA, Vidal MN, Nakano K, Bartrons R, Gottlieb E, Vousden KH (2006) TIGAR, a p53-inducible regulator of glycolysis and apoptosis. Cell 126(1):107–120. https://doi.org/10.1016/j.cell.2006.05.036
129. Schwartzenberg-Bar-Yoseph F, Armoni M, Karnieli E (2004) The tumor suppressor p53 down-regulates glucose transporters GLUT1 and GLUT4 gene expression. Cancer Res 64(7):2627–2633
130. Zhang C, Liu J, Wu R, Liang Y, Lin M, Liu J, Chan CS, Hu W, Feng Z (2014) Tumor suppressor p53 negatively regulates glycolysis stimulated by hypoxia through its target RRAD. Oncotarget 5(14):5535–5546. https://doi.org/10.18632/oncotarget.2137
131. Jiang P, Du W, Wang X, Mancuso A, Gao X, Wu M, Yang X (2011) p53 regulates biosynthesis through direct inactivation of glucose-6-phosphate dehydrogenase. Nat Cell Biol 13(3):310–316. https://doi.org/10.1038/ncb2172
132. Tavana O, Gu W (2017) Modulation of the p53/MDM2 interplay by HAUSP inhibitors. J Mol Cell Biol 9(1):45–52. https://doi.org/10.1093/jmcb/mjw049
133. Zhou G, Pantelopulos GA, Mukherjee S, Voelz VA (2017) Bridging microscopic and macroscopic mechanisms of p53-MDM2 binding with kinetic network models. Biophys J 113(4):785–793. https://doi.org/10.1016/j.bpj.2017.07.009
134. Wang L, Xiong H, Wu F, Zhang Y, Wang J, Zhao L, Guo X, Chang LJ, Zhang Y, You MJ, Koochekpour S, Saleem M, Huang H, Lu J, Deng Y (2014) Hexokinase 2-mediated Warburg effect is required for PTEN- and p53-deficiency-driven prostate cancer growth. Cell Rep 8(5):1461–1474. https://doi.org/10.1016/j.celrep.2014.07.053
135. Mostoslavsky R, Chua KF, Lombard DB, Pang WW, Fischer MR, Gellon L, Liu P, Mostoslavsky G, Franco S, Murphy MM, Mills KD, Patel P, Hsu JT, Hong AL, Ford E, Cheng HL, Kennedy C, Nunez N, Bronson R, Frendewey D, Auerbach W, Valenzuela D, Karow M, Hottiger MO, Hursting S, Barrett JC, Guarente L, Mulligan R, Demple B, Yancopoulos GD, Alt FW (2006) Genomic instability and aging-like phenotype in the absence of mammalian SIRT6. Cell 124(2):315–329. https://doi.org/10.1016/j.cell.2005.11.044
136. Kaidi A, Weinert BT, Choudhary C, Jackson SP (2010) Human SIRT6 promotes DNA end resection through CtIP deacetylation. Science 329(5997):1348–1353. https://doi.org/10.1126/science.1192049
137. Mao Z, Hine C, Tian X, Van Meter M, Au M, Vaidya A, Seluanov A, Gorbunova V (2011) SIRT6 promotes DNA repair under stress by activating PARP1. Science 332(6036):1443–1446. https://doi.org/10.1126/science.1202723
138. Sebastian C, Zwaans BM, Silberman DM, Gymrek M, Goren A, Zhong L, Ram O, Truelove J, Guimaraes AR, Toiber D, Cosentino C, Greenson JK, MacDonald AI, McGlynn L, Maxwell F, Edwards J, Giacosa S, Guccione E, Weissleder R, Bernstein BE, Regev A, Shiels PG, Lombard DB, Mostoslavsky R (2012) The histone deacetylase SIRT6 is a tumor suppressor that controls cancer metabolism. Cell 151(6):1185–1199. https://doi.org/10.1016/j.cell.2012.10.047
139. Dang CV, Semenza GL (1999) Oncogenic alterations of metabolism. Trends Biochem Sci 24(2):68–72
140. Elstrom RL, Bauer DE, Buzzai M, Karnauskas R, Harris MH, Plas DR, Zhuang H, Cinalli RM, Alavi A, Rudin CM, Thompson CB (2004) Akt stimulates aerobic glycolysis in cancer cells. Cancer Res 64(11):3892–3899. https://doi.org/10.1158/0008-5472.can-03-2904
141. Dang CV (2013) MYC, metabolism, cell growth, and tumorigenesis. Cold Spring Harb Perspect Med 3(8):a014217. https://doi.org/10.1101/cshperspect.a014217

142. Jin L, Alesi GN, Kang S (2016) Glutaminolysis as a target for cancer therapy. Oncogene 35(28):3619–3625. https://doi.org/10.1038/onc.2015.447
143. Gao P, Tchernyshyov I, Chang TC, Lee YS, Kita K, Ochi T, Zeller KI, De Marzo AM, Van Eyk JE, Mendell JT, Dang CV (2009) c-Myc suppression of miR-23a/b enhances mitochondrial glutaminase expression and glutamine metabolism. Nature 458(7239):762–765. https://doi.org/10.1038/nature07823
144. Wise DR, DeBerardinis RJ, Mancuso A, Sayed N, Zhang XY, Pfeiffer HK, Nissim I, Daikhin E, Yudkoff M, McMahon SB, Thompson CB (2008) Myc regulates a transcriptional program that stimulates mitochondrial glutaminolysis and leads to glutamine addiction. Proc Natl Acad Sci U S A 105(48):18782–18787. https://doi.org/10.1073/pnas.0810199105
145. Marbaniang C, Kma L (2018) Dysregulation of glucose metabolism by oncogenes and tumor suppressors in cancer cells. Asian Pac J Cancer Prev 19(9):2377–2390. https://doi.org/10.22034/apjcp.2018.19.9.2377
146. Maiuri MC, Tasdemir E, Criollo A, Morselli E, Vicencio JM, Carnuccio R, Kroemer G (2009) Control of autophagy by oncogenes and tumor suppressor genes. Cell Death Differ 16(1):87–93. https://doi.org/10.1038/cdd.2008.131
147. Crighton D, Wilkinson S, O'Prey J, Syed N, Smith P, Harrison PR, Gasco M, Garrone O, Crook T, Ryan KM (2006) DRAM, a p53-induced modulator of autophagy, is critical for apoptosis. Cell 126(1):121–134. https://doi.org/10.1016/j.cell.2006.05.034
148. Tasdemir E, Chiara Maiuri M, Morselli E, Criollo A, D'Amelio M, Djavaheri-Mergny M, Cecconi F, Tavernarakis N, Kroemer G (2008a) A dual role of p53 in the control of autophagy. Autophagy 4(6):810–814. https://doi.org/10.4161/auto.6486
149. Tasdemir E, Maiuri MC, Galluzzi L, Vitale I, Djavaheri-Mergny M, D'Amelio M, Criollo A, Morselli E, Zhu C, Harper F, Nannmark U, Samara C, Pinton P, Vicencio JM, Carnuccio R, Moll UM, Madeo F, Paterlini-Brechot P, Rizzuto R, Szabadkai G, Pierron G, Blomgren K, Tavernarakis N, Codogno P, Cecconi F, Kroemer G (2008b) Regulation of autophagy by cytoplasmic p53. Nat Cell Biol 10(6):676–687. https://doi.org/10.1038/ncb1730
150. Longley DB, Johnston PG (2005) Molecular mechanisms of drug resistance. J Pathol 205(2):275–292. https://doi.org/10.1002/path.1706
151. Zeller C, Dai W, Steele NL, Siddiq A, Walley AJ, Wilhelm-Benartzi CS, Rizzo S, van der Zee A, Plumb JA, Brown R (2012) Candidate DNA methylation drivers of acquired cisplatin resistance in ovarian cancer identified by methylome and expression profiling. Oncogene 31(42):4567–4576. https://doi.org/10.1038/onc.2011.611
152. Housman G, Byler S, Heerboth S, Lapinska K, Longacre M, Snyder N, Sarkar S (2014) Drug resistance in cancer: an overview. Cancer 6(3):1769–1792. https://doi.org/10.3390/cancers6031769
153. Maier P, Spier I, Laufs S, Veldwijk MR, Fruehauf S, Wenz F, Zeller WJ (2010) Chemoprotection of human hematopoietic stem cells by simultaneous lentiviral overexpression of multidrug resistance 1 and O(6)-methylguanine-DNA methyltransferase(P140K). Gene Ther 17(3):389–399. https://doi.org/10.1038/gt.2009.133
154. Valent P, Bonnet D, De Maria R, Lapidot T, Copland M, Melo JV, Chomienne C, Ishikawa F, Schuringa JJ, Stassi G, Huntly B, Herrmann H, Soulier J, Roesch A, Schuurhuis GJ, Wohrer S, Arock M, Zuber J, Cerny-Reiterer S, Johnsen HE, Andreeff M, Eaves C (2012) Cancer stem cell definitions and terminology: the devil is in the details. Nat Rev Cancer 12(11):767–775. https://doi.org/10.1038/nrc3368
155. Meacham CE, Morrison SJ (2013) Tumour heterogeneity and cancer cell plasticity. Nature 501:328. https://doi.org/10.1038/nature12624
156. Anderson K, Lutz C, van Delft FW, Bateman CM, Guo Y, Colman SM, Kempski H, Moorman AV, Titley I, Swansbury J, Kearney L, Enver T, Greaves M (2011) Genetic variegation of clonal architecture and propagating cells in leukaemia. Nature 469(7330):356–361. https://doi.org/10.1038/nature09650
157. Ding L, Ley TJ, Larson DE, Miller CA, Koboldt DC, Welch JS, Ritchey JK, Young MA, Lamprecht T, McLellan MD, McMichael JF, Wallis JW, Lu C, Shen D, Harris CC, Dooling DJ, Fulton RS, Fulton LL, Chen K, Schmidt H, Kalicki-Veizer J, Magrini VJ, Cook L, McGrath

SD, Vickery TL, Wendl MC, Heath S, Watson MA, Link DC, Tomasson MH, Shannon WD, Payton JE, Kulkarni S, Westervelt P, Walter MJ, Graubert TA, Mardis ER, Wilson RK, DiPersio JF (2012) Clonal evolution in relapsed acute myeloid leukaemia revealed by whole-genome sequencing. Nature 481:506. https://doi.org/10.1038/nature10738
158. Zahreddine H, Borden KL (2013) Mechanisms and insights into drug resistance in cancer. Front Pharmacol 4:28. https://doi.org/10.3389/fphar.2013.00028
159. Aas T, Borresen AL, Geisler S, Smith-Sorensen B, Johnsen H, Varhaug JE, Akslen LA, Lonning PE (1996) Specific P53 mutations are associated with de novo resistance to doxorubicin in breast cancer patients. Nat Med 2(7):811–814
160. Soengas MS, Alarcon RM, Yoshida H, Giaccia AJ, Hakem R, Mak TW, Lowe SW (1999) Apaf-1 and caspase-9 in p53-dependent apoptosis and tumor inhibition. Science 284(5411):156–159. https://doi.org/10.1126/science.284.5411.156
161. Berns K, Horlings HM, Hennessy BT, Madiredjo M, Hijmans EM, Beelen K, Linn SC, Gonzalez-Angulo AM, Stemke-Hale K, Hauptmann M, Beijersbergen RL, Mills GB, van de Vijver MJ, Bernards R (2007) A functional genetic approach identifies the PI3K pathway as a major determinant of trastuzumab resistance in breast cancer. Cancer Cell 12(4):395–402. https://doi.org/10.1016/j.ccr.2007.08.030
162. Dieras V, Vincent-Salomon A, Degeorges A, Beuzeboc P, Mignot L, de Cremoux P (2007) Trastuzumab (Herceptin) and breast cancer: mechanisms of resistance. Bull Cancer 94(3):259–266
163. Gottesman MM, Fojo T, Bates SE (2002) Multidrug resistance in cancer: role of ATP-dependent transporters. Nat Rev Cancer 2(1):48–58. https://doi.org/10.1038/nrc706
164. Hu T, Liu S, Breiter DR, Wang F, Tang Y, Sun S (2008) Octamer 4 small interfering RNA results in cancer stem cell-like cell apoptosis. Cancer Res 68(16):6533–6540. https://doi.org/10.1158/0008-5472.can-07-6642
165. Barkan D, Kleinman H, Simmons JL, Asmussen H, Kamaraju AK, Hoenorhoff MJ, Liu ZY, Costes SV, Cho EH, Lockett S, Khanna C, Chambers AF, Green JE (2008) Inhibition of metastatic outgrowth from single dormant tumor cells by targeting the cytoskeleton. Cancer Res 68(15):6241–6250. https://doi.org/10.1158/0008-5472.can-07-6849
166. Papa S, Choy PM, Bubici C (2019) The ERK and JNK pathways in the regulation of metabolic reprogramming. Oncogene 38(13):2223–2240. https://doi.org/10.1038/s41388-018-0582-8
167. Hanahan D, Weinberg RA (2011) Hallmarks of cancer: the next generation. Cell 144(5):646–674. https://doi.org/10.1016/j.cell.2011.02.013
168. Maher JC, Wangpaichitr M, Savaraj N, Kurtoglu M, Lampidis TJ (2007) Hypoxia-inducible factor-1 confers resistance to the glycolytic inhibitor 2-deoxy-D-glucose. Mol Cancer Ther 6(2):732–741. https://doi.org/10.1158/1535-7163.mct-06-0407
169. Simons AL, Ahmad IM, Mattson DM, Dornfeld KJ, Spitz DR (2007) 2-Deoxy-D-glucose combined with cisplatin enhances cytotoxicity via metabolic oxidative stress in human head and neck cancer cells. Cancer Res 67(7):3364–3370. https://doi.org/10.1158/0008-5472.can-06-3717
170. Floridi A, Paggi MG, D'Atri S, De Martino C, Marcante ML, Silvestrini B, Caputo A (1981) Effect of lonidamine on the energy metabolism of Ehrlich ascites tumor cells. Cancer Res 41(11 Pt 1):4661–4666
171. Cao X, Fang L, Gibbs S, Huang Y, Dai Z, Wen P, Zheng X, Sadee W, Sun D (2007) Glucose uptake inhibitor sensitizes cancer cells to daunorubicin and overcomes drug resistance in hypoxia. Cancer Chemother Pharmacol 59(4):495–505. https://doi.org/10.1007/s00280-006-0291-9
172. Chesney J (2006) 6-phosphofructo-2-kinase/fructose-2,6-bisphosphatase and tumor cell glycolysis. Curr Opin Clin Nutr Metab Care 9(5):535–539. https://doi.org/10.1097/01.mco.0000241661.15514.fb
173. Clem B, Telang S, Clem A, Yalcin A, Meier J, Simmons A, Rasku MA, Arumugam S, Dean WL, Eaton J, Lane A, Trent JO, Chesney J (2008) Small-molecule inhibition of 6-phosphofructo-2-kinase activity suppresses glycolytic flux and tumor growth. Mol Cancer Ther 7(1):110–120. https://doi.org/10.1158/1535-7163.mct-07-0482

174. Wu MC, Arimura GK, Yunis AA (1978) Mechanism of sensitivity of cultured pancreatic carcinoma to asparaginase. Int J Cancer 22(6):728–733. https://doi.org/10.1002/ijc.2910220615
175. Griffiths M, Keast D, Patrick G, Crawford M, Palmer TN (1993) The role of glutamine and glucose analogues in metabolic inhibition of human myeloid leukaemia in vitro. Int J Biochem 25(12):1749–1755
176. Narta UK, Kanwar SS, Azmi W (2007) Pharmacological and clinical evaluation of L-asparaginase in the treatment of leukemia. Crit Rev Oncol 61(3):208–221. https://doi.org/10.1016/j.critrevonc.2006.07.009
177. Enns GM, Berry SA, Berry GT, Rhead WJ, Brusilow SW, Hamosh A (2007) Survival after treatment with phenylacetate and benzoate for urea-cycle disorders. N Engl J Med 356(22):2282–2292. https://doi.org/10.1056/NEJMoa066596
178. Fuchs BC, Bode BP (2005) Amino acid transporters ASCT2 and LAT1 in cancer: partners in crime? Semin Cancer Biol 15(4):254–266. https://doi.org/10.1016/j.semcancer.2005.04.005
179. Esslinger CS, Cybulski KA, Rhoderick JF (2005) Ngamma-aryl glutamine analogues as probes of the ASCT2 neutral amino acid transporter binding site. Bioorg Med Chem 13(4):1111–1118. https://doi.org/10.1016/j.bmc.2004.11.028
180. Nicklin P, Bergman P, Zhang B, Triantafellow E, Wang H, Nyfeler B, Yang H, Hild M, Kung C, Wilson C, Myer VE, MacKeigan JP, Porter JA, Wang YK, Cantley LC, Finan PM, Murphy LO (2009) Bidirectional transport of amino acids regulates mTOR and autophagy. Cell 136(3):521–534. https://doi.org/10.1016/j.cell.2008.11.044
181. Erickson JW, Cerione RA (2010) Glutaminase: a hot spot for regulation of cancer cell metabolism? Oncotarget 1(8):734–740. https://doi.org/10.18632/oncotarget.208
182. Qin JZ, Xin H, Nickoloff BJ (2010) Targeting glutamine metabolism sensitizes melanoma cells to TRAIL-induced death. Biochem Biophys Res Commun 398(1):146–152. https://doi.org/10.1016/j.bbrc.2010.06.057
183. Luo Z, Zang M, Guo W (2010) AMPK as a metabolic tumor suppressor: control of metabolism and cell growth. Future Oncol 6(3):457–470. https://doi.org/10.2217/fon.09.174
184. Buzzai M, Bauer DE, Jones RG, Deberardinis RJ, Hatzivassiliou G, Elstrom RL, Thompson CB (2005) The glucose dependence of Akt-transformed cells can be reversed by pharmacologic activation of fatty acid beta-oxidation. Oncogene 24(26):4165–4173. https://doi.org/10.1038/sj.onc.1208622
185. Carew JS, Nawrocki ST, Kahue CN, Zhang H, Yang C, Chung L, Houghton JA, Huang P, Giles FJ, Cleveland JL (2007) Targeting autophagy augments the anticancer activity of the histone deacetylase inhibitor SAHA to overcome Bcr-Abl-mediated drug resistance. Blood 110(1):313–322. https://doi.org/10.1182/blood-2006-10-050260
186. Nelson EC, Evans CP, Mack PC, Devere-White RW, Lara PN Jr (2007) Inhibition of Akt pathways in the treatment of prostate cancer. Prostate Cancer Prostatic Dis 10(4):331–339. https://doi.org/10.1038/sj.pcan.4500974
187. Kong D, Yamori T (2008) Phosphatidylinositol 3-kinase inhibitors: promising drug candidates for cancer therapy. Cancer Sci 99(9):1734–1740. https://doi.org/10.1111/j.1349-7006.2008.00891.x
188. Guertin DA, Sabatini DM (2009) The pharmacology of mTOR inhibition. Sci Signal 2(67):pe24. https://doi.org/10.1126/scisignal.267pe24
189. Shim H, Dolde C, Lewis BC, Wu CS, Dang G, Jungmann RA, Dalla-Favera R, Dang CV (1997) c-Myc transactivation of LDH-A: implications for tumor metabolism and growth. Proc Natl Acad Sci U S A 94(13):6658–6663. https://doi.org/10.1073/pnas.94.13.6658
190. Hagland H, Nikolaisen J, Hodneland LI, Gjertsen BT, Bruserud O, Tronstad KJ (2007) Targeting mitochondria in the treatment of human cancer: a coordinated attack against cancer cell energy metabolism and signalling. Expert Opin Ther Targets 11(8):1055–1069. https://doi.org/10.1517/14728222.11.8.1055
191. Turton JL, Raab R, Rooney KB (2018) Low-carbohydrate diets for type 1 diabetes mellitus: a systematic review. PLoS One 13(3):e0194987. https://doi.org/10.1371/journal.pone.0194987

192. Buyken AE, Toeller M, Heitkamp G, Irsigler K, Holler C, Santeusanio F, Stehle P, Fuller JH (2000) Carbohydrate sources and glycaemic control in Type 1 diabetes mellitus. EURODIAB IDDM Complications Study Group. Diabet Med 17(5):351–359
193. Cheung NW, Conn JJ, d'Emden MC, Gunton JE, Jenkins AJ, Ross GP, Sinha AK, Andrikopoulos S, Colagiuri S, Twigg SM (2009) Position statement of the Australian Diabetes Society: individualisation of glycated haemoglobin targets for adults with diabetes mellitus. Med J Aust 191(6):339–344
194. Hall KD, Chung ST (2018) Low-carbohydrate diets for the treatment of obesity and type 2 diabetes. Curr Opin Clin Nutr Metab Care 21(4):308–312. https://doi.org/10.1097/mco.0000000000000470
195. Taylor R, Barnes AC (2018) Translating aetiological insight into sustainable management of type 2 diabetes. Diabetologia 61(2):273–283. https://doi.org/10.1007/s00125-017-4504-z
196. Mansoor N, Vinknes KJ, Veierod MB, Retterstol K (2016) Effects of low-carbohydrate diets v. low-fat diets on body weight and cardiovascular risk factors: a meta-analysis of randomised controlled trials. Br J Nutr 115(3):466–479. https://doi.org/10.1017/s0007114515004699
197. Leidy HJ, Clifton PM, Astrup A, Wycherley TP, Westerterp-Plantenga MS, Luscombe-Marsh ND, Woods SC, Mattes RD (2015) The role of protein in weight loss and maintenance. Am J Clin Nutr 101(6):1320s–1329s. https://doi.org/10.3945/ajcn.114.084038
198. Holmes MV, Asselbergs FW, Palmer TM, Drenos F, Lanktree MB, Nelson CP, Dale CE, Padmanabhan S, Finan C, Swerdlow DI, Tragante V, van Iperen EP, Sivapalaratnam S, Shah S, Elbers CC, Shah T, Engmann J, Giambartolomei C, White J, Zabaneh D, Sofat R, McLachlan S, Doevendans PA, Balmforth AJ, Hall AS, North KE, Almoguera B, Hoogeveen RC, Cushman M, Fornage M, Patel SR, Redline S, Siscovick DS, Tsai MY, Karczewski KJ, Hofker MH, Verschuren WM, Bots ML, van der Schouw YT, Melander O, Dominiczak AF, Morris R, Ben-Shlomo Y, Price J, Kumari M, Baumert J, Peters A, Thorand B, Koenig W, Gaunt TR, Humphries SE, Clarke R, Watkins H, Farrall M, Wilson JG, Rich SS, de Bakker PI, Lange LA, Davey Smith G, Reiner AP, Talmud PJ, Kivimaki M, Lawlor DA, Dudbridge F, Samani NJ, Keating BJ, Hingorani AD, Casas JP (2015) Mendelian randomization of blood lipids for coronary heart disease. Eur Heart J 36(9):539–550. https://doi.org/10.1093/eurheartj/eht571
199. Siri-Tarino PW, Chiu S, Bergeron N, Krauss RM (2015) Saturated fats versus polyunsaturated fats versus carbohydrates for cardiovascular disease prevention and treatment. Annu Rev Nutr 35:517–543. https://doi.org/10.1146/annurev-nutr-071714-034449
200. Lennerz BS, Barton A, Bernstein RK, Dikeman RD, Diulus C, Hallberg S, Rhodes ET, Ebbeling CB, Westman EC, Yancy WS (2018) Management of type 1 diabetes with a very low–carbohydrate diet. Pediatrics 141(6):e20173349
201. Ma S, Suzuki K (2019) Keto-adaptation and endurance exercise capacity, fatigue recovery, and exercise-induced muscle and organ damage prevention: a narrative review. Sports 7(2):40
202. Gasior M, French A, Joy MT, Tang RS, Hartman AL, Rogawski MA (2007) The anticonvulsant activity of acetone, the major ketone body in the ketogenic diet, is not dependent on its metabolites acetol, 1,2-propanediol, methylglyoxal, or pyruvic acid. Epilepsia 48(4):793–800
203. McNally MA, Hartman AL (2012) Ketone bodies in epilepsy. J Neurochem 121(1):28–35
204. Roberts MN, Wallace MA, Tomilov AA, Zhou Z, Marcotte GR, Tran D, Perez G, Gutierrez-Casado E, Koike S, Knotts TA (2017) A ketogenic diet extends longevity and healthspan in adult mice. Cell Metab 26(3):539–546
205. Chang C-K, Borer K, Lin P-J (2017) Low-carbohydrate-high-fat diet: can it help exercise performance? J Hum Kinet 56(1):81–92
206. Weber DD, Aminazdeh-Gohari S, Kofler B (2018) Ketogenic diet in cancer therapy. Aging 10(2):164
207. Morscher RJ, Aminzadeh-Gohari S, Feichtinger RG, Mayr JA, Lang R, Neureiter D, Sperl W, Kofler B (2015) Inhibition of neuroblastoma tumor growth by ketogenic diet and/or calorie restriction in a CD1-Nu mouse model. PLoS One 10(6):e0129802

208. Hrynevich SV, Waseem TV, Hébert A, Pellerin L, Fedorovich SV (2016) β-Hydroxybutyrate supports synaptic vesicle cycling but reduces endocytosis and exocytosis in rat brain synaptosomes. Neurochem Int 93:73–81
209. Gano LB, Patel M, Rho JM (2014) Ketogenic diets, mitochondria, and neurological diseases. J Lipid Res 55(11):2211–2228
210. Ghosh S, Castillo E, Frias ES, Swanson RA (2018) Bioenergetic regulation of microglia. Glia 66(6):1200–1212
211. Yang X, Cheng B (2010) Neuroprotective and anti-inflammatory activities of ketogenic diet on MPTP-induced neurotoxicity. J Mol Neurosci 42(2):145–153
212. Stephens KE, Miaskowski CA, Levine JD, Pullinger CR, Aouizerat BE (2013) Epigenetic regulation and measurement of epigenetic changes. Biol Res Nurs 15(4):373–381
213. Shimazu T, Hirschey MD, Newman J, He W, Shirakawa K, Le Moan N, Grueter CA, Lim H, Saunders LR, Stevens RD (2013) Suppression of oxidative stress by β-hydroxybutyrate, an endogenous histone deacetylase inhibitor. Science 339(6116):211–214
214. Olson CA, Vuong HE, Yano JM, Liang QY, Nusbaum DJ, Hsiao EY (2018) The gut microbiota mediates the anti-seizure effects of the ketogenic diet. Cell 173(7):1728–1741
215. Pekun TG, Lemeshchenko VV, Lyskova TI, Waseem TV, Fedorovich SV (2013) Influence of intra-and extracellular acidification on free radical formation and mitochondria membrane potential in rat brain synaptosomes. J Mol Neurosci 49(1):211–222

Unravelling the Genomic Targets of Small Molecules and Application of CRISPR-Cas 9 System for Genomic Editing in Cancer with Respective Clinical Applications

3

Muhammad Usama Tariq

3.1 Targeting of Cancer

Cancer develops as a consequence of perturbation of cell's integral pathways mainly involved in growth, proliferation, differentiation. etc. Deregulation of these pathways results in the development of hallmarks such as limitless replicative potential, insensitivity to growth signals, evading apoptosis, sustained angiogenesis, self-sufficiency in growth signals, tissue invasion, and metastasis [1]. Having deregulated at multiple levels and affecting various processes, cancer becomes a multifaceted disease. Therefore, its treatment is done accordingly.

To date, scientists are putting their efforts to develop a cure which can treat multiple cancers; however, given its nature, such treatment is not possible yet. In the past, cancer treatment has primarily been focused by the use of chemotherapy in which a chemical agent nonselectively inhibits multiple targets in a cell. With the passage of time, efforts were invested to develop more targeted strategies. Although this chapter is mainly focused on targeted inhibition at nucleic acid level, we need to know about different treatments required for curing cancers. Therefore, we will start with the most basic treatments.

M. U. Tariq (✉)
College of Health and Life Sciences, Hamad Bin Khalifa University, Education city (Qatar foundation), Doha, Al Rayyan, Qatar
e-mail: 15140020@lums.edu.pk

N. Masood, S. Shakil Malik (eds.), *'Essentials of Cancer Genomic, Computational Approaches and Precision Medicine*,
https://doi.org/10.1007/978-981-15-1067-0_3

3.2 Types of Treatments

3.2.1 Surgery

For the treatment of early stage or locally resident tumors, this method is successful because surgery utilizes the physical removal of tumor by incision of the skin and organs with the help of instruments. Theoretically, surgery cures the cancer successfully. However, this is not always the case since tumors have a capability to metastasize and spread to other regions of the body. For that, physicians cannot always tear off every organ or region of the body to remove tumors [2]. Surgery also has another limitation, for instance, if after surgery, a single cancer cell is left in the body, it has a capability to give rise to a whole tumor which we call tumor relapse. Therefore, to make surgery successful, it is usually done before and after administering other forms of treatments, e.g., chemotherapy, etc.

3.2.2 Radiation Therapy

Another treatment strategy is based on using ionizing radiations. Mechanistically, these radiations either target DNA or generate high reactivity free radicals in cancer cells which interfere with the DNA. This form of treatment is effective because the intensity of radiations can be adjusted according to the stage and location of the tumor [3]. It has been reported that cancer cells do not have a capacity to treat the faults introduced by ionizing radiation, whereas normal cells of the body, which are continuously being replaced, can avoid the damage. Despite such benefits, radiation therapy has certain drawbacks. For instance, treating cancers of later stages, a very high-intensity radiation is required, such intensity can damage non-specific locations in the body, which ultimately leads to severe side effects [3]. To kill metastasized cancers, repeated exposure to high intensity radiations is necessary, which is very harmful for the body. Moreover, radiation therapy cannot be used for treating hematologic malignancies.

3.2.3 Chemotherapy

The use of cytotoxic drugs which can destroy cancer cells is referred to as chemotherapy. In this, a drug which has multiple targets is used to cause cytotoxicity in the cells. The above mentioned strategy is effective in treating resident cancers; however, chemotherapy is effective in killing metastasized tumors because the drug spreads throughout the body. Mechanistically, chemotherapeutic drugs either have a large number of targeted proteins to inhibit or they damage DNA at excessive sites which results in killing cancer [4]. Since this treatment can spread throughout the body, therefore, along with killing cancer, it has an equal probability to kill normal cells of the body. A high dosage of chemotherapeutic drug can cause excessive toxicity in the body, which, resultantly, can lead to death of an individual. Chemotherapeutic drugs include DNA-damaging agents, multiprotein-targeting inhibitors, alkylating agents, antimetabolites, corticosteroids, etc. [4].

3.2.4 Targeted Therapy

Targeted therapy was made available some two decades ago when scientists started focusing on selectively killing cancer cells, leaving the normal cells unaffected. In this kind, the drug acts by targeting the deregulated pathway which eventually kills the cancer cell only. Since that pathway is responsible for cancer formation, therefore, its selective inhibition is beneficial for normal cells of the body [5]. Targeted drugs can either be developed through computational modelling or by screening and identifying natural compounds capable of killing cancer. As the name suggests, it does not cause excessive toxicity in the body as in the case of chemotherapy. Identification of the processes involved in cancer formation is primary to the success of this form of therapy. It can be done at levels such as inhibiting enzyme activity, manipulating specific genes or regulatory sequences, inhibiting specific pathways, manipulating the uptake of different macromolecules in the cells, etc. [6].

Despite its benefits in overcoming excessive toxicity in the body, targeted inhibition still comes with a limitation such as cancer relapse. For instance, for the treatment of FLT3 receptor tyrosine kinase mutated acute myeloid leukemia, a drug named tandutinib also known as MLN-518 was developed. Initially MLN-518 showed very potent inhibition; however, after constant exposure, AML started getting resistant leaving the drug ineffective because the cancer developed a gatekeeping mutation in FLT3 which did not let MLN-518 bind to it [7]. Recently, with the advent of next-generation sequencing technologies, selective nucleic acid-based inhibition has grabbed the attention of cancer research community because firstly, it overcomes the limitations found in the case of chemotherapy and targeted inhibition and, secondly, it can be utilized under the idea of personalized medicine.

This chapter is mainly focused on discussing the potential of nucleic acid targeting by identifying the targeted regions, techniques required for identification, and the role of CRISPR technology as an example of emerging treatments against cancer. However, to better understand this, we need to understand the levels at which targeted inhibition occurs.

3.3 Levels of Cancer Targeting for Targeted Therapy

Sugar uptake in the cells, pathway inhibition or overexpression, deregulation of genes required for controlling growth of cancer cells, posttranslational modifications, and many others are the processes which are responsible for the growth and maintenance of cancer cells. Each process, if targeted, has its importance in terms of killing cancer. Therefore, we will look deep into the levels of targeting and eventually focus on DNA targeting the most.

3.3.1 Carbohydrate Targeting

Metabolism at cellular level starts with the process of glycolysis which produces energy in the form of adenosine triphosphates (ATP). During physiological conditions, cells respire through aerobic mechanisms in which glycolysis is extended to mitochondrial oxidative phosphorylation producing excess energy. However, in cancerous conditions, metabolic pathways are adjusted which resultantly produce pyruvate converted to lactate after glycolysis through Warburg effect. Such process is not efficient in producing energy as compared to oxidative phosphorylation; however, it is essential in producing metabolites required by cancers to carry out different functions [8]. A question arises, if Warburg effect is not efficient in producing energy, how does cancer fulfill its energy requirements? Cancer adjusts its metabolic requirements and depends on the increased uptake of glucose which in turn produces required energy through the Warburg effect. Such process makes glucose an attractive therapeutic target for the treatment of cancer [8].

Since glucose is being used by every cell of the body, therefore, glucose inhibition has to be specific in tumor microenvironment for killing cancer. Recently, nanoelectrical circuits were developed; these circuits are directed toward tumor microenvironment where they chelate available glucose and kill cancer cells through starvation. On the other hand, glucose-mimicking analogs are also being used to inhibit the uptake of glucose in cancer cells. These analogs have structural similarities with glucose due to which a competition is created, and resultantly, glycolysis and other metabolic activities are halted [9]. Accumulating evidence suggests that certain glucose-mimicking analogs have also been developed which are taken up by the cells; however, they do not perform any function which results in cell death.

3.3.2 Protein Targeting

Protein targeting is a major focus of researchers around the world. Although it is the DNA which codes for proteins and primarily is mutated in cancer, proteins can additionally be modified during posttranslational modifications such as phosphorylation and contribute to cancer formation. The process of drug development is paved by the identification of protein therapeutic targets. In general, certain proteins are associated with a specific type of cancer. For instance, human epidermal growth factor receptor 2 (HER2) is deregulated in 20–25% of breast cancers, epidermal growth factor receptor in colorectal cancer, while 50% of melanoma have mutated BRAF.

Protein drug targeting has shown success for the treatment of cancer because proteins have favorable binding pockets. Such pockets are beneficial for a drug to bind and inhibit the function. A number of different inhibitors have been developed for targeting proteins. On top of the list are the inhibitors against G protein-coupled receptors (GPCR) which are mutated in a variety of cancers. Second to the list is kinase-targeting inhibitors [10]. Our genome codes for 478 kinases approximately, each performing a specific function. These kinases add a gamma phosphate group of ATP to the proteins which resultantly turn on or off them. In the case of receptor tyrosine kinases which are attached to the cell surface, autophosphorylation of receptor occurs upon ligand binding. However, in cytosol, different kinases have different substrates to phosphorylate. To summarize, a kinase domain is required to add the gamma phosphate group of ATP either on same or on a different protein which eventually turn on or off the cascade in cancer as per requirement. The kinase-targeting inhibitors specifically kill cancers by inhibiting the phosphorylation of kinases required for cancer progression [10].

To date, a large variety of such inhibitors have been approved by FDA to be used in the clinic as given in Table 3.1. The mechanisms of kinase inhibition can be categorized into different types and are given below [10]:

Type 1: Binds to the ATP-binding pocket of kinases and competes for substrate in active conformation of protein.

Type 2: Binds to inactive enzyme conformation.

Type 3: Binds to the enzyme next to ATP-binding pocket. In this way, ATP and inhibitor both bind to the enzyme simultaneously.

Type 4: Undergoes a reversible interaction outside ATP-binding pocket.

Type 5: Binds covalently to the protein kinase target.

Despite the success, protein targeting has many limitations. For instance, certain types of proteins such as transcription factors like Myc do not have a favorable binding pocket for a drug to bind. This in turn poses great challenges as these transcription factors are frequently deregulated in multiple cancers [23]. Different approaches such as targeting upstream regulatory proteins, inhibiting the crosstalk etc., have been utilized to inhibit undruggable proteins. However, this approach can disturb other pathways of the cell. Another drawback for protein targeting is the development of resistance as mentioned in protein targeting section of this chapter. To

Table 3.1 List FDA-approved kinase inhibitors and their drug targets

Drug targets	Drugs
ALK	Crizotinib, ceritinib, alectinib, brigatinib [11]
BCR–Abl	Bosutinib, dasatinib, imatinib, nilotinib, ponatinib [12]
B-Raf	Vemurafenib, dabrafenib [13]
BTK	Ibrutinib [14]
CDK family	Palbociclib, ribociclib [15]
c-Met	Crizotinib, cabozantinib [16]
EGFR family	Gefitinib, erlotinib, lapatinib, vandetanib, afatinib, osimertinib [17]
JAK family	Ruxolitinib, tofacitinib [18]
MEK1/2	Trametinib [19]
PDGFR α/β	Axitinib, gefitinib, imatinib, lenvatinib, nintedanib, pazopanib, regorafenib, sorafenib, sunitinib [20]
RET	Vandetanib [21]
Src family	Bosutinib, dasatinib, ponatinib, vandetanib [22]

overcome such limitations, nucleic acid targeting-based treatments hold greater promise.

3.3.3 Nucleic Acid Targeting

Nucleic acids are constantly exposed to genotoxic insults. The mutations introduced by a certain genotoxic agent are most frequently cleared by the DNA damage repair pathways or immune clearance; however, sometimes an escape from available defenses resultantly forms cancer. For decades, DNA targeting by the use of chemotherapeutic agents has been a prime focus for the treatment of cancers. Such strategy nonselectively targets multiple sites on DNA which resultantly cause cytotoxicity in cancer as well as normal cells. Due to excessive DNA damage, the undesired mutations in normal cells can cause side effects and eventually the death of an individual [4].

Looking at the drawbacks of treating cancers by nonselectively damaging the DNA, targeted therapy for targeting deregulated proteins was introduced. Yet, such therapy has its own limitations as described above. However, with the advent of advanced molecular techniques and high-throughput sequencing technologies, the information stored in DNA became available. Such information was analyzed by creating its relevance with cancer progression, and resultantly, genome targeting showed great promise. The information helps us design new drugs and strategies to manipulate or inhibit the genome.

Despite the progress in designing chemically designed inhibitors for specific gene targeting, the success is very limited because such process may have multiple off-target genes. The reason can be the structure of the inhibitor which may find multiple attachment sites on genome and affect the normal cells or pathways required for sustenance [24]. For this, two strategies are important, one, targeting nucleic acids by nucleic acid-based therapeutic strategies and second, by identifying genomic regions which can help us design specific gene targeting drugs.

3.4 Molecular Happenings While Targeting Genes for Cancer Treatment

For killing cancer without effecting normal cells, cancer treatments have to have selective gene delivery methods with highly specific gene expression, specific gene product activity, and, possibly, specific drug activation. For this, efficient delivery systems are available and described later in the chapter. To understand the mechanisms of gene therapy, understanding the molecular basis of cancer is very important. At molecular level, cancer develops as a result of deregulation of telomere maintenance, tumor suppressors, oncogenes, apoptosis, and DNA damage repair pathways [25]. Each process is regulated by the products of certain genes. Switching on and off of these genes in a way that contributes to cancer formation is very important. Under strict immune surveillance, the mutations in these genes are most often cleared; however, an orderly selection of mutations in genes involved in each mentioned process leads to cancer formation [25].

Since the basis of cancer deregulation is genome because mutations are being introduced there, hence, targeting identified genes is the best possible option. For this, specific genes involved in each mentioned process are therapeutically targeted using approaches described below. Alternatively, chromatin- and DNA-binding proteins are also important targets for cancer therapy owing to their role in cancer progression. Several drugs which target DNA-binding proteins including histones have been designed; however, the exact mechanism of their action still needs to be elucidated [24].

A number of factors should be considered while introducing a specific type of therapeutic agent in the cells. If the therapy is expression-based, in other words, a therapy in which DNA sequences are introduced into the cells which resultantly transcribe, then the expression of the sequence being introduced is supposed to be regulated very tightly; otherwise, it can cause harms. Using promoters to control the expression of genes is the best strategy to restrict the effect of the therapy toward tumors only [26].

A number of drug and nucleic acid-based treatments are currently being developed for targeting nucleic acids in cancer cells. Since the time required to develop and commercialize them is too long, therefore it would take some time for nucleic acid-targeting therapeutic strategies to get access to the clinic as they are being tested at different levels. However, we will look into their progress and the mechanisms through which they affect the growth of cancer cells specifically.

3.4.1 RNAi

Under physiological conditions, double-stranded RNA plays a very crucial role in regulating the genes for maintaining cellular function, posttranscriptionally. This RNA does so by the process of RNA interference (RNAi). Mechanistically, RNAi controls the expression of targeted genes by inhibiting posttranscriptional gene regulation. Certain genes are present in cells which code for RNAi-related transcripts. Such genes do not code for any protein or transcribe antisense strand of RNA. When a messenger RNA of a targeted gene to be silenced is present, available antisense strand binds to it and allows inhibition [20].

Since there is an altered expression of multiple genes in cancer cells, RNAi can be used to inhibit the targeted genes. Following are two different types of RNA, which can be used for targeting genes for inhibition, microRNA (miRNA) and small interfering RNA (siRNA). siRNA is a 21–22 nucleotides long RNA. It is produced by the cleavage of 200–500 nucleotide long double stranded RNA molecule by Dicer protein. siRNA interacts with RISC complex and controls gene silencing, viral defense, and transposon control. On the other hand miRNA, a 22 nucleotide long RNA molecule, is produced by the cleavage of imperfect RNA hairpins encoded in long primary transcripts by Dicer and Drosha. A number of

RNAi-mediated cures are currently being developed and tested in clinical trials owing to their affordability and precision as shown in Table 3.2 [20].

3.4.2 Chromatin and DNA Targeting

Chromatin is an important regulator of gene expression in cancers which comes under the umbrella of epigenetic regulation. Most cancers turn on or off the expression of required genes by epigenetic regulation through which they can be used for cancer progression. Therefore, targeting chromatin-bound proteins, e.g., histones or the proteins which are regulating them such as histone transferases, etc., for the treatment of cancer is a favorable approach. Despite the importance of these proteins, the required genomic information to use them for selective gene targeting is very limited due to which they affect additional regions in the genome. For instance, the protein might also be bound with genes which are not deregulated; therefore, its targeting will pose additional threats. Hence, such targeting poses a great challenge of target selectivity [24].

Despite the challenges, a number of such drugs are being tested in clinical trials. However, their success is very limited. Advanced drugs are required which can selectively target a specific chromatin-related protein or a gene. Using the next-generation molecular techniques, identification of the genomic targets where a specific drug binds on DNA will reveal the binding mechanisms of available drugs which eventually will help us design drugs having more specificity and efficacy [24].

3.4.3 Nucleic Acid-Based Therapeutic Strategy for Inhibition of DNA-Binding Proteins

The potential of DNA in killing cancer is not restricted to genome targeting only, but DNA can also inhibit proteins directly. For instance, a certain transcription factor such as Myc which does not have any favorable binding pocket for a chemical

Table 3.2 RNAi-mediated cancer treatments in clinical trials

Drug	Target	Vehicle	Disease	Phase
CALAA-01	RRM2	Cyclodextrin nanoparticle, TF, and PEG	Solid tumors	[27]
Atu027	PKN3	siRNA-lipoplex	Advanced solid cancer	I [28]
iPsiRNA	LMP2, LMP7, MECL1	Transfection	Metastatic melanoma	I [20]
EZN-2968	HIF-1, survivin	Nacked	Advanced solid tumor or lymphoma	I [29]
FANG vaccine	Furin and GM-CSF	Electroporation	Solid tumors	I [30]

drug to bind can be inhibited through DNA-mediated inhibition in which DNA mimetics are used. Instead of chemically designed mimetics, DNA-based sequences can also be used. Such mimetics are similar to the binding site of a specific DNA-binding protein. When this agent is present in the cell, it does not let the DNA-binding protein attach to its targeted sequence through competition [31]. Resultantly, the idle protein is inhibited. Accumulating evidence suggests that the inhibition of topoisomerase through the use of mimetics resulted in faulty replication during S-phase of the cell cycle [32].

For the success of this strategy, extensive bioinformatics analysis in identifying the binding site of a certain protein to develop a consensus sequence is required. For this, delivery of the designed construct is the rate-limiting step. Following are different delivery mechanisms which can be used for the introduction of a construct or therapeutic agent into the cells:

3.5 Mechanisms to Deliver Therapeutic Agent in Cancer Cells

3.5.1 Viral-Mediated Gene Therapy

Cancer occurs as a consequence of activation of oncogenes and repression of tumor suppressors. Specific genes are associated with specific cancers. Activation and repression occur at genomic level which in turn control the pathways required for excessive proliferation and cancer progression. Identification of such genes can help us gain insights to the cancer treatment. The genes like tumor suppressors, which are not beneficial for cancer, can be integrated in the genome at specific sites using viral vectors, and they can selectively kill cancer cells. Their use is mainly encouraged because of the precision for integration at desired region in the genome. For this, viral genome is manipulated in a way that its virulence-related genes are deleted and it is only left with the capability to transfer the gene of interest [33]. Approximately 70% of gene transfer clinical trials include the transfer using viral vectors. Although adenovirus and retrovirus are most commonly used, other viruses are also being tested in humans. Every virus has a different advantage. For instance, retroviruses have great capacity to infect dividing cells, lentiviruses have increased capacity to infect nondividing cells, adenoviruses are safe for transient gene transfer because they do not integrate their genome into the host cells, and poxviruses have inverted terminal repeats in the terminal regions of their genome which help them stably integrate the gene of interest [33].

3.5.2 Non-viral-Mediated Gene Therapy

A lot of concerns lie with viral-mediated gene therapy. On top is the ability of viruses to cause harm. Although the sequences which can cause harm are deleted from the viral genome before application, a high probability exists for it to become virulent. To overcome such problem, non-viral-mediated gene therapy is very helpful. Moreover, they are safe and have easy preparation advantages. The examples are expression and delivery vectors. These vectors are important for introduction of the construct into the cells [33]. For this, multiple options are available. Generally these options are categorized as physical and chemical approaches. Physical approaches involve particle bombardment, gene gun, electroporation, hydrodynamics, ultrasonics, etc., whereas chemical approaches include membrane fusion, receptor-mediated endocytosis, cationic lipids, cationic polymers, lipofectamine-mediated endocytosis, etc.

3.5.3 Nanotechnology-Based Gene Therapy

Another important non-viral-mediated gene transfer approach is by the use of nanotechnology-based vectors. They are important in delivering specific drugs and nucleic acid-based inhibitors to the cancer specifically. Such approach does not spread the drug to various parts of the body which resultantly reduces the toxicity [34]. For instance, a PI3 kinase-targeting inhibitor called wortmannin was developed and aborted in phase II clinical trials due to high toxicity in the body. However, subsequent studies by coating wortmannin with silver nanoparticles resulted in increased efficiency of the drug with minimum toxicity and side effects [35].

Along with chemically developed inhibitors, nanoparticle-mediated delivery is also being used to deliver DNA-based therapeutic sequences for gene therapy. The most crucial factor in using nanoparticle-based delivery systems is formulation of the nanoparticle because it reaches to the target location through the bloodstream. Therefore, the formulation should be designed keeping the effects in mind. Different nanoparticle-mediated delivery systems have been developed and shown promise during preclinical and clinical trials. For example, liposome, lipoplexes, cyclodextrin, chitosan, PLGA, calcium phosphate, carbon nanotubes, gold, quantum dots, silicon-based nanoparticles, etc. have proven to be successful in different clinical trial applications [34].

3.6 Identification of Genomic Targets

As mentioned above that small-molecule drugs nonselectively target cancer-causing genes and DNA-bound proteins; however, their importance in targeting cancer without causing major drawbacks, cannot be denied. The carried limitation by such approach can be tackled by identifying genome sequences where a specific drug binds. Doing so will reveal the information which in turn can be used to design drugs that can specifically target the cancer-causing genes. The importance of target identification at genomic level is also integral because sometimes certain noncoding genes are involved in cancer formation. Without analyzing the genomic data, such targets cannot be identified. Hence, the more we have the genomic information, the better we can develop strategies for cancer cure. With the advent of next-generation sequencing and advanced microarray technologies, the genomic information is more readily available, and the off-target effects can easily be controlled.

Moreover, identification and validation of genomic data are also very important for targeting histones and other DNA-binding proteins. Different DNA sequences have different binding efficiencies toward similar histones based on the presence of specific nucleotide sequences. When a specific gene is targeted by a certain histone-targeting drug, the drug may affect multiple genes where the same histone is bound. For this reason, availability of genomic data holds integral importance because it can be used to manipulate only the genes which are involved in cancer formation. To generate required genetic information, different strategies are used; some of these are described as follows:

3.6.1 Chem-Seq

Several genotoxic drugs have been used for decades to treat cancers; the exact mechanisms by which they operate are not fully understood. It is established that these compounds interfere with the processes of transcription and replication, thereby promoting genomic instability and cell death. As yet no genome-wide map of the binding of these drugs is available [24]. However, through Chem-seq, we can identify targets in the genome. Revealing such information can help us develop an understanding of the mechanism of their action. This method is based on chemical affinity capture and massively parallel DNA sequencing that allows investigators to identify genomic sites where small chemical molecules interact with their targets on DNA [24]. For instance, bromodomain family of proteins are deregulated in multiple myeloma and found to be associated with transcriptionally active genes. A bromodomain inhibitor called JQ1, when exposed to cells and checked for targets, showed binding with similar genes as reported for BRD family of proteins. This gave the confirmation that targeting BRD family of proteins with JQ1 can inhibit the function of BRD-bound genes which eventually introduces disturbance in the genome [36]. Through such information, more specific inhibitors targeting a single type of BRD protein can be designed.

Chem-seq can also be used for different classes of drugs. For instance, binding of AT7519, an inhibitor of CDK9 which rests at the promoter regions of the genes and is associated with transcription apparatus, was investigated. AT7519's inhibition affects the elongation process of transcription, thereby leading to faulty mRNA production. A biotinylated version of AT7519 was used in multiple myeloma cells for the identification of genomic targets. The results showed that AT7519 had similar genome coverage as of CDK9. However, a number of other target sequences were also identified which shows that other than CDK9, AT7519 may also have additional targets for inhibition [36].

Similarly, Chem-seq can also be extended to identify the genome targets of drugs which directly bind to the DNA. For instance, the targets of psoralen, a mutagen which intercalates in the DNA, were identified through Chem-seq. Recently, it has been established that psoralen intercalates to the transcriptionally active genes. Genome-wide association studies of psoralen through Chem-seq not only confirmed this finding but also showed that psoralen binds to transcription start sites of transcriptionally active genes [36].

Along with psoralen, Chem-seq can be used to identify the genomic targets of a vast range of intercalating agents such as ethidium bromide, proflavine, doxorubicin, daunorubicin, dactinomycin, etc. All we need is a biotinylated form of the chemical agent which after introduction into the cells can be used to identify the drug targets. Moreover, DNA-damaging and DNA-modifying agents such as carboplatin, cisplatin, oxaliplatin, cyclophosphamide, dacarbazine, carmustine, etc. can also be used. To date, there exists a reluctance in using these compounds for cancer treatment due to their off-target effects; however, identifying their genomic targets with the help of techniques like Chem-seq can help redesign them with altered, more efficient, and specific functions.

Mechanistically, a compound or a ligand of interest whose genomic targets are to be identified has to be biotinylated with certain agent such as polyethylene glycol spacer with appended biotin feature. This conjugate is introduced into the cells and allowed for binding with specific DNA-binding proteins/genes/DNA sequences. Resultantly, the whole genome is isolated and fragmented, and biotinylated compound-bound DNA fragments are separated. The separated DNA fragments are then sequenced to generate data that is aligned on the genome which consequently tells the genomic targets of the compound under study [36].

3.6.2 ChIP-Seq

ChIP-seq is also known as *chromatin immunoprecipitation* following high-throughput sequencing. The technique is used to identify the genome-wide localization of known proteins. The technique comes with diverse applications. For instance, in cancers, it can be used to identify the genetic sequences bound with the protein of interest. Although, the information contained in polypeptide sequence of therapeutically important proteins is important for their targeting; yet, the information about the genomic regions where these therapeutically important proteins bind would give us better insights about their roles in cancer formation [24].

In combination with Chem-seq, ChIP-seq gives reliable information to identify the genomic targets of chemical drugs. For this, ChIP-seq can be used to identify the genome-wide localization of proteins. The sequence information of genes deciphered through ChIP-seq can be used to compare the sequence information generated after studying the genome-wide localization of drug through Chem-seq [24]. For instance, suppose that apart from knowing that BRD is a DNA-bound protein, we do not have any information about it. For this, ChIP-seq can play a vital role to decipher its genome localization. It can tell the specific regions where BRD binds.

After having the information related to sequences bound with BRD in genome, next we want to know the genome-wide localization of JQ1 (BRD inhibitor). For this, we can use Chem-seq which will give information of JQ1's genome coverage. Since JQ1 is a BRD-specific inhibitor, therefore comparing ChIP-seq and Chem-seq data will confirm the genomic targets of small-molecule inhibitors [24].

Mechanistically, ChIP-seq has a minor difference with Chem-seq; however, this minor difference accounts for the different applications of both techniques. In Chem-seq, the biotinylated chemical agent, whereas in ChIP-seq, antibodies specific against the protein of interest are used. In ChIP-seq, the antibody is allowed to incubate for binding with the targets in cells. After incubation time, the antibodies bound with targeted proteins are separated from the cells. The targeted proteins are bound with the DNA sequences which are separated for sequencing which eventually gives the genomic targets of proteins under study [24].

3.7 CRISPR/Cas9 Technology

Clustered regularly interspaced short palindromic repeats (CRISPR) is the most powerful genome editing tool of this century and has revolutionized the idea of treating diseases. It has shown unprecedented potential in treating diseases without limitations and paved the path of drug discovery. Comparing CRISPR with earlier genome editing technologies such as zinc-finger nucleases (ZFNs) and transcription activator-like effector nucleases (TALENs), increased efficacy, affordability, and ease of use can be seen. CRISPR was discovered as an adaptive immune response in bacteria in response to invading viruses [37]. The most commonly used system for gene editing is the type II CRISPR/Cas system, which consists of three components: an endonuclease (Cas9), a CRISPR RNA (crRNA), and a transactivating crRNA (tracrRNA). The crRNA and tracrRNA molecules form a duplex structure called the guide RNA (gRNA) that can be replaced by a synthetic fused chimeric single gRNA (sgRNA), which simplifies the use of CRISPR/Cas9 in genome engineering. The sgRNA contains a unique 20 base-pair (bp) sequence that is designed to be complementary to the target DNA site, and this must be followed by a short DNA sequence termed the "protospacer-adjacent motif" (PAM), which is essential for compatibility with the Cas9 protein used [37].

CRISPR facilitates genome editing by allowing efficient cleavage of a desired DNA segment in the genome. The unique quality of this technique lies in its multiplexibility through which a DNA segment of interest in the genome can be manipulated. For this, availability/ways to synthesize different sgRNAs are a prerequisite. Another advantage with this technique is its flexibility. It cannot only excise or delete the DNA sequence of interest but can also do more improved functions such as gene editing, addition, knockdown, suppression, etc.

3.8 Role in Cancer

3.8.1 For Treatments

It's been decades that efforts are being invested to develop drugs and find ways to treat cancer. However, being an evolving disease, which even develops resistance against the treatments being used, cancer poses great challenges. Therefore, the introduction of CRISPR technology can help reduce the burden of cancer owing to its efficiency and promise in dealing with genome-based applications [38]. It can do so by regulating (inhibiting or activation) the altered gene expression thereby inhibiting the deregulated pathways. CRISPR-mediated cancer application can also be done through epigenetic modification in which the Cas protein, which is recruited to the DNA, can be modified by being tethered with histones and DNA-modifying enzymes. Moreover, genome-based editing through CRISPR can also be done to avoid the production of cancer markers which require extensive cancer-relevant genomic data [38].

Oncolytic viruses are important to lyse cancer cells or generate immune responses in the cells which eventually leads to cell death. The latter is also important to produce tumor antigens necessary for directing immune cells toward cancer. Through CRISPR-mediated genome editing, viruses can be engineered to allow enhanced immune responses in cancer cells. A prime example of such virus is herpes simplex virus type 1 variants with strong lytic properties, engineered by deletion of the ICP34.5 neurovirulence and ICP6 (UL39) (ribonucleotide reductase) genes. Another example of immune-based CRISPR therapies for cancer is the generation of chimeric antigen receptor (CAR) T cells. These cells are manipulated to target tumors by expressing tumor-targeting receptor [37].

3.8.2 For Research Purpose

Identification of therapeutic targets has always remained the backbone of cancer research because availability of such information is a prerequisite to the development of novel therapeutic strategies for the treatment of cancer. Such identification has been done using genetic screens by introducing specific mutations in the genome. Subsequently, novel genetic mechanisms involved in the progression of cancer are discovered. However, this process has limited success because it usually produces heterozygous mutants carrying unknown mutations. Yet, this limitation can be avoided using targeted RNAi. Interestingly, high-throughput RNAi libraries give reliable information about the genes and the pathways; however, the efficiency of knockdown is compromised, and off-target effects occur a lot. To cater to this situation, CRISPR-mediated libraries allow complete inactivation, high reproducibility, and targeting whole genome [37].

There are mainly three different types of CRISPR-based libraries:

(i) CRISPR knockout: gene knockout library based on loss of function, used for the identification of new mechanisms including drug resistance and cell survival mechanisms
(ii) CRISPRa: gene activation library, used to screen a gain of function
(iii) CRISPRi: gene inhibition library based on loss of function, used to screen for loss of function

CRISPR can be used to identify the genes involved in the development of drug resistance. This can be done by exposing drug-resistant cells to CRISPR-based genome libraries. Each cell will be exposed to a single but different gRNA from CRISPR library as compared to the other cell. Specific resistant cells would become sensitive to drug after getting exposed to the targeted gRNA from the library. The identified genes can then be used to develop therapeutic strategies to overcome the resistance. In a study for the identification of mechanisms involved in drug resistance, a CRISPR library identified that HPRT1 gene knockout results in overcoming resistance to 6-thioguanine. In other words, CRISPR library identified that HPRT1 gene is responsible for generating resistant cells to the said drug [37].

3.9 Mechanism of CRISPR Technology

CRISPR-mediated genome editing has a broad range of treatment applications which enables it to tackle the dynamicity in cancers. Owing to the great promise, different CRISPR-related treatments are currently being tested in humans for the technique to approach the clinic. These clinical trials are discussed at the end of this chapter. The exact mechanisms through which the technique is being applied in different cancers are important for understanding and described below.

The pioneering study on the application of CRISPR for cancer treatment was focused on replacing cancer-causing genes TMEM135-CCDC67 and MAN2A1-FER with cell death-promoting gene in prostate and liver cancers, respectively. The deregulation of said genes in cancer results in the formation of fusion gene which is important for tumor progression. The study was focused on delivering the gene editing tools in cancer cells using viral-mediated delivery method. Two different viruses were used, the first had CRISPR/Cas9 tool for allowing the break points in the fusion gene, while the second virus introduced DNA sequences in the created break points to hinder the functioning of fusion gene. The introduced manipulations resulted in suicide in the cells [39].

Another study for using CRISPR for the treatment of cancer employed the engineering of immune cells to trigger the immune system. This was achieved by expressing chimeric antigen receptor (CAR) on the surface of T cells. CARs are highly specific against tumor antigens. When expressed on the surface of T cells, they promote efficient killing of specific cancer cells. Under pathological conditions, CARs are either repressed or tumor cell surface antigens escape recognition by them. However, manipulating CARs with CRISPR can make T cells efficient for recognition and killing cancer. Patients with B-cell malignancies having CD19, CD20, CD22, and CD30 antigenic receptors shown promising results during clinical trials. In fact, the most efficient effect was seen in patients with B-cell-mediated acute lymphoblastic leukemia in which CD19 antigen-specific CART cells were used. The CRISPR system was used to introduce CD19 target CAR in T cells which resultantly showed very potent effects in treating patients. A relapse was observed in some patients. This relapse was the result of loss of tumor antigen on the surface of cancer cells. However, this limitation can be dealt with by using different types of CART cells, simultaneously targeting multiple tumor-specific antigens [39].

Recently, the mechanism to excise HIV1 DNA from HIV1-infected human lymphocytes has been developed using CRISPR/Cas9 technique. The success and promise of this approach is currently restricted to mouse only and is expected to be tested in humans soon. This study is indicative of treating viral-mediated malignancies such as Kaposi sarcoma-associated herpes virus (KSHV or HHV8), human T-lymphotropic virus leukemia (HTLV), and Epstein-Barr virus (EBV)-induced Burkitt lymphoma because these viruses also integrate their genome in the host cell's DNA for causing cancer [39].

3.10 Clinical Trials of CRISPR for Cancer Treatment

Based on the promising preclinical trials of CRISPR-based genome editing for the treatment of cancer, the strategy received a green signal to be tested in humans. Currently, 11 clinical trials are undergoing for diverse types of cancers in different regions of the world, and majority of them are immunotherapies [40]. It is expected that the first CRISPR-mediated treatment of cancer will be available in the clinic soon. Following are the examples of clinical trials for CRISPR:

Using CRISPR/Cas9 system, a team of researchers designed a strategy to kill cancer by targeting programmed cell death (PD1) protein. This protein is an important therapeutic target for negative regulation of immune system. Several inhibitors including the clinically approved pembrolizumab have been developed against PD1; however, the development of CRISPR/Cas9 mediated knock-out of PD1 revolutionzied the metastatic non-small cell lung cancer treatment. Currently, the clinical trials of this study are undergoing in China under the clinical trial identification number: NCT02793856. Mechanistically, cells were harvested from patients, and using CRISPR/Cas9 technique, PD1 knockouts were developed ex-vivo in harvested cells. Subsequently, CRISPR-modified cells were injected back into the patients to trigger immune responses for killing cancer. Similar PD1 knockout-dependent clinical studies for the treatment of cancers including EBV associated malignancies, prostate, bladder, esophageal, renal, T cell are also being conducted with clinical trials identification numbers: NCT03044743, NCT02867345, NCT02863913, NCT02867332, and NCT03081715 [40].

The ex vivo CRISPR-based genome editing for cancer treatment also included the generation of chimeric antigen receptor T cells as described earlier. CART cells are important for targeting tumor cells expressing specific receptor antigens. This gain-of-function approach for CRISPR is applied to target multiple cancers such as multiple myeloma, synovial sarcoma, and myxoid/round cell liposarcoma under the clinical trials' identification number: NCT03399448. CART cells targeting CD19, CD20, and CD22 on tumor cell surface were generated; however, CD19 showed most effective results during clinical trials. Unfortunately, some of the patients injected with CD19 targeting CART cells showed relapse due to the downregulation of CD19 in cancer cells. Thus other clinical trials with dual specificity CART cells (which target any two of these three CD19, CD20, CD 22) were introduced under the clinical trial identification number: NCT03398967 [40].

Another phase I clinical trial for the treatment of human papillomavirus induced-cervical cancer is currently in progress. HPV encodes E7 protein which is important to induce the malignant phenotype in cervical cancer. Targeting the production of E7 protein with relevant CRISPR/Cas9 plasmids led to the destruction of HPV-triggered cervical cancer cells during preclinical trials. This preclinical confirmation paved the way for testing this treatment for safety and efficacy studies in the clinic [40].

3.11 Conclusion

In conclusion, genome editing through CRISPR-based cancer therapeutics and related DNA-targeting strategies have a potential in treating different forms of cancer. Not only at present, such approaches can deal with newly developing cancers in the future and keep them from developing resistance. Effective techniques such as CRISPR being inexpensive and easily available can revolutionize the cancer research regardless of economic conditions. Moreover, its application is not only specific to cancers as the success has also been seen for treating other diseases as well.

References

1. Hanahan D, Weinberg Robert A (2011) Hallmarks of cancer: the next generation. Cell 144(5):646–674. https://doi.org/10.1016/j.cell.2011.02.013
2. Sabel MS, Diehl KM, Chang AE (2006) Principles of surgical therapy in oncology. In: Chang AE, Hayes DF, Pass HI et al (eds) Oncology: an evidence-based approach. Springer, New York, pp 58–72. https://doi.org/10.1007/0-387-31056-8_4
3. Kinsella T, Sohn J, Wessels B (2006) In: Chang AE et al (eds) Oncology. Springer, New York, pp 41–57. https://doi.org/10.1007/0-387-31056-8_3
4. Lundqvist EÅ, Fujiwara K, Seoud M (2015) Principles of chemotherapy. Int J Gynecol Obstet 131(S2):S146–S149. https://doi.org/10.1016/j.ijgo.2015.06.011
5. Padma VV (2015) An overview of targeted cancer therapy. Biomedicine (Taipei) 5(4):19. https://doi.org/10.7603/s40681-015-0019-4
6. Yan L, Rosen N, Arteaga C (2011) Targeted cancer therapies. Chin J Cancer 30(1):1–4. https://doi.org/10.5732/cjc.010.10553

7. Zhou J, Chng W-J (2018) Resistance to FLT3 inhibitors in acute myeloid leukemia: molecular mechanisms and resensitizing strategies. World J Clin Oncol 9(5):90–97. https://doi.org/10.5306/wjco.v9.i5.90
8. Cairns RA, Harris IS, Mak TW (2011) Regulation of cancer cell metabolism. Nat Rev Cancer 11(2):85–95. https://doi.org/10.1038/nrc2981
9. Wrodnigg TM, Steiner AJ, Ueberbacher BJ (2008) Natural and synthetic iminosugars as carbohydrate processing enzyme inhibitors for cancer therapy. Anti Cancer Agents Med Chem 8(1):77–85
10. Bhullar KS, Lagaron NO, McGowan EM, Parmar I, Jha A, Hubbard BP, Rupasinghe HPV (2018) Kinase-targeted cancer therapies: progress challenges and future directions. Mol Cancer 17(1):48. https://doi.org/10.1186/s12943-018-0804-2
11. Chan BA, Hughes BGM (2015) Targeted therapy for non-small cell lung cancer: current standards and the promise of the future. Transl Lung Cancer Res 4(1):36–54. https://doi.org/10.3978/j.issn.2218-6751.2014.05.01
12. Brehme M, Hantschel O, Colinge J, Kaupe I, Planyavsky M, Köcher T, Mechtler K, Bennett KL, Superti-Furga G (2009) Charting the molecular network of the drug target Bcr-Abl. Proc Natl Acad Sci 106(18):7414. https://doi.org/10.1073/pnas.0900653106
13. Durrant DE, Morrison DK (2018) Targeting the Raf kinases in human cancer: the Raf dimer dilemma. Br J Cancer 118(1):3–8. https://doi.org/10.1038/bjc.2017.399
14. Parmar S, Patel K, Pinilla-Ibarz J (2014) Ibrutinib (imbruvica): a novel targeted therapy for chronic lymphocytic leukemia. Pharm Ther 39(7):483–519
15. Schettini F, De Santo I, Rea CG, De Placido P, Formisano L, Giuliano M, Arpino G, De Laurentiis M, Puglisi F, De Placido S, Del Mastro L (2018) CDK 4/6 inhibitors as single agent in advanced solid tumors. Front Oncol 8:608–608. https://doi.org/10.3389/fonc.2018.00608
16. Zhang Y, Xia M, Jin K, Wang S, Wei H, Fan C, Wu Y, Li X, Li X, Li G, Zeng Z, Xiong W (2018) Function of the c-met receptor tyrosine kinase in carcinogenesis and associated therapeutic opportunities. Mol Cancer 17(1):45–45. https://doi.org/10.1186/s12943-018-0796-y
17. Mooso BA, Vinall RL, Mudryj M, Yap SA, deVere White RW, Ghosh PM (2015) The role of EGFR family inhibitors in muscle invasive bladder cancer: a review of clinical data and molecular evidence. J Urol 193(1):19–29. https://doi.org/10.1016/j.juro.2014.07.121
18. Hsu L, Armstrong AW (2014) JAK inhibitors: treatment efficacy and safety profile in patients with psoriasis. J Immunol Res 2014:283617. https://doi.org/10.1155/2014/283617
19. Banks M, Crowell K, Proctor A, Jensen BC (2017) Cardiovascular effects of the MEK inhibitor, Trametinib: a case report, literature review and consideration of mechanism. Cardiovasc Toxicol 17(4):487–493. https://doi.org/10.1007/s12012-017-9425-z
20. Mansoori B, Sandoghchian Shotorbani S, Baradaran B (2014) RNA interference and its role in cancer therapy. Adv Pharm Bull 4(4):313–321. https://doi.org/10.5681/apb.2014.046
21. Vozniak JM, Jacobs JM (2012) Vandetanib. J Adv Pract Oncol 3(2):112–116
22. Zhang S, Yu D (2012) Targeting Src family kinases in anti-cancer therapies: turning promise into triumph. Trends Pharmacol Sci 33(3):122–128. https://doi.org/10.1016/j.tips.2011.11.002
23. McKeown MR, Bradner JE (2014) Therapeutic strategies to inhibit MYC. Cold Spring Harb Perspect Med 4(10):a014266. https://doi.org/10.1101/cshperspect.a014266
24. Rodriguez R, Miller KM (2014) Unravelling the genomic targets of small molecules using high-throughput sequencing. Nat Rev Genet 15:783. https://doi.org/10.1038/nrg3796
25. Giancotti FG (2014) Deregulation of cell signaling in cancer. FEBS Lett 588(16):2558–2570. https://doi.org/10.1016/j.febslet.2014.02.005
26. Dachs GU, Dougherty GJ, Stratford IJ, Chaplin DJ (1997) Targeting gene therapy to cancer: a review. Oncol Res 9(6–7):313–325
27. Zuckerman JE, Gritli I, Tolcher A, Heidel JD, Lim D, Morgan R, Chmielowski B, Ribas A, Davis ME, Yen Y (2014) Correlating animal and human phase Ia/Ib clinical data with CALAA-01, a targeted, polymer-based nanoparticle containing siRNA. Proc Natl Acad Sci U S A 111(31):11449–11454. https://doi.org/10.1073/pnas.1411393111
28. Aleku M, Schulz P, Keil O, Santel A, Schaeper U, Dieckhoff B, Janke O, Endruschat J, Durieux B, Röder N, Löffler K, Lange C, Fechtner M, Möpert K, Fisch G, Dames S, Arnold

W, Jochims K, Giese K, Wiedenmann B, Scholz A, Kaufmann J (2008) Atu027, a liposomal small interfering RNA formulation targeting protein kinase N3 inhibits cancer progression. Cancer Res 68(23):9788. https://doi.org/10.1158/0008-5472.CAN-08-2428

29. Bianchini D, Omlin A, Pezaro C, Lorente D, Ferraldeschi R, Mukherji D, Crespo M, Figueiredo I, Miranda S, Riisnaes R, Zivi A, Buchbinder A, Rathkopf DE, Attard G, Scher HI, de Bono J, Danila DC (2013) First-in-human phase I study of EZN-4176, a locked nucleic acid antisense oligonucleotide to exon 4 of the androgen receptor mRNA in patients with castration-resistant prostate cancer. Br J Cancer 109(10):2579–2586. https://doi.org/10.1038/bjc.2013.619
30. Senzer N, Barve M, Kuhn J, Melnyk A, Beitsch P, Lazar M, Lifshitz S, Magee M, Oh J, Mill SW, Bedell C, Higgs C, Kumar P, Yu Y, Norvell F, Phalon C, Taquet N, Rao DD, Wang Z, Jay CM, Pappen BO, Wallraven G, Brunicardi FC, Shanahan DM, Maples PB, Nemunaitis J (2012) Phase I trial of "bi-shRNAi(furin)/GMCSF DNA/autologous tumor cell" vaccine (FANG) in advanced cancer. Mol Ther 20(3):679–686. https://doi.org/10.1038/mt.2011.269
31. Sun H, Zhu X, Lu PY, Rosato RR, Tan W, Zu Y (2014) Oligonucleotide aptamers: new tools for targeted cancer therapy. Mol Ther Nucleic Acids 3(8):e182–e182. https://doi.org/10.1038/mtna.2014.32
32. Ziach K, Chollet C, Parissi V, Prabhakaran P, Marchivie M, Corvaglia V, Bose PP, Laxmi-Reddy K, Godde F, Schmitter J-M, Chaignepain S, Pourquier P, Huc I (2018) Single helically folded aromatic oligoamides that mimic the charge surface of double-stranded B-DNA. Nat Chem 10(5):511–518. https://doi.org/10.1038/s41557-018-0018-7
33. Lundstrom K (2018) Viral vectors in gene therapy. Diseases 6(2):42. https://doi.org/10.3390/diseases6020042
34. Harrison EB, Azam SH, Pecot CV (2018) Targeting accessories to the crime: nanoparticle nucleic acid delivery to the tumor microenvironment. Front Pharmacol 9:307–307. https://doi.org/10.3389/fphar.2018.00307
35. Karve S, Werner ME, Sukumar R, Cummings ND, Copp JA, Wang EC, Li C, Sethi M, Chen RC, Pacold ME, Wang AZ (2012) Revival of the abandoned therapeutic wortmannin by nanoparticle drug delivery. Proc Natl Acad Sci 109(21):8230. https://doi.org/10.1073/pnas.1120508109
36. Anders L, Guenther MG, Qi J, Fan ZP, Marineau JJ, Rahl PB, Lovén J, Sigova AA, Smith WB, Lee TI, Bradner JE, Young RA (2014) Genome-wide localization of small molecules. Nat Biotechnol 32(1):92–96. https://doi.org/10.1038/nbt.2776
37. Martinez-Lage M, Puig-Serra P, Menendez P, Torres-Ruiz R, Rodriguez-Perales S (2018) CRISPR/Cas9 for cancer therapy: hopes and challenges. Biomedicine 6(4):E105. https://doi.org/10.3390/biomedicines6040105
38. Yin H, Xue W, Anderson DG (2019) CRISPR–Cas: a tool for cancer research and therapeutics. Nat Rev Clin Oncol 16(5):281–295. https://doi.org/10.1038/s41571-019-0166-8
39. Isakov N (2017) Future perspectives for cancer therapy using the CRISPR genome editing. Technology 08. https://doi.org/10.4172/2155-9899.1000e120
40. Tian X, Gu T, Patel S, Bode AM, Lee M-H, Dong Z (2019) CRISPR/Cas9 – an evolving biological tool kit for cancer biology and oncology. Npj precision. Oncology 3(1):8. https://doi.org/10.1038/s41698-019-0080-7

Genome Editing in Cancer Research and Cure

4

Sabin Aslam and Sarmad Mehmood

4.1 Introduction

Cancer is defined as a set of diseases involved in abnormal development of cells with an increased risk of dispersal to other parts of the affected body [1, 2]. Cancerous cells are regarded as neoplasms, i.e., cluster of cells with unregulated growth and ability to develop a lumpy mass, often dispersed diffusely [3, 4]. Absence of appropriate signals for optimized cell division and growth, unlimited cell divisions, escape from programmed cell death (PCD), unlimited assemblage of blood circulation vessels, tissue invasion, and metastasis formation are the characteristic features of cancerous cells [5]. These cells are considered as different from tumors which do not disperse to other body parts [4]. Initial symptoms of cancerous cells include lumpy region, unusual bleeding, continued cough, inexplicable loss in body weight, and a shift in excrement. Human body is affected by more than 100 types of cancers [6, 7].

Most obvious cause of cancer is smoking tobacco that contributes to cause more than 22% of cancers in human body. Approximately 10% of cancer is caused by body fatness, inadequate body movement/physical exercise, improper diet, and extreme alcohol drinking [7, 8]. Exposure to radiations and chemical pollutants may also be the cause of developing cancers. Most of the developing countries are at increased risk of suffering from cancers mainly due to infections of hepatitis B and

S. Aslam (✉)
Department of Plant Science, University of California, Davis, Davis, CA, USA

University of Agriculture Faisalabad, Faisalabad, Pakistan
e-mail: sabaslam@ucdavis.edu

S. Mehmood
Atta-ur-Rahman School of Applied Biosciences, National University of Sciences and Technology, Islamabad, Pakistan

Department of Pathology, CMH Institute of Medical Sciences, Bahawalpur, Pakistan
e-mail: sarmadmehmood89@yahoo.com

N. Masood, S. Shakil Malik (eds.), *'Essentials of Cancer Genomic, Computational Approaches and Precision Medicine*,
https://doi.org/10.1007/978-981-15-1067-0_4

C, *Helicobacter pylori*, human papilloma virus, human immunodeficiency syndrome, and Epstein-Barr virus [9]. These elements of developing cancer may modify the genes within the cells, thereby triggering the cells for abnormal development. Most of these genetic changes are heritable, and the chance of transferring from parents to offsprings is 5–10%.

Occurrence of different types of cancers varies in men, women, and children. The most frequently occurring cancer types in men are colorectal, lung, prostate, and stomach cancer [10]. Breast, cervical, colorectal, and lung cancers are most commonly occurring cancer types in women [1], while children are most commonly suffering from brain tumors, lymphoblastic leukemia, and non-Hodgkin lymphoma [1]. Occurrence of cancer varies with age and lifestyle. Current mortality rate due to cancer is 80% in developing countries and 66% in the United States[11].

Cancers are often detected by signs and symptoms, and medical-based screening tests are followed by a confirmation with imaging and biopsy [12].

A number of cancers can be prevented to some extent by avoiding tobacco smoking and alcohol; less exposure to sunlight; maintaining an optimized body weight; consuming fresh fruits, vegetables, and cereals; proper vaccination against infectious diseases; and avoiding red meat and processed food [13, 14].

Routine treatment of cancer involves a combination of chemotherapy, targeted therapy, irradiation, and surgery of the affected body area [15, 16].

4.2 Signs and Symptoms

At the beginning, no obvious signs of cancers can be observed on the body. Symptoms appear only when affected region develops an observable mass of cells (depending on the type and location of cancer). Only few symptoms are common to all cancer types, others being specific and vary in different individuals. Cancer is often diagnosed in individuals suffering from other infectious diseases with the symptoms commonly observed in cancerous patients; thereby it is called as a "great imitator." For instance, lung cancer can cause blockage of bronchi with the result of having cough and pneumonia; difficulty in swallowing food may result from narrowing of esophagus due to esophageal cancer; contraction of bowel may result from colorectal cancer affecting bowel movement. Bleeding occurs due to ulceration, which may lead to bleeding during cough, in bowel, and during urination, through rectum or vaginal bleeding. Initially swelling may occur in the affected area which is normally painless. Pain may occur at advanced stage of cancer. Sometimes, fluids accumulate in abdominal or chest region [17]. General symptoms include constant fever, persistent body weight loss, abrupt changes to skin, and extreme fatigue [18].

Cancer can be metastatic in nature, i.e., it is dispersed to other parts of the body away from its origin either by hematogenous spread (dispersal by blood) or lymphatic spread (dispersal by lymph to lymph nodes). Metastatic cancer may lead to enlarged lymph nodes often felt as hard nodes under the skin. It may also lead to inflamed liver or spleen with painful abdomen.

4.3 Cause

Cancer is caused by either environmental (90–95%) or genetic factors (5–10%). Environmental factors may include economical, behavioral, and physical factors that are not merely considered to be heritable.

Carcinogens may be the primary cause of developing most of cancers. For instance, smoking tobacco causes 25–30% of all the cancers. Tobacco is the leading cause of lung cancer (90%) in addition to causing neck, head, larynx, esophagus, stomach, kidney, bladder, and pancreatic cancer [19, 20]. As smoke of tobacco contains more than 50 carcinogens with nitrosamines and polycyclic aromatic hydrocarbons, thereby it is responsible for 1 out of 5 deaths due to cancer worldwide [20, 21]. Extra body weight is linked to the development of different types of cancers leading to death (14–20%) in the United States [22]. In the United Kingdom, nearly 12,000 cancer cases are reported each year due to increased body mass index which may lead to death [22].

Lack of physical exercise, obesity, and poor nutrition are also the cause of cancer (30–35%). Lack of bodily movement is associated with health effects on immune system as well as on endocrine system [22]. Overeating is also the cause of cancer than eating few fresh fruits and vegetables. Some foods have carcinogens that may cause a specific type of cancer. For example, oral cancer is caused by chewing betel nut, gastric cancer is caused by having highly salted diet, and liver cancer is caused by aflatoxin B1 [23].

Infectious diseases are causing approximately 15–20% of all the cancers. According to an estimate, 18% of cancer deaths are caused by infectious diseases (with a rate of 25% deaths in Africa and 10% in developed world) [21]. Viruses are the leading source of cancer throughout the world. Among viruses, Epstein-Barr virus, hepatitis B and C virus, human papilloma virus, human T-cell leukemia virus-I, and Kaposi's sarcoma herpesvirus are causing B-cell lymphoproliferative disease, hepatocellular carcinoma, cervical cancer, T-cell leukemia, effusion lymphomas, and Kaposi sarcoma, respectively. Some bacteria may cause certain types of cancers, for example, gastric carcinoma. Some cancers are also caused by parasites such as bladder carcinoma and cholangiocarcinoma [24–26].

Irradiation is the major cause of skin cancer (10%). Ultraviolet radiations, sunlight, radon gases, and rays emitting from medical imaging tools [27] are the leading causes of developing skin cancer. Combination of radiations with tobacco smoke and radon gas becomes a strong cause of cancer affecting almost every part of the body [26]. Almost all the cancers are nonheritable, but only a lesser percentage (0.3%) of population become carrier to this disease causing nearly 3–10% of all the cancers. For example, inherited mutations in particular genes may increase the risk of cancers (mutation in BRCA-I and BRCA-II genes may increase the risk of breast, ovarian, and non-polyposis colorectal cancer to 75%) [28]. Taller people have more tendency of developing cancers as they possess more number of cells as compared to short stature individuals [29].

Prolonged exposure to some fibrous physical substances such as asbestos, attapulgite, glass wool, rock wool, and wollastonite may also cause cancer. Some nonfibrous materials are powdered nickel, cobalt, cristobalite, quartz, and tridymite. Physical materials need to remain inside the body for long for causing cancer [30].

Hormones are the potent accelerators of carcinogenesis. For example, growth factors involved in insulin production and their associated binding proteins are potential source of developing cancer. Sex-linked cancers (breast, bone, endometrium, thyroid, testis, and ovarian cancers) are often spread by hormones [31]. Obesity is also an indirect cause of cancer due to involvement of certain hormones. Hormone replacement therapy by some individuals may lead to cancer. That's why, doing exercise may minimize the risk of developing cancer due to lesser hormone production [31].

4.4 Genome Editing

A branch of genetic engineering which involves integration, removal, replacement, or modification of DNA within genome of an organism is termed as genome engineering or genome editing. Genetic engineering is no longer a new approach. During the 1970s, it emerged as a method of introducing a unique DNA sequence into an organism's genome. Genome engineering puts forward a huge number of products with designated benefit to mankind. But major drawback of this technology was the increased risks of random insertion of transgene which may disturb adjoining genes and their expression. Scientists struggled to seek out alternative strategies for targeting foreign genes at specific location without disturbing indigenous genes, which may not only help in editing DNA sequences precisely but also help in minimizing off-target effects of the introduced gene. Site-specific genome engineering will find its way for gene therapy to cure numerous genetic disorders by introducing a functional gene and to replace it with diseased one.

Contrary to previous genome-editing strategies which rely on random gene insertions/deletions, latest genome engineering tools target insertions/deletions site specifically. These genome engineering tools are termed as molecular scissors. Since 2015, these engineered nucleases are grouped into four families: meganucleases [32], zinc finger nucleases (ZFNs) [33], transcription activator-like effector nucleases (TALENs) [34], and clustered regularly interspaced short palindromic repeats (CRISPRs) [35]. Nine editors of living organisms are reported: three DNA (TtAgo, het/exo MAGE, and RecA CAGE), two RNA (Cas9 and Group II introns), and four proteins (recombinases, meganucleases, ZFN, and TALEs) [35, 36]. By the start of 2011, meganucleases, ZFNs, and TALENs were designated as genome-editing tools of the year by *Nature Methods* [37]. A major breakthrough of 2015 was CRISPR/Cas9 system, which was considered as the most efficient genome engineering tool of the current era [38].

Integrity of genetic material is extensively vital for its function. As DNA is intrinsically unstable in living organisms, it is subjected to sheer due to extensive physical, chemical, or mechanical stress (reactive oxygen species produced by respiratory pathways or chemotherapeutic drugs) or ionizing radiations which may lead to single- or double-strand break (DSB). Such DSBs also occur during meiosis when recombination occurs between nonhomologous chromosomes during crossover or chiasma formation that allows exchange of segments between nonhomologous chromosomes. Although there is no report on how persistently a DNA damage can occur inherently without exposure to any foreign chemical, it is noticeable that a single DNA damage can cause cell death. DSB, if rendered unrepaired, can cause gene disruptions and deletion of chromosome or other chromosomal aberrations that may ultimately lead to cancer [39]. Such DSBs are repaired inherently by two mechanisms: nonhomologous end-joining (NHEJ)/illegitimate recombination and homology directed repairing/homologous recombination (HDR/HR). Apart from these repair mechanisms, DSBs can also be repaired by a single-strand annealing (SSA) mechanism, which involves removal of DNA sequences flanked between repetitive DNA elements [39].

All the DNA damages including DSB are harnessed at check points within cell cycle which may halt the cell cycle and prevent the genetic material to enter into mitotic (M) or synthetic (S) phase. This process prevents the most common errors caused by DNA damage or chromosomal loss. When the DNA damage is repaired by repair mechanisms, the cell cycle continues from where it was halted [8]. DSBs may lead to cell death/apoptosis, which result from the intolerable damage of DNA (tolerance of DNA damage by different cells within an organism varies) [39].

During homologous recombination, DNA double helix unwinds and invades into the paired homologous duplex (homologous chromosome, sister chromatid, or a homologous viral/vector genome). This DNA DSB repair is done with homologous recombination using homologous strand as a template (Fig. 4.1). Thus homologous recombination needs wide sections of homologous DNA in other duplex without having any loss of genetic material. Numerous genes responsible for homologous recombination have been reported, viz., MRE-11, RAD-50, RAD-51, RAD-52, RAD-54, RAD-55, RAD-57, and XRS-2. These genes were identified by using

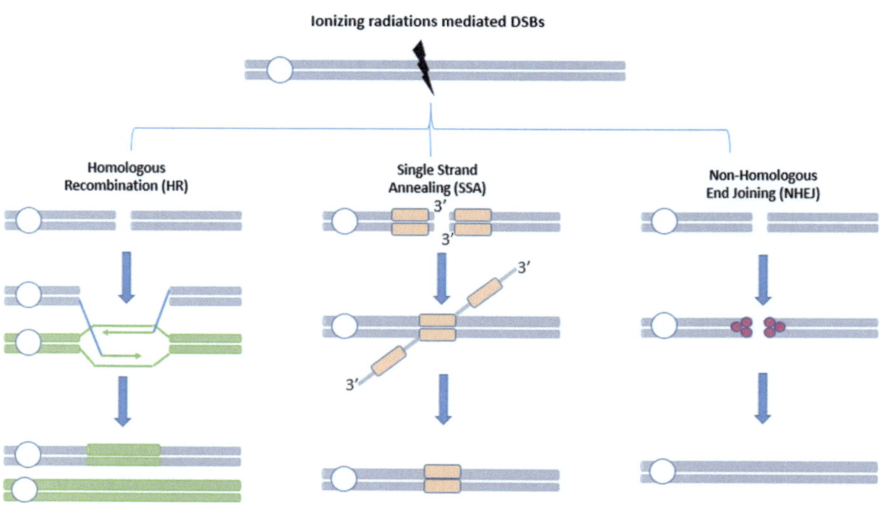

Fig. 4.1 Double-strand breaks repair

ionizing radiation-sensitive mutants during yeast genetics studies. Currently these genes have been cloned for studies in mammalian cells [39]. The DSB repair pathway is the preferred route of DNA repair in yeast. The process works by involving RAD-52, which is a binding protein for DNA ends, and RAD-51, which is a filament-forming protein around unwound strands of DNA. The process also involves DNA polymerase and DNA ligase I (DNA ends ligation). Some other proteins help in unwinding of DNA without any loss of genetic material.

Nonhomologous end joining doesn't require much homology with other DNA duplex for DSB repair (Fig. 4.1). This process joins the broken ends directly and requires a Ku protein in mammalian cells which is a DNA ends-binding protein. Ku protein forms a complex with DNA-PKcs in mammals. Other genes responsible for nonhomologous end joining are MRE-11, NBS-1, and RAD-50 and XRCC4-DNA ligase IV complex. There are chances for missing of few base pairs during repair by nonhomologous end joining [40].

Often, DSBs aren't blunt ended, but they carry single-strand overhangs. Such type of DSBs needs to be clipped by exo-/endonucleases to make them blunt ended.

4.5 Genome-Editing Tools

The phenomenon of genome editing relies on occurrence of DSBs. Most of the currently used restriction enzymes were able to cut DNA at multiple locations within genome. To address this controversy and to make DSBs repair site specific, new classes of endonuclease were introduced for site-specific genome editing. These were named as meganucleases, ZFNs, TALENs, and CRISPR/Cas system.

4.6 Meganucleases

Meganucleases were discovered in later half of 1980s. These nucleases belong to the family of endonucleases which are able to identify and cut large sequences of DNA ranging between 14 and 40 base pairs [40]. Widely characterized meganucleases are from the family of LAGLIDADG nucleases, whose name comes from a conserved sequence of amino acids. Meganucleases were first discovered in microbes with a characteristic of more than 40 base pairs long DNA recognition sequence [41, 42]. But there are no specific meganucleases that can target specific sequence of DNA. For addressing the problem of non-specificity, high-throughput screening methods were utilized to make them as specific [42, 43]. Alternate strategy was to fuse a meganuclease with another one to create a hybrid enzyme that is able to recognize a unique DNA sequence [44, 45]. A substitute method for stating the specificity of meganucleases was introduced by adjusting DNA-interacting amino acids. This method was named as rationally designed meganucleases by Smith et al. [36]. A programmed model of homing endonucleases was also proposed as an alternate strategy to assign specificity to meganucleases [46]. Moreover multiple units can be combined to make chimeric meganucleases. Chimeric enzymes can provide a wide range of applications in agriculture, health, industry, and energy sector. An example includes a commercial scale production of meganucleases that can cleave XPC gene in humans capable of developing a severe disease *Xeroderma pigmentosum*. This disease may cause skin burns leading to skin cancer by exposure to UV irradiation [47].

Meganucleases seem to be less toxic to living cells in terms of less DNA sequence specificity as compared to ZFNs and TALENs. But the construction of chimeric or sequence-specific nucleases is expensive and time-consuming. Meganucleases are also not using combinatorial properties of nuclease and binding domains as ZFNs and TALENs are using.

4.7 Zinc Finger Nucleases (ZFNs)

Contrary to meganucleases, ZFNs and TALENs technology relies on the combination of a non-specific nuclease domain and a very specific DNA-binding domain. DNA-binding domain recognizes specific proteins, i.e., zinc fingers or TALEs, and the nuclease domain causes DSB at the recognized region. For construction of engineered nucleases, a specific endonuclease is required which has both the domains (nuclease and DNA-binding domains) separate from each other. Most of the time, the nuclease domain of such enzymes is separated and is connected to DNA-recognizing sequences of high specificity (Fig. 4.2) [47].

Most of the transcription factors carry zinc finger motif which is responsible for their three-dimensional structure. Zinc finger motif is present at the junction of proteins and DNA which helps in stabilizing the interaction between DNA and protein. Each finger has C-terminal region responsible for recognizing specific DNA sequence. Each zinc finger is able to recognize short only three-base-pair DNA sequence, but combining more than 6–8 zinc fingers makes them a unique nuclease, able to recognize more than 20 bp of DNA. This strategy is reported to control the phenomenon of angiogenesis in animals [37]. ZFNs can be used in genome engineering by fusing zinc fingers with catalytic domain of restriction endonuclease for targeted DNA DSB [49]. The actual process involves the association of DNA-binding protein carrying most precisely chosen catalytic domain of FokI restriction endonuclease. FokI enzyme needs to be dimerized in order to cleave the double-stranded

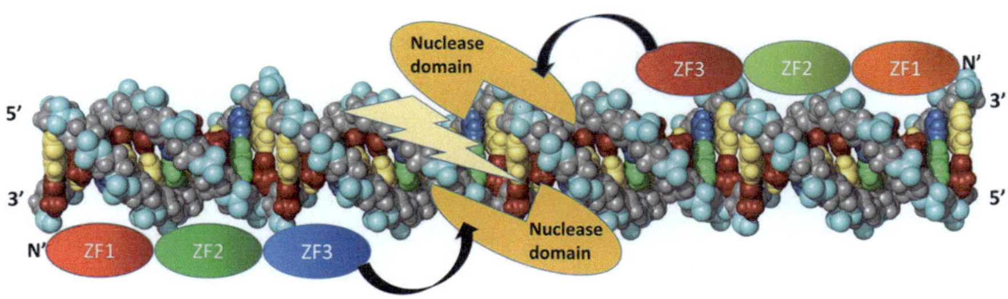

Fig. 4.2 Zinc finger nucleases (Source: Aslam et al. [48])

DNA. Both the enzymes recognize two DNA sequences which separated a few base pairs apart. Both the FokI domains come closer on interaction with their respective DNA sequences. The specificity of each zinc finger is markedly increased on dimerization and recognition of specific DNA sequence. To give them marked specificity, nuclease domain is engineered to function as heterodimer [50].

Multiple approaches are available for designing an engineered ZFN. Modular assembly involves the use of a combination of zinc finger units with known DNA sequence. Bacteria, yeast, and mammalian cells are optimized to characterize the specificity and cell tolerance of ZFNs. Genome-wide characterization of ZFNs has not yet been reported. It has been reported that only 1–2 DSBs occur as background in samples treated with ZFNs carrying a 24 bp DNA recognition site FokI nuclease domain as heterodimer [50]. Heterodimer functioning of ZFNs creates enhanced specificity of creating a DSB. Although the nuclease domain of both the TALENs and ZFNs possess the same characteristics, the only difference is in their DNA recognition domain. ZFNs are made up of Cys2-His2 zinc fingers and TALENs are made up of TALE proteins. Both the TALENs and ZFNs are constructed to maintain their natural properties of DNA recognizing domain combination. A large number of DNA interrelating proteins, i.e., transcription factors, possess Cys2-His2 zinc fingers in repeats normally three base pairs apart and in varied combinations. All the ZFNs are considered entirely independent, but the binding affinity is determined by its neighboring ZFN.

Contrary to ZFNs, each TALE is able to recognize a single base pair of the recognized region. Due to their construction in repeated pattern, varied combinations impart a wide variety to the engineering of TALENs and ZFNs [51]. Zinc fingers have been engineered to make them site specific using multiple approaches, viz., modular assembly, OPEN, and bacterial single hybrid system for screening libraries of ZFN. ZFNs are being used in R&D for genome editing in multiple laboratories. Sangamo Biosciences, a renowned company in the United States, is utilizing ZFNs for therapeutic reasons in genome engineering of stem and immune cells [52, 53]. Genetically modified T lymphocytes through ZFNs are in initial clinical trials for treatment of glioblastoma, a king of brain cancer. Engineered ZFNs are also being used in fighting against AIDS [50].

4.8 TALENs

Transcription activator-like effector nucleases (TALENs) are specific restriction enzymes designed to recognize a specific sequence of DNA. These engineered nucleases are constructed by combining DNA-binding domain (TALE) and DNA cleavage domain (FokI). Generally they are made up of 30–35 amino acids long with each amino acid capable of recognizing a single base pair. These targeted proteins are termed as molecular scissors that are capable of site-specific insertion, removal, and translocation of gene within living organisms [54]. DNA-binding domain of TALENs is obtained from TAL effectors, a specific DNA-binding protein extracted from a plant pathogenic bacterium *Xanthomonas*. TALE effectors are

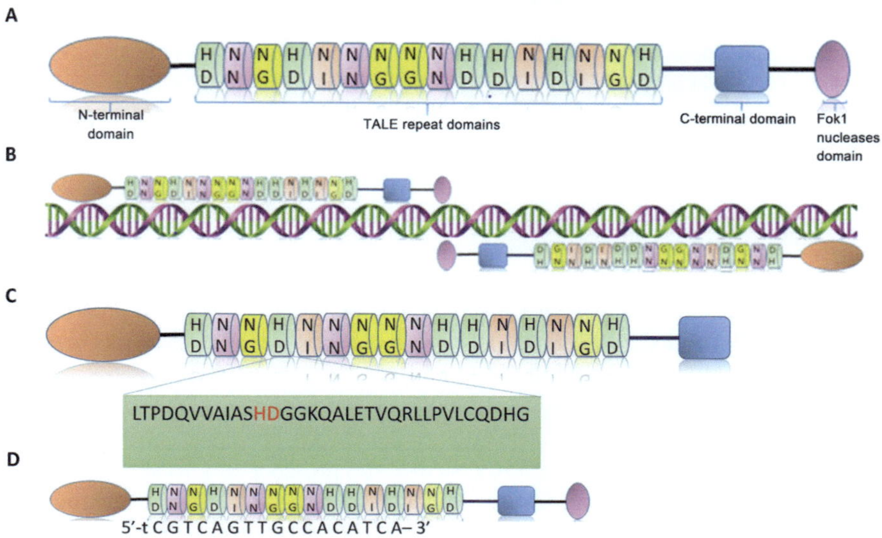

Fig. 4.3 Transcription activator-like effectors nucleases (Source: Aslam et al. [48])

composed of repeated TALE domains that consist of normally 34 amino acids, with each amino acid capable of recognizing a single base pair of the targeted DNA. Like ZFN, targeting TALENs creates DSB that can be repaired by indigenous NHEJ repair mechanism within the cell. A small integration or removal happens at the target site during the course of repair. All repeats within a TALEN are conserved except the amino acids positioned at 12th and 13th position. These specific repeats are termed as repeat variable di-residues (RVDs) whose specificity determines the DNA sequence with which that specific TALEN has to bind. The process of binding each TALE with a specific base pair at the target site is pretty straightforward as compared to ZFNs. TALEs fuse to catalytic domain of FokI restriction endonuclease to form TALENs. This combination imparts specificity to TALEN to target and cleave specific DNA site. Recognition system of TALENs is conveniently predictable than ZFNs; this convenience is due to its 30 plus base pairs recognition site. TALENs are able to bind within a range of six base pairs of any nucleotide within the entire genome of a living organism [55, 56]. TALENS are more efficient as compared to ZFNs in terms of higher specificity to bind DNA target site, lesser off-target effects, and an easier construction of DNA-binding domain (Fig. 4.3).

4.9 CRISPR/Cas System

Bacteria use a defense system called clustered regularly interspaced short palindromic repeats (CRISPR) to protect themselves against viruses [57]. CRISPR system consists of short palindromic repeat sequences originated from viral/phage genome and has been integrated into the genome of bacteria during prior viral/

phage attack. These sequences are used to disintegrate viruses/phages during subsequent attacks. These DNA sequences play a significant role in serving as a defense system of bacteria and archaea [57]. CRISPR system uses CRISPR-associated proteins (Cas9) as an enzyme to target and cleave the Cas9-recognized complementary DNA sequence. CRISPR-associated proteins are involved in processing the DNA sequence to match it according to the attacking viral sequence for specific targeting. This combination of Cas9 protein and CRISPR DNA sequences makes today's era the most remarkable technology, the CRISPR/Cas9 system [58] (Fig. 4.4).

The CRISPR/Cas9 system is an inherent immune system of bacteria/archaea to impart acquired immunity against invading genetic elements (phages/viruses/plasmids) [59–61]. Guided RNA (gRNA) having spacer sequences guides Cas9 proteins to recognize and cleave invading viral and RNA sequences [62]. CRISPR system has been reported in nearly 50% and 90% of bacterial and archaeal sequenced genomes, respectively [63].

A significant addition to CRISPR system is the presence of CRISPR-associated genes. Minor clusters of Cas genes are present adjacent to CRISPR spacer sequences. Cumulatively, 35 families containing 93 CRISPR-associated genes have been reported based on sequence homology. Among 35 Cas gene families, 11 families form the core structure of CRISPR system comprising Cas1–9 gene families. CRISPR/Cas locus must possess at least one Cas core gene for proper recognition and cleavage of the targeted sequence [64].

CRISPR/Cas system is categorized into two classes. Class I CRISPR system uses a combination of Cas genes to cleave foreign DNA sequence. This class is further subdivided into type I, III, and IV CRISPR systems. Contrary to Class I, Class II CRISPR system uses a single Cas gene for degrading foreign genetic elements. Class II is further subdivided into type II, V, and VI [65]. All the 6 CRISPR/

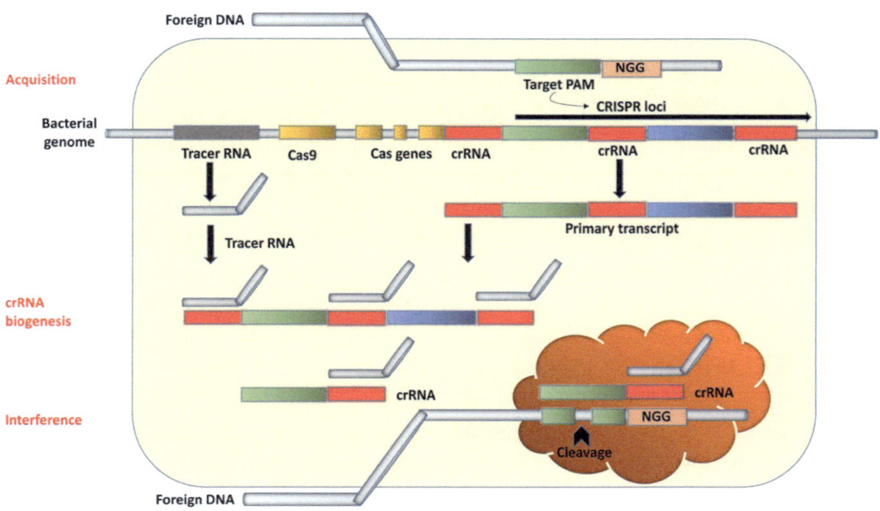

Fig. 4.4 CRISPR/Cas system (Source: Aslam et al. [48])

Cas systems are divided into 19 subtypes characterized by a specific protein unique to that specific type [66].

The mechanism of CRISPR/Cas system starts by invading a virus. As a first step in adaptive immunity, the viral sequence is captured and is inserted as spacer sequence into the CRISPR locus and cleaving of protospacer. As Cas-I and Cas-II genes are involved in spacer sequence acquisition, they are present in all types of CRISPR systems [56, 67–71]. The protospacer sequence is bound to direct repeat sequences present next to the leader sequences. Single strand extends to repair the CRISPR sequence resulting in duplication of direct repeat. The rest of the two stages in CRISPR mechanism (CrRNA processing stage and interference stage) act differentially in all the three CRISPR systems. Cas9 genes cleave primary CRISPR transcript to yield CrRNA. Type I CRISPR system uses Cas6e and Cas6f to cleave the direct repeat at the intersection of single-strand (ss) and double-strand (ds) RNA by forming a hairpin structure. Type II CRISPR system makes dsRNA by using a tracer RNA (trans-activating RNA) cut by Cas9 enzyme and RNase III. Type III CRISPR system uses a homolog of Cas6 that doesn't involve any hairpin structure for cleavage. Furthermore, types II and III systems require trimming at 5′ or 3′ position to yield fully functional CrRNAs. Interference complexes are made by combination of CrRNA and Cas proteins. For proper functioning of type I and type II CRISPR systems, association between PAM sequences and Cas proteins is required for cleaving foreign DNA. But type III system doesn't require association for PAM sites for cleavage as base pairing occurs between mRNA and CrRNA which is indirectly targeted by type IIIB system [56, 67–70].

This system is currently being used for targeting specific DNA sequences of eukaryotic genomes in multiple strategies. One strategy is to introduce a CRISPR-based plasmid-carrying Cas genes and its associated gRNA and scaffold into genome of living organisms to cut the genome at a very specific target site [70]. Numerous companies like Cellectis [72] and Editas have emerged to monetize the CRISPR/Cas system and are contributing toward gene therapies [73].

Numerous significant innovations regarding CRISPR system have been recently reported in terms of bridged nucleic acid integrated CRISPR RNA for highly precise recognition of DNA [74], highly efficient CAS9 system for homology-directed DNA repair [75], HypaCAS9 [76], xCAS9 associated with bordering PAM sites [77], and LOAD system (local accumulation of double-strand break repair) [78].

4.10 Could Genome Editing Enhance or Diminish Cancer Risk? The Big Picture

According to two independent study reports from University of Helsinki Finland and Karolinska Institute, CRISPR/Cas9 system can enhance the cancer risk. Scientists and researchers from both institutes reported that p53 protein that serves as the first aid kit of cells is activated by CRISPR/Cas system in human cells. On activation, p53 diminishes the CRISPR/Cas9 system genome-editing efficiency; thereby cells having no or lesser p53 are more likely to succeed for genome editing. The cells lacking in p53 are more likely to grow overpoweringly and turn out to be cancerous. Dr. Emma Haapaniemi at the Department of Medicine in Karolinska Institute said that the cells with successfully repaired damaged gene are more likely to lack functional p53 proteins. And if a foreign gene for a hereditary disease is transplanted into an individual in cells lacking p53, there is a high risk of cancer in those cells that can promote the biosafety regulations of CRISPR system. Dr. Bernhard from the Department of Medical Biochemistry and Biophysics from the same institute added that CRISPR/Cas system is a powerful tool but has a staggering potential for gene therapy.

Long story short, no doubt CRISPR system is a powerful tool of genome editing, but it is something that the patients and doctors must know of. It is further suggested that the there is a dire need for the work on the response of p53 CRISPR system-based gene therapies [79].

4.11 Conclusion

Genome-editing technologies have revolved out to be obligatory for scientific progressions. This may be due to their widespread applicability in both fields, i.e., basic research in understanding fundamental queries about how basic life form works and in the development of biotherapies for multifaceted diseases like cancer. However, there are still numerous challenges linked with this technology that need to be addressed. For example, the huge size of Cas9 protein makes it problematic to package the protein in low-immunogenic AAV vectors that can be used both ways, i.e., in vivo and in vitro gene delivery. For instance, Cas9 from *Staphylococcus aureus* and *Staphylococcus pyogenes* has been reported to cause infectious diseases in humans. One favorable strategy to resolve this issue is to restructure Cas9 protein or use a different protein from bacteria that is able to outflow from the immune response of the host. A CRISPR/Cas9 delivery system based on the lipid nanoparticles has been developed by Intellia Therapeutics, which was developed for gene editing of rodents and primates (nonhuman). Some ethical issues also developed with the progression of genome-editing technologies. With the reported advent of "CRISPR babies" in November 2018, scientists and researchers were liable to answer the challenges of latest genome-editing technologies potentially entering into the era of genetic inequality and its long-term consequences. Although the challenges and risks prevail, genome-editing technologies embrace vast prospective and are a prodigious addition to the genetic engineering toolbox for the development of biotherapies that can recover patients in the future permanently.

References

1. Bray F, Ferlay J, Soerjomataram I, Siegel RL, Torre LA, Jemal A (2018) Global cancer statistics 2018: GLOBOCAN estimates of incidence and mortality worldwide for 36 cancers in 185 countries. CA Cancer J Clin 68(6):394–424

2. Pan F, Pan D, Pardoll DM, Barbi J, Fu J (2019) Compositions and methods for targeting activin signaling to treat cancer. Google Patents
3. Singer M, Wang C, Cong L, Marjanovic ND, Kowalczyk MS, Zhang H, Nyman J, Sakuishi K, Kurtulus S, Gennert D (2016) A distinct gene module for dysfunction uncoupled from activation in tumor-infiltrating T cells. Cell 166(6):1500–1511.e9
4. Beloribi-Djefaflia S, Vasseur S, Guillaumond F (2016) Lipid metabolic reprogramming in cancer cells. Oncogene 5(1):e189
5. Beguin E (2018) Sonodynamic therapy of hypoxic tumours. University of Oxford, Oxford
6. Grossman DC, Curry SJ, Owens DK, Barry MJ, Davidson KW, Doubeni CA, Epling JW, Kemper AR, Krist AH, Kurth AE (2018) Screening for ovarian cancer: US preventive services task force recommendation statement. JAMA 319(6):588–594
7. Sasieni PD, Parkin DM (2018) Global perspectives surrounding cancer prevention and screening. In: Cancer prevention and screening: concepts, principles and controversies, p 1
8. Thompson R, Mitrou G, Brown S, Almond E, Bandurek I, Brockton N, Kälfors M, McGinley-Gieser D, Sinclair B, Meincke L (2018) Major new review of global evidence on diet, nutrition and physical activity: a blueprint to reduce cancer risk. Nutr Bull 43(3):269–283
9. Knoll LJ, Hogan DA, Leong JM, Heitman J, Condit RC (2018) Pearls collections: what we can learn about infectious disease and cancer. PLoS Pathog 14(3):e1006915. https://doi.org/10.1371/journal.ppat.1006915
10. Siegel RL, Miller KD, Jemal A (2019) Cancer statistics, 2019. CA Cancer J Clin 69(1):7–34
11. Fitzmaurice C, Akinyemiju TF, Al Lami FH, Alam T, Alizadeh-Navaei R, Allen C, Alsharif U, Alvis-Guzman N, Amini E, Anderson BO (2018) Global, regional, and national cancer incidence, mortality, years of life lost, years lived with disability, and disability-adjusted life-years for 29 cancer groups, 1990 to 2016: a systematic analysis for the global burden of disease study. JAMA Oncol 4(11):1553–1568
12. Doubeni CA, Gabler NB, Wheeler CM, McCarthy AM, Castle PE, Halm EA, Schnall MD, Skinner CS, Tosteson AN, Weaver DL (2018) Timely follow-up of positive cancer screening results: a systematic review and recommendations from the PROSPR consortium. CA Cancer J Clin 68(3):199–216
13. Gapstur SM, Drope JM, Jacobs EJ, Teras LR, McCullough ML, Douglas CE, Patel AV, Wender RC, Brawley OW (2018) A blueprint for the primary prevention of cancer: targeting established modifiable risk factors. CA Cancer J Clin 68(6):446–470
14. Forman D, Bauld L, Bonanni B, Brenner H, Brown K, Dillner J, Kampman E, Manczuk M, Riboli E, Steindorf K (2018) Time for a European initiative for research to prevent cancer: a manifesto for Cancer Prevention Europe (CPE). J Cancer Policy 17:15–23
15. Vargo JA, Moiseenko V, Grimm J, Caudell J, Clump DA, Yorke E, Xue J, Vinogradskiy Y, Moros EG, Mavroidis P (2018) Head and neck tumor control probability: radiation dose–volume effects in stereotactic body radiation therapy for locally recurrent previously-irradiated head and neck cancer: report of the AAPM working group. Int J Radiat Oncol Biol Phys. https://doi.org/10.1016/j.ijrobp.2018.01.044
16. Alam A, Farooq U, Singh R, Dubey V, Kumar S, Kumari R, Kumar K, Naik B, Dhar K (2018) Chemotherapy treatment and strategy schemes: a review. J Toxicol 2(7):555600. https://doi.org/10.19080/OAJT.2018.02.555600
17. Miller KD, Siegel RL, Lin CC, Mariotto AB, Kramer JL, Rowland JH, Stein KD, Alteri R, Jemal A (2016) Cancer treatment and survivorship statistics, 2016. CA Cancer J Clin 66(4):271–289
18. Perkins A, Liu G (2016) Primary brain tumors in adults: diagnosis and treatment. Am Fam Physician 93(3):211–217
19. Hecht SS, Carmella SG, Murphy SE, Stepanov I, Balbo S, Hatsukami DK, Yuan J-M, Park SL, Stram DO, Haiman C (2016) Tobacco smoke toxicant and carcinogen biomarkers and lung cancer susceptibility in smokers. J Thorac Oncol 11(2):S7–S8
20. Gazdar AF, Zhou C (2018) Lung cancer in never-smokers: a different disease. In: IASLC thoracic oncology. Elsevier, pp 23–29.e23

21. Kuper H, Adami HO, Boffetta P (2002) Tobacco use, cancer causation and public health impact. J Intern Med 251(6):455–466
22. Kushi LH, Byers T, Doyle C, Bandera EV, McCullough M, Gansler T, Andrews KS, Thun MJ (2006) American Cancer Society guidelines on nutrition and physical activity for cancer prevention: reducing the risk of cancer with healthy food choices and physical activity. CA Cancer J Clin 56(5):254–281
23. Park S, Bae J, Nam B-H, Yoo K-Y (2008) Aetiology of cancer in Asia. Asian Pac J Cancer Prev 9(3):371–380
24. Pagano JS, Blaser M, Buendia M-A, Damania B, Khalili K, Raab-Traub N, Roizman B (2004) Infectious agents and cancer: criteria for a causal relation. In: Seminars in cancer biology, vol 6. Elsevier, Amsterdam, pp 453–471
25. Sonker P, Tewari AK, Chaube SK, Kumar R, Sharma VP, Sonker A, Yadav P (2018) A study on cancer and its drugs with their molecular structure and mechanism of action: A Review. World J Pharm Sci 6(7):13–34
26. Samaras V, Rafailidis PI, Mourtzoukou EG, Peppas G, Falagas ME (2010) Chronic bacterial and parasitic infections and cancer: a review. J Infect Dev Ctries 4(05):267–281
27. Brenner DJ, Hall EJ (2007) Computed tomography—an increasing source of radiation exposure. N Engl J Med 357(22):2277–2284
28. Roukos DH (2009) Genome-wide association studies: how predictable is a person's cancer risk? Expert Rev Anticancer Ther 9(4):389–392
29. Green J, Cairns BJ, Casabonne D, Wright FL, Reeves G, Beral V, collaborators MWS (2011) Height and cancer incidence in the Million Women Study: prospective cohort, and meta-analysis of prospective studies of height and total cancer risk. Lancet Oncol 12(8):785–794
30. Forschungsgemeinschaft D (2015) Carcinogenic substances. In: List of MAK and BAT values 2015: permanent senate commission for the investigation of health hazards of chemical compounds in the work area, pp 163–181
31. Jeon S-Y, Hwang K-A, Choi K-C (2016) Effect of steroid hormones, estrogen and progesterone, on epithelial mesenchymal transition in ovarian cancer development. J Steroid Biochem Mol Biol 158:1–8
32. Breitling R, Takano E (2016) Synthetic biology of natural products. Cold Spring Harb Perspect Biol 8(10):a023994
33. Carroll D, Golic MM, Bibikova M, Drews G, Golic KG (2016) Targeted chromosomal mutagenesis using zinc finger nucleases. Google Patents
34. Forsyth A, Weeks T, Richael C, Duan H (2016) Transcription activator-like effector nucleases (TALEN)-mediated targeted DNA insertion in potato plants. Front Plant Sci 7:1572
35. Huang M, Zhou X, Wang H, Xing D (2018) Clustered regularly interspaced short palindromic repeats/Cas9 triggered isothermal amplification for site-specific nucleic acid detection. Anal Chem 90(3):2193–2200
36. Smith JJ, Jantz D, Hellinga HW (2011) Rationally-designed meganucleases with altered sequence specificity and DNA-binding affinity. Google Patents
37. Baker M (2011) Gene-editing nucleases. Nature Publishing Group, London
38. Bosley KS, Botchan M, Bredenoord AL, Carroll D, Charo RA, Charpentier E, Cohen R, Corn J, Doudna J, Feng G (2015) CRISPR germline engineering—the community speaks. Nat Biotechnol 33(5):478
39. Stoddard BL (2005) Homing endonuclease structure and function. Q Rev Biophys 38(1):49–95
40. Loong SLE (2005) Late Radiation Morbidity Incidence in a South-East Scottish cohort and investigation into abnormalities in DNA double-strand break repair and damage response. Edinburgh Medical School thesis. http://hdl.handle.net/1842/24851
41. De Souza N (2011) Primer: genome editing with engineered nucleases. Nat Methods 9(1):27
42. Smith J, Grizot S, Arnould S, Duclert A, Epinat J-C, Chames P, Prieto J, Redondo P, Blanco FJ, Bravo J (2006) A combinatorial approach to create artificial homing endonucleases cleaving chosen sequences. Nucleic Acids Res 34(22):e149–e149
43. Seligman LM, Chisholm KM, Chevalier BS, Chadsey MS, Edwards ST, Savage JH, Veillet AL (2002) Mutations altering the cleavage specificity of a homing endonuclease. Nucleic Acids Res 30(17):3870–3879

44. Chevalier BS, Kortemme T, Chadsey MS, Baker D, Monnat RJ Jr, Stoddard BL (2002) Design, activity, and structure of a highly specific artificial endonuclease. Mol Cell 10(4):895–905
45. Arnould S, Chames P, Perez C, Lacroix E, Duclert A, Epinat J-C, Stricher F, Petit A-S, Patin A, Guillier S (2006) Engineering of large numbers of highly specific homing endonucleases that induce recombination on novel DNA targets. J Mol Biol 355(3):443–458
46. Ashworth J, Taylor GK, Havranek JJ, Quadri SA, Stoddard BL, Baker D (2010) Computational reprogramming of homing endonuclease specificity at multiple adjacent base pairs. Nucleic Acids Res 38(16):5601–5608
47. Redondo P, Prieto J, Munoz IG, Alibés A, Stricher F, Serrano L, Cabaniols J-P, Daboussi F, Arnould S, Perez C (2008) Molecular basis of xeroderma pigmentosum group C DNA recognition by engineered meganucleases. Nature 456(7218):107
48. Aslam S, Khan SH, Ahmed A, Dandekar AM (2019) Genome editing tools: need of the current era. Am J Mol Biol 9(3):85–109
49. Rebar EJ, Huang Y, Hickey R, Nath AK, Meoli D, Nath S, Chen B, Xu L, Liang Y, Jamieson AC (2002) Induction of angiogenesis in a mouse model using engineered transcription factors. Nat Med 8(12):1427
50. Kim Y-G, Cha J, Chandrasegaran S (1996) Hybrid restriction enzymes: zinc finger fusions to Fok I cleavage domain. Proc Natl Acad Sci 93(3):1156–1160
51. Cox DBT, Platt RJ, Zhang F (2015) Therapeutic genome editing: prospects and challenges. Nat Med 21(2):121
52. Reik A, Zhou Y, Wagner J, Hamlett A, Mendel M, Liu P-Q, Lee G, Paschon D, Rebar E, Ando D (2008) Zinc finger nucleases targeting the glucocorticoid receptor allow IL-13 zetakine transgenic CTLs to kill glioblastoma cells in vivo in the presence of immunosuppressing glucocorticoids. AACR Annual Meeting, San Diego, CA
53. Holt N, Wang J, Kim K, Friedman G, Wang X, Taupin V, Crooks GM, Kohn DB, Gregory PD, Holmes MC (2010) Human hematopoietic stem/progenitor cells modified by zinc-finger nucleases targeted to CCR5 control HIV-1 in vivo. Nat Biotechnol 28(8):839
54. Gaj T, Gersbach CA, Barbas CF III (2013) ZFN, TALEN, and CRISPR/Cas-based methods for genome engineering. Trends Biotechnol 31(7):397–405
55. Pérez-Quintero AL, Rodriguez-R LM, Dereeper A, López C, Koebnik R, Szurek B, Cunnac S (2013) An improved method for TAL effectors DNA-binding sites prediction reveals functional convergence in TAL repertoires of Xanthomonas oryzae strains. PLoS One 8(7):e68464
56. Aliyari R, Ding SW (2009) RNA-based viral immunity initiated by the dicer family of host immune receptors. Immunol Rev 227(1):176–188
57. Barrangou R (2015) The roles of CRISPR–Cas systems in adaptive immunity and beyond. Curr Opin Immunol 32:36–41
58. Zhang F, Wen Y, Guo X (2014) CRISPR/Cas9 for genome editing: progress, implications and challenges. Hum Mol Genet 23(R1):R40–R46
59. Sternberg SH, Doudna JA (2015) Expanding the biologist's toolkit with CRISPR-Cas9. Mol Cell 58(4):568–574
60. Barrangou R, Fremaux C, Deveau H, Richards M, Boyaval P, Moineau S, Romero DA, Horvath P (2007) CRISPR provides acquired resistance against viruses in prokaryotes. Science 315(5819):1709–1712
61. Marraffini LA, Sontheimer EJ (2008) CRISPR interference limits horizontal gene transfer in staphylococci by targeting DNA. Science 322(5909):1843–1845
62. Mohanraju P, Makarova KS, Zetsche B, Zhang F, Koonin EV, Van der Oost J (2016) Diverse evolutionary roots and mechanistic variations of the CRISPR-Cas systems. Science 353(6299):aad5147
63. Hille F, Richter H, Wong SP, Bratovič M, Ressel S, Charpentier E (2018) The biology of CRISPR-Cas: backward and forward. Cell 172(6):1239–1259
64. Makarova KS, Wolf YI, Alkhnbashi OS, Costa F, Shah SA, Saunders SJ, Barrangou R, Brouns SJ, Charpentier E, Haft DH (2015) An updated evolutionary classification of CRISPR–Cas systems. Nat Rev Microbiol 13(11):722

65. Wright AV, Nuñez JK, Doudna JA (2016) Biology and applications of CRISPR systems: harnessing nature's toolbox for genome engineering. Cell 164(1–2):29–44
66. Westra ER, Dowling AJ, Broniewski JM, van Houte S (2016) Evolution and ecology of CRISPR. Annu Rev Ecol Evol Syst 47:307–331
67. Dugar G, Herbig A, Förstner KU, Heidrich N, Reinhardt R, Nieselt K, Sharma CM (2013) High-resolution transcriptome maps reveal strain-specific regulatory features of multiple Campylobacter jejuni isolates. PLoS Genet 9(5):e1003495
68. Hatoum-Aslan A, Maniv I, Marraffini LA (2011) Mature clustered, regularly interspaced, short palindromic repeats RNA (crRNA) length is measured by a ruler mechanism anchored at the precursor processing site. Proc Natl Acad Sci 108(52):21218–21222
69. Yosef I, Goren MG, Qimron U (2012) Proteins and DNA elements essential for the CRISPR adaptation process in Escherichia coli. Nucleic Acids Res 40(12):5569–5576
70. Swarts DC, Mosterd C, Van Passel MW, Brouns SJ (2012) CRISPR interference directs strand specific spacer acquisition. PLoS One 7(4):e35888
71. Mussolino C, Alzubi J, Fine EJ, Morbitzer R, Cradick TJ, Lahaye T, Bao G, Cathomen T (2014) TALENs facilitate targeted genome editing in human cells with high specificity and low cytotoxicity. Nucleic Acids Res 42(10):6762–6773
72. Rinaldo AR, Ayliffe M (2015) Gene targeting and editing in crop plants: a new era of precision opportunities. Mol Breed 35(1):40
73. Regalado A (2015) CRISPR gene editing to be tested on people by 2017, says Editas. MIT Technol Rev:1–3
74. Cromwell CR, Sung K, Park J, Krysler AR, Jovel J, Kim SK, Hubbard BP (2018) Incorporation of bridged nucleic acids into CRISPR RNAs improves Cas9 endonuclease specificity. Nat Commun 9(1):1448
75. Charpentier M, Khedher A, Menoret S, Brion A, Lamribet K, Dardillac E, Boix C, Perrouault L, Tesson L, Geny S (2018) CtIP fusion to Cas9 enhances transgene integration by homology-dependent repair. Nat Commun 9(1):1133
76. Chen JS, Dagdas YS, Kleinstiver BP, Welch MM, Sousa AA, Harrington LB, Sternberg SH, Joung JK, Yildiz A, Doudna JA (2017) Enhanced proofreading governs CRISPR–Cas9 targeting accuracy. Nature 550(7676):407
77. Hu JH, Miller SM, Geurts MH, Tang W, Chen L, Sun N, Zeina CM, Gao X, Rees HA, Lin Z (2018) Evolved Cas9 variants with broad PAM compatibility and high DNA specificity. Nature 556(7699):57
78. Sakuma T, Yamamoto T (2018) Acceleration of cancer science with genome editing and related technologies. Cancer Sci 109(12):3679
79. Haapaniemi E, Botla S, Persson J, Schmierer B, Taipale J (2018) CRISPR–Cas9 genome editing induces a p53-mediated DNA damage response. Nat Med 24(7):927

New Adsorption-Based Biosensors for Cancer Detections and Role of Nano-medicine in Its Prognosis and Inhibition

5

Naheed Bibi, Iram Taj Awan, and Almas Taj Awan

5.1 Introduction

Rise in the cancer mortality is indeed mostly accredited to the detection of cancer in its advanced stage, which sometimes makes the controlling of the disease inefficient with subsequent treatment. In order to potentially reduce cancer-related mortality, a device that is efficient and capable of diagnosing cancer at its initial stages in routine checkups can bring revolution in this debate. The possibility of tracking cancer exists well before the symptoms are expressed [1], through the identification of cancer biomarkers. According to the National Cancer Institute of the United States, biomarkers can indicate abnormalities such as cancer [2] when they are found in different tissues and body fluids. They can also indicate the type of cancer and its degree of progress by the concentration of the type of protein found in the fluid/tissue. There are specific biomarkers associated with different kinds of cancer [3]. Various biomarkers are used in treating patients and the development of new forms of diagnosis/prognosis. These biomarkers can be detected through some analytical devices of great sensitivity and selectivity [4–6] at early stage disease. Noteworthy are the proteins, the specific interaction of antibodies with antigens (AB-AG) and nucleic acids (DNA, mRNA). An example is gene p53 that is inactive in various types of tumors, e.g., leukemia, lung, gastrointestinal, breast, and adrenocortical and skin cancers [7]. This prospect has taken worldwide attention toward a huge search for appropriate biomarkers.

N. Bibi (✉)
Department of Chemistry, Shaheed Benazir Bhutto Women University (SBBWU), Peshawar, Pakistan

I. T. Awan
São Carlos Institute of Physics, University of São Paulo (IFSC-USP), São Paulo, SP, Brazil

A. T. Awan
Department of Chemistry, Federal University of São Carlos (UFSCar), São Carlos, SP, Brazil

N. Masood, S. Shakil Malik (eds.), *'Essentials of Cancer Genomic, Computational Approaches and Precision Medicine*,
https://doi.org/10.1007/978-981-15-1067-0_5

Widely, biosensors have been produced by taking in use the molecular engineering, where the synergy of the constituent material provides great sensitivity and selectivity to the sensors [8, 9]. Many devices are fabricated in a layer-by-layer manner, where a bioactive layer is placed over a suitably selected matrix [9–13]. In this regard, most methods to detect the biomarkers make use of the strategy of the specific interaction that takes place between the immobilized/stranded biomolecules on a biosensor and the biomarkers on the cells in the sample [14]. The biosensors in this way are referred to as immunosensors as they involve the interaction of antigen and antibody [14]. Performance excellence by such biosensing schemes may be specifically relevant to the early and efficient detection of cancer, which is a source of great motivation behind all the extensive work going on in this field.

Hereof, various different types of immunosensors have been made, each kind with a different principle of detection. These detection principles involve surface plasmon resonance [15–17], electrochemistry [18–20], piezoelectricity [21, 22], chemiluminescence, and impedance spectroscopy [9, 23, 24]. In this chapter, we are going to emphasize on the sensing units that are based on the models of adsorption. These units are made by incorporating nanostructured films with the aid of methods like self-assembling of monolayers (SAMs) [25] and layer-by-layer (LBL) [26, 27]. These two methods are suitable methods, as they preserve the activity of the adsorbed biomolecules.

In the case of adsorption, after the initial work from Langmuir, adsorption models have been approved from quite some time [28]. Through the Langmuir model, it can be explained and quantified how an adsorbate forms a monolayer on a surface, depending on ionic equilibrium among the solid-liquid phases [28, 29]. For instance, with a little modification, the Langmuir-Freundlich model is indeed a useful model to explain and demonstrate how adsorption takes place on heterogeneous surfaces, as it considers the possibility of successful adsorption in multilayers. Despite the simplifications that these two models possess, these are capable to be applied to explain the adsorption of macromolecules, such as to the semiconducting polymers, when they are applied in a layer-by-layer way [30]. Here we describe the working of immunosensors based on the principle of adsorption by using Langmuir and Langmuir-Freundlich models. Distinct methods have been developed and applied to verify the adsorption of biomolecules, e.g., polarization modulation-infrared reflection-absorption spectroscopy (PM-IRRAS), nano-gravimetry with a quartz crystal microbalance (QCM), and atomic force microscopy (AFM).

5.1.1 Biosensor and Cancer

A biosensor is essentially a device which is useful in the detection of any biological molecule/analyte that can be a part of the environment or present in any biological species (i.e., within living species), as shown in Fig. 5.1. A biosensor typically consists of three parts which are recognition element, signal transducer, and a signal processor that finally processes and shows a result. The recognition element tends to recognize the signal from the analyte, where the transducer is incorporated to

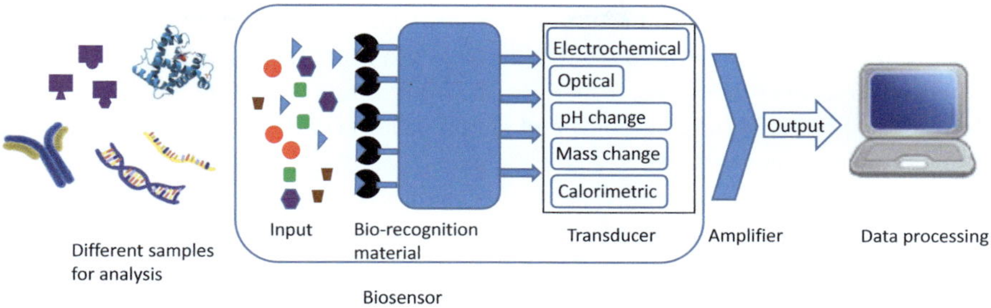

Fig. 5.1 Illustration of working of a biosensor

convert the biological signal into an electrical signal at the output [31]. Information like whether an analyte is present in a living being and up to what extent can be transduced into an electrical signal which may later be amplified, displayed, and analyzed. The analytes may include biological components, any metabolic component like glucose, nucleic acid, and proteins (such as antigen, antibodies, and enzymes).

Within the area of medicine, such biosensors can be employed to display sugar levels in diabetic patients, for detection of pathogens and for the diagnosis and monitoring of cancer. In military line, the biosensors are of potential interest to diagnose any warfare elements of chemical and biological nature in order to avoid any infections due to potential exposure. In the future biosensors would also include chip-scale devices that would be installed on the human body to detect any vital signals and for the correction of any abnormalities or even for signaling call in case of an emergency. Hence, there are unlimited ways in which biosensors can make our lives easier.

In the case of cancer, biosensors mainly detect the analyte which is held responsible for the presence of a tumor in a patient. By measuring the extent of the level of a certain protein, biosensors can diagnose the presence or absence of tumor and whether or not a certain treatment helped in curing cancer cells and so on. Since in many cancer types multiple biomarkers are involved, biosensors capable of detecting multiple analytes are effective. This ability of a biosensor to test and recognize simultaneously multiple markers not only is helpful in cancer diagnosis but is also a time-saving and a financially friendly possibility.

5.1.2 Biomarkers

According to the National Cancer Institute, biomarkers are defined as biological molecules that are found in blood or in different body fluids, or in tissues, which possess signs for any normal or abnormal condition, process, or disease. This is how biomarkers can be utilized to evaluate how a body responds to a specific disease and to a specific treatment. There can be various molecular origins for the biomarkers such as DNA (translocation, amplification, specific mutation, and loss of heterozygosity), RNA, or protein (antibody, tumor suppressor, hormone, or specific genes). In this regard, cancer biomarkers are potentially one of the valuable tools for the cancer detection. Typically, the body fluids where the biomarkers are detected are blood serum, cerebral and spinal fluid, urine, or the tumor cells [32]. Some of the cancer biomarkers with the cancer types they cause are listed here, for example, CA19-9 is potentially held responsible for the pancreatic cancer [33], CA15-3 for the breast cancer [34], Her-2/neu for the stage IV breast cancer [35], and PSA for the prostate cancer [36]. Most cancer biomarkers, however, have yet to show sufficient specificity and sensitivity regarding the monitoring of cancer treatments, which is where biosensor technology can prove itself to be of vital importance.

5.1.3 Manufacturing of a Biosensor

Fabrication of sensing units mostly possesses some metal electrodes plus nanostructured matrix and organic films containing biomolecules. The use of nanomaterial films in the bioanalytical devices has proven itself critical as it enhances the sensitivity and detection limits of devices for the detection of single molecules [37]. Besides, such biosensors are cheaper, faster, and robust alternatives to the bulky devices traditionally used for early cancer detection. Furthermore, the use of such films brings versatility in biosensors in terms of their synergy, like which nano-film to be used and with which combination of films a sensing unit can perform better. Unfortunately, there is no general rule discovered so far for this purpose. Systematic studies are needed to optimize the synergy issues in biosensing. A variety of nanomaterials are used in the build-out of biosensor immobilization; few examples are carbon nanotubes [38], titanium dioxide (TiO_2) [39], and graphene [40].

The group [9] used mainly gold electrodes that consist of 50 pairs of interdigitated electrodes with the breadth of each digit as 10 μm and spaced 10 μm away from each other. Two methods are mainly employed to put nanostructured organic films on such sensing units (the gold electrodes); these are named as (1) layer-by-layer and (2) self-assembling of monolayer. Using any of these techniques, multilayers are carefully selected and assembled sequentially over one another, on the electrodes, where the final layer of deposition is the layer of analyte (cancer antibodies). These antibodies are the biomarkers that correspond to a specific cancer type. The techniques applied to put layers on the electrodes are described as follows.

5.1.3.1 Layer-by-Layer (LBL) Scheme

Layer-by-layer is the self-assembly scheme by physical adsorption, which lets the fabrication of organized ultrathin robust films of bigger size with the film thickness and properties that can be precisely controlled in nanometer scale [41]. It is based on a relatively simple and inexpensive method, where surface modification is obtained by layer-by-layer adsorption of polyelectrolyte of opposite charges in aqueous solution. This technique allows to organize individual molecules in alternate layers with thickness control at the molecular level, which enables the planning of the final properties of the films. A wide variety of materials can be deposited by using the LBL scheme. Some materials to name are polyions, nanoparticles, metals, biological molecules, and ceramics. By using LBL, a combination of polyethyleneimine and carbon nanotubes was used to adsorb antibodies like anti-CA19-9 [38], for detecting CA19-9 antigen.

5.1.3.2 Self-Assembled Monolayers (SAMs)

When the organic molecules are self-assembled in the form of films, by the chemical adsorption of an active surfactant on a solid surface, it is called as self-assembling of monolayers (SAMs). The chemical group (the head group) present in the molecules usually has a strong affinity with the substrate, which helps to anchor the molecule to the substrate. The type of the head group is selected, depending on the application of the SAM [42]. Typically, with the head group, a molecular chain is connected to which the terminal end can be functionalized, which brings variations in the wetting and interfacial properties [43]. The most commonly used functional groups are thiols, phosphonates, and silanes, which correspond to the polar part of the molecule. An appropriate substrate is chosen to react with the head group. Substrates can be planes such as metals and silicon or curved surfaces which can be obtained by the use of nanoparticles on a surface.

By using self-assembled monolayer (SAM), 11-mercaptoundecanoic acid (11-MUA) was anchored onto gold interdigitated electrode which was used to adsorb anti-CA19-9 antibodies [44] and anti-p53 antibodies [13], for the detection of CA19-9 and p53 antigens, respectively. In another work, a combination of SAM and LBL was used to combine films of polysaccharide chitosan and the protein concanavalin A, for the tracking of CA19-9 antigen [9]. All these studies lead to the formation of adsorption-based biosensors.

5.1.4 Adsorption and Biosensing

Adsorption processes are particularly important to understand in biosensors which are built using the LBL and SAMs, as the thin films are adsorbed on the sensing surface. In general, an adsorption isotherm is a curve that describes adsorption phenomena, by describing the mobility of a substance from the aquatic environments to a solid phase, having pH and temperature as constant [45, 46]. The ratio between the adsorbed amounts with the remaining in the solution is called as an adsorption equilibrium. It is established when an adsorbate remains in contact with an adsorbent for a sufficient amount of time, where the adsorbate concentration of the bulk solution remains in dynamic balance with the interface concentration [47, 48].

In terms of three fundamental approaches, some equilibrium isotherm models have been expressed. The first of which considers the kinetics of adsorption, where the adsorption equilibrium is defined as a state of dynamic equilibrium, with the same rates of adsorption and desorption. The second approach is based on the thermodynamics and provides a framework for deriving adsorption isotherm models.

The third approach (which is mainly utilized in cancer biosensing) exploits the main idea of generating characteristic curves, which is an approach mainly used in exploring the adsorption behaviors taking place in immunosensors. However, in modeling the isotherm, derivation with more than one approach can prove interesting, as it directs to the difference in the physical interpretation of the parameters of the model. Soares et al. [44] have performed several studies where they developed cancer biosensors and proved that adsorption was the reason behind biosensing. They found that for most of their biosensors, Langmuir and Langmuir-Freundlich adsorption models worked well to explain the adsorption behaviors in their biosensors.

5.1.5 PM-IRRAS: A Means of Characterization

The sensing mechanism that arises due to the specific adsorption in immunosensors can be verified by the use of polarization modulation-infrared reflection-absorption spectroscopy (PM-IRRAS). It is a spectroscopic technique used to characterize thin films or monolayers on metal substrates as it possesses certain advantages like high surface sensitivity. For such spectroscopy, each layer in the sensor matrix (which is the principal building block of such sensors) is characterized. A spectrum is measured after adsorption of each matrix layer onto the sensor. The spectrum of the whole matrix is taken as a reference spectrum for the characterization of thin films of antibody-antigen, which gives an understanding of the interaction between both the films. Soares et al. [44] observed such spectrum, which shows the interaction between antibodies and different concentrations of CA19-9 antigens. They found bands assigned to the amide II and amide I groups. These functional groups are present in both antigen and antibody analytes and are the main responsible for the molecular interactions between the two. For their biosensor, they observed that as the analyte concentration elevated, the area under the curve and the intensity of these bands increased as well, which evidenced the process of adsorption.

5.1.6 Impedance Spectroscopy as a Method of Detection

Impedance spectroscopy is employed to detect the analyte solutions in adsorption-based biosensors. It is preferable as it does not need any reference electrodes and hence allows for the miniaturization of the electrodes/sensors. To perform the impedance spectroscopy, the sensing unit is subjected to solutions of different antigen concentrations, and the spectroscopy is performed for each analyte concentration, one by one. For that, different concentrations of antigen solution are prepared by diluting it in the PBS solution. The electrode is immersed in each solution and then left for a suitable time, so to adsorb maximum antigens on the electrode. The electrode is then cleaned with distilled water and carefully dried with a low flux of N_2 gas. Afterward, impedance behavior is recorded. For the impedance measurements, the capacitance values are recorded over a frequency range of $1–10^6$ Hz. This is done using software packages ZView 2 and ZPlot 2. An illustration of the impedance characteristics obtained for a biosensor that is more responsive at low frequencies (1–100 Hz) is shown in Fig. 5.2. For illustration purpose capacitance curves for different arbitrary antigen concentrations are shown, along with the curve of the antibody solution. The antibody curve serves as a reference for all other curves to show the interaction of different antigen solutions with the immunosensor. It is experimentally observed that the capacitance increases with the analyte concentration, until it gets saturated, which is a typical behavior for the immunosensors based on the interaction of the antigen-antibodies, as shown in Fig. 5.2. In the case of immunosensors, in addition to the different antigen solutions, the electrode is also tested against solutions like ascorbic acid, glucose, etc. These solutions are called as the negative control solutions and, therefore, are used to check the specificity of the sensor.

Such impedance measurements give information on which frequencies are more responsive to the biosensing properties of a particular sensor. Sensor [49] showed more response at low frequency, as a considerable distinction between the different curves in such frequency was observed. In other words, at low frequency, the electrical response of that particular sensing device got affected by the interaction with the analyte. Similarly, some biosensors can be more responsive in the middle frequencies that are around 1 kHz. Sensitivity at the low frequencies is owed to the changes induced by the analyte layer on the electrical double layer that existed between solid- and liquid-charged interfaces. There are studies [50, 51] that showed that the electrical responses at low frequencies around and below 100 Hz are dominated by the changes in the double layer. In the 1 kHz region, film properties remain dominant, and at high frequencies, mostly capacitance changes refer to the change in the geometrical capacitance. That's the reason the intermediate frequencies are given more importance and then the low frequencies are given at the second place while accessing sensing response of a sensing unit.

Once the best frequencies are obtained for a biosensor, a capacitance versus concentration curve can be achieved, also termed as a calibration curve, by considering the capacitance values for different analyte concentrations at the ideal frequency.

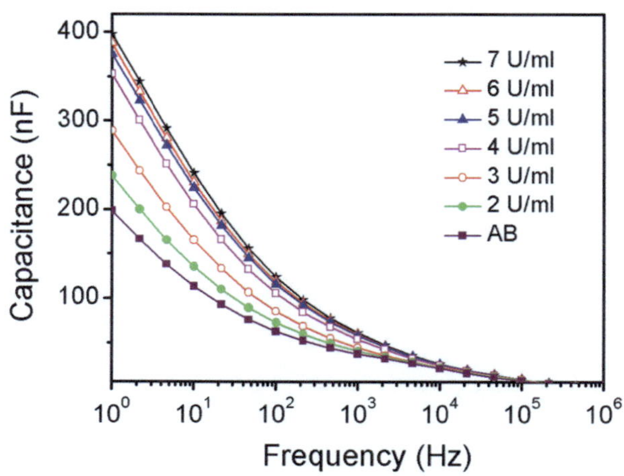

Fig. 5.2 Illustration of the impedance characteristics obtained when a sensing unit is exposed to the solution of antibody and various antigen concentrations

The calibration curve in adsorption-based biosensors is important as this data can be fitted with any suitable adsorption model. Mostly Langmuir or Langmuir-Freundlich adsorption models give best fittings to such curves, showing the nature of adsorption that takes place in such immunosensors [44].

5.1.7 Determining the Limit of Detection

In order to check the sensitivity of a cancer biosensor, it is vital to investigate on the limit of detection (LD) that refers to the lowest amount of antigen detected by a sensor. LD is determined using the IUPAC method:

$$\mathrm{LD} = \frac{3 \times \mathrm{SD}}{\alpha}$$

where SD is the standard deviation and α is the slope of the curve, which can be measured by taking the initial part of the curve and approximating a straight line [38]. In immunosensors, the lowest amount of antigen detected means the highest the sensitivity the sensor has [38].

5.1.8 Information Visualization for Biosensing

Statistical methods such as principal component analysis (PCA) [52] are commonly used to treat the biosensing data. However, optimization of the biosensing performance may be obtained by using information visualization methods that makes possible to evaluate the data in detail, especially when the examination of a selective feature is desired. This is particularly relevant for the sensors that are explored through impedance spectroscopy, as the electrical response of the analytes varies significantly with the frequency of the applied field, where the sensing event may arise at only specific frequency range. Indeed, the low-frequency region (100 Hz or less) is the most relevant, particularly when the sensing of a sensor depends on the variations in the electrical double layer, which is formed at the interface of the solid and liquid, on a charged surface. In such cases, the capacitance spectra are proceeded using a free software suite named Pex sensors [53], which is an information visualization software used to treat the impedance data. The projection technique it uses is called an Interactive Document Mapping (IDMAP) [54], which takes into account the interactive maps in 2-D(IDMAP) and parallel coordinates (PC) to project the capacitance or the impedance data. It considers the Euclidean distances to perform mapping of the data points.

Suppose that the impedance versus frequency curves can be represented by $X = \{x1, x2, \ldots, xn\}$, where the dissimilarity between the two samples (i and j) is given by $\delta\,(xi, xj)$ and the distance between the two projected data points (yi and yj) is given by $d(yi - yj)$. The data through IDMAP is projected on a 2D space, using an injective function f: $X \rightarrow Y$, which minimizes the so-called cost or error function, $| \delta(xi, xj) - d(yi - yj) \; \forall \; xi, xj \in X$, defined with the following equation. [54]:

$$\text{SIDMAP} = \frac{\delta(xi,xj) - \delta_{\min}}{\delta_{\max} - \delta_{\min}} - d(yi - yj)$$

where $\delta_{\max}$ and $\delta_{\min}$ are the maximum and the minimum distances between the data instances measured in the original space. In this way, a visual representation of the data is generated that reveals the distribution of data and its correlations.

The importance of using such visualization technique owes from the fact that when sensing through a biosensor is performed for multiple varieties of samples, it is almost impossible to get some useful information by plotting the data in mere x–y plots. The conversion of such information with the help of a multidimensional technique, in a way to check the similarity relationships among the different data instances, is indeed very helpful. In this regard, IDMAP is a nonlinear mapping which has been proved to be the best strategy that can be adapted to represent the biosensor data.

5.1.9 Specificity of the Detection of a Sensor

One of the challenges is to avoid the non-specific adsorption, onto the immunosensors, to obtain them with a highly selective nature. A highly selective nature of a biosensor translates that the principles of detection of the sensor only gets affected by the interaction of that specific antigen and antibody pair, for which the sensor is made. For this purpose, experimental procedures are adopted to guarantee the selectivity of a certain immunosensor. The reactivity of a sensor that is made to respond to the reaction of only one specific antigen-antibody pair is tested against various other antigens and non-specific analytes which are part of the blood samples taken from the patients. As an example, an immunosensor made for the detection of anti-p53-BSA [13] was verified against various other antigens and analytes like HCV antigen (responsible for hepatitis C), p24 antigen (for the HIV), glucose, uric acid, and ascorbic acid, respectively. In this regard, all the analytes and antigen solutions tested were made in commercially prepared PBS solutions. It was observed from the plot of charge transfer resistance calculated from the impedance data for the film (when exposed to each analyte) that the only solution which gave visibly different values from the PBS buffer solution was the solution of antigen p53. The rest of all other analytes showed Rct values very similar to that of the PBS buffer, with the anomaly for the ascorbic acid that showed some effect on the immunosensor, yet it was also effortlessly identifiable from the large effect caused by the p53 antigen, for whose detection the sensor was made. This testing method is sufficient to evidence the selectivity of any biosensor.

Such kind of subsidiary experiments with cell lines and possible interferents is always important to interpret the selectivity of an immunosensor so as to avoid false positives and false negatives.

5.1.10 Data Analysis: Use of Pex Sensors

The impedance data can also be visualized by the use of a visualization technique that is a multidimensional projection technique described in Sect. 5.1.9. With the aid of such technique, it is possible to plot a large set of samples in a small space, which aids in easy and simple analysis of a huge number of samples altogether, where the dissimilar samples lie far from each other and the samples that show similar behavior with the immunosensor lie close to each other in space.

For this purpose, different categories of solutions are prepared; here we will discuss about three categories: (1) the ones with different concentrations of cell line lysates that contain the specific cancer biomarker (referred to as the positive samples), (2) the ones with different concentrations of cell line lysates that do not contain any cancer biomarker (referred to as negative samples), and (3) the ones which are obtained by mixing specific antigen with commercially acquired PBS buffer solution (instead of the cell line lysates) to obtain the different concentrations of solutions (referred to as the standard samples). The first two categories can also be termed as the real samples, as they are diluted in the bovine serum albumin (BSA) solution and not in the PBS. These all three categories of solutions were tested against the specific immunosensor, and the impedance responses were observed by [13]. Such impedance versus frequency responses were plotted using the technique of IDMAP. The IDMAP shows data obtained for each sample as a point in the 2D space. It was noted that the standard and the real samples lied near to each other in the plot and showed the same tendency with increasing concentration. However, the negative samples lied far and lacked to show any specific pattern in terms of concentration, since for such samples the variations recorded in the electrical properties were much smaller, which usually instigate from the fluctuations due to sample dispersion. In this case, what really matters is the relative distance between the data points, and showing axis has no physical meaning, so the axis is usually not mentioned in the IDMAP plots. Subsequently, only the samples containing the specific biomarker can guarantee a positive response from the immunosensor, which confirms the immunosensor is sensitive toward a specific biomarker. For this very reason, the choice of an appropriate data analysis method is crucial in terms of enhancing the selectivity and sensitivity of sensors.

Once the tumor is detected, the focus shifts to advanced targeted therapies.

5.2 Advanced Targeted Therapies in Cancer

For cancers, surgery and radiotherapy are considered the most effective treatments. However, they are not efficient when cancer is transmitted throughout a human body. For treating metastatic cancer, it is important to have a treatment that can reach throughout the body using bloodstream. Therefore, the use of different drugs that serve for chemo-, hormonal, and biological therapies is common these days [55].

Chemotherapy deals with the usage of drugs that forbids fast proliferation of cancer cells although there are numerous side effects due to inhibition of rapid growth of healthy cells like those linked to hair follicles, bone marrow, etc. [55]. For many years, chemotherapeutic drugs that led to the indiscriminate destruction of cells were the only effective treatment of metastatic cancer even if this was not ideal and unspecific.

Discovery of cell signaling networks changed the way cancer was treated. Cell signaling constitutes a communication process to run and coordinate basic cell activities. This function is the basis of development, repairing damaged tissues and the immune system. In mammals, the interaction of cell signaling pathways forms networks [56]. The combination of experimental and computational/theoretical approaches is required for understanding cell signaling networks [57]. Research in the area of cell signaling networks further allowed drugs designing that were specific in their action toward specific networks, thus opening a new form of cancer treatment based on targeted therapy back in the late 1990s [55].

5.2.1 Targeted Therapies

Targeted therapies inhibit specific cellular pathways or protein molecules linked to tumor growth and disease progression. For instance, those protein molecules are the main targets that are found overexpressed/mutated in comparison to normal tissues. Such therapy works by either acting on one or more of the following functions [58]:

a. By blocking respective signals, to stop malignant cells from growing and dividing uncontrollably
b. By initiating apoptosis to cause the death of tumor cells
c. By stimulating the immune system
d. By chemotherapeutic drugs targeting specifically tumor cells, avoiding the mortality/injury of healthy cells [55, 59]

5.2.2 Types of Targeted Therapies

The kind of therapy that brings changes in cell signaling events is called the direct approach of targeted therapy [60], while the indirect approach involves targeting molecules expressed exceptionally on the exterior part of tumor cells. The indirect approach deals with cytotoxic molecules that are induced and later pair up with monoclonal antibodies through a chemical linker or involve nanocarriers that bring specificity compared to the conventional chemotherapy [61, 62].

Monoclonal antibodies are designed for connecting with specific proteins in cancer cells that are later recognized by the immune system to fight against and as a result lead to the death of such cells [58]. They also have the capability of preventing mitogenic signals by blocking the docking sites of growth factors [63]. In 1997, the very first monoclonal antibody was authorized by the FDA. It was named as rituximab and was used in targeted therapy [64]. Signaling pathways linked to abnormal cancer cell activities can also be blocked by small-molecule inhibitors mostly designed to interrupt tyrosine kinases [60, 65]. Angiogenic proteins produce new blood vessels' network that feeds the tumor. Such unwanted proteins can be attacked by monoclonal antibodies as well as small inhibitor molecular species [66]. The specificity of monoclonal antibodies coupled with chemotherapeutic drugs forms antibody-drug conjugates [58]. In recent years research has proved cytotoxic peptide conjugates as better alternatives to antibody-drug conjugates. Cytotoxic peptide conjugates can be 100 times smaller and have low cytotoxicity in comparison to antibody-drug conjugates [58].

5.2.2.1 Nanocarriers: Indirect Form of Target Therapy

Nanocarriers are used in the indirect form of target therapy. They are as submicron (<1 μm)/nanoscale colloidal systems with the ability to transport anticancer agents. Such agents can be small molecules of drugs or macromolecules such as proteins. Just as antibodies and peptide-drug conjugates act, nanocarriers are selective in targeting just cancer cells and avoiding normal cells, thus, in contrast to the free drugs, reducing toxicity for the rest of the body as side effects of therapy [58].

After entering the body, nanocarriers release the drug by swelling, degradation, erosion, or simply by diffusion [67].

5.2.3 Technological Advantages of Nanocarriers

The technological advantages of nanocarriers are as follows [67]:

a. High stability that protects drug degradation.
b. Renal clearance reduces, while their half-life in the blood flow increases.
c. Elevate carrier capacity of cytotoxic drugs, and many drug molecules can be carried in a single matrix.
d. Enable controlled release of the anticancer drugs from the matrix.
e. Viability of various routes of drug intake, such as oral and inhalation.
f. Ease of accepting both hydrophilic and hydrophobic substances.

5.2.3.1 Composition of Nanocarriers

Nanocarriers mainly include polymeric therapeutics and particulate drug nanocarriers as explained below:

5.2.3.2 Polymeric Therapeutics

In polymeric therapeutics, the anticancer drug or protein is covalently attached to the polymeric structure. They include polymer-protein and polymer-drug conjugates. They are aqua-soluble linear macromolecular structures with cleavable bonds. These structures are very stable during transportation while, once they arrive at the tumor site, the drug is released [68]. However, as the drug is released after the breakage of the linker between polymer and drug due to chemical or biological enzymatic degradation, it's also a bit difficult to control the drug release [58].

In 1994, the FDA approved the first polymer-protein conjugate known as pegaspargase for treating acute lymphoblastic leukemia [69, 70]. However, no polymer-drug conjugates are yet available commercially although clinical trials have increased many folds in the last few years [71]. Currently, around 20 polymer-drug conjugates are in clinical trials for cancer treatment [71–73].

5.2.3.3 Particulate Drug Nanocarriers

Such nanocarriers have drugs physically bagged inside the molecular assemblies composed of a variety of materials, thus providing physical protection to the anti-cancer drug from the outside environment and macrophages, for example, polymers, lipids, or organometallic compounds [58]. The following are some details about their types:

Liposomes

They are lipid-bilayered colloidal vesicles made up of amphiphilic phospholipids that can host encapsulation of both hydrophilic and hydrophobic agents using its aqueous or hydrophobic cores/membranes, respectively [74, 75]. They possess long circulation time in blood. They are biocompatible and almost inert by not causing any kind of reaction in the most number of patients as reported.

They have some limitations such as low drug loading, difficulty in sterilization, problems with stability, commercial reproducibility, phospholipid oxidation, and drug release kinetics [76–78].

Up to now, the FDA has approved only five liposome-based drugs linked to cancer treatment [58]. Recently, some new approaches in liposomal research have been evolved, and chemotherapeutic drugs coupled with stimuli-responsive release strategies have been part of clinical research [79, 80].

Carbon Nanotubes

They are tubelike hydrophobic networks. They are composed of carbon atoms. Their diameter is in the range of 1–4 nm (based on graphene layers), and length is 1–100 μm. They have unique chemical and physical properties [81, 82]. Although insoluble in all solvents, when chemical modifications are applied to them, they undergo structural transformation which makes them water-soluble carriers. This transformation helps in increasing the biocompatibility and decreasing their toxicity in living systems [83–85].

They have the capacity to include different anticancer drugs on their surface [86] or in their inner cavity [87, 88]. On the account of their vast surface area, they can accommodate high payload on their surface. They can easily enter the cancerous cells by passing through the plasma membrane by penetrating just like a thin needle or by the process of endocytosis [89, 90].

Although in vitro and in vivo passive targeting preclinical results are satisfactory in cancer treatment demonstrating that carbon nanotubes are promising nanocarriers, FDA has not yet approved any of the carbon nanotubes, neither are there any clinical trials in the process [58, 86, 88, 91].

Polymeric Nanocarriers

They are polymer-based nanocarriers of anticancer agents with a variety of structures. Liposomes have numerous advantages proven by their clinical validation; however, they have many problems with their stability and also limited control over the kinetics of the drug once they enter the system. For overcoming these liposomal limitations, polymeric nanocarriers present more stable in vivo studies. They proved high circulation times, increased loadings, and are capable of better controlled and targeted anticancer drug release control within in vivo literature studies [92, 93]. One of their examples is in the form of capsules/particles called polymeric nanoparticles.

5.3 Polymeric Nanoparticles in Targeted Therapy

Using biodegradable and biocompatible polymers (either natural or synthetic) allows controlled release of active agents from polymer nanoparticles by mechanisms of diffusion, erosion, or degradation [94, 95]. Such sustained long-term drug release is more effective compared to the pulse supply of agents in high concentration by chemotherapy [96].

In 1976, first-time polymeric systems were indicated for cancer treatment based on controlled release system [97]. Couvreur and colleagues in 1979 used polymeric nanoparticles for in vitro and in vivo studies. Polyalkylcyanoacrylate was the polymeric nanoparticles that were used for releasing doxorubicin [98].

Later, researchers continued to explore diverse options such as by advancements in polymer sciences; they developed biodegradable polymeric nanoparticles that are effective carriers for chemotherapy [58]. The last 10 years are very important in the advancement of scientific research in this area of polymeric nanoparticles. Few most promising preclinical studies in this area linked to active and passive cancer treatment are discussed in detail below:

5.3.1 Passive Targeting Polymeric Nanoparticles (NPs)

Due to enhanced permeability of the cancer cells, NPs accumulate in them due to the angiogenic process. As mentioned earlier, the tumor contains highly permeable blood vessels that allow nanoparticle accumulation, and thus the cytotoxic drug is released in the vicinity of tumor cells. The following are few examples of formulations of polymeric NPs that use passive targeting for cancer treatment.

5.3.1.1 Polymeric NPs Loaded with Cisplatin

Literature studies show that cisplatin when loaded upon gelatin-poly(acrylic acid) NPs (100 nm), drug release pattern was slow and controlled. This high-loaded drug showed stability and in vivo activity was enhanced in tumor cells. High drug accumulation was also found in the vicinity of liver cancer tumor when applied to the model of infected mice [99].

5.3.1.2 Polymeric NPs Loaded with Doxorubicin

Literature studies show that antitumor activity was increased in rat glioblastoma model when the doxorubicin-based lecithin containing poly(D,L-lactide-co-glycolic) acid/human serum albumin (PLGA/HAS) also covered with poloxamer 188 was used [100].

5.3.1.3 Polymeric NPs with Paclitaxel

Taxol is the commercial formulation of paclitaxel used in chemotherapy. Encapsulated paclitaxel into PEGylated (polyethylene glycol) PCL (polycaprolactone), PLGA nanoparticles, has shown an increase in the in vitro and in vivo cytotoxic effect [101]. Studies linked to human cervix carcinoma cells (HeLa) also proved greater anticancer activity when compared to Taxol. The in vivo studies linked to TLT (transplantable liver tumors) revealed that when the paclitaxel-loaded nanoparticles were used, tumor growth was inhibited in mice. For eradicating hypoxic tumor cells as well, paclitaxel encapsulation to poly(D,L-lactide-co-glycolic) acid (PLGA) nanoparticles is a promising formulation [58].

5.3.1.4 Polymeric NPs Loaded with Curcumin

Curcumin-loaded nanoparticles are around 80.9 nm in size and are biodegradable. Compared to sole curcumin, the in vivo effects such as anti-invasive, antitumor, and antiangiogenic activities are enhanced by encapsulating curcumin. Encapsulation helped to suppress proliferation in various forms of cancer cell lines [58].

5.3.1.5 Polymeric NPs That Incorporate Macromolecules

Macromolecules such as genes or proteins can also be incorporated in polymeric nanoparticles. For instance, during the angiogenic process, the main integrin that is involved is alfaV-beta3. When the RGD peptide was encapsulated by Kim et al. [102] that targets the alfaV-beta3 integrin, antitumor efficacy of the peptide was enhanced. In this study, self-assembled GCN (glycol chitosan nanoparticles) with 230 nm size were used that increased half-life of RGD involved in the in vivo studies. This led to a considerable increase in antitumoral and antiangiogenic effect. Therefore, free peptide activity was enhanced by encapsulation, and its intratumoral administration improved growth inhibition in cancer cells [58].

5.3.2 Active Targeting Polymeric Nanoparticles (NPs)

Active targeting involves functionalization of polymer NP surface. It refines the therapeutic efficacy of antitumor medicines and shows active targeting characteristics. It also helps in overcoming MDR (multidrug resistance) [103, 104]. Active targeting NPs involve specific ligands connected to the basic structure of NPs. They are capable of recognizing different overexpressed antigens or other receptors present on the exterior area of the cancer cell. The selectivity factor that comes with such recognition ability increases the anticancer effect in cancer cells while reducing many counter-effects due to other nonselective drugs [105].

5.3.2.1 Albumin-Based Targeting

Besides accumulating in the cancer site by enhanced permeability and retention (EPR) effect, albumin-based NPs stick with glycoprotein 60 receptor. This combination helps in endothelial transcytosis. The albumin nanoparticles are capable of binding to the BM-40 (SPARC, osteonectin) that is the albumin-binding protein overexpressed in the cancer cell and thus easily taken inside the tumor by endocytosis [106, 107].

5.3.2.2 Hyaluronic Acid-Based Targeting

The hyaluronic acid (HA) is biodegradable and biocompatible. It is capable of targeting cells where the glycoprotein CD44 receptor is overexpressed [108]. Amphiphilic HA nanoparticles are known to bind CD44 receptor in cancer cells [109]. Investigations by Cho et al. [110] show that hyaluronic acid ceramide conjugate and Pluronic P85 are nontoxic and can be used for transporting docetaxel. The <150 nm particle size allows the intravenous delivery of docetaxel both by active and passive targeting.

5.3.2.3 Biotin-Based Targeting

Biotin or vitamin H is effective against tumors. This vitamin is fast in proliferation for cancer cells that's why higher amounts are required [111]. For the targeted delivery of methotrexate to tumor cells, Taheri et al. [112, 113] investigated human serum albumin (HSA) nanoparticles. In their experiments, biotin was used as targeting ligand. In vitro results from their study proved increased cytotoxicity compared to non-functionalized particles.

5.3.2.4 Folate-Based Targeting

Folate or folic acid binds selectivity to the folate receptors present on the exterior part of the cell. Folate receptors are overexpressed in case of epithelial cancers, in hematologic cancers, as well as in sarcomas [114, 115]. The folate-based NPs once target the folate receptors on cancer cells become internalized and release the cytotoxic drug into the cytoplasm.

5.3.2.5 Transferrin-Based Targeting

Transferrin helps in transporting iron to growing cells. It is actually a membrane glycoprotein [116]. Transferrin receptors (TfRs) are present in high quantity on the exterior part of tumor tissues as the demand of iron increases. The formulations involving drug agents attached to transferrin that targets the TfRs on the cancer cells and, after endocytosis, release the drug inside infected cells [103].

5.3.2.6 Aptamer-Based Targeting

They are nucleic acid-based ligands, short in length. They are effective ligands just like folate and transferrin and are specific in targeting [117]. Literature study has shown that the prostate-specific membrane antigen (PSMA) aptamer-based NPs are 80 times more cytotoxic when applied to prostate cancer cells compared to the free drug [118].

5.3.2.7 Peptidic Targeting

Just like antibodies, peptides are utilized as ligands. They are less expensive and a bit complex compared to antibodies. As discussed earlier, integrin alfaV-beta3 is overexpressed on the exterior area of cancer cells, to easily get targeted by peptide ligands [119, 120].

5.4 Coordination Compounds as Anticancer Drugs

With the advent of cisplatin in chemotherapy, a whole new field of metal-based chemotherapeutics unfolded, and since then various metal complexes have been synthesized aiming at treating cancer [121]. Medicinal inorganic chemistry is extensively devoted to designing therapeutic agents for curing ailments not easily accessed by organic molecules [122]. Being positively charged, metal centers are capable of binding with the negatively charged biomolecules, whereas the constituents of biomolecules may serve as ligands for the metal center. Metal complexes have variable oxidation states, number and nature of the ligands attached, and flexibility of coordination geometries that allows them to be used as drugs. Their redox properties and ligand substitution reactions before reaching the site of action make them suitable candidates as "prodrugs." An important step in developing anticancer drugs is to control and manipulate the aforementioned processes/properties using thermodynamics and kinetics and devise a suitable mechanism for drug delivery.

Deposition of metal ions may have deleterious effects on the body; due to this reason, before using metal complexes as drugs, a vast study of their bio-distribution, clearance, and pharmacological specificity is carried out. Before entering clinical trials, the physiological effect of the potential drugs is investigated in vitro and in vivo on the related biomolecules.

For use as anticancer drugs, metal complexes are well-known for their effects on cellular processes like cell division and gene expression which get altered with cancer. In chemotherapy, the main focus is the destruction of cancerous cells, avoiding harm to the normal functioning cells.

5.4.1 Platinum Complexes as Anticancer Agents

A huge number of platinum compounds have been synthesized and subjected to tests and trials for their anticancer activity. However after the iconic mainstream cisplatin, carboplatin, and oxaliplatin, it has not been easy for new platinum-based chemotherapeutic agents to enter trials in clinics. Other three drugs, namely, heptaplatin, nedaplatin, and lobaplatin, have been tested and are in use in some countries [123]. The most well-known and extensively studied anticancer platinum compound "cisplatin" displays antitumor properties; however, its *trans* form does not show such behavior. Some of its derivatives have been proved to inhibit growth and contain N-H functionality, conferring donor properties which assist in the transport of the agent to the target. Anticancer platinum compounds are generally of *cis* geometry with the formula $[PtX_2(NHR_2)_2]$, where X is the leaving group and R is the alkyl or aromatic group. Many Pt(II) coordination compounds are known today that exhibit activity against cancerous cells, including a few examples of the *trans* isomers too. The exact mechanism of action of these compounds is elusive; however, it is evident that such compounds with other metals are not necessarily working against tumors [124]. The main reasons why platinum is more effective lie in the ligand exchange kinetics. The Pt-ligand bonding has less strength than covalent bonds; however, the ligand exchange phenomenon is very slow. This gives the compounds an extra kinetic stability, and the ligand exchange is slow to occur, taking long durations from minutes to days, contrary from other metal complexes that take seconds or even fraction of second. Pt(II) has an affinity for bonding to S-donor groups, making it harder to reach DNA helix due to the presence of many competing S-containing donor ligands in the cytosol. Another important property worth noting is the *trans* effect in Pt complexes [125, 126].

Cisplatin, despite its success story, has strong side effects like renal damage, hearing loss, anemia, etc. To counter these adverse effects because of non-selectivity of the therapeutic agent, modified or substituted cisplatin was introduced, leading to the second and third generations of the drug like oxaliplatin and carboplatin. Carboplatin, a second-generation Pt(II) drug with the formula $[Pt(C_6H_6O_4)(NH_3)_2]$, has lesser toxicity and is not highly reactive which allows administration of high dosage. Carboplatin is mainly used in ovarian cancer, and oxaliplatin serves best for colon cancer therapy [123]. Tumor cells pose a spontaneous drug resistance after being treated with these anticancer drugs which is a serious limitation of chemotherapy. This challenge has been countered by designing and developing new amines containing drugs that lack conventional *cis*-diamine and two leaving groups and hence giving rise to the third-generation Pt(II) drugs. Another approach to deal with resistance and side effects is to use a combination of different drugs that has a synergistic effect.

Cisplatin, which has the formula *cis*-$[PtCl_2(NH_3)_2]$, was introduced in the mid-1840s; however, its anticancer activity was not known till 1964. Its therapeutic properties have played wonders in solid tumors, especially ovarian, bladder, cerebral, and testicular tumors. The drug is given intravenously due to solubility issues, which transports by the process of diffusion through the cell membrane to the cytoplasm. An equilibrium establishes because the intracellular chloride ions are lesser in concentration than across the cell walls. Square planar geometry of the complex undergoes associative ligand substitution, where water molecule replaces a chloride in the formula, developing a positively charged platinum complex *cis*-$[Pt(NH_3)_2Cl(H_2O)]^+$. Water substitution of the chloride ions is suppressed in the bloodstream because of the greater quantity of Cl^- ions, but substitution is favored in the cytoplasm where Cl^- is in low concentration. The cation is easily trapped by the cell and is easily enticed to DNA in the nucleus where water molecule is replaced by DNA base [127–129]. Extensive research during the past decades has suggested DNA to be the functional target of these drugs; however, there is enough evidence to support other interactions with proteins and RNA as modes of action as well. The N7 sites on deoxyguanosine residues in DNA are highly vulnerable and most nucleophilic positions to be platinated. ^{195}PtNMR spectroscopic monitoring evidenced the formation of single covalent bond to DNA initially, followed by a distant reaction showing the loss of another chloride ion and substitution with guanine of the DNA [130]. This forms a cross-link between bases on the same or nearby strands. Similar cross-links arise when other drugs are administered; however, the proportion of intrastrand and interstrand cross-links differ. These cross-links cause severe distortion in DNA, leading to unwinding and disruption of the helical structure. These damaged cells then try to repair themselves during the cell cycle at G2/M transition. The cisplatin-bound parts are removed through the repair mechanism; enhanced repairing process leads the cells to develop resistance against platinum drugs. The high-mobility group box proteins found in the nucleus have a high affinity for intrastrand cross-links, which upon binding to these disrupted DNA lesions provide shielding against the cellular repair; this makes certain cancerous cells more susceptible to cisplatin. If the cells fail to repair themselves, transcription is inhibited across the lesion which prompts proapoptotic proteins, triggering apoptosis which is programmed cell death [131].

Researchers have put tremendous efforts in designing and investigating new anticancer agents with immense changes in the typical molecular skeleton, with an aim at unraveling different modes of actions that are efficacious versus a vast spectrum of cancers. Such efforts to design a drug which works as "magic bullet" that pursue the target cells on its own aim at attacking the receptors on cell surface, targeting the tumorous tissues as a whole by seeking characteristic proteins and allowing action in acidic media specific to cancer cells [132]. Enhanced uptake of sugar by the cancerous cells can also be exploited for targeting. A class of targeted drugs uses steroid units incorporated in the non-leaving groups which direct the drug to the tissues with steroid receptors. For example, for administering drugs to breast cancer cells, estrogen receptor which is overly expressed in this particular case is targeted. Similarly, drugs conjugated to bile acids in an effort to target liver cells are used [133].

Some *trans* complexes and their analogs like diamminedichloroplatinum(II) have dissipated the common notion that only *cis* Pt complexes are anticancer. These *trans* compounds may contain heteroaromatic, iminoether, or asymmetric aliphatic ligands giving rise to three separate sub-types. Substitution of ammines of the *trans* complex diamminedichloroplatinum(II) by the aforementioned ligands alters their cytotoxic properties, and their mode of action significantly differs from the other common drugs [134, 135].

Besides the Pt(II) complexes, Pt(IV) compounds are potential cytotoxic agents; however, their physicochemical characteristics differ from the Pt(II) complexes. They, usually, adopt octahedral geometries and do not allow substitution with ease contrary to the Pt(II) complexes, which helps in avoiding side reactions before binding to DNA. The extra two ligands in this geometry assist in attaining certain properties like lipophilicity, stability, and target specificity. Examples of platinum(IV) complexes include *cis*, trans, *cis*-dichlororidodihydroxidobis(isopropylamine)platinum(IV) which is commonly known as iproplatin [136] and *trans,cis,cis*-bis(acetato)amminecyclohexylaminedichloroplatinum(IV), also known as satraplatin [124].

5.4.2 Gold Complexes as Anticancer Agents

Au(III) being isoelectronic with Pt(II) which is d^8 with a square planar geometry of its complexes should, in principle, have antitumor activity. Despite many similarities, a very limited data is present in literature that shows the anticancer activity of Au(III) complexes. From direct analogy with Pt(II) complexes and some previous data, a similar course of action is hypothesized which involves binding with DNA [137, 138]. Gold(I) complexes known for their applications in treating rheumatoid arthritis also exhibit anticancer behavior. A number of these compounds such as auranofin analogues have been analyzed for their cytotoxicity contra P388 leukemia and B16 melanoma cells [139]. The drugs were also tested for in vivo activity against leukemia in rats. Gold(I) thiosugar compounds with phosphine were found to be efficient antitumor in both in vivo and in vitro. Gold(I) compounds of tetrahedral geometry having 1,2-bis(diphenylphosphino)ethane (DPPE) and 1,2-bis(dipyridylphosphino) ethane were observed to be active in vivo, particularly in cisplatin-resistant tumors. Contrary to that of cisplatin, the course of action does not involve DNA targeting in these complexes, but their cytotoxicity proceeds with hindrance in cellular function like that of mitochondria and inhibition of protein synthesis. Gold(I)-phosphine complexes with aromatic cations were studied, and direct dependence of cellular uptake on the lipophilicity of drugs was found [140]. Since therapeutic agent uptake increased with its lipophilicity, efforts were put in optimizing lipophilicity, and the mode of action in vitro was studied. The drug was found to be concentrated in mitochondria of the cells which induced apoptosis. The study of a complex $[(AuCl)_2(DPPE)]$ revealed loss of the chloride ions on reaction with DPPE and closure of the ring to form a tetrahedral cation $[Au(DPPE)_2]^+$ with different counterions which showed great stability in solution [141]. The extracted cation with chloride as counterion was found to improve the life expectancy of rats having leukemia cells up to ~85% at optimum dose of 2–3 μmol/kg/day for a period of 5 days. Similarly, a 60% improvement in life span was observed for mice infected with i.p. M5076 reticulum cell sarcoma. Tumorous tissues with cisplatin-resistant subline were found to be cross-resistant to the gold(I) complex; a combination of cisplatin and gold(I) complex proved to be advantageous. The compound has cytotoxic activity in tumor cell lines which is slightly inhibited by serum and works by cross-linking DNA. The cross-linking inhibits replication of DNA and also affects protein synthesis. The compound was found to be stable in serum by ^{31}PNMR spectroscopic studies.

Ligand DPPE, complex $[(AuCl)_2DPPE]$, and bis[trichlorogold(III)] $[DPPE(AuCl_3)_2]$ exhibit in vivo activity as well. To investigate the effects of metal bonding with DPPE in situ, the activity of DPPE, $DPPE(AuCl)_2$, and $[DPPE(AuCl_3)_2]$, as well as mixtures of the ligand and metal salts, was analyzed. The cytotoxicity improved tenfold both in vitro and in vivo than the DPPE alone. P338/DPPE cells can be used to monitor and evaluate the efficiency of drugs that follow the mitochondrial pathway to apoptosis. An Au(I) compound of monophosphine, diphosphine, and chloride ligand has proven to show a good cytotoxicity level against a number of tumor cells. Another complex tetrakis-((tris(hydroxymethyl))phosphine) gold(I) also displayed considerable cytotoxicity by restricting cell growth through

G1 phase elongation. Chlorotriethylphosphine gold(I) was discovered to exhibit cytotoxicity by inducing decomposition of lipids in cellular membranes in rat hepatocytes. Electron microscopy of the hepatocytes showed dense precipitates in mitochondria preceding apoptosis [142].

Gold(III) coordination compounds with metal center to be isoelectronic with Pt(II) and very likely to be cytotoxic have been investigated. The Au(III) compounds usually show good cytotoxicity, but they are not highly stable in physiological conditions. Some new gold(III) drugs have been designed for this purpose with considerable physiological stability in vitro and cytotoxicity in vitro against tumors, offering lesser resistance as opposed to platinum complexes. Initial studies suggested the interactions between Au(III) and DNA to be weaker. Some complexes with ligands ethylenediamine and *N*-benzyl-*N*,*N*-dimethylamine were tested too [143]. Bipyridine complexes with Au(III), for example, $[Au(bipy)(OH)_2]PF_6$, were effective against various tumor cell lines, with DNA as their primary target [137]. Complexes of Au(III) with *N*-methylimidazole, 2-methylbenzoxazole, and 5-dimethylbenzoxazole have been tested and found effective against leukemia cells and ovarian carcinoma [144]. In general, significant success has been achieved with gold complexes in fighting cancerous cells resistant to cisplatin; however, a better understanding in attaining physiological stability is required to develop efficient drugs.

5.4.3 Copper Complexes as Anticancer Agents

Copper-free ions, being harmful, have a regulated concentration in the human body; many pathological conditions like Alzheimer's disease, Parkinson's disease, and various cancer tissues (breast, prostate, etc.) involve an elevated level of these ions. In case of breast cancer, copper levels in serum rise to 1.67 μg/ml which is unreasonably elevated than the normal levels (0.99 μg/ml) found in healthy beings [145, 146]. Detailed investigation of how the increase in copper ion level occurs is not carried out yet; however, some researchers attribute it to the role copper plays in angiogenesis, invasion, and metastasis [147]. Coordination complexes of copper(I) and copper(II) are more common, whereas Cu(III) complexes are relatively lesser in number. Copper(I) coordinates to ligands with soft donors like C, P, thioether S, aromatic amines, etc. and is tetrahedral, whereas for Cu(II), square planar, trigonal bipyramidal, and octahedral geometries are possible. Different kinds of S-donor systems mainly thiosemicarbazones (TSCs) [148], thiosemicarbazides, dithiocarbamates (DTCs), thioureas [149], and dithiolates [150] coordinate to copper imparting different characteristics. Copper-TSC with a number of subclasses has been investigated to be active against viral, fungal, and bacterial infections, as well as cancerous cells. Complexes with thiosemicarbazides and substituted thiosemicarbazides containing donor atoms like O, S, and N are usually formed by loss of hydrazinic hydrogen atom. Recently efforts have been invested in designing a drug with glycosyl saccharide derivative which confers stability as well as binding environment. This approach aims at providing freedom to the pendant moiety to communicate with carbohydrate transport mechanism and metabolic ways of the cells and hinder the normal functioning. Thioureas are known to form complexes with Cu(I) that shows the cytotoxic activity of the same moderate level as cisplatin. Some complexes with O-donor ligands and κ^2O,O-donor systems have been synthesized and shown to have antiproliferative activity. Complexes with N,O-donor systems and N-donor systems such as imidazoles, triazoles, etc. have been widely investigated in the literature. Copper complexes with Schiff base systems, polydentate and/or macrocyclic systems, P-donor phosphines, N-N diamines, and C-donor N-heterocyclic carbenes have also been widely studied, and detailed discussion would be out of the scope of this chapter.

In general, copper complexes exhibit a wide range of activity and low toxicity than cisplatin. Also, some of these complexes break the resistance offered to cisplatin treatment. They display distinct and unique mode of action compared to corresponding Pt complexes; however, scarce knowledge is available in this regard. Copper complexes form non-covalent interactions with DNA, instead of coordinated adducts. New approaches other than interaction with DNA have been investigated, such as targeting cellular constituents like those of proteasome multiprotein complex. Other modes of actions include groove binding, oxidative cleavage, hydrolytic cleavage, topoisomerase inhibition, and proteasome inhibition.

5.4.4 Cobalt Complexes as Anticancer Agents

Cobalt is a trace element with crucial functions in biological systems, predominantly found in vitamin B12 or cobalamin which is essential to RBC formation, DNA synthesis, and functioning of the central nervous system. Cobalamin has an important function in the metabolism of biomolecules like fatty acids and amino acids [151]. Usually, cobalt is found in +1 oxidation state, with an ability to further oxidize to +2 and +3 states, and is relatively less toxic when compared with Pt and hence less toxic complexes than those of Pt. Cobalt complex with bis(acetylacetone) ethylenediamine (acacen), generally known as Doxovir, has toxic activity against herpes virus, and the accurate mode of action is unexplored yet. However, researchers believe that its activity is based on covalent interaction with histidine residues found in the enzymes of the herpes virus, which blocks the active site crucial to the replication of the virus [152]. Hurtado et al. investigated that histidine residues in proteins can be used as a target for inhibition of cancer cell growth. This was achieved by attaching specific nucleotides and peptides to Doxovir core. Hence, a number of Co(III) Schiff bases and their conjugates were synthesized in an attempt to find an anticancer agent with less toxicity to the normal cells. In this regard, Co(II) and Co(III) Schiff bases exhibit antitumor properties. Co(II) complex with 4-(4-aminophenyl) morpholine did not show considerable activity against liver carcinoma cells, whereas Co(II) complex with 2,6-bis(2,6-diethylphenyliminomethyl) pyridine displayed activity against colorectal and cervix adenocarcinoma cells [153]. Against breast cancer cells, another Co(III) complex of a tridentate Schiff base was found effective. Co(III) with [2-(2-hydroxybenzylideneamino) phenol] also inhibited colorectal adenocarcinoma cells [154]. A coordination polymer of Co(II) with 2-oxo-1,2-dihydroquinoline-3-carbaldehyde (isonicotinic) hydrazine exhibited cytotoxicity to a set of cancerous cell lines of the liver and rectum; interestingly, healthy cells were not affected which proved lower toxicity against normal cells in mouse embryonic tissues [155]. Cobalt complexes with typical ligands like bipyridine and phenanthroline were anticancer when tested. Compounds showing surfactant-like properties induce cell death through DNA cross-bonding. Dicobalt(0) hexacarbonyl complexes coordinated to ethinylestradiol are employed to surveil steroid interaction with estrogen receptors. An α-cation forms near dicobalt(0) hexacarbonyl moiety which assists covalent bonding to the active sites in estrogen receptors. Such an approach to damage cancerous cell DNA motivated researchers to study cytotoxicity of $[Co_2(CO)_6]$-acetylene compounds [156]. Studies showed that aspirin derivative with alkyne substitution was a highly efficient cytotoxic agent. These aspirin-containing drugs [157] induce apoptosis and angiogenesis by blocking cyclooxygenase enzymes. Cobalt(II) complexes attached to naproxen, mefenamic acid, and tolfenamic acid via carboxylate oxygen and pyridine/other pyridyl ligands were found to interact with biological components of the cells. These conjugations exhibit strong affinity for DNA and hence high cytotoxicity. Hypoxic cancerous tissues are immune to chemotherapy; hence, prodrugs are used which get activated by certain stimuli. Cobalt(III) prodrugs with octahedral geometry have been synthesized that get activated in hypoxic regions in tumors, by undergoing intracellular reduction to Co(II). Co(III) complexes are inert, whereas Co(II) complexes being high spin (d^7) are reactive because of lability due to susceptibility to substitution. Typical hypoxia-activated substances are oxidized back to their inert states in healthy cells which protects them from their harmful effects. Normal cells can have hypoxic conditions too; therefore, to avoid harm to the healthy cells, the activation threshold for these prodrugs should be set high. For this purpose, different ligands can be used to fine-tune reduction potentials of the Co(III) prodrugs ranging from 0 mV to −1400 mV [158].

5.4.5 Ruthenium Complexes as Anticancer Agents

Many ruthenium complexes have been prepared with varying properties and great deal of applications; interrelationships have been developed among properties and characteristics of the binding groups attached to the central metal ion. Ruthenium sulfoxide is known to have catalytic as well as chemotherapeutic properties. Ruthenium(II) complexes with polypyridyl and other aromatic ligands [159] have garnered much attention due to their fascinating spectroscopic and electrochemical properties that find their applications in various molecular electronic devices, solar cells, and DNA-disrupting agents.

Ruthenium complexes have been found to display low cytotoxicity, and also less toxic than cisplatin, hence requiring a higher dose to function. Despite low cytotoxicity, it has been evidenced that they increase life expectancy in cancer patients. Ruthenium(III) complexes convert to Ru(II) compounds in low pH and oxygen levels, conditions characteristic of cancer cells. This explains the selective toxicity of Ru(III) complexes. To activate "in vivo," a reduction potential is required which can be fine-tuned using different ligands. Another approach to explain the cytotoxic activity of ruthenium compounds is the fact that they interact readily with transferrin receptors. Hence, this interaction/binding can be manipulated for targeting transferrin receptors located on cancer cells. Cancer cells have high levels of iron and hence more transferrin receptors. Both ruthenium(II) and ruthenium(III) coordination compounds have been found to exhibit antitumor properties in vitro. It has been observed that ruthenium complexes show better interaction with cancerous cells as compared to healthy cells. Some ruthenium complexes have been tested in different sets of cancerous cells, including those resistant to cisplatin, and it was discovered that Ru(III) compounds showed better results. Ru(III) complexes even showed activity against autochthonous colorectal carcinoma of rats which is quite interesting because there is no satisfactory drug for rectal cancers of humans that lead to high mortality. Solubility can be a serious issue as was observed for a class of Ru(III) complexes with monocyclic or multicyclic basic heterocycles [160]. They were tested on leukemia, melanoma, and autochthonous carcinoma of colon cells and had satisfactory performance. They could be employed for treatment of prostate, ovarian, stomach, and breast cancer and many others but difficult to dissolve in water which hindered their use as they could not be lyophilized. Conjugation of ruthenium anticancer therapeutic agents with serum proteins is crucial because it ensures drug delivery and distribution in the body and also affects cytotoxicity. Experiments in mice showed HInd *trans*-$[RuCl_4(ind)_2]$ (ind = indazole) to be less toxic with higher antitumor activity as compared to HIm *trans*-$[RuCl_4(im)_2]$ (where Im is imidazole) because of better binding with protein [161]. Another pathway is through interaction with cytochrome c, oligonucleotides, and polynucleotides. Certain intertwining of DNA occurs during replication and transcription which can be corrected by topoisomerases. These enzymes are crucial to the survival of cells and can be poisoned when targeted with anticancer ruthenium drugs.

Many palladium and zinc complexes have also been investigated for anticancer activity. For example, Pd(II) complex with sugar-conjugated triazoles was synthesized by Yano et al. [162]. Zinc(II) with Schiff base complexes containing 4-(4-aminophenyl) morpholine derivatives was prepared and studied for antimicrobial and antitumor activity [153].

5.5 Conclusion

It can be concluded that the progress of such biosensors relies on parameters like harmlessness, sensitivity, specificity, identification of tiny molecules, and cost-friendliness. Ideally, the most outstanding feature that a commercial biosensor can possess aside from its cheap and portable nature is its efficiency in detection. Through surface engineering, using nanomaterials, it's possible to enhance and achieve highly efficient biosensors. A better combination of bioelectronic principles will guarantee the successful development of powerful biosensors for the modern era. Various advanced targeted therapies have been employed that use functionalization of nanocarriers and polymeric nanoparticles with specific ligands to recognize and interact with target cells. This approach improves the anticancer effects of drugs and has been in vogue from the last three decades. As for therapeutic agents or drugs, coordination metal complexes have provided a flexible scaffold to tweak and adjust their characteristic properties by changing or substituting ligands or metal itself. A huge amount of quality research literature has been developed in a struggle to find an anticancer drug with minimum harm to the normal cells and high cytotoxicity to the cancer cells. A number of coordination complexes of Pt(II), Pt(IV), Au(I), Au(III), Cu(I), Co(II), Co(III), Ru(II), Ru(III), Pd(II), and Zn(II) have been found to show cytotoxicity to cancerous cells. Some complexes and their activity have been discussed in this chapter to introduce the readers to a general idea of the use of metal complexes as anticancer agents and the course of their action.

References

1. Wu C-C, Hsu C-W, Chen C-D, Yu C-J, Chang K-P, Tai D-I, Liu H-P, Su W-H, Chang Y-S, Yu J-S (2010) Candidate serological biomarkers for cancer identified from the secretomes of 23 cancer cell lines and the human protein atlas. Mol Cell Proteomics 9:1100–1117. https://doi.org/10.1074/mcp.M900398-MCP200
2. Henry NL, Hayes DF (2012) Cancer biomarkers. Mol Oncol 6:140–146
3. Kearney AJ, Murray M (2009) Breast cancer screening recommendations: is mammography the only answer? J Midwifery Womens Health 54:393–400. https://doi.org/10.1016/j.jmwh.2008.12.010
4. Du D, Yan F, Liu S, Ju H (2003) Immunological assay for carbohydrate antigen 19-9 using an electrochemical immunosensor and antigen immobilization in titania sol-gel matrix. J Immunol Methods 283:67–75. https://doi.org/10.1016/j.jim.2003.08.014
5. Li L, Zhang L, Yu J, Ge S, Song X (2015) All-graphene composite materials for signal amplification toward ultrasensitive electrochemical immunosensing of tumor marker. Biosens Bioelectron 71:108–114. https://doi.org/10.1016/j.bios.2015.04.032
6. Zhang Q, Chen X, Tang Y, Ge L, Guo B, Yao C (2014) Amperometric carbohydrate antigen 19-9 immunosensor based on three dimensional ordered macroporous magnetic Au film coupling direct electrochemistry of horseradish peroxidase. Anal Chim Acta 815:42–50. https://doi.org/10.1016/j.aca.2014.01.033
7. Muller PAJ, Vousden KH (2014) Mutant p53 in cancer: new functions and therapeutic opportunities. Cancer Cell 25:304–317. https://doi.org/10.1016/j.ccr.2014.01.021
8. Oliveira ON, Iost RM, Siqueira JR, Crespilho FN, Caseli L (2014) Nanomaterials for diagnosis: challenges and applications in smart devices based on molecular recognition. ACS Appl Mater Interfaces 6:14745–14766. https://doi.org/10.1021/am5015056
9. Soares AC, Soares JC, Shimizu FM, Melendez ME, Carvalho AL, Oliveira ON (2015) Controlled film architectures to detect a biomarker for pancreatic cancer using impedance spectroscopy. ACS Appl Mater Interfaces 7:25930–25937. https://doi.org/10.1021/acsami.5b08666
10. Moraes ML, Rodrigues VC, Soares JC, Ferreira M, de Souza NC, Oliveira ONJ (2014) Immunosensor for HIV-1 diagnostics based on immobilization of the antigenic peptide p24-3 into liposomes. J Nanosci Nanotechnol 14:6638–6645
11. Raymundo-Pereira PA, Shimizu FM, Coelho D, Piazzeta MHO, Gobbi AL, Machado SAS, Oliveira ONJ (2016) A Nanostructured bifunctional platform for sensing of glucose bio-

marker in artificial saliva: synergy in hybrid Pt/Au surfaces. Biosens Bioelectron 86:369–376. https://doi.org/10.1016/j.bios.2016.06.053
12. Soares JC, Shimizu FM, Soares AC, Caseli L, Ferreira J, Oliveira ON (2015) Supramolecular control in nanostructured film architectures for detecting breast cancer. ACS Appl Mater Interfaces 7:11833–11841. https://doi.org/10.1021/acsami.5b03761
13. Soares JC, Soares AC, Pereira PAR, da Rodrigues VC, Shimizu FM, Melendez ME, Scapulatempo Neto C, Carvalho AL, Leite FL, Machado SAS, Oliveira ON (2016) Adsorption according to the Langmuir–Freundlich model is the detection mechanism of the antigen p53 for early diagnosis of cancer. Phys Chem Chem Phys 18:8412–8418. https://doi.org/10.1039/C5CP07121F
14. Luppa PB, Sokoll LJ, Chan DW (2001) Immunosensors--principles and applications to clinical chemistry. Clin Chim Acta 314:1–26
15. Ishihara S, Labuta J, Van Rossom W, Ishikawa D, Minami K, Hill JP, Ariga K (2014) Porphyrin-based sensor nanoarchitectonics in diverse physical detection modes. Phys Chem Chem Phys 16:9713–9746. https://doi.org/10.1039/c3cp55431g
16. Law W-C, Yong K-T, Baev A, Prasad PN (2011) Sensitivity improved surface plasmon resonance biosensor for cancer biomarker detection based on plasmonic enhancement. ACS Nano 5:4858–4864. https://doi.org/10.1021/nn2009485
17. Yang M, Yi X, Wang J, Zhou F (2014) Electroanalytical and surface plasmon resonance sensors for detection of breast cancer and Alzheimer's disease biomarkers in cells and body fluids. Analyst 139:1814–1825. https://doi.org/10.1039/C3AN02065G
18. Chikkaveeraiah BV, Bhirde AA, Morgan NY, Eden HS, Chen X (2012) Electrochemical immunosensors for detection of cancer protein biomarkers. ACS Nano 6:6546–6561. https://doi.org/10.1021/nn3023969
19. Tang CK, Vaze A, Rusling JF (2014) Paper-based electrochemical immunoassay for rapid, inexpensive cancer biomarker protein detection. Anal Methods 6:8878–8881. https://doi.org/10.1039/C4AY01962H
20. Warsinke A, Benkert A, Scheller FW (2000) Electrochemical immunoassays. Fresenius J Anal Chem 366:622–634
21. Loo L, Capobianco JA, Wu W, Gao X, Shih WY, Shih W-H, Pourrezaei K, Robinson MK, Adams GP (2011) Highly sensitive detection of HER2 extracellular domain in the serum of breast cancer patients by piezoelectric microcantilevers. Anal Chem 83:3392–3397. https://doi.org/10.1021/ac103301r
22. Su L, Zou L, Fong C-C, Wong W-L, Wei F, Wong K-Y, Wu RSS, Yang M (2013) Detection of cancer biomarkers by piezoelectric biosensor using PZT ceramic resonator as the transducer. Biosens Bioelectron 46:155–161. https://doi.org/10.1016/j.bios.2013.01.074
23. Soares AC, Soares JC, Rodrigues VC, Follmann HDM, Arantes LMRB, Carvalho AC, Melendez ME, Fregnani JHTG, Reis RM, Carvalho AL, Oliveira ONJ (2018) Microfluidic-based genosensor to detect human papillomavirus (HPV16) for head and neck cancer. ACS Appl Mater Interfaces 10:36757–36763. https://doi.org/10.1021/acsami.8b14632
24. Xie Y, Chen A, Du D, Lin Y (2011) Graphene-based immunosensor for electrochemical quantification of phosphorylated p53 (S15). Anal Chim Acta 699:44–48. https://doi.org/10.1016/j.aca.2011.05.010
25. Wink T, van Zuilen SJ, Bult A, van Bennekom WP (1997) Self-assembled monolayers for biosensors. Analyst 122:43R–50R. https://doi.org/10.1039/a606964i
26. Decher G, Hong JD, Schmitt J (1992) Buildup of ultrathin multilayer films by a self-assembly process: III. Consecutively alternating adsorption of anionic and cationic polyelectrolytes on charged surfaces. Thin Solid Films 210:831–835. https://doi.org/10.1016/0040-6090(92)90417-A
27. Rydzek G, Ji Q, Li M, Schaaf P, Hill JP, Boulmedais F, Ariga K (2015) Electrochemical nanoarchitectonics and layer-by-layer assembly: from basics to future. Nano Today 10:138–167. https://doi.org/10.1016/j.nantod.2015.02.008
28. Langmuir I (1918) The adsorption of gases on plane surfaces of glass, mica and platinum. J Am Chem Soc 40:1361–1403. https://doi.org/10.1021/ja02242a004

29. Jeppu GP, Clement TP (2012) A modified Langmuir-Freundlich isotherm model for simulating pH-dependent adsorption effects. J Contam Hydrol 129–130:46–53. https://doi.org/10.1016/j.jconhyd.2011.12.001
30. Raposo M, Oliveira ON (2000) Energies of adsorption of poly(o-methoxyaniline) layer-by-layer films. Langmuir 16:2839–2844. https://doi.org/10.1021/la990945y
31. Bohunicky B, Mousa SA (2010) Biosensors: the new wave in cancer diagnosis. Nanotechnol Sci Appl 4:1–10. https://doi.org/10.2147/NSA.S13465
32. Tothill IE (2009) Biosensors for cancer markers diagnosis. Semin Cell Dev Biol 20:55–62. https://doi.org/10.1016/j.semcdb.2009.01.015
33. Yamaguchi K, Nagano M, Torada N, Hamasaki N, Kawakita M, Tanaka M (2004) Urine diacetylspermine as a novel tumor marker for pancreatobiliary carcinomas. Rinsho Byori 52:336–339
34. Ciambellotti E, Coda C, Lanza E (1993) Determination++ of CA 15-3 in the control of primary and metastatic breast carcinoma. Minerva Med 84:107–112
35. Cook GB, Neaman IE, Goldblatt JL, Cambetas DR, Hussain M, Luftner D, Yeung KK, Chan DW, Schwartz MK, Allard WJ (2001) Clinical utility of serum HER-2/neu testing on the Bayer Immuno 1 automated system in breast cancer. Anticancer Res 21:1465–1470
36. Gann PH, Hennekens CH, Stampfer MJ (1995) A prospective evaluation of plasma prostate-specific antigen for detection of prostatic cancer. JAMA 273:289–294
37. Turner APF (2013) Biosensors: sense and sensibility. Chem Soc Rev 42:3184–3196. https://doi.org/10.1039/c3cs35528d
38. Thapa A, Soares AC, Soares JC, Awan IT, Volpati D, Melendez ME, Fregnani JHTG, Carvalho AL, Oliveira ON (2017) Carbon nanotube matrix for highly sensitive biosensors to detect pancreatic cancer biomarker CA19-9. ACS Appl Mater Interfaces 9:25878–25886. https://doi.org/10.1021/acsami.7b07384
39. Mavri T, Ben M, Imani R, Junkar I, Valant M, Kralj-igli V (2018) Electrochemical biosensor based on TiO2 nanomaterials for cancer diagnostics. Adv Biomembr Lipid Self-Assembly 27:63–105. https://doi.org/10.1016/bs.abl.2017.12.003
40. Aschberger K, Gottardo S (2016) Nanomaterials based biosensors for cancer biomarker detection. J Phys Conf Ser 704:1. https://doi.org/10.1088/1742-6596/704/1/012011
41. Sim J-B, Yang H-H, Lee M-J, Yoon J-B, Choi S-M (2012) Transparent conducting hybrid thin films fabricated by layer-by-layer assembly of single-wall carbon nanotubes and conducting polymers. Appl Phys A Mater Sci Process 108:305–311. https://doi.org/10.1007/s00339-012-6920-8
42. Love JC, Estroff LA, Kriebel JK, Nuzzo RG, Whitesides GM (2005) Self-assembled monolayers of thiolates on metals as a form of nanotechnology. Chem Rev 105:1103–1169
43. Madou MJ (2002) Fundamentals of microfabrication: the science of miniaturization. CRC Press, Boca Raton, p 49
44. Soares AC, Soares JC, Shimizu FM, Rodrigues V da C, Awan IT, Melendez ME, Piazzetta MH de O, Gobbi AL, Reis RM, Fregnani JHTG, Carvalho AL, Oliveira ON Jr (2018) A simple architecture with self-assembled monolayers to build immunosensors for detecting the pancreatic cancer biomarker CA19-9. Analyst 143(14):3302–3308. https://doi.org/10.1039/C8AN00430G
45. Allen SJ, Mckay G, Porter JF (2004) Adsorption isotherm models for basic dye adsorption by peat in single and binary component systems. J Colloid Interface Sci 280:322–333. https://doi.org/10.1016/j.jcis.2004.08.078
46. Limousin G, Gaudet JP, Charlet L, Szenknect S, Barths V, Krimissa M (2007) Sorption isotherms: a review on physical bases, modeling and measurement. Appl Geochem 22:249–275
47. Ghiaci M, Abbaspur A, Kia R, Seyedeyn-Azad F (2004) Equilibrium isotherm studies for the sorption of benzene, toluene, and phenol onto organo-zeolites and as-synthesized MCM-41. Sep Purif Technol 40:217–229. https://doi.org/10.1016/j.seppur.2004.03.001
48. Vasanth Kumar K, Sivanesan S (2007) Sorption isotherm for safranin onto rice husk: comparison of linear and non-linear methods. Dyes Pigments 72:130–133. https://doi.org/10.1016/j.dyepig.2005.07.020

49. Soares JC, Iwaki LEO, Soares AC, Rodrigues VC, Melendez ME, Fregnani JHTG, Reis RM, Carvalho AL, Correa DS, Oliveira ON (2017) Immunosensor for pancreatic cancer based on electrospun nanofibers coated with carbon nanotubes or gold nanoparticles. ACS Omega 2:6975–6983. https://doi.org/10.1021/acsomega.7b01029
50. Riul A, Soto AMG, Mello SV, Bone S, Taylor DM, Mattoso LHC (2003) An electronic tongue using polypyrrole and polyaniline. Synth Met 132:109–116. https://doi.org/10.1016/S0379-6779(02)00107-8
51. Taylor DM, Macdonald AG (1987) AC admittance of the metal/insulator/electrolyte interface. J Phys D Appl Phys 20:1277
52. Riul AJ, Dantas CAR, Miyazaki CM, Oliveira ONJ (2010) Recent advances in electronic tongues. Analyst 135:2481–2495. https://doi.org/10.1039/c0an00292e
53. Paulovich FV, Moraes ML, Maki RM, Ferreira M, Oliveira ON Jr, de Oliveira MCF (2011) Information visualization techniques for sensing and biosensing. Analyst 136:1344–1350. https://doi.org/10.1039/C0AN00822B
54. Paulovich FV (2008) Mapeamento de dados multi-dimensionais – integrando mineração e visualização. USP, São Paulo
55. Chabner BA, Roberts TG (2005) Chemotherapy and the war on cancer. Nat Rev Cancer 5:65–72. https://doi.org/10.1038/nrc1529
56. Feher J (2017) Cell signaling. In: Quantitative human physiology: an introduction, 2nd edn. Academic Press. https://doi.org/10.1016/B978-0-12-800883-6.00019-7
57. Eungdamrong N, Iyengar R (2004) Modeling cell signaling networks. Biol Cell 96:355–362. https://doi.org/10.1016/j.biolcel.2004.03.004
58. Pérez-Herrero E, Fernández-Medarde A (2015) Advanced targeted therapies in cancer: drug nanocarriers, the future of chemotherapy. Eur J Pharm Biopharm 93:52–79. https://doi.org/10.1016/j.ejpb.2015.03.018
59. Hanahan D, Weinberg RA (2011) Hallmarks of cancer: the next generation. Cell 144:646–674. https://doi.org/10.1016/j.cell.2011.02.013
60. Wu H-C, Chang D-K, Huang C-T (2006) Targeted therapy for cancer. J Cancer Mol 2(2):57–66
61. Danhier F, Feron O, Préat V (2010) To exploit the tumor microenvironment: passive and active tumor targeting of nanocarriers for anti-cancer drug delivery. J Control Release 148:135–146. https://doi.org/10.1016/j.jconrel.2010.08.027
62. Hughes B (2010) Antibody–drug conjugates for cancer: poised to deliver? Nat Rev Drug Discov 9:665–667. https://doi.org/10.1038/nrd3270
63. Jungbluth AA, Stockert E, Huang HJS, Collins VP, Coplan K, Iversen K, Kolb D, Johns TJ, Scott AM, Gullick WJ, Ritter G, Cohen L, Scanlan MJ, Cavanee WK, Old LJ (2003) A monoclonal antibody recognizing human cancers with amplification/overexpression of the human epidermal growth factor receptor. Proc Natl Acad Sci 100:639–644. https://doi.org/10.1073/pnas.232686499
64. Scott SD (1998) Rituximab: a new therapeutic monoclonal antibody for non-Hodgkin's lymphoma. Cancer Pract 6:195–197
65. Cohen P (1999) The development and therapeutic potential of protein kinase inhibitors. Curr Opin Chem Biol 3:459–465. https://doi.org/10.1016/S1367-5931(99)80067-2
66. Zogakis TG, Libutti SK (2001) General aspects of anti-angiogenesis and cancer therapy. Expert Opin Biol Ther 1:253–275. https://doi.org/10.1517/14712598.1.2.253
67. Gelperina S, Kisich K, Iseman MD, Heifets L (2005) The potential advantages of nanoparticle drug delivery systems in chemotherapy of tuberculosis. Am J Respir Crit Care Med 172:1487–1490. https://doi.org/10.1164/rccm.200504-613PP
68. Duncan R (2006) Polymer conjugates as anticancer nanomedicines. Nat Rev Cancer 6:688–701. https://doi.org/10.1038/nrc1958
69. Dinndorf PA, Gootenberg J, Cohen MH, Keegan P, Pazdur R (2007) FDA drug approval summary: pegaspargase (Oncaspar(R)) for the first-line treatment of children with acute lymphoblastic leukemia (ALL). Oncologist 12:991–998. https://doi.org/10.1634/theoncologist.12-8-991

70. Masetti R, Pession A (2009) First-line treatment of acute lymphoblastic leukemia with pegasparaginase. Biologics 3:359–368
71. Canal F, Sanchis J, Vicent MJ (2011) Polymer–drug conjugates as nano-sized medicines. Curr Opin Biotechnol 22:894–900. https://doi.org/10.1016/j.copbio.2011.06.003
72. Banerjee SS, Aher N, Patil R, Khandare J (2012) Poly(ethylene glycol)-prodrug conjugates: concept, design, and applications. J Drug Deliv 2012:1–17. https://doi.org/10.1155/2012/103973
73. Egusquiaguirre SP, Igartua M, Hernández RM, Pedraz JL (2012) Nanoparticle delivery systems for cancer therapy: advances in clinical and preclinical research. Clin Transl Oncol 14:83–93. https://doi.org/10.1007/s12094-012-0766-6
74. Blanco E, Hsiao A, Mann AP, Landry MG, Meric-Bernstam F, Ferrari M (2011) Nanomedicine in cancer therapy: innovative trends and prospects. Cancer Sci 102:1247–1252. https://doi.org/10.1111/j.1349-7006.2011.01941.x
75. Malam Y, Loizidou M, Seifalian AM (2009) Liposomes and nanoparticles: nanosized vehicles for drug delivery in cancer. Trends Pharmacol Sci 30:592–599. https://doi.org/10.1016/j.tips.2009.08.004
76. Kono K, Ozawa T, Yoshida T, Ozaki F, Ishizaka Y, Maruyama K, Kojima C, Harada A, Aoshima S (2010) Highly temperature-sensitive liposomes based on a thermosensitive block copolymer for tumor-specific chemotherapy. Biomaterials 31:7096–7105. https://doi.org/10.1016/j.biomaterials.2010.05.045
77. Schroeder A, Honen R, Turjeman K, Gabizon A, Kost J, Barenholz Y (2009) Ultrasound triggered release of cisplatin from liposomes in murine tumors. J Control Release 137:63–68. https://doi.org/10.1016/j.jconrel.2009.03.007
78. Simões S, Moreira JN, Fonseca C, Düzgüneş N, de Lima MC (2004) On the formulation of pH-sensitive liposomes with long circulation times. Adv Drug Deliv Rev 56:947–965. https://doi.org/10.1016/j.addr.2003.10.038
79. Dicko A, Mayer LD, Tardi PG (2010) Use of nanoscale delivery systems to maintain synergistic drug ratios in vivo. Expert Opin Drug Deliv 7:1329–1341. https://doi.org/10.1517/17425247.2010.538678
80. May JP, Li S-D (2013) Hyperthermia-induced drug targeting. Expert Opin Drug Deliv 10:511–527. https://doi.org/10.1517/17425247.2013.758631
81. Nagai H, Okazaki Y, Chew SH, Misawa N, Yamashita Y, Akatsuka S, Ishihara T, Yamashita K, Yoshikawa Y, Yasui H, Jiang L, Ohara H, Takahashi T, Ichihara G, Kostarelos K, Miyata Y, Shinohara H, Toyokuni S (2011) Diameter and rigidity of multiwalled carbon nanotubes are critical factors in mesothelial injury and carcinogenesis. Proc Natl Acad Sci 108:E1330–E1338. https://doi.org/10.1073/pnas.1110013108
82. Sinha N, Yeow JT-W (2005) Carbon nanotubes for biomedical applications. IEEE Trans Nanobioscience 4:180–195. https://doi.org/10.1109/TNB.2005.850478
83. Ali-Boucetta H, Al-Jamal KT, Müller KH, Li S, Porter AE, Eddaoudi A, Prato M, Bianco A, Kostarelos K (2011) Cellular uptake and cytotoxic impact of chemically functionalized and polymer-coated carbon nanotubes. Small 7:3230–3238. https://doi.org/10.1002/smll.201101004
84. Bianco A, Kostarelos K, Prato M (2011) Making carbon nanotubes biocompatible and biodegradable. Chem Commun 47:10182–10188. https://doi.org/10.1039/c1cc13011k
85. Vardharajula S, Ali SZ, Tiwari PM, Eroğlu E, Vig K, Dennis VA, Singh SR (2012) Functionalized carbon nanotubes: biomedical applications. Int J Nanomedicine 7:5361–5374. https://doi.org/10.2147/IJN.S35832
86. Wu W, Li R, Bian X, Zhu Z, Ding D, Li X, Jia Z, Jiang X, Hu Y (2009) Covalently combining carbon nanotubes with anticancer agent: preparation and antitumor activity. ACS Nano 3:2740–2750. https://doi.org/10.1021/nn9005686
87. Ajima K, Murakami T, Mizoguchi Y, Tsuchida K, Ichihashi T, Iijima S, Yudasaka M (2008) Enhancement of in vivo anticancer effects of cisplatin by incorporation inside single-wall carbon nanohorns. ACS Nano 2:2057–2064. https://doi.org/10.1021/nn800395t

88. Hampel S, Kunze D, Haase D, Krämer K, Rauschenbach M, Ritschel M, Leonhardt A, Thomas J, Oswald S, Hoffmann V, Büchner B (2008) Carbon nanotubes filled with a chemotherapeutic agent: a nanocarrier mediates inhibition of tumor cell growth. Nanomedicine 3:175–182. https://doi.org/10.2217/17435889.3.2.175
89. Kam NWS, Liu Z, Dai H (2006) Carbon nanotubes as intracellular transporters for proteins and DNA: an investigation of the uptake mechanism and pathway. Angew Chem Int Ed 45:577–581. https://doi.org/10.1002/anie.200503389
90. Kostarelos K, Lacerda L, Pastorin G, Wu W, Wieckowski S, Luangsivilay J, Godefroy S, Pantarotto D, Briand J-P, Muller S, Prato M, Bianco A (2007) Cellular uptake of functionalized carbon nanotubes is independent of functional group and cell type. Nat Nanotechnol 2:108–113. https://doi.org/10.1038/nnano.2006.209
91. Fabbro C, Ali-Boucetta H, Da Ros T, Kostarelos K, Bianco A, Prato M (2012) Targeting carbon nanotubes against cancer. Chem Commun 48:3911–3926. https://doi.org/10.1039/c2cc17995d
92. Zamboni WC (2008) Concept and clinical evaluation of carrier-mediated anticancer agents. Oncologist 13:248–260. https://doi.org/10.1634/theoncologist.2007-0180
93. Zheng S, Chang S, Lu J, Chen Z, Xie L, Nie Y, He B, Zou S, Gu Z (2011) Characterization of 9-nitrocamptothecin liposomes: anticancer properties and mechanisms on hepatocellular carcinoma in vitro and in vivo. PLoS One 6:e21064. https://doi.org/10.1371/journal.pone.0021064
94. Panyam J, Dali MM, Sahoo SK, Ma W, Chakravarthi SS, Amidon GL, Levy RJ, Labhasetwar V (2003) Polymer degradation and in vitro release of a model protein from poly(d,l-lactide-co-glycolide) nano- and microparticles. J Control Release 92:173–187. https://doi.org/10.1016/S0168-3659(03)00328-6
95. Panyam J, Labhasetwar V (2003) Biodegradable nanoparticles for drug and gene delivery to cells and tissue. Adv Drug Deliv Rev 55:329–347. https://doi.org/10.1016/S0169-409X(02)00228-4
96. Feng S-S (2004) Nanoparticles of biodegradable polymers for new-concept chemotherapy. Expert Rev Med Devices 1:115–125. https://doi.org/10.1586/17434440.1.1.115
97. Langer R, Folkman J (1976) Polymers for the sustained release of proteins and other macromolecules. Nature 263:797–800. https://doi.org/10.1038/263797a0
98. Couvreur P, Kante B, Roland M, Speiser P (1979) Adsorption of antineoplastic drugs to polyalkylcyanoacrylate nanoparticles and their release in calf serum. J Pharm Sci 68:1521–1524. https://doi.org/10.1002/jps.2600681215
99. Ding D, Zhu Z, Liu Q, Wang J, Hu Y, Jiang X, Liu B (2011) Cisplatin-loaded gelatin-poly(acrylic acid) nanoparticles: Synthesis, antitumor efficiency in vivo and penetration in tumors. Eur J Pharm Biopharm 79:142–149. https://doi.org/10.1016/j.ejpb.2011.01.008
100. Wohlfart S, Khalansky AS, Gelperina S, Maksimenko O, Bernreuther C, Glatzel M, Kreuter J (2011) Efficient chemotherapy of rat glioblastoma using doxorubicin-loaded PLGA nanoparticles with different stabilizers. PLoS One 6:e19121. https://doi.org/10.1371/journal.pone.0019121
101. Danhier F, Lecouturier N, Vroman B, Jérôme C, Marchand-Brynaert J, Feron O, Préat V (2009) Paclitaxel-loaded PEGylated PLGA-based nanoparticles: in vitro and in vivo evaluation. J Control Release 133:11–17. https://doi.org/10.1016/j.jconrel.2008.09.086
102. Kim J-H, Kim Y-S, Park K, Kang E, Lee S, Nam HY, Kim K, Park JH, Chi DY, Park R-W, Kim I-S, Choi K, Chan Kwon I (2008) Self-assembled glycol chitosan nanoparticles for the sustained and prolonged delivery of antiangiogenic small peptide drugs in cancer therapy. Biomaterials 29:1920–1930. https://doi.org/10.1016/j.biomaterials.2007.12.038
103. Sahoo SK, Ma W, Labhasetwar V (2004) Efficacy of transferrin-conjugated paclitaxel-loaded nanoparticles in a murine model of prostate cancer. Int J Cancer 112:335–340. https://doi.org/10.1002/ijc.20405
104. Wang X, Li J, Wang Y, Koenig L, Gjyrezi A, Giannakakou P, Shin EH, Tighiouart M, Chen Z, Nie S, Shin DM (2011) A folate receptor-targeting nanoparticle minimizes drug resistance in a human cancer model. ACS Nano 5:6184–6194. https://doi.org/10.1021/nn200739q

105. Steichen SD, Caldorera-Moore M, Peppas NA (2013) A review of current nanoparticle and targeting moieties for the delivery of cancer therapeutics. Eur J Pharm Sci 48:416–427. https://doi.org/10.1016/j.ejps.2012.12.006
106. Desai NP, Trieu V, Hwang LY, Wu R, Soon-Shiong P, Gradishar WJ (2008) Improved effectiveness of nanoparticle albumin-bound (nab) paclitaxel versus polysorbate-based docetaxel in multiple xenografts as a function of HER2 and SPARC status. Anti-Cancer Drugs 19:899–909. https://doi.org/10.1097/CAD.0b013e32830f9046
107. Frei E (2011) Albumin binding ligands and albumin conjugate uptake by cancer cells. Diabetol Metab Syndr 3:11. https://doi.org/10.1186/1758-5996-3-11
108. Choi KY, Saravanakumar G, Park JH, Park K (2012) Hyaluronic acid-based nanocarriers for intracellular targeting: interfacial interactions with proteins in cancer. Colloids Surf B Biointerfaces 99:82–94. https://doi.org/10.1016/j.colsurfb.2011.10.029
109. Choi KY, Chung H, Min KH, Yoon HY, Kim K, Park JH, Kwon IC, Jeong SY (2010) Self-assembled hyaluronic acid nanoparticles for active tumor targeting. Biomaterials 31:106–114. https://doi.org/10.1016/j.biomaterials.2009.09.030
110. Cho H-J, Yoon HY, Koo H, Ko S-H, Shim J-S, Lee J-H, Kim K, Chan Kwon I, Kim D-D (2011) Self-assembled nanoparticles based on hyaluronic acid-ceramide (HA-CE) and Pluronic® for tumor-targeted delivery of docetaxel. Biomaterials 32:7181–7190. https://doi.org/10.1016/j.biomaterials.2011.06.028
111. Na K, Bum Lee T, Park K-H, Shin E-K, Lee Y-B, Choi H-K (2003) Self-assembled nanoparticles of hydrophobically-modified polysaccharide bearing vitamin H as a targeted anti-cancer drug delivery system. Eur J Pharm Sci 18:165–173. https://doi.org/10.1016/S0928-0987(02)00257-9
112. Taheri A, Dinarvand R, Atyabi F, Nouri F, Ahadi F, Ghahremani MH, Ostad SN, Borougeni AT, Mansoori P (2011) Targeted delivery of methotrexate to tumor cells using biotin functionalized methotrexate-human serum albumin conjugated nanoparticles. J Biomed Nanotechnol 7:743–753. https://doi.org/10.1166/jbn.2011.1340
113. Taheri A, Dinarvand R, Nouri FS, Khorramizadeh MR, Borougeni AT, Mansoori P, Atyabi F (2011) Use of biotin targeted methotrexate-human serum albumin conjugated nanoparticles to enhance methotrexate antitumor efficacy. Int J Nanomedicine 6:1863–1874. https://doi.org/10.2147/IJN.S23949
114. Hilgenbrink AR, Low PS (2005) Folate receptor-mediated drug targeting: from therapeutics to diagnostics. J Pharm Sci 94:2135–2146. https://doi.org/10.1002/jps.20457
115. Sudimack J, Lee RJ (2000) Targeted drug delivery via the folate receptor. Adv Drug Deliv Rev 41:147–162. https://doi.org/10.1016/S0169-409X(99)00062-9
116. Ponka P, Lok CN (1999) The transferrin receptor: role in health and disease. Int J Biochem Cell Biol 31:1111–1137. https://doi.org/10.1016/S1357-2725(99)00070-9
117. Gu FX, Karnik R, Wang AZ, Alexis F, Levy-Nissenbaum E, Hong S, Langer RS, Farokhzad OC (2007) Targeted nanoparticles for cancer therapy. Nano Today 2:14–21. https://doi.org/10.1016/S1748-0132(07)70083-X
118. Dhar S, Gu FX, Langer R, Farokhzad OC, Lippard SJ (2008) Targeted delivery of cisplatin to prostate cancer cells by aptamer functionalized Pt(IV) prodrug-PLGA-PEG nanoparticles. Proc Natl Acad Sci 105:17356–17361. https://doi.org/10.1073/pnas.0809154105
119. Brooks PC, Montgomery AMP, Rosenfeld M, Reisfeld RA, Hu T, Klier G, Cheresh DA (1994) Integrin αvβ3 antagonists promote tumor regression by inducing apoptosis of angiogenic blood vessels. Cell 79:1157–1164. https://doi.org/10.1016/0092-8674(94)90007-8
120. Byrne JD, Betancourt T, Brannon-Peppas L (2008) Active targeting schemes for nanoparticle systems in cancer therapeutics. Adv Drug Deliv Rev 60:1615–1626. https://doi.org/10.1016/j.addr.2008.08.005
121. Rosenberg B, Vancamp L, Trosko JE, Mansour VH (1969) Platinum compounds: a new class of potent antitumour agents. Nature 222:385–386. https://doi.org/10.1038/222385a0
122. Cohen SM, Lippard SJ (2001) Cisplatin: from DNA damage to cancer chemotherapy. Prog Nucleic Acid Res Mol Biol 67:93–130

123. Johnstone TC, Suntharalingam K, Lippard SJ (2016) The next generation of platinum drugs: targeted Pt(II) agents, nanoparticle delivery, and Pt(IV) prodrugs. Chem Rev 116:3436–3486. https://doi.org/10.1021/acs.chemrev.5b00597
124. Kelland LR, Abel G, McKeage MJ, Jones M, Goddard PM, Valenti M, Murrer BA, Harrap KR (1993) Preclinical antitumor evaluation of bis-acetato-ammine-dichloro-cyclohexyl-amine platinum(IV): an orally active platinum drug. Cancer Res 53:2581–2586
125. Grunicke H, Doppler W, Helliger W, Hermann BJ, Hofmann J, Lindner H, Puschendorf B (1986) Tumor biochemistry as basis for advances in tumor chemotherapy. Arch Geschwulstforsch 56:193–201
126. Zhukova OS, Dobrynin IV (2001) Current results and perspectives of the use of human tumor cell lines for antitumor drug screening. Vopr Onkol 47:706–709
127. Di Pasqua AJ, Goodisman J, Kerwood DJ, Toms BB, Dubowy RL, Dabrowiak JC (2006) Activation of carboplatin by carbonate. Chem Res Toxicol 19:139–149. https://doi.org/10.1021/tx050261s
128. Frey U, Ranford JD, Sadler PJ (1993) Ring-opening reactions of the anticancer drug carboplatin: NMR characterization of cis-[Pt(NH3)2(CBDCA-O)(5'-GMP-N7)] in solution. Inorg Chem 32:1333–1340. https://doi.org/10.1021/ic00060a005
129. Junker A, Roy S, Desroches M-C, Moussay C, Berhoune M, Bellanger A, Fernandez C, Farinotti R (2009) Stability of oxaliplatin solution. Ann Pharmacother 43:390–391
130. Bancroft DP, Lepre CA, Lippard SJ (1990) Platinum-195 NMR kinetic and mechanistic studies of cis- and trans-diamminedichloroplatinum(II) binding to DNA. J Am Chem Soc 112:6860–6871. https://doi.org/10.1021/ja00175a020
131. Todd RC, Lippard SJ (2009) Inhibition of transcription by platinum antitumor compounds. Metallomics 1:280–291. https://doi.org/10.1039/b907567d
132. Ziegler CJ, Silverman AP, Lippard SJ (2001) High-throughput synthesis and screening of platinum drug candidates. JBIC 5:774–783
133. Tannock IF, Rotin D (1989) Acid pH in tumors and its potential for therapeutic exploitation. Cancer Res 49:4373–4384
134. Cleare MJ, Hoeschele JD (1973) Studies on the antitumor activity of group VIII transition metal complexes. Part I. Platinum (II) complexes. Bioinorg Chem 2:187–210. https://doi.org/10.1016/S0006-3061(00)80249-5
135. Farrell N (1996) Current status of structure-activity relationships of platinum anticancer drugs: activation of the trans geometry. Met Ions Biol Syst 32:603–639
136. Pendyala L, Cowens JW, Chheda GB, Dutta SP, Creaven PJ (1988) Identification of cis-dichloro-bis-isopropylamine platinum(II) as a major metabolite of iproplatin in humans. Cancer Res 48:3533–3536
137. Marcon G, Carotti S, Coronnello M, Messori L, Mini E, Orioli P, Mazzei T, Cinellu MA, Minghetti G (2002) Gold(III) complexes with bipyridyl ligands: solution chemistry, cytotoxicity, and DNA binding properties. J Med Chem 45:1672–1677. https://doi.org/10.1021/jm010997w
138. Messori L, Orioli P, Tempi C, Marcon G (2001) Interactions of selected gold(III) complexes with calf thymus DNA. Biochem Biophys Res Commun 281:352–360. https://doi.org/10.1006/bbrc.2001.4358
139. Mirabell CK, Johnson RK, Hill DT, Faucette LF, Girard GR, Kuo GY, Sung CM, Crooke ST (1986) Correlation of the in vitro cytotoxic and in vivo antitumor activities of gold(I) coordination complexes. J Med Chem 29:218–223. https://doi.org/10.1021/jm00152a009
140. McKeage MJ, Berners-Price SJ, Galettis P, Bowen RJ, Brouwer W, Ding L, Zhuang L, Baguley BC (2000) Role of lipophilicity in determining cellular uptake and antitumour activity of gold phosphine complexes. Cancer Chemother Pharmacol 46:343–350. https://doi.org/10.1007/s002800000166
141. Berners-Price SJ, Mirabelli CK, Johnson RK, Mattern MR, McCabe FL, Faucette LF, Sung CM, Mong SM, Sadler PJ, Crooke ST (1986) In vivo antitumor activity and in vitro cytotoxic properties of bis[1,2-bis(diphenylphosphino)ethane]gold(I) chloride. Cancer Res 46:5486–5493

142. Rush GF, Smith PF, Alberts DW, Mirabelli CK, Snyder RM, Crooke ST, Sowinski J, Jones HB, Bugelski PJ (1987) The mechanism of acute cytotoxicity of triethylphosphine gold(I) complexes. I. Characterization of triethylphosphine gold chloride-induced biochemical and morphological changes in isolated hepatocytes. Toxicol Appl Pharmacol 90:377–390
143. Buckley RG, Elsome AM, Fricker SP, Henderson GR, Theobald BR, Parish RV, Howe BP, Kelland LR (1996) Antitumor properties of some 2-[(dimethylamino)methyl]phenylgold(III) complexes. J Med Chem 39:5208–5214. https://doi.org/10.1021/jm9601563
144. Cossu F, Matovic Z, Radanovic D, Ponticelli G (1994) Cytotoxic activity of some gold(III) complexes. Farmaco 49:301–302
145. Labbe S, Thiele DJ (1999) Pipes and wiring: the regulation of copper uptake and distribution in yeast. Trends Microbiol 7:500–505
146. Milne DB (1998) Copper intake and assessment of copper status. Am J Clin Nutr 67:1041S–1045S. https://doi.org/10.1093/ajcn/67.5.1041S
147. Brewer GJ (2001) Copper control as an antiangiogenic anticancer therapy: lessons from treating Wilson's disease. Exp Biol Med 226:665–673. https://doi.org/10.1177/153537020222600712
148. Beraldo H, Gambino D (2004) The wide pharmacological versatility of semicarbazones, thiosemicarba-zones and their metal complexes. Mini Rev Med Chem 4:31–39
149. Bolos CA, Chaviara AT, Mourelatos D, Iakovidou Z, Mioglou E, Chrysogelou E, Papageorgiou A (2009) Synthesis, characterization, toxicity, cytogenetic and in vivo antitumor studies of 1,1-dithiolate Cu(II) complexes with di-, tri-, tetra- amines and 1,3-thiazoles. Structure–activity correlation. Bioorg Med Chem 17:3142–3151. https://doi.org/10.1016/j.bmc.2009.02.059
150. Balzarini J, Keyaerts E, Vijgen L, van der Meer F, Stevens M, De Clercq E, Egberink HF, Van Ranst M (2006) Pyridine N-oxide derivatives are inhibitory to the human SARS and feline infectious peritonitis coronavirus in cell culture. J Antimicrob Chemother 57(3):472–481
151. Dwyer FP, Gyarfas EC, Wright RD, Shulman A (1957) Effect of inorganic complex ions on transmission at a neuromuscular junction. Nature 179:425–426. https://doi.org/10.1038/179425a0
152. Hurtado RR, Harney AS, Heffern MC, Holbrook RJ, Holmgren RA, Meade TJ (2012) Specific inhibition of the transcription factor Ci by a Cobalt(III) schiff base–DNA conjugate. Mol Pharm 9:325–333. https://doi.org/10.1021/mp2005577
153. Dhahagani K, Mathan Kumar S, Chakkaravarthi G, Anitha K, Rajesh J, Ramu A, Rajagopal G (2014) Synthesis and spectral characterization of Schiff base complexes of Cu(II), Co(II), Zn(II) and VO(IV) containing 4-(4-aminophenyl)morpholine derivatives: antimicrobial evaluation and anticancer studies. Spectrochim Acta A Mol Biomol Spectrosc 117:87–94. https://doi.org/10.1016/j.saa.2013.07.101
154. Ghosh P, Chowdhury AR, Saha SK, Ghosh M, Pal M, Murmu NC, Banerjee P (2015) Synthesis and characterization of redox non-innocent cobalt(III) complexes of a O,N,O donor ligand: radical generation, semi-conductivity, antibacterial and anticancer activities. Inorg Chim Acta 429:99–108. https://doi.org/10.1016/j.ica.2015.01.029
155. Raja DS, Bhuvanesh NSP, Natarajan K (2012) A novel water soluble ligand bridged cobalt(II) coordination polymer of 2-oxo-1,2-dihydroquinoline-3-carbaldehyde (isonicotinic) hydrazone: evaluation of the DNA binding, protein interaction, radical scavenging and anticancer activity. Dalton Trans 41:4365–4377. https://doi.org/10.1039/c2dt12274j
156. Schmidt K, Jung M, Keilitz R, Schnurr B, Gust R (2000) Acetylenehexacarbonyldicobalt complexes, a novel class of antitumor drugs. Inorg Chim Acta 306:6–16. https://doi.org/10.1016/S0020-1693(00)00139-0
157. Vane JR (1971) Inhibition of prostaglandin synthesis as a mechanism of action for aspirin-like drugs. Nat New Biol 231:232–235
158. Schafer FQ, Buettner GR (2001) Redox environment of the cell as viewed through the redox state of the glutathione disulfide/glutathione couple. Free Radic Biol Med 30:1191–1212
159. Bibi N, Guerra RB, Huamaní LESC, Formiga ALB (2018) Crystal structure, electrochemical and spectroscopic investigation of mer -tris-[2-(1 H-imidazol-2-yl-κN(3))pyrimidine-κN(1)]

ruthenium(II) bis(hexafluoridophosphate) trihydrate. Acta Crystallogr Sect E Crystallogr Commun 74:874–877. https://doi.org/10.1107/S2056989018007995
160. Keppler B (1989) United States Patent, US 7,589,084 B2. http://intezyne.com/assets/patents-and-publications/patents/IT-139/6-IT-139-US7589084.pdf
161. Kratz F, Hartmann M, Keppler B, Messori L (1994) The binding properties of two antitumor ruthenium(III) complexes to apotransferrin. J Biol Chem 269:2581–2588
162. Yano S, Ohi H, Ashizaki M, Obata M, Mikata Y, Tanaka R, Nishioka T, Kinoshita I, Sugai Y, Okura I, Ogura S, Czaplewska JA, Gottschaldt M, Schubert US, Funabiki T, Morimoto K, Nakai M (2012) Syntheses, characterization, and antitumor activities of platinum(II) and palladium(II) complexes with sugar-conjugated triazole ligands. Chem Biodivers 9:1903–1915. https://doi.org/10.1002/cbdv.201100426

Part II

Genomic Instability and Cancer Metastasis

6

Hira Gull and Nosheen Masood

6.1 Introduction

DNA play a vital role in maintenance of healthy body in a sense that genes encode products after transcription and translation in the form of either proteins or enzymes that regulate normal body functions. But there are many agents (genotoxic) that can damage our DNA to certain extent. These toxic agents can be present inside cells (intracellular) or in environment [1]. ROS (reactive oxygen species) are the by-product of those metabolic processes that take place in our body, and these are produced intracellular, whereas ionizing radiations, UV light, etc. are produced in the environment. These radiations and ROS are the DNA-damaging toxic agents. These agents can cause gene mutations, that is, the change in the sequence of DNA bases inside cell. These mutations are collectively called GIN (genome instability).

In normal cells, DNA repair pathways including BER (base excision repair) and NER (nucleotide excision repair) and cell cycle checkpoints act as a cell caretaker that strictly regulates the genome maintenance, minimizes the GIN, and ensures the integrity and survival of genome. Defects in these caretakers may lead toward the initiation of many severe human diseases, e.g., cancer development, NGC (neurodegenerative conditions) and NPT (neoplastic transformations), etc. [2].

6.2 Genomic Instability in Cancer

Cancer is one of the prevalent and lethal genetic diseases. It is caused by mutations ranging from single nucleotide change to severe alterations in chromosomes. These mutations promote GIN by boosting cell division and inhibiting cell death and

H. Gull · N. Masood (✉)
Microbiology and Biotechnology Research Lab, Department of Biotechnology, Fatima Jinnah Women University, Rawalpindi, Pakistan

N. Masood, S. Shakil Malik (eds.), *'Essentials of Cancer Genomic, Computational Approaches and Precision Medicine*,
https://doi.org/10.1007/978-981-15-1067-0_6

hence become the reason of disturbing cellular machinery [3]. On the basis of type and degree of genetic changes, GIN can be divided into three groups [2]:

1. MSI or MIN (microsatellite instability)
2. NIN (nucleotide instability)
3. CIN (chromosomal instability)

6.2.1 MSI or MIN (Microsatellite Instability)

Those bases or nucleotides that are accidently mismatched or impaired either by alkylating agents or by DNA polymerase are repaired by MMR (mismatch repair) pathway [1]. Two to six basepair tandem repeats of short DNA that is present widely in genome is called MSI (microsatellites). Instability in microsatellite DNA occurs due to disruption in DNA mismatch repair system. MMR first identifies the mismatch bases and then binds with it, and then it excises the mismatch nucleotide and repairs the DNA damage caused by the mismatch [4]. This type of MSI is responsible for variety of cancers like ovarian, colorectal (CRC), lung, and gastric cancers [2].

6.2.2 NIN (Nucleotide Instability)

Insertion, deletion, and substitution of bases in the sequence of DNA are termed as NIN [5]. Dysfunctions in DNA repair machinery, e.g., BER or NER, and errors during replication of DNA result in these types of alterations. mtDNA (mitochondrial DNA) also show NIN instability [5]. In 80% of pancreatic tumor, missense mutation was seen in K-ras gene [6]. In lung, CRC, and gastric cancers, mtDNA instability is common [7].

6.2.3 CIN (Chromosomal Instability)

Changes in part of or in entire chromosome in terms of number or structure including inversion, deletion, translocation, insertion, amplification, homozygous deletions, and LOH (loss of heterozygosity) are termed as CIN. These alterations may result in the conditions called aneuploidy, polyploidy, and formation of chimeric chromosome [5]. CIN alters the genomic expression in tumor cells [8]. CIN is seen in 90% of tumors and is the most prevalent one among others like NIN and MIN [9]. PTEN is the tumor suppressor gene and is inactivated in glioblastomas due to the loss of tenth chromosome [10].

6.3 Repair Pathways for Suppression of Tumor and Fidelity of Genome

Cross-linking, oxidation, dimerization, strand breaks in DNA, and alkylation are the main processes that contribute in damaging DNA. So in order to protect the body from diseases, there is DNA repair mechanism that enables to maintain the integrity of whole genome. DNA repair pathways that are responsible for tumor suppression and genetic fidelity are divided into two categories [11]:

1. Excision repair pathways
2. DSB (double-strand break repair)

6.3.1 Excision Repair Pathways (ERP)

ERP is divided into three types in order to repair SSDNA (single-stranded DNA) damage [11]:

(a) NER (nucleotide excision repair)
(b) BER (base excision repair)
(c) DNA MMR (mismatch repair)

6.3.1.1 NER (Nucleotide Excision Repair)

DNA damage like helix-distorting lesions, bulky structures that are induced by oxidizing or alkylating agents, ultraviolet radiations, and chemotherapeutic drugs, is repaired by NER pathway [12]. TCNER (transcriptionally coupled NER) and GGNER (global genome NER) are two sub-pathways in nucleotide excision repair pathway [13]. Transcriptionally active genes are repaired, and TCNER and GGNER repair both DNA strands regardless of whether genes are transcribed actively or not [14]. To identify the deformation in double helix, GGNER uses XPC-RAD23 homolog B HR23B (xeroderma pigmentosum complementation group C) and DDB1-DDB2/XPE protein (DNA damage-binding protein 1), whereas TCNER is stalled on the location where DNA polymerase is present. Severe skin cancer called xeroderma pigmentosum is associated with the polymorphism in gene products of NER [15].

6.3.1.2 BER (Base Excision Repair)

Damaged bases of DNA are fixed by BER pathway. Glycosidic bond that is formed between the damage bases of DNA and sugar molecule of DNA backbone is cleaved by enzyme named DNA glycosylase. First identification and then removal of lesions are being done by BER pathway. Mutations in these enzymes may lead toward the onset of diseases like diabetes and cancer [16].

6.3.1.3 DNA MMR (Mismatch Repair)

Machinery of MMR and replication enzyme DNA polymerase did proofreading activity in series. Either large deletion or insertion loops or base-to-base mispair is the prime target for DNA MMR machinery [17]. G2/M cycle checkpoints in cell cycle are activated by MMR machinery after identification of damaged DNA [11].

6.3.1.4 DSB (Double-Strand Break Repair)

Double-strand break repair is the most life-threatening form of DNA damage [18]. As it is involve in variety of genomic changes, e.g., deletion, translocation, and amplification, these changes result in heritable cellular GIN that can lead to malignancy of tumor cells [19]. NHEJ and HR are two types of repair pathways. In G2 phase of cell cycle, HR repair pathway is present, and on the other hand, NHEJ is present throughout the cell cycle. HR is error-free repair because it joins broken DNA by identifying DNA sequence homology [20]. NHEJ is considered as error-prone repair because without identifying DNA sequence homology, it joins the broken ends of DNA [21]. BRCA1 and BRCA2 are genes that are involved in maintaining the stability of DNA and in suppression of cancer cells. These genes are the players of HR repair pathway [22].

6.4 EPGIN (Epigenomic Instability) in Cancer

An inherited change that modifies the expression of genes without affecting the basic sequence of DNA, e.g., remodeling of chromatin and methylation of DNA, is termed as EPG (Epigenetics). The most commonly known EPG processes are histone modification and DNA methylation. It is clear that the main feature in the case of cancer is EPGIN, but it is not still certain that these inherited alterations are either the cause or consequences of cancer formation [2].

6.4.1 DNAmet (Methylation) in Cancer

Process in which methyl group is added to cytosine nucleotide at the position 5 of carbon through the group of DNMT (DNA methyltransferase) enzyme is termed as DNA methylation. DNAmet results in silencing of genes and situated in heterochromatin at CpG island [23]. These methylation patterns are specific for every individual cell and thus play an important role in establishment of tissue-specific expression of genes. In cancer two epimutations, site-specific hyper- and global DNA hypomethylations, occur. Site-specific hypermethylation promotes cancer development by silencing the transcription of tumor suppressor genes, e.g., p16, Rb, and BRCA1 [24]. On the other hand, global DNA hypomethylation causes the overexpression of oncogenes, e.g., S-100 in colon and R-Ras in gastric cancers [25]. Thus, it is directly related to malignancy in many cancers such as brain, cervix, and breast [26].

6.4.2 Histone Modification (HM) in Cancer

Modification of four histones such as (H2A, H2B, H3, and H4) at the chromatin level is responsible for the regulation of expression of genes. Phosphorylation, acetylation, methylation, deacetylation, and ubiquitination are all modifications of histones. Gene transcription and formation of euchromatin are promoted by acetylation of H4 and H3, while transcription repression and formation of heterochromatin are promoted by H3K9 (H3 lysine9), H3K27, H4K20, and R2 methylation (H3 arginine 2) [27].

A change in modification of histones is used as markers (prognostic), but loss of function of H4K16ac and H4K20me3 is responsible for all types of human cancers [28]. Histone deacetylases, lysine methyltransferases, and acetyltransferases are all modifying enzymes (histones) that can catalyze these epigenetic markers [27]. Dysfunction of DNA is caused by changes in modification of histones that is the result of abnormal expression of these enzymes. Chromatin structure changes with the change in the patterns of histone modification and directly increases the level of chromosome breakage and random transposons translocation [2].

6.4.3 NR (Nucleosome Remodeling) in Cancer

Regulatory sequences of transcription factors and the structure of chromatin are determined by the specific shape and particular design of nucleosomes as they are the primary and significant units of DNA folding or packaging. An alternation in the content of histone proteins within nucleosomes and the repositioning of nucleosome is termed as NR (nucleosome remodeling). Genetic expression and accessibility to chromatin are determined by incorporation of new and removal of old nucleosomes in cancer epigenome [29].

6.5 Mechanisms for GS and EPGS (Genome and Epigenome Stability)

In normal body cells, genome is duplicated accurately, and the genetic material is distributed between two daughter cells. While duplication mechanisms play an important role in order to maintain integrity of genome. During S phase duplication of DNA occurs at high fidelity. Proper and accurate separation of chromosomes during mitosis is important. DNA repair during whole cell cycle is monitored, and checkpoints that control progression of cell cycle are also controlled [2].

6.5.1 Replication of DNA (Error-Free)

RI (replication licensing) is the process that regulates the replication of DNA and control the copy number during S phase of cell cycle. CDK (cyclin-dependent

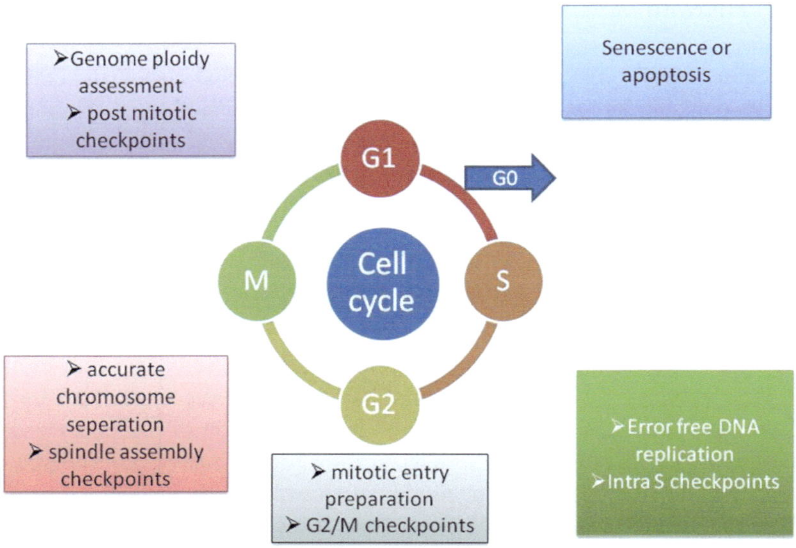

Fig. 6.1 Mechanism to prevent GIN throughout cell cycle

kinases) regulates RI [30]. To ensure the completion of replication, replication fork, during extension phase, often pauses and restarts. Failure in restart of these forks will result in single-stranded, double-stranded DNA breaks, and this all is solved by DNA damage repair pathway before entering to mitotic phase [31]. Figure 6.1 explains the mechanism of cell cycle to prevent genome instability.

6.6 CCCPTS (Cell Cycle Checkpoints)

Cell cycle checkpoints play an important role in maintaining normal genome and in preventing damage of DNA. Abnormal structures of chromosome and lesions of DNA are recognized by G1/S and G2/M checkpoints. Interaction between spindle fibers and chromosomes is monitored by spindle assembly checkpoints [2]. Multiple functions of cell cycle checkpoints are described in Fig. 6.2.

If G1/S phase recognizes the mutation or damaged DNA, then it will halt the replication of DNA. This postmitotic checkpoint is dependent on p53 and is mutated in cancerous genes [32].

A G2/M checkpoint identifies the damage DNA and promotes repair by stopping its mitotic entry. Mitosis-promoting complex cyclin B1/cdc2 kinase is inhibited by these checkpoints. If problem arises in these checkpoints, then the damaged DNA or chromosome will enter in mitosis phase and result in chromosomal rearrangements [33].

SACP (spindle assembly checkpoints) play an important role in taking the preventive measures against GIN. Cohesion complex keeps two sister chromatids close

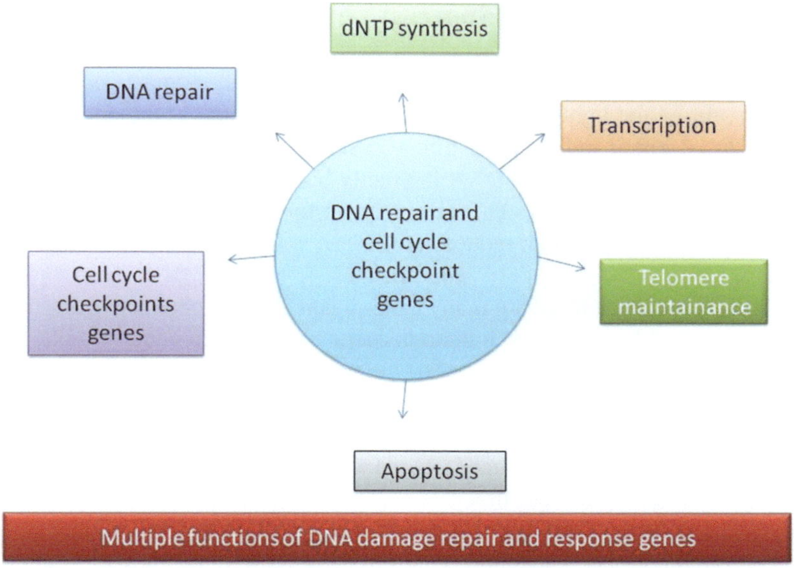

Fig. 6.2 Multiple functions of DNA damage repair and response genes

to each other during mitosis [34]. This complex is broken down by cyclosomes (anaphase-promoting complex). Tension is generated across the sister chromatids due to the accurate bipolar attachment of chromosomes [35]. Wait signal is generated by the SACP in order to check the incorrect attachments, e.g., (monotelic) situation when only one chromatid is attached and (syntelic) when on same pole both sister chromatids are attached [36]. On activation of assembly checkpoints, cyclosome (anaphase-promoting complex) is inhibited, and it allows the cell to correct the miss-attachment of chromosome [34].

Cascade of signaling pathways is generated by SACP just to check the miss-attachments, correct attachment errors, and segregation of chromosomes [37], e.g., Aurora kinase A do not detect miss-attachments, but it overrides the checkpoints and enters in anaphase phase [38]; on the other hand, Aurora kinase B stops the cell cycle once it detects miss-attachment of chromosomes [39].

6.7 Prognosis, Detection, and Prevention of GIN (Genome Instability)

Risk of cancer development can be reduced by preventing GIN and DNA damage. In order to limit the risk of cancer and to reduce the exposure to non-inherited sources, measures on vast scale are taken, but there is no way to prevent genomic damage [2].

6.7.1 NIS (Non-inherited Sources)

On daily basis people are exposed to solar radiations and the most common one is UV light (ultraviolet light). UV-A and UV-B are considered as the main cause that damages DNA either indirectly or directly. Skin cancer is caused by UV-induced DNA damage. UV-A damages DNA indirectly by producing ROS species and free radical, while UV-B damages DNA directly by forming the pyrimidine dimmers. Use of sunscreen or sunblock reduces the risk of skin damage by UV-A and UV-B radiations [40].

In our environment, there are many carcinogens that are chemical in nature, and they are responsible for several human diseases. Air pollution and cigarette smoke can cause GIN [41]. In blood cancer or in leukemia, a prevalent carcinogen, benzene, is recognized that is responsible for DNA damage, alteration in chromosome structure and number, and thus GIN [42].

Diet is also linked to GIN and DNA damage. Due to the deficiency of dietary folate, rather than thymidine, uracil is incorporated into genome [43]. It induces damage in excision repair pathway and breaks in chromosomal strands. Risk of cancer development becomes more with the increase in deficiency of vitamin B6, whereas deficiency of folic acid is directly related to DNA hypomethylation, micronuclei formation, and chromosomal breaks [44]. Increased GIN is associated with low dietary intake of vitamin E, folic acid, calcium, retinol, and B carotene, and increased intake of riboflavin and biotin is linked with GIN. Maximum intake of B carotene helps in reducing the risk of CC (colon cancer) [45].

6.7.2 Diagnosis of GIN in Cancer

Genome instability is quantified by the gene expression, genome sequence, and the chromosome structure [20]. We can diagnose large-scale and small-scale alternations by using different techniques. Array CGH, FISH (fluorescence in situ hybridization), flow cytometry, and karyotype are techniques that are used in determining large alternations in sequence of DNA. AP-PCR (arbitrarily primed), ISSR-PCR (inter-simple sequence repeats), genome sequencing, and SNP (single nucleotide polymorphism) array are used for detecting small alternations that lead toward GIN [46].

6.7.3 GIN and CP (Genetic Instability and Cancer Prognosis)

Poor prognosis is directly related to GIN. Better prognosis is seen in CRC patients having microsatellite instable cancers [47]. Negative impact of GIN is seen in biological fitness.

6.8 Conclusion

All mutations that become the reason for change in the sequence of DNA come under the umbrella of genome instability. Different factors like diet, ROS species, air pollution, and cigarette smoke and endogenous and exogenous factors are considered as the prime cause of genetic instability. These factors act like toxic agents that damaged our DNA. Nucleotides, chromosomes, and microsatellite DNA are damaged by these genotoxic agents. But, in spite of environmental and intracellular agents, there are some inherited specific patterns that, if become unstable, play an important role in promoting different diseases and specifically tumorigenesis. So in order to protect the body from toxic effects of these agents and to ensure the survival and integrity of DNA, there are cell cycle checkpoints, repair pathways, and damage-responding genes. The cell cycle checkpoints strictly regulate the replication of DNA in S phase and try to maintain equal number of chromosomes distributed between two sister chromatids during mitosis. Damage-recognizing genes recognize the damage in DNA, and then they trigger the repairing pathways NER, BER, double-streak break repair to ensure the stability of genome. But the mutation in these checkpoints or in repairing genes can lead toward the prevalent and lethal disease *cancer*. Therapeutic opportunities provide us the mean to determine the prognosis and to diagnose small-scale and large-scale aberrations in cells, DNA, and chromosome of individual. FISH, AP-PCR, ISSR-PCR, array CGH, etc. are the diagnosis techniques that help us in diagnosing and thus become a mean to control and save the life of individuals from *cancer* metastasis.

References

1. Broustas CG, Lieberman HB (2014) DNA damage response genes and the development of cancer metastasis. Radiat Res 181(2):111–130
2. Chen H, Maxwell C, Connell M (2015) The generation, detection, and prevention of genomic instability during cancer progression and metastasis. In: Genomic instability and cancer metastasis. Springer, Cham, pp 15–38
3. Futreal PA, Coin L, Marshall M, Down T, Hubbard T, Wooster R, Rahman N, Stratton MR (2004) A census of human cancer genes. Nat Rev Cancer 4(3):177
4. Halling KC, Harper J, Moskaluk CA, Thibodeau SN, Petroni GR, Yustein AS, Tosi P, Minacci C, Roviello F, Piva P (1999) Origin of microsatellite instability in gastric cancer. Am J Pathol 155(1):205–211
5. Lengauer C, Kinzler KW, Vogelstein B (1998) Genetic instabilities in human cancers. Nature 396(6712):643
6. Almoguera C, Shibata D, Forrester K, Martin J, Arnheim N, Perucho M (1988) Most human carcinomas of the exocrine pancreas contain mutant c-K-ras genes. Cell 53(4):549–554
7. Lee HC, Yin PH, Lin JC, Wu CC, Chen CY, Wu CW, Chi CW, Tam TN, Wei YH (2005) Mitochondrial genome instability and mtDNA depletion in human cancers. Ann N Y Acad Sci 1042(1):109–122
8. Jefford CE, Irminger-Finger I (2006) Mechanisms of chromosome instability in cancers. Crit Rev Oncol Hematol 59(1):1–14
9. Gagos S, Irminger-Finger I (2005) Chromosome instability in neoplasia: chaotic roots to continuous growth. Int J Biochem Cell Biol 37(5):1014–1033

10. Wang SI, Puc J, Li J, Bruce JN, Cairns P, Sidransky D, Parsons R (1997) Somatic mutations of PTEN in glioblastoma multiforme. Cancer Res 57(19):4183–4186
11. Ferguson LR, Chen H, Collins AR, Connell M, Damia G, Dasgupta S, Malhotra M, Meeker AK, Amedei A, Amin A (2015) Genomic instability in human cancer: molecular insights and opportunities for therapeutic attack and prevention through diet and nutrition. Semin Cancer Biol 35:S5–S24
12. Aguilera A, Gómez-González B (2008) Genome instability: a mechanistic view of its causes and consequences. Nat Rev Genet 9(3):204
13. Houtgraaf JH, Versmissen J, van der Giessen WJ (2006) A concise review of DNA damage checkpoints and repair in mammalian cells. Cardiovasc Revasc Med 7(3):165–172
14. Sancar A, Lindsey-Boltz LA, Ünsal-Kaçmaz K, Linn S (2004) Molecular mechanisms of mammalian DNA repair and the DNA damage checkpoints. Annu Rev Biochem 73(1):39–85
15. Hanawalt PC, Spivak G (2008) Transcription-coupled DNA repair: two decades of progress and surprises. Nat Rev Mol Cell Biol 9(12):958
16. Thoms KM, Kuschal C, Emmert S (2007) Lessons learned from DNA repair defective syndromes. Exp Dermatol 16(6):532–544
17. Albertson TM, Ogawa M, Bugni JM, Hays LE, Chen Y, Wang Y, Treuting PM, Heddle JA, Goldsby RE, Preston BD (2009) DNA polymerase ε and δ proofreading suppress discrete mutator and cancer phenotypes in mice. Proc Natl Acad Sci 106(40):17101–17104
18. Ciccia A, Elledge SJ (2010) The DNA damage response: making it safe to play with knives. Mol Cell 40(2):179–204
19. Helleday T, Lo J, van Gent DC, Engelward BP (2007) DNA double-strand break repair: from mechanistic understanding to cancer treatment. DNA Repair 6(7):923–935
20. Wan T, Ma ES (2012) Molecular cytogenetics: an indispensable tool for cancer diagnosis. Chang Gung Med J 35(2):96–110
21. Moynahan ME, Jasin M (2010) Mitotic homologous recombination maintains genomic stability and suppresses tumorigenesis. Nat Rev Mol Cell Biol 11(3):196
22. Hall JM, Lee MK, Newman B, Morrow JE, Anderson LA, Huey B, King M-C (1990) Linkage of early-onset familial breast cancer to chromosome 17q21. Science 250(4988):1684–1689
23. Miller OJ, Schnedl W, Allen J, Erlanger BF (1974) 5-Methylcytosine localised in mammalian constitutive heterochromatin. Nature 251(5476):636
24. Sharma S, Kelly TK, Jones PA (2010) Epigenetics in cancer. Carcinogenesis 31(1):27–36
25. Wilson AS, Power BE, Molloy PL (2007) DNA hypomethylation and human diseases. Biochim Biophys Acta 1775(1):138–162
26. Ehrlich M (2002) DNA methylation in cancer: too much, but also too little. Oncogene 21(35):5400
27. Kouzarides T (2007) Chromatin modifications and their function. Cell 128(4):693–705
28. Fraga MF, Ballestar E, Villar-Garea A, Boix-Chornet M, Espada J, Schotta G, Bonaldi T, Haydon C, Ropero S, Petrie K (2005) Loss of acetylation at Lys16 and trimethylation at Lys20 of histone H4 is a common hallmark of human cancer. Nat Genet 37(4):391
29. Mavrich TN, Ioshikhes IP, Venters BJ, Jiang C, Tomsho LP, Qi J, Schuster SC, Albert I, Pugh BF (2008) A barrier nucleosome model for statistical positioning of nucleosomes throughout the yeast genome. Genome Res 18(7):1073–1083
30. Shen Z (2011) Genomic instability and cancer: an introduction. J Mol Cell Biol 3(1):1–3
31. Aguilera A, García-Muse T (2013) Causes of genome instability. Annu Rev Genet 47:1–32
32. Vogelstein B (1990) Cancer. A deadly inheritance [news; comment]. Nature 348:681–682
33. Kommajosyula N, Rhind N (2006) Cdc2 tyrosine phosphorylation is not required for the S-phase DNA damage checkpoint in fission yeast. Cell Cycle 5(21):2495–2500
34. Maresca TJ, Salmon E (2010) Welcome to a new kind of tension: translating kinetochore mechanics into a wait-anaphase signal. J Cell Sci 123(6):825–835
35. Lara-Gonzalez P, Westhorpe FG, Taylor SS (2012) The spindle assembly checkpoint. Curr Biol 22(22):R966–R980
36. de Medina-Redondo M, Meraldi P (2011) The spindle assembly checkpoint: clock or domino? In: Cell cycle in development. Springer, Berlin, pp 75–91

37. Lens SM, Voest EE, Medema RH (2010) Shared and separate functions of polo-like kinases and aurora kinases in cancer. Nat Rev Cancer 10(12):825
38. Anand S, Penrhyn-Lowe S, Venkitaraman AR (2003) AURORA-A amplification overrides the mitotic spindle assembly checkpoint, inducing resistance to Taxol. Cancer Cell 3(1):51–62
39. Foley EA, Kapoor TM (2013) Microtubule attachment and spindle assembly checkpoint signalling at the kinetochore. Nat Rev Mol Cell Biol 14(1):25
40. Jhappan C, Noonan FP, Merlino G (2003) Ultraviolet radiation and cutaneous malignant melanoma. Oncogene 22(20):3099
41. Hecht SS (1999) Tobacco smoke carcinogens and lung cancer. J Natl Cancer Inst 91(14):1194–1210
42. Orjuela M, Castaneda VP, Ridaura C, Lecona E, Leal C, Abramson DH, Orlow I, Gerald W, Cordon-Cardo C (2000) Presence of human papilloma virus in tumor tissue from children with retinoblastoma: an alternative mechanism for tumor development. Clin Cancer Res 6(10):4010–4016
43. Blount BC, Mack MM, Wehr CM, MacGregor JT, Hiatt RA, Wang G, Wickramasinghe SN, Everson RB, Ames BN (1997) Folate deficiency causes uracil misincorporation into human DNA and chromosome breakage: implications for cancer and neuronal damage. Proc Natl Acad Sci 94(7):3290–3295
44. Fenech M (2001) The role of folic acid and vitamin B12 in genomic stability of human cells. Mutat Res 475(1–2):57–67
45. Satia JA, Keku T, Galanko JA, Martin C, Doctolero RT, Tajima A, Sandler RS, Carethers JM (2005) Diet, lifestyle, and genomic instability in the North Carolina Colon Cancer Study. Cancer Epidemiol Biomarkers Prev 14(2):429–436
46. Mol BM, Massink MP, van der Hout AH, Dommering CJ, Zaman JM, Bosscha MI, Kors WA, Meijers-Heijboer HE, Kaspers GJ, Riele H (2014) High resolution SNP array profiling identifies variability in retinoblastoma genome stability. Genes Chromosom Cancer 53(1):1–14
47. Mettu RK, Wan Y-W, Habermann JK, Ried T, Guo NL (2010) A 12-gene genomic instability signature predicts clinical outcomes in multiple cancer types. Int J Biol Markers 25(4):219–228

DNA Damage Response Pathways in Cancer Predisposition and Metastasis

7

Saima Shakil Malik and Iqra

7.1 Introduction

DNA is perpetually damaged by various genotoxic agents produced either in the cell-like reactive oxygen species (ROS) or in the environment such as ionizing radiations and UV light [1]. In normal cells, genome integrity is safeguarded by a very systematic and robust DNA damage response (DDR) [2] including different DNA repair pathways and specialized cell cycle checkpoints [3], whereas cancer cells are formed as a result of several genetic alterations leading to survival compensations and growth [4].

Impairment of DNA repair features either gain or loss can enhance genomic instability and DNA errors promoting immune deficiencies [5, 6], ageing [7], neurodegenerative disorders [8] and predominantly cancer [9]. Epigenetic silencing and somatic mutations in DDR genes without any inherent genetic link are commonly observed among different cancers [10], whereas germline mutations of DNA repair or cell cycle checkpoint genes can cause predisposition to hereditary cancers [11]. DNA repair genes intricated in mismatch repair (MMR) [12], nucleotide excision repair (NER) [13], homologous recombination (HR) and non-homologous end joining (NHEJ) [14] can persuade several types of cancer.

DNA repair gene's dysregulation affects the normal and cancerous cells' response towards DNA-damaging anticancer treatment [15]. Upregulated repair pathways

S. S. Malik (✉)
Fatima Jinnah Women University, Rawalpindi, Pakistan

Armed Forces Institute of Pathology, Rawalpindi, Pakistan
e-mail: Saimamalik.afip@numspak.edu.pk

Iqra
Microbiology & Biotechnology Research Lab, Fatima Jinnah Women University, Rawalpindi, Pakistan

N. Masood, S. Shakil Malik (eds.), *'Essentials of Cancer Genomic, Computational Approaches and Precision Medicine*,
https://doi.org/10.1007/978-981-15-1067-0_7

result in resistance to chemotherapeutic and radiotherapeutic treatment; therefore, inhibitors of these DNA repair pathways can possibly sensitize cancer cells against these agents [16]. On the other hand, cancer cells that do not have proper repair mechanism and are merely dependent on some alternative repair mechanism become susceptible to functional pathway targeting by synthetic lethality, whereas normal healthy cells with two functional repair mechanisms would establish resistance [17, 18].

Recently, with the advanced technology, increasing evidence has been observed about the additional cellular roles of DDR genes other than repairing DNA damage and controlling cell cycle checkpoints, for example, chromatin remodelling, transcriptional regulation and programmed cell death [19]. Acceptable balance between mutations avoidance by DNA repair and various other cellular responses to DNA damage which affects the formation and obstinacy of genetic alterations and stability as shown in Fig. 7.1. Current chapter highlights the role of DNA damage response genes in not only cancer initiation but progression and metastasis as well.

7.2 Cancer Initiation and DNA Repair Genes

Most of the human malignancies are the consequence of genomic instability and thought as cancer cells hallmark [20]. Downregulation of DDR pathways, for instance, those regulated by ataxia telangiectasia mutated (ATM) and ataxia

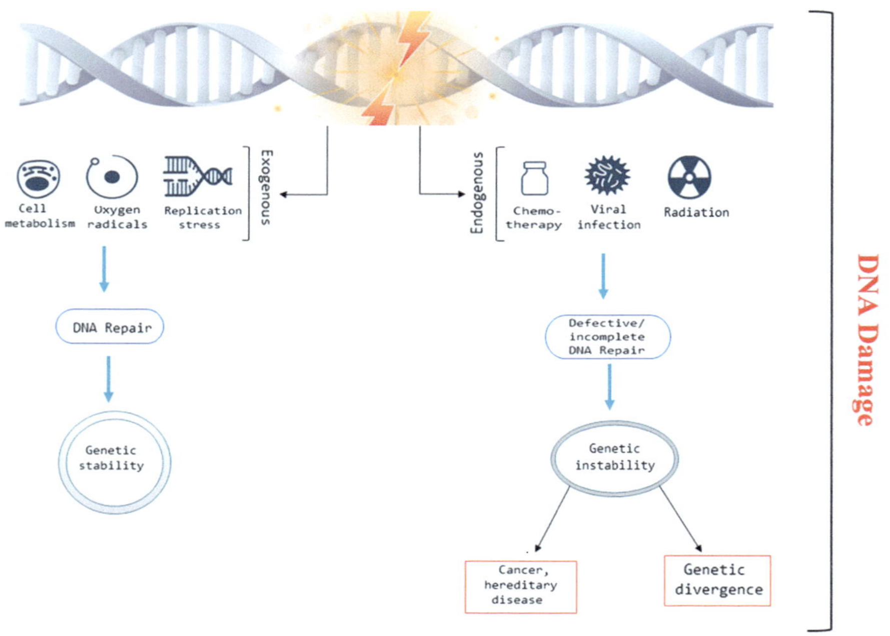

Fig. 7.1 Acceptable balance between mutation avoidance by DNA repair and various other cellular responses to DNA damage

telangiectasia Rad3-related protein (ATR) kinases and p53, can lead to genomic instability [21]. Alternatively, tumours with altered genome can ascend from damages in any one of the repair pathways, base excision repair (BER), NER, MMR, HR and NHEJ [19]. The link between tumorigenesis and DNA repair damages is emphasized by the fact that inherently damaged DNA repair mechanisms that cause enhanced ageing syndromes, like Nijmegen, Bloom, Werner and Rothmund–Thomson, along with ataxia telangiectasia, trichothiodystrophy and xeroderma pigmentosum also have increased cancer risk [22].

Besides DDR gene alterations, either somatic or inherited, epigenetic gene silencing might also promote carcinogenesis. Epigenetic inactivation of DNA repair genes has been reported in different cancers and found to be linked with various DNA repair pathways [23]. Epigenetic silencing of a gene such as BRCA1 or FANCF via methylation of the promoter region is the most commonly observed mechanism among sporadic cancers [24]. Epigenetic silencing of certain DNA repair genes, for example, MLH1, BRCA1, BRCA1, FANCF and WRN, can promote genomic instability and enhance mutation rates in cancerous cells [25]. The current chapter briefly describes the relationship between definite aberrant alterations in DNA repair pathways and malignancies.

7.2.1 Direct Repair

Direct repair or reversal of any lesion is the easiest form of DNA repair [26] and can be achieved with the help of MGMT (O6-methylguanine-DNA methyltransferase). It is also meant to be involved in cancer treatment by conferring resistance to DNA-alkylating agents [27] and repairs O6-alkylated guanine residues. O6-Methylguanine gets paired with thymine and results in G to A transition if left unrepaired in DNA replication [28]. Epigenetic silencing of MGMT is reported in different tumour including lung cancer [29], glioblastoma [30], head and neck cancer [31], colorectal cancer [32], breast cancer [33] and gastric cancer [34].

7.2.2 Nucleotide Excision Repair (NER)

The NER pathway is a fundamental DNA repair process involved in protecting and maintaining the genome integrity by repairing several DNA modifications, specifically bulky helix-distorting damage [35]. However, recently researchers have reported that some of the NER proteins possess diverse roles other than DNA repair such as histone ubiquitylation, nucleosome remodelling and gene's transcriptional activation which are responsible for stem cell reprogramming, nuclear receptor signalling and post-natal mammalian growth [36]. Tumours with damaged NER pathway developed an innate resistance to radio- and chemotherapy and paved to continued tumour growth and metastasis even after treatment [37, 38].

NER encompasses 30 unlike genes with diverse functions. Among these 30, 7 were xeroderma pigmentosum (XP) complementation groups executing several critical roles in NER pathway [39–41]. XPC is responsible for initiating the recognition of DNA damage followed by DNA unwinding with various enzymes [42]. Afterwards XPG incise the damaged DNA leading to the removal of roughly 25–30 nucleotides followed by the gap filling and joining of ends by DNA polymerase and DNA ligase, respectively [40, 43].

Researchers have revealed that less reductions in NER at polymorphic frequencies among general population may be attributed to the risk of lung and breast cancers. Many researchers emphasize on assessing the role of single nucleotide polymorphisms of these genes and cancer risk [43–47]. It is thought that tobacco serves as an "internal sun" especially in cancer cases, engendering lesions that require to be repaired by NER pathway. It was a well-known fact that XP follows an autosomal recessive mode of inheritance, whereas heterozygous carriers were thought to be phenotypically normal [48].

Loss of XPA gene was reported in testicular germ cell tumours [49]. XPC another important global genome NER component is meant to be regulated by promoter methylation in bladder carcinoma [50]. ERCC1 was also reported to be inactivated in glioma cancers via promoter methylation [23]. Furthermore, mutations of XPA–XPG have been reported in different cancers like testicular [51], skin [52], breast [35] and lung cancer [44].

7.2.3 Mismatch Repair

Mismatch repair (MMR) pathway performs essential role in identifying insertion/deletion loop (IDL) and repairing newly synthesized DNA with inaccurate genetic material, produced during replication. MMR protect cells from various spontaneous mutations, like microsatellite instability (MSI) [53]. MMR pathway functions with the help of three heterodimers: "MutSα (MSH2 and MSH6), MutSβ (MSH2 and MSH3) and MutLα (MLH1 and PMS2)". Two of the heterodimers, MutSα or MutSβ, were involved in recognizing IDLs in DNA strand formed due to polymerase slippage in replication [54, 55]. HEK36me3 (epigenetic histone marker) was found to assist MutSα recruitment to chromatin by interrelating with MSH6 PWWP (DNA-binding domain). It is plentifully available in S and G1 phases and guaranteed MutSα enhancement on chromatin prior mismatch introduction in replication. Lack of H3K36 trimethyltransferase SETD2 leads to spontaneous mutations and MSI, basic hallmarks of MMR deficiency. This phenomenon highlighted the potential relationship of MMR deficiency and various cancers owning MS1 [56, 57].

MutSα/MutSβ distinguishes mismatch and recruits MutLα heterodimer in an ATP-dependent reaction [58]. It also repairs accidentally introduced nucleotides after administrating chemotherapeutic drugs such as alkylating agents [59]. MSI high tumours ascend from an epigenetic defect in sporadic cancers. MLH1 promoter region methylation was found to be associated with decreased activity in sporadic colon and lung cancer [60–63]. Moreover, aberrant methylation also controls MLH1 functioning in sporadic endometrial [64] and gastric carcinoma [65].

7.2.4 Base Excision Repair

The BER pathway is responsible for protecting the genome from devastating effects of reactive oxygen species exposure. BER not only eradicates damaged basis from the DNA but also is meant to repair single-strand breaks in DNA [26]. This repair pathway comprises of variant of enzymes such as endonucleases {flap structure-specific endonuclease 1 (FEN1), apurinic/apyrimidinic endonuclease 1 (APE1)} [66], DNA glycosylases {human homolog of the *E. coli* mutY gene (MUTYH), 8-oxoguanine DNA glycosylase (OGG1)}, DNA ligase III, DNA polymerase b (Polb), PARP-1 and XRCC1 (X-ray repair complementing defective repair 1) [67]. Inherited mutations are rarely observed in BER genes. However, literature has confirmed the genetic linkage of APE1, XRCC1 and OGG1 gene polymorphisms with different cancers [68] such as breast [69, 70], lung [71, 72], head and neck [73, 74], bladder [75, 76], gastric [77], oral [78] and colorectal carcinoma [79–81]. Biallelic germline mutations of MUTYH were the first ever reported alterations in the BER pathway. These mutations were found in individuals with predisposition to numerous colorectal carcinomas and adenomas [82, 37, 83]. OGG1 is responsible for repairing oxidatively damaged guanine (G) bases of DNA and found to be involved in carcinogenesis as well [84, 85]. TDG gene is a thymine DNA glycosylase, and its expression levels decrease in various multiple myeloma cells by promoter methylation in tissue culture experiments when compared with normal plasma cells [86]. APE1 work by following the DNA glycosylases in BER pathway, and their increased production has been observed in germ cell tumours [87], whereas APE1 greater protein levels have demonstrated association with higher resistance to radiation exposure and drugs [88]. Overexpression of Polb, which fills the gap with nucleotides formed by APE1, was reported in breast, prostate and colon cancer cells [89–91]. Furthermore, elevated Polb levels can cause genomic instability via accumulating DNA single- and double-strand breaks [92, 93].

7.2.5 Homologous Recombination

DNA double-strand breaks cause most damaging threat among all the genotoxic attacks to cell survival and are meant to be repaired by either HR or NHEJ [94]. HR was found to be disrupted among ovarian and breast carcinomas [95]. Researchers have illustrated genetic alterations of two key HR genes BRCA1 and BRCA2 in early onset of breast cancer [96], ovarian cancer [97, 98], pancreatic carcinoma [99, 100] and prostatic carcinoma [101].

Loss of BRCA1 expression was also observed in nonhereditary ovarian and breast carcinoma by promoter hypermethylation [102, 103]. Furthermore, gene responsible for encoding NBSI and constituting a heterotrimeric complex of RAD50 and MRE11 meant for sensing DNA double-strand breaks was found to be frequently altered in lymphomas [104]. Expressional loss of NBS1 gene was also demonstrated in prostatic carcinoma [105]. Moreover, RAD50 frameshift mutations also lead to a truncated protein resulting in gastrointestinal cancers [106].

7.2.6 Non-homologous End Joining

NHEJ is predominantly responsible for repairing DNA double-strand breaks [107]. Gene meant to encode DNA ligase IV is the key mediator of NHEJ and responsible for leukaemia [108], whereas Artemis is altered in lymphoma also known as Omenn syndrome [109]. Researchers have also reported the expressional loss of Ku70 in colorectal, cervical and breast carcinomas [110–113], whereas decreased Ku86 expression is found in rectal carcinoma [114].

7.3 Role of DNA Repair Machinery in Cancer Metastasis

Metastasis is major cause of cancer-related deaths as 90 percent of them are due to lack of local control. Tumour metastasis comprises a list of complex steps that must be accomplished in order to give rise to detectable tumours at positions far away from organs where primary tumours initiate [115, 116]. A wide range of studies showed abnormal expression patterns of various genes responsible for different kinds of cancer- and tumour-related functions like kinase activation, angiogenesis, etc. [117]. Anyhow evidences confirmed that DNA repair genes are directly involved in tumorigenesis and their deficiencies are considered to be involved in inherent disposition to cancer [118, 119]. However, there is still a need to explore direct relation of DNA repair in the aetiology of metastasis. Presently, DNA repair role in aetiology of metastasis has been estimated by two different ways. First is DNA gene expression microarray analysis and the other is in vitro assays that are considered as an alternative for in vivo metastasis phenotypes [120]. Certain number of genes are overexpressed with the advancement of tumour, while some others are downregulated with tumour stage and metastasis progression. There is still a need to explore how these genes control the process of metastasis either by their part in cell cycle control, DNA repair and regulation of genomic stability or by some other novel functions like involvement in transcriptional regulation, acting as transcription factors, etc. [19, 121, 122].

Oncomine analysis revealed that various cancers, like pancreas, brain, head and neck, kidney and cervix, exhibited overexpressed DNA repair proteins [123]. Additionally, elevated levels of DNA repair proteins were observed in metastatic than in primary tumours among melanoma cases [124]. However, only HR and NER but not BER genes were found to be upregulated in melanomas determined by immunohistochemical and gene expression microarray analysis [125–127]. Genomic stability gives rise to distant metastasis from a melanoma cell [128, 129]. Therefore, most of the neoplastic cells (present in melanoma cells) have tendency to metastasize, as they have upregulated genes for effective repair producing genetically stable cells that have ability to metastasize [130, 131]. On the basis of these findings, it was hypothesized that genomic instability is useful in the initial stages of tumour development. However, metastatic and late-stage tumours upregulate series of DNA repair genes to certify lowest of genomic stability [132]. This activation and deactivation mode of DNA repair genes helps in estimating sensitivity or resistance of chemotherapy. Experiments have revealed that DNA repair pathway might not work properly in early carcinogenesis resulting in genetic instability; however, respective secondary variations confer a selective benefit to tumour [133–135]. Consequently, reactivation of repair pathway occurs [136].

Many genes that play a role in DNA damage-induced checkpoints and DNA repair by different means like upregulation (*PARP1*, *RAD9*), downregulation or mutation (BRCA1, TP53) have been found to be linked with metastasis checked by immunohistochemistry and various in vitro assays [37, 137–139]. Various genes among them along with their probable association with metastasis are discussed here. For example, RAD9 is a multiplex protein that helps in various cell functions along with cell cycle checkpoint activation. Some of these functions are dNTP biosynthesis, transcriptional regulation of genes, DNA repair, apoptosis and telomere maintenance [140]. It plays role in every DNA repair pathway except non-homologous end joining [141]. Telomere instability is also related with faulty DNA repair and RAD9 effects [142]. In addition, chromosome end-to-end association is also associated with genomic instability and resulting carcinogenesis [3, 143, 144]. An increase in chromosome end-to-end association and frequency in telomere loss can be seen when RAD9 is not in its active form [145]. Along with all these mentioned roles, RAD9 also helps in apoptosis. RAD9 sometimes neutralizes anti-apoptotic BclXL and Bcl-2 activity and induces pro-apoptotic Bax activity [146, 147]. One of the most important and less studied RAD9 activities is its potential to act as transcription factor and regulate various downstream target genes. It has also been identified as coregulator in prostate cancer cell lines that can suppress androgen-androgen receptor transactivation [142] (Table 7.1).

7.4 Conclusion

Recently, it has become evident that several genes play vital role in DNA repair and are responsible for tumorigenesis along with cancer metastasis. However, underlying molecular mechanisms are not fully explored yet. Genome profiling of primary in comparison with metastatic tumours and immunohistochemical analysis of tumour samples have confirmed the involvement of DNA repair genes. Moreover, results from in vitro experimentation evidenced the potential linkage of DNA repair genes with increased tumour invasion, migration, anchorage-independent growth and anoikis resistance. DNA repair proteins are multifunctional performing biochemical, cellular and gene regulatory roles. Nevertheless, which of the manifold roles of DNA repair proteins is required for metastases regulation is not completely known. However, from a practical perception, exploration of the molecular mechanisms involved is pivotal in facilitating the design of DNA-targeted therapies via proteins as innovative anticancer agents.

Table 7.1 Repair genes and functional roles of DNA damage response

Role in DDR	Gene	Other functions	References
DNA damage response	*ATM*	Cell metabolism	[148]
	H2AX	Apoptosis, TR	[149]
	NBSI		[150]
	RAD17	Cell cycle checkpoint	[151]
	TP53	TF, apoptosis	[152]
	TIP60	DSBR	[153]
Homologous recombination repair	*BRCA1*	Cell cycle checkpoint	[154]
	BRCA2		
	MCPH1/ BRIT1	Apoptosis	[155]
	PARP-1		[154]
	RAD9	dNTP synthesis, telomere maintenance, TF, apoptosis	[154]
	RAD51		[156]
Cell cycle checkpoint	*14-3-3δ*	Centrosome regulation, apoptosis, TR, chromatin remodelling	[157]
	BRCA1		[158]
	BRCA2	Centrosome duplication, TR	
	CDC25A		[159]
	RAD9	dNTP synthesis, TF, telomere maintenance, apoptosis	[160]
	RAD17		
Nucleotide excision repair	*GADD45a*	Apoptosis, TR	[106, 161]
	NM23	Nucleoside diphosphate kinase	[162]
	RAD9	TF, apoptosis, telomere maintenance, dNTP synthesis	[163]
	XRCC3	TF, apoptosis	[164]
Base excision repair	*PARP-1*	Apoptosis, TR	[165]
Mismatch repair	*RAD9*	Telomere maintenance, dNTP synthesis, apoptosis, TF	[166]
Double-strand break repair	*TIP60*		[167]
	H2AX	Apoptosis, TR	[168]

References

1. Srivastava R, Mishra N, Singh UM, Srivastava R (2016) Genotoxicity: mechanisms and its impact on human diseases. Octa J Biosci 2016:4
2. Tian H, Gao Z, Li H, Zhang B, Wang G, Zhang Q, Pei D, Zheng J (2015) DNA damage response–a double-edged sword in cancer prevention and cancer therapy. Cancer Lett 358(1):8–16
3. Jeggo PA, Pearl LH, Carr AM (2016) DNA repair, genome stability and cancer: a historical perspective. Nat Rev Cancer 16(1):35
4. Topalian SL, Taube JM, Anders RA, Pardoll DM (2016) Mechanism-driven biomarkers to guide immune checkpoint blockade in cancer therapy. Nat Rev Cancer 16(5):275
5. Schwertman P, Bekker-Jensen S, Mailand N (2016) Regulation of DNA double-strand break repair by ubiquitin and ubiquitin-like modifiers. Nat Rev 17(6):379
6. Nakad R, Schumacher B (2016) DNA damage response and immune defense: links and mechanisms. Front Genet 7:147
7. Gorbunova V, Seluanov A (2016) DNA double strand break repair, aging and the chromatin connection. Mutat Res 788:2–6

8. Maynard S, Fang EF, Scheibye-Knudsen M, Croteau DL, Bohr VA (2015) DNA damage, DNA repair, aging, and neurodegeneration. Cold Spring Harb Perspect Med 5(10):a025130
9. Tubbs A, Nussenzweig A (2017) Endogenous DNA damage as a source of genomic instability in cancer. Cell 168(4):644–656
10. Baylin SB, Jones PA (2016) Epigenetic determinants of cancer. Cold Spring Harb Perspect Biol 8(9):a019505
11. Nielsen FC, van Overeem Hansen T, Sørensen CS (2016) Hereditary breast and ovarian cancer: new genes in confined pathways. Nat Rev Cancer 16(9):599
12. Malik SS, Masood N, Asif M, Ahmed P, Shah ZU, Khan JS (2019) Expressional analysis of MLH1 and MSH2 in breast cancer. Curr Probl Cancer 43(2):97–105
13. Li Q, Damish AW, Frazier Z, Liu D, Reznichenko E, Kamburov A, Bell A, Zhao H, Jordan EJ, Gao SP (2019) ERCC2 helicase domain mutations confer nucleotide excision repair deficiency and drive cisplatin sensitivity in muscle-invasive bladder cancer. Clin Cancer Res 25(3):977–988
14. Murfuni I, Rass U (2016) Targeting homologous recombination repair in cancer. In: DNA repair in cancer therapy. Elsevier, London, pp 225–275
15. O'Connor MJ (2015) Targeting the DNA damage response in cancer. Mol Cell 60(4):547–560
16. Goldstein M, Kastan MB (2015) The DNA damage response: implications for tumor responses to radiation and chemotherapy. Annu Rev Med 66:129–143
17. Kelley MR, Logsdon D, Fishel ML (2014) Targeting DNA repair pathways for cancer treatment: what's new? Future Oncol 10(7):1215–1237
18. Jdey W, Thierry S, Russo C, Devun F, Al Abo M, Noguiez-Hellin P, Sun J-S, Barillot E, Zinovyev A, Kuperstein I (2017) Drug-driven synthetic lethality: bypassing tumor cell genetics with a combination of AsiDNA and PARP inhibitors. Clin Cancer Res 23(4):1001–1011
19. Gorgoulis VG, Pefani DE, Pateras IS, Trougakos IP (2018) Integrating the DNA damage and protein stress responses during cancer development and treatment. J Pathol 246(1):12–40
20. Smith MT, Guyton KZ, Gibbons CF, Fritz JM, Portier CJ, Rusyn I, DeMarini DM, Caldwell JC, Kavlock RJ, Lambert PF (2015) Key characteristics of carcinogens as a basis for organizing data on mechanisms of carcinogenesis. Environ Health Perspect 124(6):713–721
21. Roos WP, Thomas AD, Kaina B (2016) DNA damage and the balance between survival and death in cancer biology. Nat Rev Cancer 16(1):20
22. Tiwari V, Wilson DM (2019) DNA damage and associated DNA repair defects in disease and premature aging. Am J Hum Genet 105(2):237–257
23. Llinas-Arias P, Esteller M (2017) Epigenetic inactivation of tumour suppressor coding and non-coding genes in human cancer: an update. Open Biol 7(9):170152
24. Knijnenburg TA, Wang L, Zimmermann MT, Chambwe N, Gao GF, Cherniack AD, Fan H, Shen H, Way GP, Greene CS (2018) Genomic and molecular landscape of DNA damage repair deficiency across The Cancer Genome Atlas. Cell Rep 23(1):239–254
25. Gao D, Herman JG, Guo M (2016) The clinical value of aberrant epigenetic changes of DNA damage repair genes in human cancer. Oncotarget 7(24):37331
26. Bauer NC, Corbett AH, Doetsch PW (2015) The current state of eukaryotic DNA base damage and repair. Nucleic Acids Res 43(21):10083–10101
27. Malaiyandi LM, Potempa LA, Marschalk N, Jungsuwadee P, Dineley KE (2018) Alkylating-agent cytotoxicity associated with O^6-methylguanine. In: Apoptosis and beyond: the many ways cells die. Wiley, Hoboken, pp 427–431
28. Samavarchi Tehrani S, Mahmoodzadeh Hosseini H, Yousefi T, Abolghasemi M, Qujeq D, Maniati M, Amani J (2019) The crosstalk between trace elements with DNA damage response, repair, and oxidative stress in cancer. J Cell Biochem 120(2):1080–1105
29. Hiddinga BI, Pauwels P, Janssens A, van Meerbeeck JP (2017) O6-methylguanine-DNA methyltransferase (MGMT): a drugable target in lung cancer? Lung Cancer 107:91–99
30. Rapkins RW, Wang F, Nguyen HN, Cloughesy TF, Lai A, Ha W, Nowak AK, Hitchins MP, McDonald KL (2015) The MGMT promoter SNP rs16906252 is a risk factor for MGMT methylation in glioblastoma and is predictive of response to temozolomide. Neuro-Oncology 17(12):1589–1598

31. Misawa K, Mochizuki D, Imai A, Endo S, Mima M, Misawa Y, Kanazawa T, Carey TE, Mineta H (2016) Prognostic value of aberrant promoter hypermethylation of tumor-related genes in early-stage head and neck cancer. Oncotarget 7(18):26087
32. Kuroiwa-Trzmielina J, Wang F, Rapkins RW, Ward RL, Buchanan DD, Win AK, Clendenning M, Rosty C, Southey MC, Winship IM (2016) SNP rs16906252C> T is an expression and methylation quantitative trait locus associated with an increased risk of developing MGMT-methylated colorectal cancer. Clin Cancer Res 22(24):6266–6277
33. Paydar P, Asadikaram G, Nejad HZ, Akbari H, Abolhassani M, Moazed V, Nematollahi MH, Ebrahimi G, Fallah H (2019) Epigenetic modulation of BRCA-1 and MGMT genes, and histones H4 and H3 are associated with breast tumors. J Cell Biochem 120(8):13726–13736
34. Yu D, Cao T, Han Y-D, Huang F-S (2016) Relationships between MGMT promoter methylation and gastric cancer: a meta-analysis. OncoTargets Ther 9:6049
35. Malik SS, Mubarik S, Masood N, Khadim MT (2018) An insight into clinical outcome of XPG polymorphisms in breast cancer. Mol Biol Rep 45(6):2369–2375
36. Spivak G (2015) Nucleotide excision repair in humans. DNA Repair 36:13–18
37. Broustas CG, Lieberman HB (2014) DNA damage response genes and the development of cancer metastasis. Radiat Res 181(2):111–130
38. Gavande NS, VanderVere-Carozza PS, Hinshaw HD, Jalal SI, Sears CR, Pawelczak KS, Turchi JJ (2016) DNA repair targeted therapy: the past or future of cancer treatment? Pharmacol Ther 160:65–83
39. Dexheimer TS (2013) DNA repair pathways and mechanisms. In: Mathews LA, Cabarcas SM, Hurt EM (eds) DNA repair of cancer stem cells. Springer, Dordrecht, pp 19–32. https://doi.org/10.1007/978-94-007-4590-2_2
40. Melis JP, van Steeg H, Luijten M (2013) Oxidative DNA damage and nucleotide excision repair. Antioxid Redox Signal 18(18):2409–2419
41. Sollier J, Stork CT, García-Rubio ML, Paulsen RD, Aguilera A, Cimprich KA (2014) Transcription-coupled nucleotide excision repair factors promote R-loop-induced genome instability. Mol Cell 56(6):777–785
42. Nemzow L, Lubin A, Zhang L, Gong F (2015) XPC: going where no DNA damage sensor has gone before. DNA Repair 36:19–27
43. Marteijn JA, Lans H, Vermeulen W, Hoeijmakers JH (2014) Understanding nucleotide excision repair and its roles in cancer and ageing. Nat Rev 15(7):465
44. Song X, Wang S, Hong X, Li X, Zhao X, Huai C, Chen H, Gao Z, Qian J, Wang J (2017) Single nucleotide polymorphisms of nucleotide excision repair pathway are significantly associated with outcomes of platinum-based chemotherapy in lung cancer. Sci Rep 7(1):11785
45. Mucha B, Markiewicz L, Cuchra M, Szymczak I, Przybylowska-Sygut K, Dziki A, Majsterek I, Dziki L (2017) Nucleotide excision repair capacity and XPC, XPD gene polymorphism modulate colorectal cancer risk. Clin Colorectal Cancer 17:e435–e441
46. Li Y-L, Wei F, Li Y-P, Zhang L-H, Bai Y-Z (2017) A case-control study on association of nucleotide excision repair polymorphisms and its interaction with environment factors with the susceptibility to non-melanoma skin cancer. Oncotarget 8(46):80994
47. Romanowicz H, Strapagiel D, Słomka M, Sobalska-Kwapis M, Kępka E, Siewierska-Górska A, Zadrożny M, Bieńkiewicz J, Smolarz B (2017) New single nucleotide polymorphisms (SNPs) in homologous recombination repair genes detected by microarray analysis in Polish breast cancer patients. Clin Exp Med 17(4):541–546
48. Bailey MH, Ding L (2018) Genomic and molecular landscape of DNA damage repair deficiency across The Cancer Genome Atlas. Cell Rep 23(1):239–254
49. Shenoy N, Dronca R, Quevedo F, Boorjian SA, Cheville J, Costello B, Kohli M, Witzig T, Pagliaro L (2017) Low hypoxia inducible factor-1α (HIF-1α) expression in testicular germ cell tumors—a major reason for enhanced chemosensitivity? Chin J Cancer Res 29(4):374
50. Sankhwar M, Sankhwar SN, Bansal SK, Gupta G, Rajender S (2016) Polymorphisms in the XPC gene affect urinary bladder cancer risk: a case-control study, meta-analyses and trial sequential analyses. Sci Rep 6:27018

51. Awuah SG, Riddell IA, Lippard SJ (2017) Repair shielding of platinum-DNA lesions in testicular germ cell tumors by high-mobility group box protein 4 imparts cisplatin hypersensitivity. Proc Natl Acad Sci 114(5):950–955
52. Le May N, Calmels N, Abiayad Y, Boukli L, Semer M (2018) Xeroderma pigmentosum groups C and A in Algerian patients with deregulation of both transcription and DNA repair. J Case Rep Stud 6(4):401
53. Jiricny J (2006) The multifaceted mismatch-repair system. Nat Rev 7(5):335
54. Naidu MD, Mason JM, Pica RV, Fung H, Peña LA (2010) Radiation resistance in glioma cells determined by DNA damage repair activity of Ape1/Ref-1. J Radiat Res 51(4):393–404
55. Groothuizen FS, Sixma TK (2016) The conserved molecular machinery in DNA mismatch repair enzyme structures. DNA Repair 38:14–23
56. Li F, Mao G, Tong D, Huang J, Gu L, Yang W, Li G-M (2013) The histone mark H3K36me3 regulates human DNA mismatch repair through its interaction with MutSα. Cell 153(3):590–600
57. Li G-M (2014) New insights and challenges in mismatch repair: getting over the chromatin hurdle. DNA Repair 19:48–54
58. Reyes GX, Schmidt TT, Kolodner RD, Hombauer H (2015) New insights into the mechanism of DNA mismatch repair. Chromosoma 124(4):443–462
59. Xie C, Sheng H, Zhang N, Li S, Wei X, Zheng X (2016) Association of MSH6 mutation with glioma susceptibility, drug resistance and progression. Mol Clin Oncol 5(2):236–240
60. Zauber P, Marotta S, Sabbath-Solitare M (2017) Molecular genetic changes in benign colorectal tumors synchronous with microsatellite unstable carcinomas do not support a field defect. Int J Mol Epidemiol Genet 8(3):27
61. Zarandi A, Irani S, Savabkar S, Chaleshi V, Ghavideldarestani M, Mirfakhraie R, Khodadoostan M, Nazemalhosseini-Mojarad E, Aghdaei HA (2017) Evaluation of promoter methylation status of MLH1 gene in Iranian patients with colorectal tumors and adenoma polyps. Gastroenterol Hepatol Bed Bench 10(Suppl 1):S117
62. Tarancón-Diez M, Büttner R, Friedrichs N (2019) Enhanced tumoral MLH1-expression in MLH1-/PMS2-deficient colon cancer is indicative of sporadic colon cancer and not HNPCC. Pathol Oncol Res. https://doi.org/10.1007/s12253-018-00571-3
63. Ma Y, Chen Y, Petersen I (2017) Expression and promoter DNA methylation of MLH1 in colorectal cancer and lung cancer. Pathol Res Pract 213(4):333–338
64. Fan Y, Wang Y, Fu S, Yang L, Lin S, Fan Q, Wen Q (2018) The diagnostic role of DNA methylation in sporadic endometrial cancer: a systematic review and meta-analysis. Oncotarget 9(9):8642
65. Hu G, Qin L, Zhang X, Ye G, Huang T (2018) Epigenetic silencing of the MLH1 promoter in relation to the development of gastric cancer and its use as a biomarker for patients with microsatellite instability: a systematic analysis. Cell Physiol Biochem 45(1):148–162
66. Jaiswal A, Williamson E, Patel B, Srinivasan G, Kong K, Lomelino C, Narayan S, Hromas R (2019) Splicing component ISY1 interacts with APE1 and regulates base excision repair. AACR, Philadelphia
67. Maynard S, Schurman SH, Harboe C, de Souza-Pinto NC, Bohr VA (2008) Base excision repair of oxidative DNA damage and association with cancer and aging. Carcinogenesis 30(1):2–10
68. Norjmaa B, Tulgaa K, Saitoh T (2016) Base excision repair pathway and polymorphisms of xrcc1 gene. J Mol Pathol Epidemiol 1(1):1–4
69. Seibold P, Behrens S, Schmezer P, Helmbold I, Barnett G, Coles C, Yarnold J, Talbot CJ, Imai T, Azria D (2015) XRCC1 polymorphism associated with late toxicity after radiation therapy in breast cancer patients. Int J Radiat Oncol 92(5):1084–1092
70. AlMutairi F, Ali Khan Pathan A, Alanazi M, Shalaby M, Alabdulkarim HA, Alamri A, Al Naeem A, Elrobh M, Shaik JP, Khan W (2015) Association of DNA repair gene APE1 Asp148Glu polymorphism with breast cancer risk. Dis Markers 2015:869512

71. Du Y, He Y, Mei Z, Qian L, Shi J, Jie Z (2016) Association between genetic polymorphisms in XPD and XRCC1 genes and risks of non-small cell lung cancer in East Chinese Han population. Clin Respir J 10(3):311–317
72. Han B, Guo Z, Ma Y, Kang S, Wang Y, Wei Q, Wu X (2015) Association of GSTP1 and XRCC1 gene polymorphisms with clinical outcome of advanced non-small cell lung cancer patients with cisplatin-based chemotherapy. Int J Clin Exp Pathol 8(4):4113
73. Dylawerska A, Barczak W, Wegner A, Golusinski W, Suchorska WM (2017) Association of DNA repair genes polymorphisms and mutations with increased risk of head and neck cancer: a review. Med Oncol 34(12):197
74. Huang S-F, Chien H-T, Liao C-T, Wang H-M, Wang Y-H (2019) Roles of XRCC1 genetic polymorphism in head and neck cancer patients receiving radiation therapy in Taiwan. AACR, Philadelphia
75. Feki-Tounsi M, Khlifi R, Louati I, Fourati M, Mhiri M-N, Hamza-Chaffai A, Rebai A (2017) Polymorphisms in XRCC1, ERCC2, and ERCC3 DNA repair genes, CYP1A1 xenobiotic metabolism gene, and tobacco are associated with bladder cancer susceptibility in Tunisian population. Environ Sci Pollut Res 24(28):22476–22484
76. Zhong J-H, Zhao Z, Liu J, Yu H-L, Zhou J-Y, Shi R (2016) Association between APE1 Asp148Glu polymorphism and the risk of urinary cancers: a meta-analysis of 18 case–control studies. OncoTargets Ther 9:1499
77. Jin E-H, Kim J, Lee S-I, Hong JH (2015) Association between polymorphisms in APE1 and XRCC1 and the risk of gastric cancer in Korean population. Int J Clin Exp Med 8(7):11484
78. Huang HI, Chen CH, Wang SH, Wang LH, Lin YC (2019) Effects of APE1 Asp148Glu polymorphisms on OPMD malignant transformation, and on susceptibility to and overall survival of oral cancer in Taiwan. Head Neck 41(6):1557–1564
79. Das S, Nath S, Bhowmik A, Ghosh SK, Choudhury Y (2016) Association between OGG1 Ser326Cys polymorphism and risk of upper aero-digestive tract and gastrointestinal cancers: a meta-analysis. Springerplus 5(1):227
80. Zhou P-T, Li B, Ji J, Wang M-M, Gao C-F (2015) A systematic review and meta-analysis of the association between OGG1 Ser326Cys polymorphism and cancers. Med Oncol 32(2):31
81. Lai C-Y, Hsieh L-L, Tang R, Santella RM, Chang-Chieh CR, Yeh C-C (2016) Association between polymorphisms of APE1 and OGG1 and risk of colorectal cancer in Taiwan. World J Gastroenterol 22(12):3372
82. Nielsen M, Hes F, Nagengast F, Weiss M, Mathus-Vliegen E, Morreau H, Breuning M, Wijnen J, Tops C, Vasen H (2007) Germline mutations in APC and MUTYH are responsible for the majority of families with attenuated familial adenomatous polyposis. Clin Genet 71(5):427–433
83. Tanskanen T (2018) Genetic predisposition to colorectal cancer in young patients and in the general population
84. Shinmura K, Yokota J (2001) The OGG1 gene encodes a repair enzyme for oxidatively damaged DNA and is involved in human carcinogenesis. Antioxid Redox Signal 3(4):597–609
85. Cadet J, Davies KJ (2017) Oxidative DNA damage & repair: an introduction. Free Radic Biol Med 107:2–12
86. Peng B, Hurt EM, Hodge DR, Thomas SB, Farrar WL (2006) DNA hypermethylation and partial gene silencing of human thymine-DNA glycosylase in multiple myeloma cell lines. Epigenetics 1(3):138–145
87. Maher RL, Wallace SS, Pederson DS (2019) The lyase activity of bifunctional DNA glycosylases and the 3′-diesterase activity of APE1 contribute to the repair of oxidized bases in nucleosomes. Nucleic Acids Res 47(6):2922–2931
88. Ferreira J, Ramos AA, Almeida T, Azqueta A, Rocha E (2018) Drug resistance in glioblastoma and cytotoxicity of seaweed compounds, alone and in combination with anticancer drugs: a mini review. Phytomedicine 48:84–93
89. Poletto M, Lirussi L, Antoniali G, Tell G (2017) The abasic endonuclease APE1: much more than a DNA repair enzyme. In: The base excision repair pathway: molecular mechanisms and role in disease development and therapeutic design. World Scientific, Singapore, pp 219–251

90. Malfatti MC, Gerratana L, Dalla E, Isola M, Damante G, Di Loreto C, Puglisi F, Tell G (2019) APE1 and NPM1 protect cancer cells from platinum compounds cytotoxicity and their expression pattern has a prognostic value in TNBC. J Exp Clin Cancer Res 38(1):309
91. Starcevic D, Dalal S, Sweasy JB (2004) Is there a link between DNA polymerase beta and cancer? Cell Cycle 3(8):996–999
92. Sobol RW (2012) Genome instability caused by a germline mutation in the human DNA repair gene POLB. PLoS Genet 8(11):e1003086
93. Koturbash I, Baker M, Loree J, Kutanzi K, Hudson D, Pogribny I, Sedelnikova O, Bonner W, Kovalchuk O (2006) Epigenetic dysregulation underlies radiation-induced transgenerational genome instability in vivo. Int J Radiat Oncol 66(2):327–330
94. Mladenov E, Magin S, Soni A (2016) Iliakis G DNA double-strand-break repair in higher eukaryotes and its role in genomic instability and cancer: cell cycle and proliferation-dependent regulation. In: Seminars in cancer biology. Elsevier, Amsterdam, pp 51–64
95. Sullivan MR, Prakash R, Mihalevic MJ, Baird JM, Jasin M, Bernstein KA (2018) Abstract A08: a novel system determines the functional significance of ovarian tumor mutations in the homologous recombination gene RAD51C. AACR, Philadelphia
96. Majidinia M, Yousefi B (2017) DNA repair and damage pathways in breast cancer development and therapy. DNA Repair 54:22–29
97. Arts-de Jong M, de Bock GH, van Asperen CJ, Mourits MJ, de Hullu JA, Kets CM (2016) Germline BRCA1/2 mutation testing is indicated in every patient with epithelial ovarian cancer: a systematic review. Eur J Cancer 61:137–145
98. Norquist BM, Harrell MI, Brady MF, Walsh T, Lee MK, Gulsuner S, Bernards SS, Casadei S, Yi Q, Burger RA (2016) Inherited mutations in women with ovarian carcinoma. JAMA Oncol 2(4):482–490
99. Lal G, Liu G, Schmocker B, Kaurah P, Ozcelik H, Narod SA, Redston M, Gallinger S (2000) Inherited predisposition to pancreatic adenocarcinoma: role of family history and germ-line p16, BRCA1, and BRCA2 mutations. Cancer Res 60(2):409–416
100. Kaufman B, Shapira-Frommer R, Schmutzler RK, Audeh MW, Friedlander M, Balmaña J, Mitchell G, Fried G, Stemmer SM, Hubert A (2015) Olaparib monotherapy in patients with advanced cancer and a germline BRCA1/2 mutation. J Clin Oncol 33(3):244
101. Kerr L, Rewhorn MJ, Longmuir M, Fraser S, Walsh S, Andrew N, Leung HY (2016) A cohort analysis of men with a family history of BRCA1/2 and Lynch mutations for prostate cancer. BMC Cancer 16(1):529
102. Prakash R, Zhang Y, Feng W, Jasin M (2015) Homologous recombination and human health: the roles of BRCA1, BRCA2, and associated proteins. Cold Spring Harb Perspect Biol 7(4):a016600
103. Ceccaldi R, Rondinelli B, D'Andrea AD (2016) Repair pathway choices and consequences at the double-strand break. Trends Cell Biol 26(1):52–64
104. Nowak J, Świątek-Kościelna B, Kałużna EM, Rembowska J, Dzikiewicz-Krawczyk A, Zawada M, Januszkiewicz-Lewandowska D (2017) Effect of irradiation on DNA synthesis, NBN gene expression and chromosomal stability in cells with NBN mutations. AMS 13(2):283
105. Cybulski C, Gorski B, Dębniak T, Gliniewicz B, Mierzejewski M, Masojć B, Jakubowska A, Matyjasik J, Złowocka E, Sikorski A (2004) NBS1 is a prostate cancer susceptibility gene. Cancer Res 64(4):1215–1219
106. Kim N-G, Choi YR, Baek MJ, Kim YH, Kang H, Kim NK, Min JS, Kim H (2001) Frameshift mutations at coding mononucleotide repeats of the hRAD50 gene in gastrointestinal carcinomas with microsatellite instability. Cancer Res 61(1):36–38
107. Takata M, Sasaki MS, Sonoda E, Morrison C, Hashimoto M, Utsumi H, Yamaguchi-Iwai Y, Shinohara A, Takeda S (1998) Homologous recombination and non-homologous end-joining pathways of DNA double-strand break repair have overlapping roles in the maintenance of chromosomal integrity in vertebrate cells. EMBO J 17(18):5497–5508

108. O'Driscoll M, Cerosaletti KM, Girard P-M, Dai Y, Stumm M, Kysela B, Hirsch B, Gennery A, Palmer SE, Seidel J (2001) DNA ligase IV mutations identified in patients exhibiting developmental delay and immunodeficiency. Mol Cell 8(6):1175–1185
109. Pannicke U, Hönig M, Schulze I, Rohr J, Heinz GA, Braun S, Janz I, Rump EM, Seidel MG, Matthes-Martin S (2010) The most frequent DCLRE1C (ARTEMIS) mutations are based on homologous recombination events. Hum Mutat 31(2):197–207
110. Komuro Y, Watanabe T, Hosoi Y, Matsumoto Y, Nakagawa K, Saito S, Ishihara S, Kazama S, Tsuno N, Kitayama J (2003) Prediction of tumor radiosensitivity in rectal carcinoma based on p53 and Ku70 expression. J Exp Clin Cancer Res 22(2):223–228
111. Ramzan Z, Nassri AB, Huerta S (2014) Genotypic characteristics of resistant tumors to pre-operative ionizing radiation in rectal cancer. World J Gastrointest Oncol 6(7):194
112. Komuro Y, Watanabe T, Hosoi Y, Matsumoto Y, Nakagawa K, Tsuno N, Kazama S, Kitayama J, Suzuki N, Nagawa H (2002) The expression pattern of Ku correlates with tumor radiosensitivity and disease free survival in patients with rectal carcinoma. Cancer 95(6):1199–1205
113. Agboola AO, Ebili HO, Iyawe VO, Banjo AA, Salami BA, Rakha EA, Nolan CC, Ellis IO, Green AR (2017) Clinicopathological and molecular characteristics of Ku 70/80 expression in Nigerian breast cancer and its potential therapeutic implications. Pathol Res Pract 213(1):27–33
114. Takada Y, Someya M, Matsumoto Y, Satoh M, Nakata K, Hori M, Saito M, Hirokawa N, Tateoka K, Teramoto M (2016) Influence of Ku86 and XRCC4 expression in uterine cervical cancer on the response to preoperative radiotherapy. Med Mol Morphol 49(4):210–216
115. Hanahan D, Weinberg RA (2011) Hallmarks of cancer: the next generation. Cell 144(5): 646–674
116. Allen S (2018) Understanding mechanisms of metastasis of aggressive breast cancers via microfluidic means
117. Ronca R, Benkheil M, Mitola S, Struyf S, Liekens S (2017) Tumor angiogenesis revisited: regulators and clinical implications. Med Res Rev 37(6):1231–1274
118. Aslan C, Maralbashi S, Salari F, Kahroba H, Sigaroodi F, Kazemi T, Kharaziha P (2019) Tumor-derived exosomes: implication in angiogenesis and antiangiogenesis cancer therapy. J Cell Physiol 234(10):16885–16903
119. Jackson M, Marks L, May GH, Wilson JB (2018) The genetic basis of disease. Essays Biochem 62(5):643–723
120. Gutschner T, Hämmerle M, Eißmann M, Hsu J, Kim Y, Hung G, Revenko A, Arun G, Stentrup M, Groß M (2013) The noncoding RNA MALAT1 is a critical regulator of the metastasis phenotype of lung cancer cells. Cancer Res 73(3):1180–1189
121. Malumbres M, Barbacid M (2009) Cell cycle, CDKs and cancer: a changing paradigm. Nat Rev Cancer 9(3):153
122. Mallick B (2019) AGO-driven non-coding RNAs: codes to decode the therapeutics of diseases. Academic, London
123. Phan NN, Wang CY, Chen CF, Sun Z, Lai MD, Lin YC (2017) Voltage-gated calcium channels: novel targets for cancer therapy. Oncol Lett 14(2):2059–2074
124. Zakaria R, Platt-Higgins A, Rathi N, Crooks D, Brodbelt A, Chavredakis E, Lawson D, Jenkinson MD, Rudland PS (2016) Metastasis-inducing proteins are widely expressed in human brain metastases and associated with intracranial progression and radiation response. Br J Cancer 114(10):1101
125. Mocellin S, Bertazza L, Benna C, Pilati P (2012) Circumventing melanoma chemoresistance by targeting DNA repair. Curr Med Chem 19(23):3893–3899
126. Dogrusöz M, Ruschel Trasel A, Cao J, Çolak S, van Pelt SI, Kroes WG, Teunisse AF, Alsafadi S, van Duinen SG, Luyten GP (2019) Differential expression of DNA repair genes in prognostically-favorable versus unfavorable uveal melanoma. Cancer 11(8):1104
127. Kaplan AR, Glazer PM (2019) Impact of hypoxia on DNA repair and genome integrity. Mutagenesis. gez019, https://doi.org/10.1093/mutage/gez019
128. Grichnik JM (2006) Genomic instability and tumor stem cells. J Investig Dermatol 126(6): 1214–1216

129. Kauffmann A, Rosselli F, Lazar V, Winnepenninckx V, Mansuet-Lupo A, Dessen P, Van den Oord J, Spatz A, Sarasin A (2008) High expression of DNA repair pathways is associated with metastasis in melanoma patients. Oncogene 27(5):565
130. Joyce JA, Pollard JW (2009) Microenvironmental regulation of metastasis. Nat Rev Cancer 9(4):239
131. Quail DF, Joyce JA (2013) Microenvironmental regulation of tumor progression and metastasis. Nat Med 19(11):1423
132. Robinson DR, Wu Y-M, Lonigro RJ, Vats P, Cobain E, Everett J, Cao X, Rabban E, Kumar-Sinha C, Raymond V (2017) Integrative clinical genomics of metastatic cancer. Nature 548(7667):297
133. Gupta GP, Massagué J (2006) Cancer metastasis: building a framework. Cell 127(4):679–695
134. Bodmer W (2008) Genetic instability is not a requirement for tumor development. Cancer Res 68(10):3558–3561
135. Lord CJ, Ashworth A (2012) The DNA damage response and cancer therapy. Nature 481(7381):287
136. Chirnomas D, Taniguchi T, de la Vega M, Vaidya AP, Vasserman M, Hartman A-R, Kennedy R, Foster R, Mahoney J, Seiden MV (2006) Chemosensitization to cisplatin by inhibitors of the Fanconi anemia/BRCA pathway. Mol Cancer Ther 5(4):952–961
137. Ta HQ, Gioeli D (2014) The convergence of DNA damage checkpoint pathways and androgen receptor signaling in prostate cancer. Endocr Relat Cancer 21(5):R395–R407
138. Attari MMA, Ostadian C, Saei AA, Mihanfar A, Darband SG, Sadighparvar S, Kaviani M, Samadi H, Yousefi B, Majidinia M (2019) DNA damage response and repair in ovarian cancer: potential targets for therapeutic strategies. DNA Repair 80:59–84
139. Alblihy A, Mesquita KA, Sadiq MT, Madhusudan S (2019) Development and implementation of precision therapies targeting base-excision DNA repair in BRCA1-associated tumors. Exp Rev Precis Med Drug Dev 4(1):11–25
140. Doak SH (2018) Exposure to engineered nanomaterials: impact on DNA repair pathways. Int J Mol Sci 18:1515
141. Liu T, Huang J (2016) DNA end resection: facts and mechanisms. Genomics Proteomics Bioinformatics 14(3):126–130
142. Lieberman HB, Panigrahi SK, Hopkins KM, Wang L, Broustas CG (2017) p53 and RAD9, the DNA damage response, and regulation of transcription networks. Radiat Res 187(4):424–432
143. Mavragani I, Nikitaki Z, Souli M, Aziz A, Nowsheen S, Aziz K, Rogakou E, Georgakilas A (2017) Complex DNA damage: a route to radiation-induced genomic instability and carcinogenesis. Cancer 9(7):91
144. Vodicka P, Musak L, Vodickova L, Vodenkova S, Catalano C, Kroupa M, Naccarati A, Polivkova Z, Vymetalkova V, Försti A (2018) Genetic variation of acquired structural chromosomal aberrations. Mutat Res 836:13–21
145. Lazzerini-Denchi E, Sfeir A (2016) Stop pulling my strings—what telomeres taught us about the DNA damage response. Nat Rev 17(6):364
146. Lieberman HB (2006) Rad9, an evolutionarily conserved gene with multiple functions for preserving genomic integrity. J Cell Biochem 97(4):690–697
147. Lieberman HB, Rai AJ, Friedman RA, Hopkins KM, Broustas CG (2018) Prostate cancer: unmet clinical needs and RAD9 as a candidate biomarker for patient management. Transl Cancer Res 7(Suppl 6):S651
148. Shiloh Y, Ziv Y (2013) The ATM protein kinase: regulating the cellular response to genotoxic stress, and more. Nat Rev 14(4):197
149. Economopoulou M, Langer HF, Celeste A, Orlova VV, Choi EY, Ma M, Vassilopoulos A, Callen E, Deng C, Bassing CH (2009) Histone H2AX is integral to hypoxia-driven neovascularization. Nat Med 15(5):553
150. Wan R, Crowe DL (2012) Haploinsufficiency of the Nijmegen breakage syndrome 1 gene increases mammary tumor latency and metastasis. Int J Oncol 41(1):345–352

151. Bozko P, Scholta T, Bui K, Toulany M, Rodemann H, Malek N (2018) Notch1-Cyclin E-p27kip1 and RAD17 form a network of proteins which control cellular proliferation and DNA damage response in cholangiocarcinoma. Z Gastroenterol 56(1):A4
152. Williams AB, Schumacher B (2016) p53 in the DNA-damage-repair process. Cold Spring Harb Perspect Med 6(5):a026070
153. Soliman S, Orlacchio A, Tessari A, Capece M, Visone R, Croce C, Palmieri D, Coppola V (2019) RANBP9 presence affects levels of Tip60 and activated p53 in lung cancer cells in response to DNA damage. AACR, Philadelphia
154. Brill E, Yokoyama T, Nair J, Yu M, Ahn Y-R, Lee J-M (2017) Prexasertib, a cell cycle checkpoint kinases 1 and 2 inhibitor, increases in vitro toxicity of PARP inhibition by preventing Rad51 foci formation in BRCA wild type high-grade serous ovarian cancer. Oncotarget 8(67):111026
155. Alsiary R, Brownhill SC, Brüning-Richardson A, Hutson R, Griffin N, Morrison EE, Bond J, Burchill SA, Bell SM (2018) Expression analysis of the MCPH1/BRIT1 and BRCA1 tumor suppressor genes and telomerase splice variants in epithelial ovarian cancer. Gene 672:34–44
156. Lim PX, Sutherland J, Noonan R, Dananberg A, Holloman W, Smogorzewska A, Jasin M (2017) Abstract A27: assessing somatic tumor-associated RAD51 mutations and screening for novel dominant-interfering RAD51 proteins. AACR, Philadelphia
157. Yamamoto Y, Koma H, Yagami T (2015) Localization of 14-3-3δ/ξ on the neuronal cell surface. Exp Cell Res 338(2):149–161
158. Takaoka M, Miki Y (2018) BRCA1 gene: function and deficiency. Int J Clin Oncol 23(1): 36–44
159. Gabrielli B, Burgess A (2016) Cdc25 family phosphatases in cancer. In: Protein tyrosine phosphatases in cancer. Springer, New York, pp 283–306
160. Nyberg KA (2003) Analysis of RAD9 functions: roles in the checkpoint response, DNA damage processing, and prevention of genomic instability. The University of Arizona
161. Kim YJ, Kim H-J, Kim HL, Kim HJ, Kim HS, Lee TR, Shin DW, Seo YR (2017) A protective mechanism of visible red light in normal human dermal fibroblasts: enhancement of GADD45A-Mediated DNA repair activity. J Investig Dermatol 137(2):466–474
162. Sheng Y, Xu M, Li C, Xiong Y, Yang Y, Kuang X, Wang D, Yang X (2018) Nm23-H1 is involved in the repair of ionizing radiation-induced DNA double-strand breaks in the A549 lung cancer cell line. BMC Cancer 18(1):710
163. Maga G, Hubscher U (2008) Repair and translesion DNA polymerases as anticancer drug targets. Anti Cancer Agents Med Chem 8(4):431–447
164. Bu D, Tomlinson G, Lewis CM, Zhang C, Kildebeck E, Euhus DM (2006) An intronic polymorphism associated with increased XRCC1 expression, reduced apoptosis and familial breast cancer. Breast Cancer Res Treat 99(3):257–265
165. Xu P, Cai X, Zhang W, Li Y, Qiu P, Lu D, He X (2016) Flavonoids of Rosa roxburghii Tratt exhibit radioprotection and anti-apoptosis properties via the Bcl-2 (Ca 2+)/Caspase-3/PARP-1 pathway. Apoptosis 21(10):1125–1143
166. Hwang B-J, Shi G, Lu A-L (2014) Mammalian MutY homolog (MYH or MUTYH) protects cells from oxidative DNA damage. DNA Repair 13:10–21
167. Radhakrishnan R, Li Y, Xiang S, Yuan F, Yuan Z, Telles E, Fang J, Coppola D, Shibata D, Lane WS (2015) Histone deacetylase 10 regulates DNA mismatch repair and may involve the deacetylation of MutS homolog 2. J Biol Chem 290(37):22795–22804
168. Moeglin E, Desplancq D, Conic S, Oulad-Abdelghani M, Stoessel A, Chiper M, Vigneron M, Didier P, Tora L, Weiss E (2019) Uniform widespread nuclear phosphorylation of histone H2AX is an indicator of lethal DNA replication stress. Cancer 11(3):355

Adapting the Foreign Soil: Factors Promoting Tumor Metastasis

8

Ramish Riaz, Shah Rukh Abbas, and Maria Shabbir

Around 90% of the deaths among cancer patients occur due to metastasis. Treatment of metastasis remains a challenge for oncologists. Metastasis can appear even decades after the removal of primary tumor. Tumors can remain dormant for years and develop metastasis when conditions become suitable. This period of latency is referred to as tumor dormancy. Disease is usually detected when tumor is already in advance stage. Detection of disseminated cancer cells and controlling the mechanisms contributing in development of overt metastasis might decrease the mortality associated with it [1].

Metastasis occurs via multistep process. Cancer cells first undergo epithelial to mesenchymal transition (EMT) which allows them to disseminate from primary tumor. Attainment of mesenchymal traits helps the cancer cells to gain motile properties. Physiologically, EMT occurs during embryogenesis and wound healing in response to signals received from neighboring cells. In carcinogenic process, EMT starts in response to signals originated from tumor microenvironment. Most common signaling pathways involved include TGF β, Notch, and WNT signaling pathways. Many growth factors including epidermal growth factor (EGF),

Shah Rukh Abbas and Maria Shabbir contributed equally with all other contributors.

R. Riaz (✉)
Atta Ur Rahman School of Applied Biosciences, NUST, Islamabad, Pakistan

Pakistan Institute of Medical Sciences, Islamabad, Pakistan
e-mail: ramish_exclusive@hotmail.com

S. R. Abbas
Department of Industrial Biotechnology, Atta Ur Rahman School of Applied Biosciences, NUST, Islamabad, Pakistan
e-mail: sabbas@asab.nust.edu.pk

M. Shabbir
Department of Healthcare Biotechnology, Atta Ur Rahman School of Applied Biosciences, NUST, Islamabad, Pakistan
e-mail: mshabbir@asab.nust.edu.pk

N. Masood, S. Shakil Malik (eds.), *'Essentials of Cancer Genomic, Computational Approaches and Precision Medicine*,
https://doi.org/10.1007/978-981-15-1067-0_8

hepatocyte growth factor (HGF), fibroblast growth factor (FGF), insulin growth factor (IGF), and platelet-derived growth factor (PDGF) play an important role in induction of EMT [2]. Hypoxia promoting HIF1α activation and release of proinflammatory cytokines like IL-1β, TNF-α, NF-κβ also promotes EMT. Induction of EMT helps cancer cells to lose cell-to-cell connection and invade the extracellular matrix (ECM). However, once inside blood vessels, factors inducing EMT are no longer present. Here platelet-derived multiple growth factors play an important role in maintaining mesenchymal state. Upon reaching the foreign soil, disseminated cells maintain their mesenchymal state by the support of premetastatic niches. These niches are rich in myeloid cells, hematopoietic progenitor cells, and a variety of factors including VEGF-1, MMP2, MMP9, COX2, as well as WNT5A which promote the maintenance of mesenchymal state [3].

Next step for disseminated cells is to invade the neighboring tissue by degrading ECM. ECM degradation is necessary for invasion and intravasation. It is tightly regulated by tissue inhibitors of matrix metalloproteases (TIMPs) and metalloproteases (MMPs). MMPs are activated in response to inflammatory cytokines like IL-1, IL-6, and TNF-α, growth factors like EGF, PDGF, and TGF in addition to proteases like elastases, chymosin, and plasmin. Most notable MMPs that play an important role in invasion are MMP1, MMP2, MMP8, and MMP9. By degrading basement membrane, MMPs not only support intravasation but also promote migration of endothelial cells, thereby supporting the process of angiogenesis. MMP9 and MMP2 also secrete vascular endothelial growth factor (VEGF) which is a mitogen factor for endothelial cells and an important promoter of angiogenesis [4].

Disseminated tumor cells (DTCs) metastasize to distant sites via vascular or lymphatic route. By degrading basement membrane, cells enter the circulation. Here they survive via escaping the immune responses and reach the distant sites [5]. Upon extravasation in foreign tissue, tumors have to adapt the microenvironment and evade immune surveillance to establish macro-metastasis. They remain there in dormant stage till they alter themselves sufficiently to develop overt metastasis. Mechanisms involving the tumor dormancy and overt growth are poorly understood and are still under research [6]. Current chapter reviews the mechanisms involving tumor dormancy, microenvironmental control, immunomodulation, mechano-transduction, and exit of dormancy and their possible role in establishing cancer metastasis.

8.1 Metastatic Tumor Dormancy

In response to stress or harmful stimuli, cells enter a dormant or nondividing stage. This helps the cell or microorganism to survive the hostile environment. Cellular dormancy is an evolutionary conserved phenomenon observed in cells and microorganism to help them in adapting stress [5, 7]. Different microorganisms like viruses (HIV, HBV) and bacteria (*Mycobacterium tuberculosis*) survive in host by entering into latent, dormant state [8]. Similarly mammalian stem cells as well as immune cells also remain in quiescent state until they receive proliferative signals [9]. Tumor dormancy refers to existence of cancerous cells without manifestation of disease.

This was identified on random autopsy of prostate tissues of population without any cancer. Postmortem reports have revealed up to 27% of the autopsies having carcinoma in prostate specimen. Similarly 39% of the histologic breast tissues upon postmortem studies have revealed carcinoma in situ [10]. This tumor dormancy occurs before the onset of primary tumor. Hadfield defined tumor dormancy as mitotic arrest at G0-G1 phase, i.e., establishment of equilibrium state between cellular division and apoptosis [11].

Metastasis has been long thought as late event resulting as a result of stepwise sequence of primary tumor spread to regional lymph nodes as well as distant organs. However, occurrence of metastasis without evidence of primary tumor changed the classical understanding of metastasis. Recent studies have revealed that tumors as small as <5 mm can develop distant metastasis. In most of the cases, metastasis appears after the onset of primary tumor, but sometimes it is detectable even before the manifestation of primary tumor. Metastasis can appear years even after the resection of primary tumor. This latent stage is usually referred to as metastatic tumor dormancy in which DTCs stay in dormant stage for years [12]. These DTCs show lack of both proliferative (Ki67) and apoptotic markers. Most common site homing DTCs is the bone marrow. Another subgroup of DTCs is circulating tumor cells (CTCs) which circulate in the blood. Detection of CTCs in peripheral blood is considered to be hallmark of advanced disease. However due to very low amount of CTCs in blood, their detection requires ultrasensitive bio-sensing devices. During latent period DTCs and CTCs alter them or equip them with necessary functions required for development of tumor at secondary site [13].

8.1.1 Mechanism of Metastatic Dormancy

Metastatic dormancy could occur as single cell or solitary dormancy or tumor mass dormancy. Several mechanisms are thought to promote metastatic dormancy including intracellular signaling mechanisms, extracellular factors, and immunological and angiogenic processes [14].

8.1.1.1 Intracellular Signaling Mechanisms

Crosstalk between mitogen-activated signals and stress-induced signals controls cellular dormancy. Among intracellular signals, mitogen-activated protein kinase (MAPK) signaling cascade is the most important signaling pathway regulating dormancy in addition to proliferation. P38α MAPK negatively regulates cellular proliferation and promotes DTCs dormancy, whereas extracellular signal-regulated kinase (ERK1/2) is a promoter of proliferation. ERK1/2 to MAPK38 ratio is an important indicator of dormancy and proliferation. Upregulation of urokinase plasminogen activator receptor (uPAR) and MAPK 38 results in activation of unfolded protein response which promotes transcription of ATF6 resulting in growth arrest [15].

ATF6 promotes the survival of dormant cells by activating RheB and mTOR independent of AKT [16]. MAPK38 pathway also promotes the activity of p53 and p16 and decreases the activity of cyclin D thereby promoting cellular dormancy [17].

Reduction in PI3K-AKT signaling also promotes autophagy and quiescence under deprived nutritional conditions. PI3K-AKT inhibits FOXO, increasing MDM2 resulting in inhibition of cell cycle arrest. Inhibition of AKT relieves FOXO and MDM2-mediated p53 inhibition resulting in quiescence and cell cycle arrest [18].

Autophagy also plays an important role in dormancy. Factors promoting autophagy promotes dormant state. Aplasia ras homolog member1 (ARH1) induces dormancy in ovarian cancer by promoting autophagy via inhibition of PI3K/AKT/mTOR signaling pathway. ARH1 interacts with BECN1 α to form autophagosome. It is reported that ARH1 promotes dormancy in vivo and cell death in vitro. Autophagy is also promoted under conditions of cellular stress. Accumulation of misfolded proteins results in unfolded protein response via protein kinase R-like endoplasmic reticulum kinase-eIF2α-activating transcription factor 4-alpha (PERK-eIF2α-ATF4) signaling axis. The axis has been found to promote dormancy in head and neck cancer [19].

8.1.1.2 Extracellular Signaling Mechanisms

Among extracellular signals transforming growth factor β (TGF β) family plays an important role in regulating dormancy. TGF β is one of the largest families of cytokines which regulate a variety of functions including angiogenesis, cellular proliferation, epithelial to mesenchymal transition, and quiescence. TGF β1 act as an inhibitor of proliferation in precancerous state and as promoter in advanced stages. TGF β3 also act as promoter of proliferation; however TGF β2 act as inhibitor of proliferation by inducing metastatic suppressor DEC (differentially expressed in chondrocyte). DEC suppresses CDK and induces p27 thereby promoting tumor dormancy [13]. TGF β promotes dormancy by both canonical, i.e., via activation of SMAD4 and noncanonical pathways independent of SMAD4. In canonical pathway, oligomerization of receptor leads to phosphorylation of SMAD2/3 which interacts with SMAD4 to directly promote transcription of dormancy associated genes. However, in noncanonical pathway, TGF β promotes dormancy by promoting MAPK38 activity [20].

Bone morphogenic proteins (BMPs) and growth arrest-specific 6 (GAS6) genes are other important extracellular signals promoting tumor dormancy. They have dual role in dormancy; some members like BMP4 and BMP7 promote dormancy, while BMP2 supports proliferation. BMP7 activates NGDR1 present downstream of N-myc which results in activation of MAPK 38 and p21 resulting in cell cycle arrest [21]. BMP4 promotes dormancy via SMAD1/5 signaling [20].

Cytoskeletal organization also has an impact on dormancy status. Stress fiber formation promotes exiting dormancy and entering proliferative stage. β1 integrin causes phosphorylation of myosin light chain by activating myosin light chain kinase MLCK. Inhibition of β1 integrin is also reported to promote dormancy in breast cancer cell lines by inhibiting myosin light chain kinase (MLCK) [16].

8.1.1.3 Immunological Mechanisms

Immune system plays an important role in preventing tumorigenesis and its progression. Tumor cells are surrounded by a variety of immune cells including lymphocytes, macrophages, natural killer cells, fibroblasts, and neutrophils which interact via a variety of signaling pathways mediated by cytokines, lymphokines, and cellular adhesion molecules which suppress its proliferation. For a cell to proliferate, it has to bypass all these signaling pathways or escape this immune surveillance. Immune system confines metastatic spread of tumor by establishing dormancy in tumor cells [22]. Natural killer cells and cytotoxic T cells play an important role in controlling overt metastasis. CD8+ T cells promote cell cycle inhibition via IFN-γ- and TNF-mediated signaling. To circumvent immune targeting, the metastatic cells have to undergo necessary alterations during dormancy [23, 24].

During dormancy, cells avoid CTL-mediated death by overexpressing B1 and B7-H1. Via paracrine signaling and secreting cytokines like IL-13, they avoid apoptosis. Also they activate JAK/STAT pathway by inhibiting SOCS1, a negative regulator of JAK/STAT pathway [25]. Inflammatory response or other perturbations in this equilibrium cause cancer cells to exit dormancy and develop overt metastasis [22].

Interleukins IL-12 and IL-23 are important interleukins secreted by dendritic cells and antigen-presenting cells. In tumor microenvironment, ratio of IL-12 and IL-23 can shape the environment to become tumor supportive or tumor repressive. IL-12 is found to activate IFN-γ and has tumor repressive function. It also promotes T-cell activity, while IL-23 is protumorigenic and causes upregulation of MMP9 and VEGF thereby promoting angiogenesis and metastasis [26].

8.1.1.4 Angiogenic Mechanisms

Tumor cells are unable to grow beyond 2 mm without new vessel formation. To get nutrients, they initiate program of angiogenesis by secreting angiogenic factors like vascular endothelial growth factor (VEGF) which recruits endothelial cells [14]. Angiogenesis is regulated by angiogenic promoters like VEGF and inhibitors like angiostatin and thrombospondin-1 (TSP1). Lack of proangiogenic factors and upregulation of antiangiogenic factors result in tumor dormancy. Upregulation of thrombospondin-1, an angiogenic inhibitor induces tumor dormancy in DTCs in osteosarcoma, glioblastoma, liposarcoma, and breast cancer [27]. Thrombospondin-1 is also produced by CD8 and CD4 T cells resulting in inhibition of angiogenesis. It promotes EMT as well as survival of dormant resistant cells. It also promotes activation of TGF β which both favor dormancy in addition to tumorigenesis by upregulating VEGF and hence play an important role in oncogenesis. Shift toward angiogenesis by VEGF helps in exiting dormancy and developing overt metastasis [28].

Downregulation of HSP27 is also found to induce tumor dormancy in breast cancer. HSP27 promotes angiogenesis by inducing angiogenic promoters. Its upregulation is linked with exit from dormancy and tumor spread [29]. Similarly VEGF, periostin, and TGF β promote neovasculature sprouting in return promoting micrometastatic outgrowth [30].

8.1.1.5 Hypoxia

Hypoxia occurs in majority of the solid malignancies and is associated with invasiveness and poor survival. Hypoxia causes activation of hypoxia-associated transcription factors including hypoxia-inducible factor HIF1α, stress-related proteins, mTOR1 complex, and stabilization of VEGF. Hypoxia is both promoter of dormancy and also helps the cells in exiting dormancy. Its role in tumor dormancy is still ambiguous. Dormancy due to hypoxia is usually attributed to its role in inducing autophagy which causes tumor cells to remain in quiescent stage for longer period and stay unresponsive to radiotherapy as well as chemotherapy [13]. Severe hypoxia also leads to the activation of PP2A which promotes growth inhibition and tumor dormancy [13, 31]. Dormancy markers like NR2F1, DEC, and p27 are upregulated in hypoxia [27]. Hypoxic factors that promote proliferation include HIFα and LOXL2. LOXL2 is involved in epithelial to mesenchymal transition and drives these cells to express cancer stem cell-like properties, thereby promoting invasion and metastasis [32]. Also for survival of cell during hypoxic state, cell must have to save its energy resources. Consumption of oxygen, glucose, and ATP is decreased during the state of dormancy; therefore it supports cancer cell survival during nutrient deprivation and hypoxic conditions. However, hypoxia also induces transcription of HIF1α which upregulates VEGF thereby promoting angiogenesis. Switch of cells toward angiogenic state helps in exiting from dormant stage [33].

8.1.1.6 Cancer Stem Cells

Cancer stem cells are the stem cells of the tumor which have full capability to initiate and support tumor at any site. Like other progenitor cells, these cells mostly remain in quiescent state and are largely resistant to therapies which mostly target rapidly dividing cells. After removal of stress or treatment, the stem cells start dividing, exit dormancy, and develop metastatic growth [34]. It has been reported that noncancer stem cells can also convert to cancer stem cells following survival mechanism [35].

Autophagy is an evolutionary conserved mechanism in stem cells. CSCs can initiate autophagy by activating LKB1-AMPK. Autophagy establishes long latency program in DTCs. However, this dormancy program is usually transient, whenever conditions become suitable; CSCs promotes epithelial to mesenchymal transition and metastasis [36].

Tumor microenvironment also helps CSCs in maintaining dormancy. Mesenchymal stem cells (MSCs) present in metastatic niches interact with disseminated CSCs to promote quiescent state. Interaction between MSCs and CSCs occur via secretion of mRNA exosomes. Presence of gap junctions allows sharing of miRNAs between MSCs and CSCs. In breast cancer stem cells, miRNAs 127,129, 222, and 223 are reported to induce quiescence by decreasing CXCL12. Bone is one of the common sites of metastasis. Bone microenvironment promotes dormancy by secreting soluble factors like TGF β and is rich in MSCs. As CSCs prefer hypoxic environment for their survival in dormant state, they also secrete stress signals. These stress proteins like clausterin bind with IGF and inhibit PI3K-AKT pathway thereby promoting dormancy [37] (Table 8.1).

Table 8.1 Factors playing role in dormancy

Mechanisms	Promoters of dormancy	Inhibitors of dormancy
Intracellular	MAPK, ATF6, ARH1, PERK-eIF2α-ATF4	ERK1/2, PI3K-AKT
Extracellular	TGF β2, BMP4, BMP7,GAS-6	TGF β3, BMP2, MLCK
Immunological	CD8 T cells, JAK/STAT, IL-12, IFN	IL-1, IL-10,IL-13,IL-23, TAM, Treg
Angiogenic	Thrombospondin-1, angiostatin	VEGF, HSP27
Stem cell based	LKB-1-AMPK; miRNAs 127,129, 222, and 223; clausterin	SDF-1, OPN, LOX, MMPs

8.2 Tumor Microenvironment

In 1889, Stephen Paget gave his famous "seed and soil" hypothesis, according to which malignant cells need receptive environment to implant its cells in distant organ. In 1930, James Ewing opposed his theory by proposing that pattern metastatic dissemination is dependent upon hematogenous flow. Isaiah Josh Fidler demonstrated that although tumor cells utilize blood flow to reach distant organ, their implantation is organ specific. His finding revived Paget's theory of need of receptive soil for successful engraftment. Research focused on pathophysiology of receptive microenvironment or niches have given the detail account of molecular mechanism that contributes in making soil receptive for metastasis [38].

8.2.1 Premetastatic Niche

Niche refers to a place or status where person is most satisfied. Similarly, in cancer biology premetastatic niche refers to microenvironment which supports the implantation and proliferation of disseminated cancer cells. Premetastatic niche in comparison to metastatic niche is devoid of cancer cell; it is site of future implantation. It evolves as a result of secretion of soluble factors and extracellular vesicles which signal the tumor-associated cells to cluster at premetastatic site to create an environment that is receptive for tumor invasion. Other factors which contribute to its evolution include pathophysiological conditions like inflammation and aging which make microenvironment conductive to colonization [39].

8.2.1.1 Initiators of Premetastatic Niche

Hematopoietic cells of myeloid origin expressing VEGF receptor 1 are considered to be key component of premetastatic niche. They arrive and cluster at the site even before the arrival of disseminated cells. These receptors also upregulate the expression of VLA-4 and fibronectin. Colonized myeloid cells and stromal fibronectin act as attractive implantation site for disseminated tumor cells. Growth factors like PIGF, inflammatory chemokines, and angiogenic factors (VEGF) secreted by tumor cells are considered to be recruiters of hematopoietic cells at premetastatic niche [40, 41].

Liver is a common site of metastasis in many malignancies. Premetastatic niche in liver is promoted by secretion of exosomes expressing macrophage migration inhibitory factors by primary tumor from Kupffer cells. TGF β promotes ECM remodeling and recruits bone marrow-derived macrophages [42]. Bone is another common site of metastasis. Depending upon the type of primary tumor and secretory factors, lesions could be osteoblastic or osteolytic. In case of osteoblastic lesions, primary tumors or circulating tumor cell secretes vascular endothelial growth factor VEGF1, bone morphogenic proteins BMPs, prostate-specific antigen PSA, insulin growth factor IGF, and endothelin-1 which together promote osteoblastic activity. Endothelin-1 suppresses DKK which act as negative regulator of WNT which is usually high in prostate cancer. However, in case of osteolytic lesion (e.g., breast cancer), extracellular matrix-modifying enzymes like lysyl oxidase are secreted. Other factors released include parathyroid hormone, matrix metalloproteases, and interleukins IL-11 and IL1, which are usually osteoblastic but by promoting RANK with concomitant decrease of OPG activates osteoclast precursors. Parathyroid hormone is the most important secretory factor expressed in 90% of the bone metastasis which reacts with parathyroid hormone receptor to promote (RANK). TGF β is another important inducer of bone resorption [43].

8.2.1.2 Establishment of Premetastatic Niche and Promotion of Engraftment

Release of secretory factors from primary tumor leads to stepwise progression of premetastatic niche establishment and tumor engraftment. Major steps in this progression are as follows.

Hyper-permeability of Vasculature

Tumor secretory factors via various mechanisms increase the vascular permeability at the site of premetastatic niche. This is manifested as increased permeability, altered morphology of endothelium, and increased basement membrane breakdown. Increased permeability is caused by release of secretory factors like EGF, MMP1, MMP2, and COX1 which promote circulating tumor cells (CTCs) extravasation. Downregulation of these factors in breast cancer cell lines had shown impaired ability of metastasis. Angiopoietin 2, MMP3, MMP9, and MMP10 are found to be associated with increased permeability in premetastatic niche of the lung in patients with breast cancer. Myeloid suppressor cells at premetastatic niche are thought to be inducer of MMP 9 which is involved in extracellular remodeling, immunosuppression, and inflammation thereby promoting an environment inductive for metastasis. Genetic ablation of MMP9 is found to be associated with decreased lung metastasis [44]. Altered endothelium causes increase in expression of VEGF-A which induces endothelial focal adhesion kinase resulting in upregulation of E-selectin. Increased expression of E-selectin promotes CTCs engraftment and proliferation [45]. VEGF-A secretion is also promoted by CCL-2 secretion from tumor cells and monocytes expressing CCR-2 in the stroma in breast cancer models. Decrease in monocytes will decrease metastasis [46].

Premetastatic niches are also associated with formation of clots. Thromboembolism is one of the reasons of death among cancer patients. Mechanism of clot formation is still ambiguous; however tissue factor playing a role in niche formation can result in clot formation. In early metastatic niches, platelets are required for MMP9 as well as CD11. Platelets play an important role in cancer-associated coagulopathies [47].

Activation of Stromal Components

Secretory factors from primary tumor causes activation of tissue stroma at site of premetastatic niche. Fibroblasts play an important role in ECM remodeling and promoting invasion. Exosomal vesicles increase the expression of S100 family members of pulmonary fibroblasts in premetastatic niche of the lung [48]. S100A4 member of this family promotes secretion of proinflammatory molecules thereby promoting metastasis. S100A4 also causes upregulation of SAA3 and SAA1 which increases tumor adhesion to fibronectin [49]. Other stromal components activated in niche formation are tissue-resident macrophages. Exosomes from pancreatic cell lines rich in macrophage-initiating factors stimulate liver Kupffer cells to increase fibronectin production from hepatic stellate cells which leads to fibrotic environment. This environment promotes BMDC recruitment and premetastatic niche formation [50]. In the lungs, alveolar macrophages inhibit TH1 response thereby promoting inflammatory environment supporting metastasis [51].

ECM Remodeling

Remodeling of extracellular matrix is necessary for CTCs or DTCs engraftment and proliferation. Degradation of existing ECM and deposition of new ECM occur at the site of premetastatic niche in response to systemic factors released from primary tumor. MMPs are upregulated at niches to promote degradation of ECM supporting tumor infiltration and releasing growth factors thereby recruiting progenitor and tumor cells [39].

In mouse melanoma and pancreatic models, fibronectin deposition mediated by stromal fibroblasts has been reported. This promotes adhesion of BMDCs [40]. Secretion of TGF β from primary tumor causes release of periostin from stromal fibroblast which in turn increases the expression of vimentin and actin. Secretion of periostin is important as it plays a key role in establishment of niche. Periostin increases WNT signaling thereby promoting infiltration [52, 53]. It also interacts with NOTCH, BMPs, and Type I collagens to engage integrins, i.e., $\alpha_v\beta_3$ and $\alpha_v\beta_5$, to promote cellular motility. It also promotes immunosuppressive functions of MDSCs making environment conducive for metastasis [54]. CD11 myeloid cell-derived veriscan is ECM preoteoglycan which promotes inflammation at premetastatic niche [55].

Lysyl oxidases (LOX) are enzymes whose expression is upregulated at premetastatic niches by hypoxic tumor cells. LOX family plays role in cross-linking collagen which provide platform for myeloid cell adhesion. Increased HIF-1 expression is associated with increased expression of LOX. Apart from hypoxic tumor cells, it is also secreted from activated fibroblasts [56, 57].

Change in mechanical properties of ECM, i.e., matrix stiffness and tissue elasticity, has direct impact on proliferation. ECM remodeling that results in change in mechanical properties such as collagen cross-linking leads to increased stiffness which supports tumor engraftment and metastatic outgrowth [58].

Formation of Immunosuppressive Environment
Metastasis is an inefficient process as new soil for disseminated cell could be deadly. These DTCs are vulnerable to immune surveillance. To make environment receptive for arriving DTCs, BMDCs and HPCs alter the microenvironment of premetastatic niche making it proinflammatory and immunosuppressive [39].

MDSCs promote immunosuppression by suppressing interferon-mediated immune responses and disrupting major immune responses, i.e., antigen presentation via dendritic cells, macrophage polarization, and inhibition of NK cytotoxicity and T-cell activation. It also makes environment inflammatory by secreting proinflammatory cytokines, interleukins, and SDF [59]. SDF recruits more BMDCs which further increases immunosuppression and inflammation. SDF also promotes neutrophils to premetastatic niche [60]. However in absence of interferon γ, they have diminished cytotoxicity [61]. Neutrophils secrete leukotrienes which make environment more inflammatory and supportive for metastasis. Increase in CD11b+ cells at premetastatic niche also reduces NK cell-induced cytotoxicity in turn promoting survival of metastatic cells [62].

In the brain, astrocytes secrete plasminogen activator (PA) which converts inactive plasminogen to plasmin. Plasminogen activates FasL cytokine which binds to incoming DTCs and induces apoptosis. Brain metastatic cells from lung adenocarcinomas and breast produce neuroserpin and serpin B2 which are plasminogen inhibitors, thereby avoiding apoptotic death [63].

8.2.2 Perivascular Niche

Perivascular niches support cancer cells which extravasate and spread near capillary basement cell membrane. The CTCs remain near the endothelium and receives paracrine signaling [64]. Perivascular niches are rich in hematopoietic stem as well as progenitor cells (HSPCs). Other cells in perivascular niches include mesenchymal stromal cells which secrete stem cell factor (SCF) and CXCL playing an important role in maintaining niche [65].

Endothelial cells maintain the proliferation of hematopoietic cells by secreting CFU-$S_{8.}$ SCF from endothelial cells is required for hematopoietic progenitor cells. Knockout of SCF resulted in decrease of hematopoietic stem cells [66]. Cancer cells need angiogenesis and lymphangiogenesis for their growth and survival. Environment with leaky vasculature and inflammatory cytokines is receptive for cancer stem cells. Paracrine factors like VEGF and EGF increase permeability in perivascular niches [67]. It has been noted in case of glioblastoma multiforme which is highly vascular tumor. In GBM, vascular endothelial cells maintain brain tumor cells in continuous stemlike state thereby increasing invasiveness. These stem cells in positive feedback form secrete VEGF promoting vasculogenesis [68, 69].

Perivascular cells like pericytes when cultured for longer time have shown to differentiate into mesenchymal cells. This could be one of the reasons of high expression of mesenchymal cell markers in perivascular niche. Analysis of pericytes in in vitro cultures and in vivo has shown its ability to differentiate into mineralized nodules and adipocytes. MSCs also secrete TGF β, hedgehog signal, and CXCL2 which promote hematopoietic stem cell maintenance [69].

8.2.3 Metastatic and Cancer Stem Cell Niche

When DTCs or CTCs got engrafted in premetastatic or perivascular niches, they are called as metastatic niches [38]. Cancer stem cell niche is specifically referred to a niche that supports cancer stem cell proliferation. Cancer stem cells are the self-renewing cells having tumor initiating and long-term repopulation potential. CSC niche is rich in factor promoting angiogenesis, recruiting CSC, immunomodulation, and factors to promote metastasis. CSCs release multiple factors which activate MSCs for secreting cytokine supportive for CSCs, release HIF1α to promote vasculogenesis, as well as secrete TGF β to convert fibroblasts into cancer-associated fibroblasts to promote stemness and thereby metastasis [70].

When DTCs land in different soil, they are faced with challenging environment where immune cells are in search of foreign cells to destroy them. To adapt to this environment and develop overt metastasis, cancer cells have to escape this immune response and make environment friendly to them. Both metastatic niche and DTCs play a role in modulating the immune microenvironment. DTCs remain in dormant stage till the environment become supportive in establishing overt metastasis. During dormancy MSCs support dormancy of CSCs by secreting various miRNAs [37]. Niches are rich in MDSCs and HSCs, which play essential role in modulating the immune environment. Once the environment becomes immunosuppressive and angiogenic, CSCs exit dormancy and develop overt metastasis [14].

8.3 Immunomodulation

8.3.1 Cancer Cell-Based Responses

8.3.1.1 Escaping the Immune Response

Tumor cells escape the immune response both by camouflaging themselves, i.e., hiding the foreign antigens, and by showing normal antigens, i.e., disguising the immune cells. For CTL response to occur, antigen presentation via MHC-1 class molecules is necessary. Fetal cells in mother also survive the immune responses of mother by similar mechanisms. They show lower expression of MHC-1 molecules. Cancer cells also show an altered expression of MHC-1 which helps them camouflage the immune surveillance. The altered expression is usually due to defects in antigen processing pathway. Also cancer cells produce certain immunosuppressive molecules which lower the MHC-1 expression thereby evading the CTL responses [71].

Even with low expression of MHC-1, a cell can get killed by natural killer cells via binding to polymorphic determinants of MHC-1 through binding with KIRs (Killer cell Inhibitory Receptors). MHC-1 interacts with KIRs and inhibits them. Upon downregulation of MHC-1, they are free to kill the tumor cells. In order to escape killing by NK cells, tumor cells have adapted a mechanism, i.e., adapted in maternal-fetal immune interaction. Tumor cells start expressing HLA-G molecule which is a nonclassical MHC-1 molecule and have immune-inhibitory effects via interacting with three KIRS. HLA-G expression has been found in a variety of cancers including melanomas, glioblastomas, ovarian cancer, and lung cancer [72].

8.3.1.2 Immunomodulatory Effects

Apart from immune escape mechanisms, cancer cells alter the immune response to survive in hostile environment. During activation and recruitment to the site, immune cells interact with each other. The process of migration is tightly controlled in which immune cells adhere and detach via release of different adhesion molecules and proteases. ICAM-1 (intercellular cell adhesion molecule) is one of the adhesion molecules which is expressed on the surface and plays significant role in interaction between NK cells and cancer cells. Cancer cells disrupt this cell-to-cell interaction by producing MMP9 which causes ICAM-1 shedding thereby preventing NK cell-mediated killing [73].

Another mechanism adapted by cancer cells to escape T-cell response is by inducing apoptosis of activated T and B cells. B7H1 induces apoptosis of T cells by binding to PD-1, a negative regulatory receptor of T cells [74]. Another member of this family B7H4 inhibits T-cell proliferation and cell cycle progression in addition to cytokine production. B7H4 expression is not found in normal tissues; however 85% of the ovarian tumors and 31% of the lung tumors express it [75].

For activation of T cells, full maturation of dendritic cells (DCs) is required. For this all three signals, i.e., 1, 2, and 3, are needed to elicit Th1-based response. If signal 1 is delivered in absence of signal 2 and 3 or in presence of immunosuppressive cytokines, Th2 response will be initiated [76]. Th1-based responses are immunosuppressive, while Th2 responses are tumor supportive. CD40 is one of the costimulatory molecule which causes dendritic cell maturation via interacting with CD40L (ligand). Loss of CD40L with continued expression of CD40 has been found to be associated with immune evasion and tumorigenesis in oral squamous cell carcinoma [77].

Also tumor cells combined with metastatic niche release molecules or recruit cell which secrete cytokines which promotes Th2 type of response. Key players of TH-2 response are MDSCs (myeloid-derived suppressor cell) and TAMs (tumor-associated macrophages). MDSCs inhibit T-cell function both directly and indirectly by recruiting T-regulatory cells (Treg cells). Treg cells are CD4 type of T cells which secrete TGF β resulting in inhibition of T-cell proliferation. Also these cells secrete immunosuppressive cytokines like IL-1, IL-10, IL-4, and IL-5 which inhibit CTL responses [78].

8.3.1.3 Promotion of Chronic Inflammatory State

Ralph Virchow in 1863 proposed that cancer develops as a result of unresolved inflammation. It has now been accepted that 25% of the tumors develop as a result of chronic inflammation. Chronic inflammation promotes epithelial to mesenchymal transition and alters the immune environment leading to carcinogenesis [79].

Neutrophils are the first to get recruited toward the damaged site and are first line of defense in innate immune system and are recruited by chemokines like CXCL8 and cognate receptors like CXCR1 and CXCR2. Neutrophils secrete multiple different chemokines and cytokine which promote development of chronic inflammatory state. They also secrete multiple soluble factors like HGF, VEGF, TGFα, and FGF and cytokines like IL1, CXCL1, CXCL 8, CXCL9, CXCL 10, CCL3, and CCL4 in addition to enzymes like MMPs which promote chronic inflammation, ECM remodeling, and angiogenesis consequently metastasis [80].

Initiation of Th2 response results in development of chronic inflammatory stage. TAMS are crucial drivers of chronic inflammation. They also promote lymphangiogenesis, angiogenesis, and immunosuppression [78]. TAMs also secrete multiple factors including interleukin-1 that has been found to be raised in variety of tumors such as melanomas, lung, head and neck, colon, and breast cancer. IL-1 also activates signal transduction pathways such as NF-κβ, JNK, p38MAPK, and AP1. NF-κβ provide a link between inflammation and carcinogenesis. It is a major regulator of apoptosis, angiogenesis, and invasion. IL-1 also activates NALP inflammasome which promote sustained inflammation. IL-1-mediated inflammation has been found to be associated with development and progression of melanoma [81].

Tumor microenvironment is a rich source of growth factors which can activate RAS by binding to RTKs like EGFR and activate downstream PI3K-AKT-mTOR and RAF-MAPK-ERK pathway. PI3K-AKT pathway promotes inflammatory state by activating NF-κβ pathway [82]. NF-κβ in turn promotes transcription of more than 60 genes involved in inflammatory responses. Apart from increasing production of proinflammatory cytokines like IL1, IL2, IL6, IL8, IL12, and TNFα, it also promotes production of chemokines like MCP-1, MIP2, IL-18, CXCL10, and CXCL11, thereby promoting angiogenesis. It promotes production of adhesion molecules like ICAM, VCAM, MMPs, and selectin which support antiapoptotic and invasive properties. It encourages cell survival by increasing cyclins, BCL-2 members, and survivin. Therefore, activation of NF-κβ pathway is considered to be a hallmark of invasion and metastasis [83].

8.3.2 Tumor Microenvironment in Immunomodulation

Tumor microenvironment at site of metastasis or metastatic niches undergoes dynamic changes during the process of metastasis to support cancer cells engraftment, progression, and development of overt metastasis. It not only provides the DTCs with necessary factors for growth but also prevents them from harsh immune environment. It alters the immune responses by secreting a variety of cytokines in addition to other factors promoting DTCs survival [84].

8.3.2.1 Role of MSCs in Immunomodulation

Mesenchymal stem cells are the stromal cells recruited in large amount in cancer stem cell and metastatic niches where they promote immunosuppressive environment to support exit from dormancy and development of overt metastasis. MSCs are recruited to stem cell niches via different signaling axes including SDF-1, chemokines signal (CXCR3, CXCL10), and TGF β. Once at site they secrete different cytokines, chemokines, and ECM components which promote immune alteration, act as chemoattractant, promote angiogenesis, and support metastatic development [85].

Naïve MSCs usually have both immune-protective and immune-suppressive function. Type of function depends upon its polarization via different stimuli. LPS through TLR4 stimulation promote MSC1 phenotype which promotes T-cell activation and has repressive effect on tumorigenesis. This is the reason; they are being employed in stem cell therapeutic approaches. In tumor microenvironment, mostly MSCs via poly i:c through TLR3 induction promote MSCs type two which are immunosuppressive and causes upregulation of CCL5, TGF β, and IL-10 which promote carcinogenesis [85].

MSCs in presence of IL-1, TNF, IFN-γ, and hypoxia release immunosuppressive factors including platelet-derived growth factor (PDGF), epidermal growth factor (EGF), vascular endothelial growth factor (VEGF), fibroblast growth factor (FGF), IL-6, and IL8. MSCs cause shift in polarization of TNFα secreting M1 to IL-10 phenotype. In pancreatic neoplasms MSCs have shown to induce M2 macrophages which are immunosuppressive in nature [86].

MSCs have inhibitory action on NK cells function via different mechanisms. In the adipose tissue, umbilical cord, and bone marrow, they inhibit activation of CD56 subset of natural killer cells. By increasing the expression of cytokine signaling three axes, they inhibit the proliferation of natural killer cells. Also MSCs isolated from leukemic patients had shown that decrease in amount of IL-6 and IL-8 decreases functioning of NK cells [87].

By secreting IL-10, MSCs are found to suppress dendritic cells (DCs). Also they decrease functioning of DCs by activating signal transduction and activator of transcription (STAT). Within TME, MSCs decrease cysteine production via STAT; this results in decrease in activation of DC mediated T-cell actions [88].

MSCs isolated from patients suffering from chronic myelogenous leukemia have shown increased recruitment of Treg population which have potent immunosuppressive functions [89]. By ligating PD-1/PD-1, MSCs inhibit B-cell activity, proliferation, and differentiation. They inhibit CD8 T cells by inducing nitric oxide production in proinflammatory environment [85].

8.3.2.2 Role of NO in Immunomodulation

Nitric oxide is synthesized physiologically by a variety of tissues via catabolism of L-arginine to L-citrulline. The reaction is catalyzed by nitric oxide synthase (NOS) expressed in low levels by neuronal and endothelial cells regulated by intracellular calcium levels. Another form of NOS is called as inducible nitric oxide synthase (iNOS) which is independent of calcium levels but induced by proinflammatory cytokines, hypoxia, endotoxins, and oxidative stress [90].

High levels of NO are implicated in pathophysiology of many malignant diseases. In most of the solid and hematological malignancies, iNOS expression has found to be substantially higher [91]. While in brain malignancies, increased expression of neuronal NOS is considered to be the reason behind high levels of nitric oxide [92].

In TME, NO is produced by a variety of cells including epithelial cells, keratinocytes, fibroblasts, chondrocytes, and some immune cells where it exerts both autocrine and paracrine effects. iNos is highly expressed by M1 macrophages where it works in autocrine manner and acts as negative regulator of M1 differentiation. High levels of NO produced by macrophages inhibit T-cell infiltration as well as endothelial cell activation; however at lower concentrations effect is opposite [93].

NO also supports evasion of T-cell-mediated immune response by nitrosylating CCL2, a chemoattractant chemokine, thereby eliminating its ability to attract CD8 T cells to cancer cells [94]. In squamous cell carcinomas, MDSCs are found to produce NO resulting in downregulation of E-selectin, thereby restricting T-cell recruitment [95]. In melanomas, iNOS expression by IL-12 is found to be associated with recruitment of MDSCs and Treg cell making environment immunosuppressive [96]. NO also plays role in metabolic reprogramming and increased immunosuppression [97].

8.3.2.3 Metabolic Reprogramming and Immunomodulation

Tumor microenvironment is characterized by hypoxia, low perfusion, fatty acid metabolism, and lactic acidosis. Cancer cells prefer glycolysis over oxidative phosphorylation even in presence of oxygen, phenomenon referred to as Warburg effect. Acidic environment on one side restricts T-cell and NK cytotoxic response and on other side recruits MDSCs and Tregs which further suppress the immune response [98].

Lactic acidosis impairs MCT-1 resulting in impaired CD8 T-cell function, increased apoptosis, and reduced IFN and IL-2 production. In vitro experimentation on melanoma cell lines showed pH of 6.5 resulted in decreased expression of T-cell receptor components like ζ chain and CD23 expression along with decreased IFN, TNFα, and IL-2 secretion [99]. Loss of NK cell activity has been noted in leukemia and colorectal cancer [100, 101]. Low pH also affects dendritic cell functioning as immature dendritic cells require OXPHOS for maturation [102].

The most potent immunosuppressive response by TME is exerted via recruitment of MDSCs. How TME attracts MDSCs is poorly understood. It is reported that upregulation of selectins play a central role in attracting MDSCs [103]. Low pH is also associated with release of proinflammatory cytokines and iNOS which in turn recruits MDSCs [104]. Increased expression of chemokines like CCL-28, CCL-17, and SDF are associated with recruitment of Treg cells [105, 106].

All these events help DTCs to escape immune response and make environment friendly for their proliferation and developing overt metastasis.

8.4 Mechano-transduction and Metastasis

Tumor has long been diagnosed as palpable mass due to its stiffer nature than normal tissue. However, it was not until the last decade, studies focused on inside mechanisms of tissue rigidity, tumor mechanics, and its effect on invasion and metastasis. Studies have shown association between increased stiffness and metastasis as well as poor survival. Diagnostic approaches like ultrasound and MR elastography help in differentiating benign versus malignant diseases of breast, liver, and kidney via measuring lesion rigidity. Matrix stiffness regulates various cellular pathways. Increase in stiffness leads to activation of various biochemical pathways which lead to cell-cycle progression, cellular proliferation, epithelial to mesenchymal transition, and cell motility. The section is focused on describing how matrix stiffness occurs and how mechano-transduction derives metastasis [107].

8.4.1 Matrix Stiffness

Remodeling of ECM stimulated by tumor microenvironment as well as tumor cells themselves leads to stiffened matrices which in turn support cancer cells. Tumor cells that have undergone EMT play vital role in changing mechanical properties of matrix. EMT causes increased fibrillin expression and deposition which is one of the major components of microfibrils [107].

Cancer cells with high metastatic potential have higher expression of lysyl oxidase (LOX) and fibronectin in addition to other ECM remodeling proteins. LOS is involved in promoting actin-myosin contractibility. LOX is also secreted by cancer-associated fibroblasts (CAFs) present in metastatic niche. Here it promotes increased cross-linking of collagen thereby promoting matrix stiffness. Hypoxia also encourages collagen deposition by upregulating LOX [108].

TWIST protein plays an important role in stabilization of myosin II and development of supracellular actin-myosin meshwork generating tissue-wide tension. It also causes activation of stress fiber formation and provides integrity to tissue [109]. High expression of TWIST is found in many tumors including breast cancer and is associated with metastasis and poor survival. It plays an important role in EMT. Its expression induces Rac-1-mediated increased cellular tension and rigidity. CAFs also promote matrix stiffening via caveolin-1. Caveolin-1 plays a role in organization of stromal architecture and promotes directional migration of cells. Its upregulation is linked with increased invasion and metastasis [107].

YAP and TAZ are transcriptional factors associated with increased invasion and metastasis. They act in a positive feedback way by supporting matrix stiffness which in turn upregulates its expression. YAP/TAZ regulate actin-myosin cytoskeleton by controlling different genes involved in ECM remodeling. YAP also regulates maintenance of CAFs which play an important role in tumor stiffness [110].

Another important regulator of cytoskeleton tension is Rho family of GTPases. Most of the functions are mediated by Rho kinases (ROCK). Rho regulates myosin phosphorylation and controls cytoskeletal contractility. Tumors with increased Rho expression are associated with increased stiffness. ROCK also promotes loss of adherens junctions (AJ), loss of polarity, and remodeling of ECM thereby promoting invasion and metastasis [111, 112].

8.4.2 Mechano-sensing and Transduction Mechanisms

Mechano-transduction refers to sensing mechanical cues and translating them into biochemical or cellular pathways leading to change in characteristic of tissues and cells. Change in mechanical stress leads to change in geometry of tissue, and this leads to change in cellular behavior [113].

There are many mechano-sensing and transduction mechanisms. Focal adhesion complexes are the most important system that sense the change in biomechanical properties. Focal adhesion complex consists of many proteins including integrins and multiple adapter in addition to signaling proteins like vinculin and talin. These proteins undergo conformational change upon application of physical force resulting in either stabilization of protein-protein interaction as in case of integrin and fibronectin or can reveal the binding site of molecules like talin. Vinculin binding to talin leads to clustering of integrins resulting in activation of signaling molecules at intracellular face of adhesion [114].

Different cell surface receptors also respond to mechanical cues including integrins, cadherins, and ephrin. Ephrin receptor 2A binds to ligand Ephrin1 and regulates cellular migration, growth, and proliferation. EGFR signaling is also found to be associated with mechanical cues. Receptor organization is determined by actin organization. Therefore change in actin organization will also effect receptor organization [115].

Mechano-sensing usually works in a positive feedback way. Change in cell surface receptors by stiffened matrices leads to stabilization of integrins, allowing focal adhesion to mature. Integrins control cell motility and spread by binding to actin-binding protein filamin A [116, 117]. This links intracellular actin cytoskeletal signaling to outside integrin signaling. In addition to integrin, discoid domain receptors (DDR) also play a role in mechano-sensing. DDR1 and DDR2 are expressed by epithelial and mesenchymal cells and are regulated by EMT. They facilitate metastasis by increasing the expression of SNAIL2. DDR2 expression has been found in many ductal breast carcinomas [118].

8.4.3 Mechano-transduction and Dissemination of Cancer Cells

For cancer cells to disseminate, first step is epithelial to mesenchymal transition (EMT). During EMT, cell loses its epithelial properties, i.e., adherens junctions and apical basal polarity, and gains mesenchymal properties, i.e., ability to migrate. EMT is defined as loss of E-cadherin and upregulation of mesenchymal markers, i.e., vimentin, fibronectin, and N-cadherin. Matrix stiffness has been found to be potent driver of EMT [119, 120]. Increased stiffness leads to nuclear translocation of EMT transcription factor TWIST. TWIST along with TGF β drives EMT [121]. Cadherins act as mechano-sensors. Switch of E-cadherin to N-cadherin leads to loss of adherens junction, i.e., cell-to-cell contact. Tissue tension leads to loss of adherent junction and drives β-catenin pathway promoting EMT [122, 123]. Increase in cytoskeleton tension has also been reported to induce epithelial to mesenchymal transition by promoting nuclear translocation of MRTF-A [124]. Tissue specimen from breast cancer patients showed increased stiffened matrices with weak adherens junctions, while normal mammary epithelium is characterized by intact adherens junctions and compliant matrix [125].

Matrix stiffness is largely characterized by deposition and modification of extracellular matrix proteins. Dense clusters of collagen fibrils and fibroblasts are usually present in stiffened matrices. Fibrotic tissues are linked with 50-fold more rigidity than normal parenchyma. Presence of fibrosis is associated with increased metastasis and poor progression in breast cancer [126]. Also fibrotic tissues are more prone to development of cancer. Approximately 80% of the hepatocellular cancers develop as a result of liver fibrosis [127].

8.4.4 Mechano-transduction and CSCs

CSCs are regulated by both intrinsic and extrinsic stimuli. Among extrinsic stimuli, mechanical cues from ECM or CSCs niche play chief role in regulating cell growth, behavior, and fate. CXCR1 causes downregulation of FAK/PI3k/AKT resulting in depletion of stem cells. Mechano-transduction by stiffened matrices can upregulate CSCs. Mechano-transduction is initiated by integrins followed by actin-myosin cytoskeleton, focal adhesion complexes, and myosin motors. Increased tension in cytoskeleton leads to activation of FAK/PI3k/AKT which promotes CSC [128].

EMT also supports of CSCs traits. Studies have shown that EMT is required for early seeding of tumor. However, for metastasis outgrowth, reverse process, i.e., mesenchymal to epithelial transition (MET), is necessary. To explain this, bipotent model was proposed. According to this model, hybrid state is present in small fraction of tumor cells to promote CSCs population [129].

8.5 Exiting the Dormancy: Development of Overt Metastasis

Cancer cells could remain in dormant stage for years till conditions become suitable for their survival. Both metastatic niches or TME and soluble factors released from tumors help in modulating the environment for establishment of overt metastasis. Changes within the microenvironment, i.e., immunomodulation, increased matrix stiffness, and genetic instability, support survival of cancer stem cells. Hence, play an important role in exiting dormancy and developing overt metastasis [24].

Remodeling of ECM, i.e., increased expression of MMPs, also helps in exiting dormancy and promotion of metastasis. Release of other tumor-supporting factors

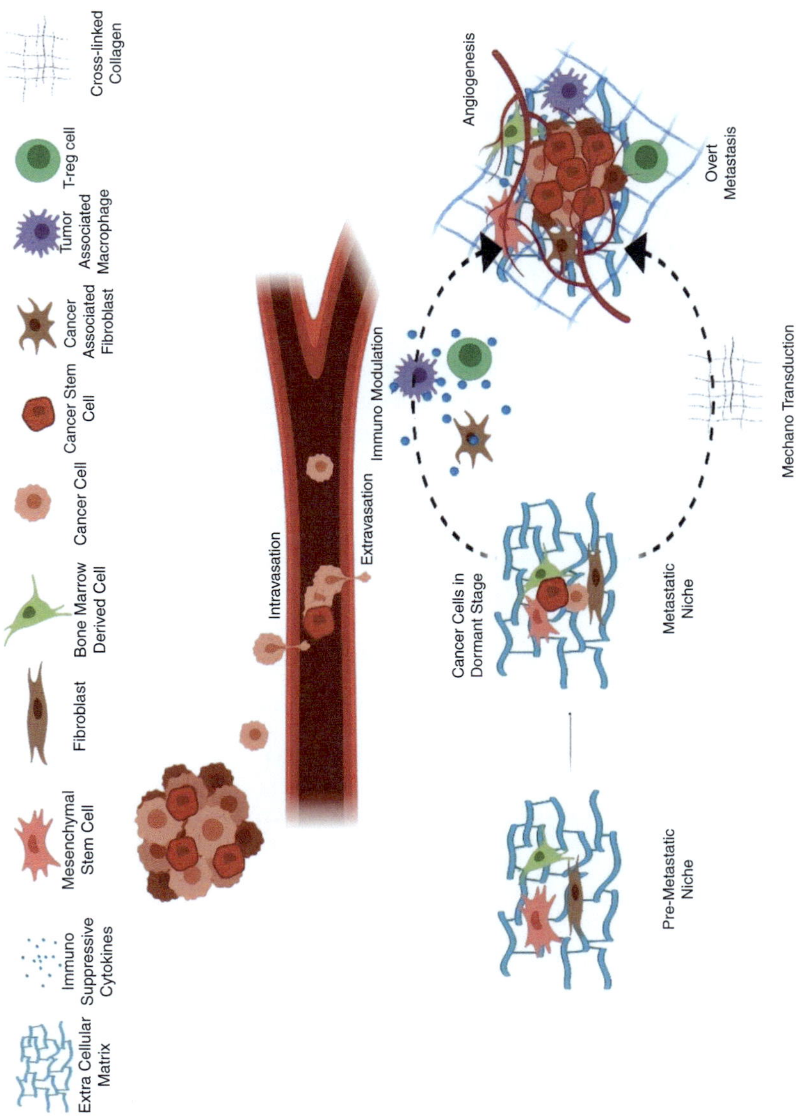

Fig. 8.1 Schematic representation of molecular mechanisms leading to metastasis

like SDF-1, OPN, LOX, activation PI3-AKT, Src, TGF β, and VEGF promotes development of metastasis. Factors supporting chronic inflammation including interleukins, NF-κβ, JNK, p38MAPK, TAM, and Treg cells also help in escaping the immune response resulting in development of metastasis [130].

Among mechano-transduction mechanisms, cancer cells engaging with FAK, integrins, and SRC pathway are successful in establishing metastasis. Study on mammary cells showed inability of cancer cells to engage with FAK, integrins, and SRC pathway resulted in quiescent state [131].

Similarly, all the mechanisms which contribute to EMT and survival of CSCs promote development of overt metastasis. As tumors cannot survive beyond 2–3 mm without blood supply, proangiogenic factors like VEGF also promotes exiting from dormancy. Metabolic reprogramming supporting immunomodulation and genesis also have supporting effect on metastasis [1].

Metastatic cells as a result of this immune modulated, rich in inflammatory cytokines and stiffened matrix are usually resistant to conventional treatments. Strategies to control these molecular mechanisms promoting metastasis are currently under study, and few drugs have been developed. Drugs controlling development of metastasis or targeting them in dormant stage in the future might be helpful in decreasing the morbidity and mortality associated with metastasis [27].

Figure 8.1 depicts the summary of all the events leading to development of overt metastasis.

References

1. Patel P, Chen EI (2012) Cancer stem cells, tumor dormancy, and metastasis. Front Endocrinol 3:125
2. Smith BN, Bhowmick NA (2016) Role of EMT in metastasis and therapy resistance. J Clin Med 5(2):E17
3. Chaffer CL, San Juan BP, Lim E, Weinberg RA (2016) EMT, cell plasticity and metastasis. Cancer Metastasis Rev 35(4):645–654
4. Jablonska-Trypuc A, Matejczyk M, Rosochacki S (2016) Matrix metalloproteinases (MMPs), the main extracellular matrix (ECM) enzymes in collagen degradation, as a target for anticancer drugs. J Enzyme Inhib Med Chem 31(suppl 1):177–183
5. Jiang WG, Sanders AJ, Katoh M, Ungefroren H, Gieseler F, Prince M et al (2015) Tissue invasion and metastasis: molecular, biological and clinical perspectives. Semin Cancer Biol 35(Suppl):S244–SS75
6. Lambert AW, Pattabiraman DR, Weinberg RA (2017) Emerging biological principles of metastasis. Cell 168(4):670–691
7. Aguirre-Ghiso JA (2007) Models, mechanisms and clinical evidence for cancer dormancy. Nat Rev Cancer 7(11):834–846
8. Lipworth S, Hammond RJ, Baron VO, Hu Y, Coates A, Gillespie SH (2016) Defining dormancy in mycobacterial disease. Tuberculosis 99:131–142
9. Sosa MS, Bragado P, Aguirre-Ghiso JA (2014) Mechanisms of disseminated cancer cell dormancy: an awakening field. Nat Rev Cancer 14(9):611–622
10. Manjili MH (2017) Tumor dormancy and relapse: from a natural byproduct of evolution to a disease state. Cancer Res 77(10):2564–2569
11. Hadfield G (1954) The dormant cancer cell. Br Med J 2(4888):607–610

12. Hosseini H, Obradovic MMS, Hoffmann M, Harper KL, Sosa MS, Werner-Klein M et al (2016) Early dissemination seeds metastasis in breast cancer. Nature 540(7634):552–558
13. Gao XL, Zhang M, Tang YL, Liang XH (2017) Cancer cell dormancy: mechanisms and implications of cancer recurrence and metastasis. Onco Targets Ther 10:5219–5228
14. Gomis RR, Gawrzak S (2017) Tumor cell dormancy. Mol Oncol 11(1):62–78
15. Aguirre-Ghiso JA, Estrada Y, Liu D, Ossowski L (2003) ERK(MAPK) activity as a determinant of tumor growth and dormancy; regulation by p38(SAPK). Cancer Res 63(7):1684–1695
16. Gay LJ, Malanchi I (2017) The sleeping ugly: tumour microenvironment's act to make or break the spell of dormancy. Biochim Biophys Acta Rev Cancer 1868(1):231–238
17. Sosa MS, Avivar-Valderas A, Bragado P, Wen HC, Aguirre-Ghiso JA (2011) ERK1/2 and p38alpha/beta signaling in tumor cell quiescence: opportunities to control dormant residual disease. Clin Cancer Res 17(18):5850–5857
18. Jo H, Jia Y, Subramanian KK, Hattori H, Luo HR (2008) Cancer cell-derived clusterin modulates the phosphatidylinositol 3′-kinase-Akt pathway through attenuation of insulin-like growth factor 1 during serum deprivation. Mol Cell Biol 28(13):4285–4299
19. Vera-Ramirez L (2019) Cell-intrinsic survival signals. The role of autophagy in metastatic dissemination and tumor cell dormancy. Semin Cancer Biol. https://doi.org/10.1016/j.semcancer.2019.07.027. [Epub ahead of print]
20. Prunier C, Baker D, ten Dijke P, Ritsma L (2019) TGF-β family signaling pathways in cellular dormancy. Trends Cancer 5(1):66–78
21. Kobayashi A, Okuda H, Xing F, Pandey PR, Watabe M, Hirota S et al (2011) Bone morphogenetic protein 7 in dormancy and metastasis of prostate cancer stem-like cells in bone. J Exp Med 208(13):2641–2655
22. Seidi K, Manjili MH, Jahanban-Esfahlan R, Javaheri T (2018) Tumor cell dormancy: threat or opportunity in the fight against cancer. Cancer 11(8):1207
23. Wang H-F, Wang S-S, Huang M-C, Liang X-H, Tang Y-J, Tang Y-L (2019) Targeting immune-mediated dormancy: a promising treatment of cancer. Front Oncol 9:498
24. Osisami M, Keller ET (2013) Mechanisms of metastatic tumor dormancy. J Clin Med 2(3):136–150
25. Saudemont A, Hamrouni A, Marchetti P, Liu J, Jouy N, Hetuin D et al (2007) Dormant tumor cells develop cross-resistance to apoptosis induced by CTLs or imatinib mesylate via methylation of suppressor of cytokine signaling 1. Cancer Res 67(9):4491–4498
26. Zhou Y, Su Y, Zhu H, Wang X, Li X, Dai C et al (2019) Interleukin-23 receptor signaling mediates cancer dormancy and radioresistance in human esophageal squamous carcinoma cells via the Wnt/Notch pathway. J Mol Med 97(2):177–188
27. Yadav AS, Pandey PR, Butti R, Radharani NNV, Roy S, Bhalara SR et al (2018) The biology and therapeutic implications of tumor dormancy and reactivation. Front Oncol 8:72
28. Senft D, Ze Ronai A (2016) Immunogenic, cellular, and angiogenic drivers of tumor dormancy-a melanoma view. Pigment Cell Melanoma Res 29(1):27–42
29. Straume O, Shimamura T, Lampa MJ, Carretero J, Oyan AM, Jia D et al (2012) Suppression of heat shock protein 27 induces long-term dormancy in human breast cancer. Proc Natl Acad Sci U S A 109(22):8699–8704
30. Ghajar CM, Peinado H, Mori H, Matei IR, Evason KJ, Brazier H et al (2013) The perivascular niche regulates breast tumour dormancy. Nat Cell Biol 15(7):807–817
31. Hofstetter CP, Burkhardt JK, Shin BJ, Gursel DB, Mubita L, Gorrepati R et al (2012) Protein phosphatase 2A mediates dormancy of glioblastoma multiforme-derived tumor stem-like cells during hypoxia. PLoS One 7(1):e30059
32. Weidenfeld K, Schif-Zuck S, Abu-Tayeh H, Kang K, Kessler O, Weissmann M et al (2016) Dormant tumor cells expressing LOXL2 acquire a stem-like phenotype mediating their transition to proliferative growth. Oncotarget 7(44):71362–71377
33. Endo H, Inoue M (2019) Dormancy in cancer. Cancer Sci 110(2):474–480
34. Alison MR, Islam S, Wright NA (2010) Stem cells in cancer: instigators and propagators? J Cell Sci 123(Pt 14):2357–2368

35. Chaffer CL, Brueckmann I, Scheel C, Kaestli AJ, Wiggins PA, Rodrigues LO et al (2011) Normal and neoplastic nonstem cells can spontaneously convert to a stem-like state. Proc Natl Acad Sci U S A 108(19):7950–7955
36. Liang J, Shao SH, Xu ZX, Hennessy B, Ding Z, Larrea M et al (2007) The energy sensing LKB1-AMPK pathway regulates p27(kip1) phosphorylation mediating the decision to enter autophagy or apoptosis. Nat Cell Biol 9(2):218–224
37. Sinha G, Sherman LS, Sandiford OA, Williams LM, Ayer S, Walker ND et al (2016) Mesenchymal stem cell-breast cancer stem cell: relevance to dormancy. J Cancer Stem Cell Res 4:1
38. Psaila B, Lyden D (2009) The metastatic niche: adapting the foreign soil. Nat Rev Cancer 9(4):285–293
39. Peinado H, Zhang H, Matei IR, Costa-Silva B, Hoshino A, Rodrigues G et al (2017) Pre-metastatic niches: organ-specific homes for metastases. Nat Rev Cancer 17(5):302–317
40. Kaplan RN, Riba RD, Zacharoulis S, Bramley AH, Vincent L, Costa C et al (2005) VEGFR1-positive haematopoietic bone marrow progenitors initiate the pre-metastatic niche. Nature 438(7069):820–827
41. Liu Y, Cao X (2016) Characteristics and Significance of the pre-metastatic Niche. Cancer Cell 30(5):668–681
42. Costa-Silva B, Aiello NM, Ocean AJ, Singh S, Zhang H, Thakur BK et al (2015) Pancreatic cancer exosomes initiate pre-metastatic niche formation in the liver. Nat Cell Biol 17(6):816–826
43. Guise T (2010) Examining the metastatic niche: targeting the microenvironment. Semin Oncol 37(Suppl 2):S2–S14
44. Gupta GP, Nguyen DX, Chiang AC, Bos PD, Kim JY, Nadal C et al (2007) Mediators of vascular remodelling co-opted for sequential steps in lung metastasis. Nature 446(7137):765–770
45. Hiratsuka S, Goel S, Kamoun WS, Maru Y, Fukumura D, Duda DG et al (2011) Endothelial focal adhesion kinase mediates cancer cell homing to discrete regions of the lungs via E-selectin up-regulation. Proc Natl Acad Sci U S A 108(9):3725–3730
46. Qian BZ, Li J, Zhang H, Kitamura T, Zhang J, Campion LR et al (2011) CCL2 recruits inflammatory monocytes to facilitate breast-tumour metastasis. Nature 475(7355):222–225
47. Labelle M, Begum S, Hynes RO (2014) Platelets guide the formation of early metastatic niches. Proc Natl Acad Sci U S A 111(30):E3053–E3061
48. Hoshino A, Costa-Silva B, Shen TL, Rodrigues G, Hashimoto A, Tesic Mark M et al (2015) Tumour exosome integrins determine organotropic metastasis. Nature 527(7578):329–335
49. Lukanidin E, Sleeman JP (2012) Building the niche: the role of the S100 proteins in metastatic growth. Semin Cancer Biol 22(3):216–225
50. Lu X, Kang Y (2007) Organotropism of breast cancer metastasis. J Mammary Gland Biol Neoplasia 12(2-3):153–162
51. Sharma SK, Chintala NK, Vadrevu SK, Patel J, Karbowniczek M, Markiewski MM (2015) Pulmonary alveolar macrophages contribute to the premetastatic niche by suppressing antitumor T cell responses in the lungs. J Immunol 194(11):5529–5538
52. Malanchi I, Santamaria-Martinez A, Susanto E, Peng H, Lehr HA, Delaloye JF et al (2011) Interactions between cancer stem cells and their niche govern metastatic colonization. Nature 481(7379):85–89
53. Deng X, Ao S, Hou J, Li Z, Lei Y, Lyu G (2019) Prognostic significance of periostin in colorectal cancer. Chin J Cancer Res 31(3):547–556
54. Kudo A (2011) Periostin in fibrillogenesis for tissue regeneration: periostin actions inside and outside the cell. Cell Mol Life Sci 68(19):3201–3207
55. Kim S, Takahashi H, Lin WW, Descargues P, Grivennikov S, Kim Y et al (2009) Carcinoma-produced factors activate myeloid cells through TLR2 to stimulate metastasis. Nature 457(7225):102–106
56. Erler JT, Bennewith KL, Cox TR, Lang G, Bird D, Koong A et al (2009) Hypoxia-induced lysyl oxidase is a critical mediator of bone marrow cell recruitment to form the premetastatic niche. Cancer Cell 15(1):35–44

57. Xiong A, Liu Y (2017) Targeting hypoxia inducible factors-1α as a novel therapy in fibrosis. Front Pharmacol 8:326
58. Cox TR, Bird D, Baker AM, Barker HE, Ho MW, Lang G et al (2013) LOX-mediated collagen crosslinking is responsible for fibrosis-enhanced metastasis. Cancer Res 73(6):1721–1732
59. Ahn GO, Brown JM (2008) Matrix metalloproteinase-9 is required for tumor vasculogenesis but not for angiogenesis: role of bone marrow-derived myelomonocytic cells. Cancer Cell 13(3):193–205
60. Casbon A-J, Reynaud D, Park C, Khuc E, Gan DD, Schepers K et al (2015) Invasive breast cancer reprograms early myeloid differentiation in the bone marrow to generate immunosuppressive neutrophils. Proc Natl Acad Sci U S A 112(6):E56–E75
61. Wu CF, Andzinski L, Kasnitz N, Kroger A, Klawonn F, Lienenklaus S et al (2015) The lack of type I interferon induces neutrophil-mediated pre-metastatic niche formation in the mouse lung. Int J Cancer 137(4):837–847
62. Wculek SK, Malanchi I (2015) Neutrophils support lung colonization of metastasis-initiating breast cancer cells. Nature 528(7582):413–417
63. Valiente M, Obenauf AC, Jin X, Chen Q, Zhang XH, Lee DJ et al (2014) Serpins promote cancer cell survival and vascular co-option in brain metastasis. Cell 156(5):1002–1016
64. Massague J, Obenauf AC (2016) Metastatic colonization by circulating tumour cells. Nature 529(7586):298–306
65. Oh M, Nor JE (2015) The perivascular niche and self-renewal of stem cells. Front Physiol 6:367
66. Ding L, Saunders TL, Enikolopov G, Morrison SJ (2012) Endothelial and perivascular cells maintain haematopoietic stem cells. Nature 481(7382):457–462
67. Celia-Terrassa T, Kang Y (2018) Metastatic niche functions and therapeutic opportunities. Nat Cell Biol 20(8):868–877
68. Borovski T, De Sousa EMF, Vermeulen L, Medema JP (2011) Cancer stem cell niche: the place to be. Cancer Res 71(3):634–639
69. Doherty MJ, Ashton BA, Walsh S, Beresford JN, Grant ME, Canfield AE (1998) Vascular pericytes express osteogenic potential in vitro and in vivo. J Bone Miner Res 13(5):828–838
70. Plaks V, Kong N, Werb Z (2015) The cancer stem cell niche: how essential is the niche in regulating stemness of tumor cells? Cell Stem Cell 16(3):225–238
71. Ting Koh Y, Luz García-Hernández M, Martin Kast W (2006) Tumor immune escape mechanisms. In: Teicher BA (ed) Cancer drug resistance. Humana Press, Totowa, pp 577–602
72. Johansen LL, Lock-Andersen J, Hviid TVF (2016) The pathophysiological impact of HLA class Ia and HLA-G expression and regulatory T cells in malignant melanoma: a review. J Immunol Res 2016:6829283
73. Fiore E, Fusco C, Romero P, Stamenkovic I (2002) Matrix metalloproteinase 9 (MMP-9/gelatinase B) proteolytically cleaves ICAM-1 and participates in tumor cell resistance to natural killer cell-mediated cytotoxicity. Oncogene 21(34):5213–5223
74. Dong H, Strome SE, Salomao DR, Tamura H, Hirano F, Flies DB et al (2002) Tumor-associated B7-H1 promotes T-cell apoptosis: a potential mechanism of immune evasion. Nat Med 8(8):793–800
75. Choi IH, Zhu G, Sica GL, Strome SE, Cheville JC, Lau JS et al (2003) Genomic organization and expression analysis of B7-H4, an immune inhibitory molecule of the B7 family. J Immunol 171(9):4650–4654
76. Garg AD, Coulie PG, Van den Eynde BJ, Agostinis P (2017) Integrating next-generation dendritic cell vaccines into the current cancer immunotherapy landscape. Trends Immunol 38(8):577–593
77. Loro LL, Ohlsson M, Vintermyr OK, Liavaag PG, Jonsson R, Johannessen AC (2001) Maintained CD40 and loss of polarised CD40 ligand expression in oral squamous cell carcinoma. Anticancer Res 21(1a):113–117
78. Disis ML (2010) Immune regulation of cancer. J Clin Oncol 28(29):4531–4538
79. Gonzalez H, Hagerling C, Werb Z (2018) Roles of the immune system in cancer: from tumor initiation to metastatic progression. Genes Dev 32(19-20):1267–1284

80. Albini A, Bruno A, Noonan DM, Mortara L (2018) Contribution to tumor angiogenesis from innate immune cells within the tumor microenvironment: implications for immunotherapy. Front Immunol 9:527
81. Multhoff G, Molls M, Radons J (2011) Chronic inflammation in cancer development. Front Immunol 2:98
82. Yan C, Theodorescu D (2018) RAL GTPases: biology and potential as therapeutic targets in cancer. Pharmacol Rev 70(1):1–11
83. Liu T, Zhang L, Joo D, Sun S-C (2017) NF-κB signaling in inflammation. Signal Transduct Target Ther 2:17023
84. Liu J, Lin PC, Zhou BP (2015) Inflammation fuels tumor progress and metastasis. Curr Pharm Des 21(21):3032–3040
85. Rivera-Cruz CM, Shearer JJ, Figueiredo Neto M, Figueiredo ML (2017) The immunomodulatory effects of mesenchymal stem cell polarization within the tumor microenvironment niche. Stem Cells Int 2017:4015039
86. Bouchlaka MN, Hematti P, Capitini CM (2017) Therapeutic purposes and risks of ex vivo expanded mesenchymal stem/stromal cells. In: Mesenchymal stromal cells as tumor stromal modulators. Elsevier, Amsterdam
87. Ribeiro A, Laranjeira P, Mendes S, Velada I, Leite C, Andrade P et al (2013) Mesenchymal stem cells from umbilical cord matrix, adipose tissue and bone marrow exhibit different capability to suppress peripheral blood B, natural killer and T cells. Stem Cell Res Ther 4(5):125
88. Liu WH, Liu JJ, Wu J, Zhang LL, Liu F, Yin L et al (2018) Retraction: novel mechanism of inhibition of dendritic cells maturation by mesenchymal stem cells via interleukin-10 and the JAK1/STAT3 signaling pathway. PLoS One 13(3):e0194455
89. Zhao ZG, Xu W, Sun L, Li WM, Li QB, Zou P (2012) The characteristics and immunoregulatory functions of regulatory dendritic cells induced by mesenchymal stem cells derived from bone marrow of patient with chronic myeloid leukaemia. Eur J Cancer 48(12):1884–1895
90. Knowles RG, Moncada S (1994) Nitric oxide synthases in mammals. Biochem J 298(Pt 2):249–258
91. Choudhari SK, Chaudhary M, Bagde S, Gadbail AR, Joshi V (2013) Nitric oxide and cancer: a review. World J Surg Oncol 11:118
92. Eyler CE, Wu Q, Yan K, MacSwords JM, Chandler-Militello D, Misuraca KL et al (2011) Glioma stem cell proliferation and tumor growth are promoted by nitric oxide synthase-2. Cell 146(1):53–66
93. Lu G, Zhang R, Geng S, Peng L, Jayaraman P, Chen C et al (2015) Myeloid cell-derived inducible nitric oxide synthase suppresses M1 macrophage polarization. Nat Commun 6:6676
94. Molon B, Ugel S, Del Pozzo F, Soldani C, Zilio S, Avella D et al (2011) Chemokine nitration prevents intratumoral infiltration of antigen-specific T cells. J Exp Med 208(10):1949–1962
95. Gehad AE, Lichtman MK, Schmults CD, Teague JE, Calarese AW, Jiang Y et al (2012) Nitric oxide-producing myeloid-derived suppressor cells inhibit vascular E-selectin expression in human squamous cell carcinomas. J Invest Dermatol 132(11):2642–2651
96. Douguet L, Bod L, Lengagne R, Labarthe L, Kato M, Avril MF et al (2016) Nitric oxide synthase 2 is involved in the pro-tumorigenic potential of gammadelta17 T cells in melanoma. Oncoimmunology 5(8):e1208878
97. Salimian Rizi B, Achreja A, Nagrath D (2017) Nitric oxide: the forgotten child of tumor metabolism. Trends Cancer 3(9):659–672
98. Huber V, Camisaschi C, Berzi A, Ferro S, Lugini L, Triulzi T et al (2017) Cancer acidity: an ultimate frontier of tumor immune escape and a novel target of immunomodulation. Semin Cancer Biol 43:74–89
99. Nakagawa Y, Negishi Y, Shimizu M, Takahashi M, Ichikawa M, Takahashi H (2015) Effects of extracellular pH and hypoxia on the function and development of antigen-specific cytotoxic T lymphocytes. Immunol Lett 167(2):72–86
100. Lotzova E, Savary CA, Herberman RB (1987) Induction of NK cell activity against fresh human leukemia in culture with interleukin 2. J Immunol 138(8):2718–2727

101. Rocca YS, Roberti MP, Arriaga JM, Amat M, Bruno L, Pampena MB et al (2013) Altered phenotype in peripheral blood and tumor-associated NK cells from colorectal cancer patients. Innate Immun 19(1):76–85
102. Dong H, Bullock TN (2014) Metabolic influences that regulate dendritic cell function in tumors. Front Immunol 5:24
103. Cao TM, Takatani T, King MR (2013) Effect of extracellular pH on selectin adhesion: theory and experiment. Biophys J 104(2):292–299
104. Bellocq A, Suberville S, Philippe C, Bertrand F, Perez J, Fouqueray B et al (1998) Low environmental pH is responsible for the induction of nitric-oxide synthase in macrophages. Evidence for involvement of nuclear factor-kappa B activation. J Biol Chem 273(9):5086–5092
105. Kinoshita H, Yashiro M, Fukuoka T, Hasegawa T, Morisaki T, Kasashima H et al (2015) Diffuse-type gastric cancer cells switch their driver pathways from FGFR2 signaling to SDF1/CXCR4 axis in hypoxic tumor microenvironments. Carcinogenesis 36(12):1511–1520
106. Ohue Y, Nishikawa H (2019) Regulatory T (Treg) cells in cancer: can Treg cells be a new therapeutic target? Cancer Sci 110(7):2080–2089
107. Wei SC, Yang J (2016) Forcing through tumor metastasis: the interplay between tissue rigidity and epithelial-mesenchymal transition. Trends Cell Biol 26(2):111–120
108. El-Haibi CP, Bell GW, Zhang J, Collmann AY, Wood D, Scherber CM et al (2012) Critical role for lysyl oxidase in mesenchymal stem cell-driven breast cancer malignancy. Proc Natl Acad Sci U S A 109(43):17460–17465
109. Riaz M, Sieuwerts AM, Look MP, Timmermans MA, Smid M, Foekens JA et al (2012) High TWIST1 mRNA expression is associated with poor prognosis in lymph node-negative and estrogen receptor-positive human breast cancer and is co-expressed with stromal as well as ECM related genes. Breast Cancer Res 14(5):R123
110. Calvo F, Ege N, Grande-Garcia A, Hooper S, Jenkins RP, Chaudhry SI et al (2013) Mechanotransduction and YAP-dependent matrix remodelling is required for the generation and maintenance of cancer-associated fibroblasts. Nat Cell Biol 15(6):637–646
111. Hebner C, Weaver VM, Debnath J (2008) Modeling morphogenesis and oncogenesis in three-dimensional breast epithelial cultures. Annu Rev Pathol 3:313–339
112. Northcott JM, Dean IS, Mouw JK, Weaver VM (2018) Feeling stress: the mechanics of cancer progression and aggression. Front Cell Dev Biol 6:17
113. Broders-Bondon F, Nguyen Ho-Bouldoires TH, Fernandez-Sanchez ME, Farge E (2018) Mechanotransduction in tumor progression: the dark side of the force. J Cell Biol 217(5):1571–1587
114. DuFort CC, Paszek MJ, Weaver VM (2011) Balancing forces: architectural control of mechanotransduction. Nat Rev Mol Cell Biol 12(5):308–319
115. Kou C-TJ, Kandpal RP (2018) Differential expression patterns of Eph receptors and ephrin ligands in human cancers. Biomed Res Int 2018:23
116. Ehrlicher AJ, Nakamura F, Hartwig JH, Weitz DA, Stossel TP (2011) Mechanical strain in actin networks regulates FilGAP and integrin binding to filamin A. Nature 478(7368):260–263
117. Iwamoto DV, Calderwood DA (2015) Regulation of integrin-mediated adhesions. Curr Opin Cell Biol 36:41–47
118. Zhang K, Corsa CA, Ponik SM, Prior JL, Piwnica-Worms D, Eliceiri KW et al (2013) The collagen receptor discoidin domain receptor 2 stabilizes SNAIL1 to facilitate breast cancer metastasis. Nat Cell Biol 15(6):677–687
119. Tsai JH, Yang J (2013) Epithelial-mesenchymal plasticity in carcinoma metastasis. Genes Dev 27(20):2192–2206
120. Scott LE, Weinberg SH, Lemmon CA (2019) Mechanochemical signaling of the extracellular matrix in epithelial-mesenchymal transition. Front Cell Dev Biol 7:135
121. Yang J, Mani SA, Donaher JL, Ramaswamy S, Itzykson RA, Come C et al (2004) Twist, a master regulator of morphogenesis, plays an essential role in tumor metastasis. Cell 117(7):927–939

122. Scarpa E, Szabo A, Bibonne A, Theveneau E, Parsons M, Mayor R (2015) Cadherin switch during EMT in neural crest cells leads to contact inhibition of locomotion via repolarization of forces. Dev Cell 34(4):421–434
123. Basu S, Cheriyamundath S, Ben-Ze'ev A (2018) Cell-cell adhesion: linking Wnt/β-catenin signaling with partial EMT and stemness traits in tumorigenesis. F1000Res 7:488
124. Gomez EW, Chen QK, Gjorevski N, Nelson CM (2010) Tissue geometry patterns epithelial-mesenchymal transition via intercellular mechanotransduction. J Cell Biochem 110(1):44–51
125. Zanetti D, Llenbach R, Plodinec M, Oertle P, Redling K et al (2018) Length scale matters: real-time elastography versus nanomechanical profiling by atomic force microscopy for the diagnosis of breast lesions. Biomed Res Int 2018:12
126. Lopez JI, Kang I, You WK, McDonald DM, Weaver VM (2011) In situ force mapping of mammary gland transformation. Integr Biol 3(9):910–921
127. Affo S, Yu LX, Schwabe RF (2017) The role of cancer-associated fibroblasts and fibrosis in liver cancer. Annu Rev Pathol 12:153–186
128. Panera N, Crudele A, Romito I, Gnani D, Alisi A (2017) Focal adhesion kinase: insight into molecular roles and functions in hepatocellular carcinoma. Int J Mol Sci 18(1):99
129. Celià-Terrassa T, Kang Y (2016) Distinctive properties of metastasis-initiating cells. Genes Dev 30(8):892–908
130. Valastyan S, Weinberg RA (2011) Tumor metastasis: molecular insights and evolving paradigms. Cell 147(2):275–292
131. Cooper J, Giancotti FG (2019) Integrin signaling in cancer: mechanotransduction, stemness, epithelial plasticity, and therapeutic resistance. Cancer Cell 35(3):347–367

Part III

MicroRNAs in Cancer: From Diagnosis to Therapeutics

9

Kanisha Shah and Rakesh M. Rawal

9.1 Introduction

MicroRNAs (miRNAs/miRs) are small, intrinsic, non-coding RNAs, which are 18–24 nucleotides (nts) long stretches, that possess a vital role in modulating gene expression at the post-transcriptional phase. The miRNAs fundamentally function by the activity of Dicer, an RNase that acts on pre-miRNAs which are hairpin-structured precursors which further mature into miRNAs [1]. miRNAs possess the property of post-transcriptionally repressing the gene expression by distinguishing complementary target sites at the 3′untranslated region (UTR) of the particular target mRNAs [2]. Ambros and colleagues found the first miRNA called the lin-4 in *Caenorhabditis elegans* species (*C. elegans*). The miRNA was recognized as a small non-coding stretch of RNA that influences the development by controlling the expression of lin-14 protein. Another miRNA let-7 has also been reported in *C. elegans* that negatively regulates the lin-41 gene in a sequence-explicit RNA-RNA interaction pattern at the 3′-UTR of the mRNA [3]. Later in 2001 different independent teams found that miRNAs were abundantly present in both vertebrates and invertebrates. Additionally it was observed that certain miRNAs were immensely conserved, suggesting that miRNA-modulated post-transcriptional regulation is a specific regulatory function found in different species [4]. Moreover, the past two decades has shed intense light on the crucial functions of miRNAs in the control of various cellular events, such as cell proliferation, differentiation, invasion, migration, stress response, apoptosis as well as metabolism [5]. However, it has been seen that miRNAs have been associated as important modulators in the advancement of various diseases [6, 7], such as cancer. At present, a total of 1872 elucidated human

K. Shah · R. M. Rawal (✉)
Department of Life Science, School of Sciences, Gujarat University, Ahmedabad, Gujarat, India

N. Masood, S. Shakil Malik (eds.), *'Essentials of Cancer Genomic, Computational Approaches and Precision Medicine*,
https://doi.org/10.1007/978-981-15-1067-0_9

miRNA precursor genes are transformed into ~ 2578 mature miRNA arrays (http://www.mirbase.org); however, the role of certain miRNAs is not yet known [2, 8].

Moreover, in humans, it has been observed that nearly one third of miRNAs are orderly structured in cluster patterns. Further, it is thought that a particular cluster might be a unique transcriptional complex indicating a synchronized control of miRNAs in these clusters. Additionally, computational analysis uncovered that a fraction of the clusters contain two or more than two miRNAs with identical sequences [9]. However, a rare event that has been observed is that miRNAs with similar mature sequence are rarely replicated in a cluster. The indicated genomic assembly leads to concurrent expression of analogous miRNAs, probably inducing conjugation distinction along with synergism of the biological functions. Nonetheless, miRNAs are regulated post-transcriptionally owing to the fact that similar and/or equal expression levels are not observed from all miRNAs belonging to a single transcriptional cluster. In addition, a notable finding is that a convincing proportion of miRNAs are either protein-coding or non-coding transcription entities located in the intronic region [10]; however, a small population of miRNAs are also mapped onto repeated sequences such as LINEs (long interspersed nuclear elements) [8, 11].

Studies have reported that >50% of miRNA genes are situated in tumour-affiliated genomic regions and were the fundamental nodal points in tumour formation and progression cascades [12], indicating that miRNAs may be associated with the pathogenesis of varied tumours. The imbalance of miRNAs may have an indispensable role in the commencement, dissemination, invasion and progression of a number of tumours. Calin et al. principally confirmed this hypothesis in chronic lymphocytic leukaemia (CLL) and validated that there was a preponderance of deletion or loss of miR-15a and miR-16-1 in approximately 90% of patients with CLL [13].

The present challenge is to uncover the complex role of miRNAs that participate in the pathogenesis of various tumours. Earlier studies depicted that miRNAs participate in regulating various molecular as well as signalling pathways in tumours by targeting different oncogenes and tumour suppressors for tumours maintenance, aggressiveness, disease progression, angiogenesis, drug resistance, epithelial-mesenchymal (EMT) transition as well as tumour metastasis. miRNAs are widely spread over the entire genome and are known to regulate nearly >50% of the human genes [14]. Studies have reported that an alteration in certain cancer-associated miRNA expression might change the plausible oncogenic or anti-oncogenic protein expression indicating that miRNAs may function as therapeutic tools for tumour treatment [15, 16].

Thus this section encompasses the functions of miRNAs and its biogenesis and regulation in humans. Furthermore, the review elucidates the processes through which miRNA expression is impaired in different tumours. Also how miRNAs are directly linked to the cancer hallmarks, acting either as oncogenes or tumour suppressors, and their role in the underlying mechanisms of various cancers have been illustrated. Lastly, we have highlighted the miRNA potentiality as predictive markers for diagnosis, prognosis as well as treatment of tumours and also the threats involved in miRNA research and applications.

9.1.1 Biogenesis, Regulation and Mechanism of miRNA Action

The miRNA biogenesis process commences with the amalgamation of a pri-miRNA that is 3′ poly-adenylated and 5′ capped structure (Fig. 9.1). The pri-miRNAs preserve features similar to mRNA such as 3′ poly(A) tail and 5′ cap structure and are transcribed by RNA polymerase II. However, other pathways govern the transcription of genomic repeats in certain minor sets of miRNAs. For example, it is observed that RNA polymerase III governs the miRNA transcription in Alu repeats [17].

Inside the nucleus, Drosha (an RNase III enzyme) along with its collaborating partner DGCR8 directs the formation of pre-miRNA from pri-miRNA [17–19]. DGCR8 identifies the stem region and the flanking single-stranded RNA (ssRNA). It further acts as an important internal component for Drosha to nick the stem nearly 11 nucleotides (nts) from the stem-ssRNA region causing liberation of the pre-miRNA [17]. Under other circumstances a subset of miRNAs (miRtrons) undertake an alternative pathway apart from the Drosha requirement, leading to the derivation of pre-miRNAs as a by-product of the splicing action [18, 19]. The exportin-5/Ran/GTP complex later exports pre-miRNA to the cytoplasm and converts it to a mature duplex miRNA by the support of an RNase III enzyme—Dicer [8, 19]. As the duplex uncoils, the mature miRNA assimilates and forms a protein complex known as RNA-induced silencing complex (RISC) which further directs RISC to target the mRNA [10]. The entire biogenesis process is tightly regulated at various steps, including transcription of miRNAs, processing by Dicer and Drosha, RISC binding, miRNA transportation and miRNA degeneration. For instance, SMAD protein and DEAD-box RNA helicases are known to participate in miRNA maturation governed by Drosha [20]. Moreover, another factor, called the KH-type splicing regulatory protein (KHSP), acts as an integral element of Drosha and Dicer networks causing the regulation of biogenesis pathway of a subpopulation of miRNAs in mammalian cells [21]. Recently, another molecule called the methyltransferase-like 3 is also identified as a miRNA biogenesis regulator as it methylates pri-miRNAs and exhibits the identification and processing by DGCR8 for generation of a mature miRNA [22].

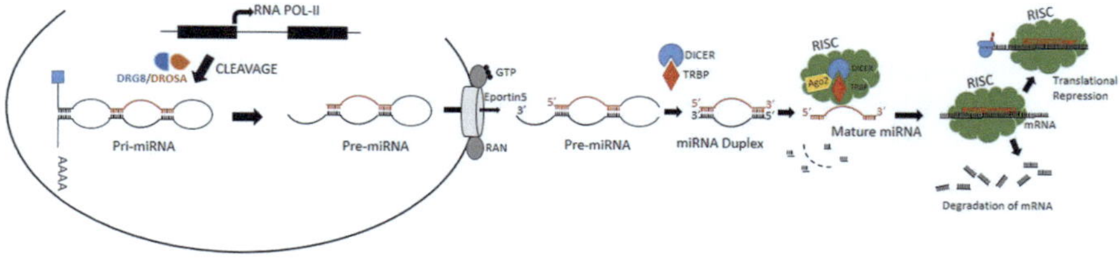

Fig. 9.1 Diagrammatic representation of microRNA biogenesis and regulation pathway

In addition, miRNA post-transcriptionally suppresses the target mRNA expression by predominantly leading to the interaction of mRNA with the 3′UTR region as depicted in Fig. 9.1. Nonetheless, the explicit functioning of miRNAs on their mRNA targets is still not known. Also it has been observed that there are bulges and mismatches in major sites of miRNA target unlike the perfect sequence complementarity that is seen among siRNA and mRNA. Earlier studies have revealed that a comparison between siRNA and miRNA indicates that mRNA destabilization occurs through siRNA, whereas mRNA translation inhibition is owing to miRNA but without affecting the levels of the messenger RNA. Therefore, an important factor that separates the two processes is the extent of complementarity among the short RNA and its target [8].

Despite the translational repression functioning for certain miRNAs is still true, it has been observed in several studies that the amount of mRNA target may be decreased even though their might be constrained sequence complementarity among the miRNA and mRNA [23]. The degradation of an mRNA by a miRNA might be elucidated by RNA processing bodies called P-bodies, which are the locus for RNA degeneration [24]. Probably, the target mRNA translation is inhibited by miRNAs which are further segregated to P-bodies ultimately leading to degradation. However, another mechanism through which miRNAs cause the degeneration of the target mRNAs is independent of requisition to P-bodies [25, 26]. During explicit events miRNA inhibits the mRNA translation, but levels are maintained, and thus sequestration of mRNAs to P-bodies may prove to be ineffective. However, it should be considered that there are varied possibilities that numerous mechanisms apply depending on the independent miRNA-mRNA interactions [8].

9.2 Mechanism of miRNA in Cancer

Dr. Croce and his group discovered the first documentation of miRNA association in human during the identification of tumour suppressors at chromosome 13q14 region in B-cell chronic lymphocytic leukaemia [13]. Moreover, it was observed that this particular region was often deleted in CLL, and later two genes, miR-15a and miR-16-1, were found in that particular region. Both these genes were either deleted or lost in majority of CLL cases. Additionally, another study demonstrated that miR-15 and miR-16-1 promote programmed cell death by supressing Bcl-2 that is generally upregulated in non-dividing tumour B cells as well as other solid malignancies [6, 27].

However, in mice the deletion/removal of miR-15 and miR-16-1 cluster causes phenotypic changes similar to CLL that were seen in humans demonstrating a crucial tumour suppression function of these miRNAs [7]. Later, miRNA sequencing and profiling showed plausible documentation that expression of miRNAs is impaired in tumours and hence might be useful for tumour classification, differentiation, tumour diagnosis and early prognosis [8]. The tumour suppressor gene expression is known to be lower in tumour cells, whereas the tumour suppressor miRNAs negatively suppress the oncogenes that regulate cell differentiation and/or apoptosis, consequently preventing tumour formation, aggressiveness and invasion.

For example, miRNA let-7 is known as tumour suppressor gene, and its expression is decreased in different types of tumours that is further associated with poor overall survival in cancer patients [28]. Moreover, the overexpression of let-7 has been correlated with decreased lung cancer cell growth in vitro [29]. Conversely in lung cancer cells, it has been observed that the decreased let-7 expression enhances RAS expression—a pro-oncogene [29–31]. Moreover, in prostate cancer the loss of miR-34a expression, another tumour suppressor, is linked with tumour progression, recurrence and metastasis, whereas its re-expression is linked to tumour cell clonogenicity, tumour invasion, migration, apoptosis, cellular stimulation of chemotherapy as well as radiation therapy in pancreatic tumours. Various other studies confirmed that the miR-34 family is responsible for the mutation and expression of p53, whereas particularly miR-34b and miR-34c target the proto-oncogene MYC [32–34]. A loss in expression of miR-34 family members mitigated p38-mitogen-activated protein kinase-dependent and p53-dependent response to DNA damage causing carcinogenesis [35].

Moreover, it was previously considered that 'oncomirs'—those miRNAs that were overexpressed in tumours—had a role in promoting tumour formation by negatively controlling genes especially those regulating cell differentiation, proliferation, apoptosis as well as tumour suppressor genes. There are different oncomirs in the tumour genome, out of which only a small fraction has been characterized, such as miR-21 [36] and the miR-17-92 cluster [37]. miR-21 is known to be overexpressed in a number of tumours such as leukaemia; lymphoma; lung, pancreatic, breast and colorectal cancer; glioblastoma; and neuroblastoma. It alters proliferation, differentiation, invasion, migration and apoptosis of tumour cells in vitro and has also been linked with in vivo overall survival of patients by targeting a tumour suppressor gene [36]. Likewise, the miR-17-92 cluster is a polycistronic transcript located at chromosome 13q31 and comprises of miRNAs 17, 18a, 19a, 19b-1, 20a and 92a-1 that are drastically upregulated in tumours such as lymphomas and lung cancer [38]. However, c-Myc stimulates and controls the miR-17-92 cluster to further regulate the E2F1 expression and inhibits c-Myc-mediated apoptosis via p53 signalling cascade [36, 38]. In addition, miR-17-92 hinders genes such as phosphatase and tensin homolog and RB2 [39] by stimulating protein kinase B signalling network that promotes tumour-cell survival. In human testicular germ cell tumour, miR-372 and miR-373 promote cell proliferation and carcinogenesis by targeting the large tumour suppressor kinase 2 [16, 40] and thus nullifying p53-modulated cyclin-dependent kinase inhibition.

9.3 Mechanisms Leading to MicroRNA Dysregulation in Cancer

In the previous decade, researchers have proved that expression of miRNAs is impaired in human carcinomas. The basic processes encompass genomic alterations, transcriptional regulatory developments, epigenetic variations and deformities in the miRNA biogenesis and processing system.

9.3.1 Deletion or Amplification of miRNA Genes/Genomic Alterations/Abnormalities

Carcinogenesis is frequently complemented by chromosomal impairments including deletion, amplification, translocation, point mutations, etc. Bioinformatic analyses have demonstrated that an important subset of miRNAs is linked with cancer-associated fragile sites or genomic regions in human as well as mice [41]. In several comparative studies comprising of array CGH (comparative genomic hybridization) and miRNA expression data, the miRNA levels have been compared with differences in copy number at the genomic loci [42, 43]. In lung cancer, downregulation of both miR-143 and miR-145 is due to the deletion of the 5q33 region that harbours both miRNAs [44]. Conversely, miR-17-92 gene cluster amplification is reported in B-cell lymphomas along with lung tumours, and the translocation of this cluster has been recorded in T-cell acute lymphoblastic leukaemia (ALL) causing upregulation of miRNAs in different cancers [42]. The elevated percentage of numerous genomic variations in miRNA loci was substantiated by techniques such as high-resolution array-based comparative genomic hybridization in approximately 227 samples from different human tumours like the ovarian and breast and melanoma [45]. Additionally, genome-wide analysis demonstrated that various miRNA genes are known to be located in the cancer-associated genomic domains. Moreover, these domains could encompass an essential region of loss of heterozygosity, which could harbour tumour suppressor genes; a marginal region of amplification, which may consist of various oncogenes; or numerous fragile sites/common breakpoint regions [46]. Overall, these findings prompt towards the idea that atypical miRNA expression in tumour cells could result owing to the amplification or deletion of explicit genomic regions comprising of miRNA genes.

9.3.2 Transcriptional Regulation of miRNA

Transcription factors might play a vital role in inducing miRNAs by triggering the pri-miRNA transcription. They activate tissue-specific miRNAs throughout the process of differentiation, and this mechanism has been observed in various malignancies. However, a wide range of effect of transcription factors is seen in principal cellular processes like proliferation, differentiation, etc. It has recently become clear that several tumour suppressor and/or oncogenes act as transcription factors such as p53, c-Myc, E2F, etc. [2]. Later it was found that c-Myc is repeatedly overexpressed in various tumours leading to control of tumour cell proliferation, apoptosis and transcriptional stimulation of the oncogenic miR-17-92 cluster by binding with E-box elements in the miR-17-92 promoter region [47]. Moreover, another important finding was that c-Myc inhibits the transcriptional stimulation of tumour-suppressive miRNAs including mir-15a, miR-26, miR-29 and mir-30 along with let-7 family which is consistent with its oncogenic function [48]. Ghoshal et al. discovered the complementary control of c-Myc and miR-122 in primary liver tumours where c-Myc inhibits miR-122 expression by linking to its promoter and in turn miR-122 indirectly supresses c-Myc transcription by targeting E2f1 and Tfdp2 factors. Thus, for hepatocellular carcinoma development, it is of utmost importance that there is an alteration in the feedback loop consisting of miR-122 and c-Myc [49]. In addition, c-Myc binds and suppresses the expression of the miR-148a-5p/miR-363-3p gene promoters, encouraging hepatocellular carcinoma by promoting progression of G1 to S phase. Consecutively, miR-148a-5p hinders the gene expression of c-Myc, while miR-363-3p destabilizes c-Myc by unequivocally targeting ubiquitin-specific proteases 28 [50]. Another example of transcriptional factors that regulate and mediate tumour-suppressive function is of the p53-miR-34 regulatory axis [51]. p53, a tumour suppressor, is the most frequently mutated gene in human tumours and is encoded by the TP53 gene. p53 forms a complex network and controls various gene expressions, including miRNA genes, and consecutively regulates cell cycle progression and apoptosis. Similarly, miR-34 family encompassing miR-34a/b/c stimulates cell cycle arrest, cell senescence and programmed cell death in different malignancies [52], implying the fact that p53 and miR-34 are connected and are in the same regulatory network. This speculation was further substantiated, and it was revealed that p53 can influence the expression of miR-34a that triggers apoptosis by binding directly to the mir-34a gene promoter. Sequentially, miR-34a induces p53 expression by deacetylation of SIRT1, which is a negative regulator of p53 [53]. Further other studies have indicated that p53 regulates the expression of a range of miRNAs, including miR-605, miR-1246 and miR-107 [54–56]. In addition to c-Myc and p53, several transcriptional factors are reported to regulate the miRNA expression. Another miRNA, miR-223, is differently expressed in the haematopoietic network with vital role in myeloid lineage developmental progression, and its expression is repressed in multiple tumours including hepatocellular carcinoma (HCC) and acute myeloid leukaemia (AML) [57–60]. It has been observed that the expression of miR-223 gene is directed by the myeloid transcription factors PU.1 and C/EBPs [61]. Moreover, Fazi et al. discovered that miR-223 and transcription factors NFI-A and C/EBPα form a mini network that controls human granulocytic differentiation [62]. These two transcription factors compete for binding to the miR-223 promoter through a mechanism such as NFI-A maintains miR-223 at low levels, whereas the retinoic acid-induced C/EBPα replaces NFI-A to upregulate miR-223 expression. Thus, miRNA expression is finely modified by multiple factors to maintain normal transcription, and its dysregulation leads to carcinogenesis and aggressiveness [8].

9.3.3 Changes in Epigenetic Factors

The changes in epigenetic regulators are established trait in cancer, which include global abnormal DNA hyper-methylation of CpG islands in promoter regions and genomic DNA hypo-methylation, along with separation of histone modification arrangements. It is understood that analogous to protein-coding genes, miRNAs are quite receptive to epigenetic modulations [63, 64].

Moreover, gene silencing owing to DNA methylation is a close event associated with histone modification. Computational analysis has demonstrated that CpG islands are present adjacent to various miRNAs [65]. The overexpression of many miRNAs is caused due to the exposure of different cells to 5-aza-2′-deoxycytidine (a demethylating agent), mutations in DNMTs (DNA methyltransferases) and/or HDAC (histone deacetylase) inhibitor treatment [65–67]. In comparison to normal tissues, it has been further identified certain miRNAs are inhibited by CpG hyper-methylation in various tumours. For instance, miR-9-1 in breast tumour [65] and miR-124a in CRC (colorectal cancer) have been reported [66]. Moreover, miR-124a hyper-methylation is thought to be tumour-specific, as there have been no reported evidences of methylation in neuroblastoma. The epigenetic suppression of a miRNA is also believed to be associated with specific tissue type. For illustration, miR-124a is generally vastly expressed in neuronal tissues but is commonly repressed epigenetically in colorectal carcinoma. Evidences state that CpG methylation is frequently halted as a result of various miRNA expressions. For instance, miR-29 targets various DNA methyltransferases such as Dnmt3A and -3B. In association to this, heterotrophic miR-29 expression caused an overall repression in DNA methylation, consequently leading to expression of certain tumour suppressor genes that had undergone silencing owing to promoter methylation in tumour cells [68]. Fazi et al. also found that epigenetic modification in a common AML-associated fusion protein AML1/ETO leads to miR-223 silencing through CpG methylation [69]. However, it was reported that 17 out of 313 human miRNAs were nearly threefold or more over-expressed in T24 bladder tumour cells post combinatorial therapy comprising of histone acetylation and DNA methylation inhibitors [70]. Furthermore, miR-127 expression that is present in a CpG island and is lost in tumour cells had appreciably increased expression posttreatment, along with downregulation in BCL6—a proto-oncogene. Conclusively these findings indicate that histone deacetylase inhibition and DNA demethylation can cause stimulation of miRNAs expression that might act as tumour suppressors. On the basis of previous findings, Lujambio et al. observed that miR-148a and miR-34b/c cluster causes distinct hyper-methylation-attributed silencing in tumour cells [71]. Besides, re-expression of miRNAs in tumour cells restricted their movement, decreased tumour progression and constrained metastasis development in vivo. Correspondingly, low expression of miR-124a, miR-9-1 and miR-145-5p can be associated with DNA hyper-methylation in lung, breast and colon carcinomas, respectively [65, 72, 73]. Thus, these studies highlight the function of epigenetic governance in miRNA expression during carcinogenesis, indicating that abnormal DNA methylation and histone acetylation of miRNAs might serve as beneficial markers for tumour diagnosis and prognostication.

9.3.4 Dysregulation of MicroRNA Biogenesis and Regulation Mechanism

As stated previously, the biogenesis process is a complexly governed event that involves numerous enzymes and regulatory proteins, including Dicer, Drosha,

DGCR8, Argonaute proteins and exprotin 5, allowing accurate maturation of miRNAs from their primary precursors. Hence, alteration, dysregulation and/or abnormal expression of different factors involved in the miRNA biogenesis event might cause an aberrant miRNA expression. However, two key RNase III endonucleases, Drosha and Dicer, are involved in miRNA maturation and are accountable for consummating the pre-miRNA and miRNA duplex. It has been observed that both Drosha and Dicer are dysregulated in certain tumours. Moreover, it has been discovered that an enormous section of miRNAs is governed at the Drosha-processing phase, and this plays a crucial role in the expression of miRNA during embryogenesis as well as carcinogenesis [74]. DGCR8 and Drosha are known to have either single-nucleotide substitution or deletion in approximately 15–20% of Wilms' tumours, causing significant reduced expression of mature let-7a and miR-200 family [75]. However, it has been observed that in regard to Dicer dysregulation, Dicer1 deterioration in colorectal tumour cells stimulates the attainment of a higher efficiency for tumour growth and progression and ultimately leads to cancer metastasis [76]. In ovarian cancer, elevated Dicer and Drosha mRNA levels are attributed to greater median survival, and conversely, lower Dicer expression has been seen to correlate with poor patient survival [77–80]. Karube et al. discovered an effective interrelationship among reduced Dicer mRNA levels and decreased let-7 expression with lower postoperative survival in patients having lung carcinomas. Argonaute proteins are known to possess a critical role in RNA-silencing processes and are essential catalytic components of RISC [78]. Like Dicer and Drosha, deregulation of Argonaute proteins has been reported in different tumours. In Wilms' tumour of the kidney, human EIF2C1/hAgo1 gene has been often reported to have an aberrant expression [81]. Moreover, human Argonaute proteins (AGO) expression is controlled in a cell-dependent approach. For example, the expression levels of AGO2 are lower in melanoma compared to their primary melanocyte, whereas in gastric cancer and their lymph node metastases the expression is remarkably elevated as compared to healthy controls [82, 83]. It has been observed that exportin 5 (XPO5), a double-stranded RNA-binding protein, arbitrates nuclear export of pre-miRNA directly in the cytoplasm. Further it was reported that XPO5 possesses certain inactivating mutations with microsatellite instability in a subset of human tumours. Moreover, in colorectal carcinoma cell lines like HCT-15 and DLD-1, it has been seen that an insertion of an 'A' in exon 32 produces a premature termination codon, causing a frameshift mutation leading to an assembly of a truncated protein. The truncated XPO5 fails to export pre-miRNAs that further is captured in the nucleus, subsequently culminating in decreased miRNA processing. The restoration of XPO5 properties reverses the damaged export of pre-miRNAs and also possesses the tumour suppressor features [84]. Further it was reported that XPO5's failure to transport pre-miRNAs from nucleus to cytoplasm was triggered by ERK kinase in hepatocellular carcinoma to phosphorylate XPO5 [8]. Along with the transcription rate of pri-miRNA, the stable level of mature miRNA is known by the processing productivity of its precursors and their stability. It is frequently seen that miRNAs demonstrate a discrepancy in expression between the mature form and its precursor [85, 86]. Although it is a known fact that miRNAs in a genomic cluster have a common origin from a pri-miRNA, but the expression levels of individual miRNAs in the cluster may not be inevitably comparable [87]. For instance, after the induction of pri-miR-21 in a time-course experiment, it was revealed that there was a delayed kinetics in aggregation of mature miR-21 [88]. Together, these results prompt towards the fact that miRNA processing and stability are crucial factors that regulate miRNA expression levels. A comprehensive analysis of expression data has highlighted this mechanism in different tumours [74]. In instances where a miRNA exists within a gene, the host genes can be considered as the pri-miRNA. A comparative study of the microarray data of mRNA and miRNA illustrated that decrease in miRNA expression in tumours is inadequately associated with reduced target gene expression. Abnormal expression of miRNAs during carcinogenesis can be linked to variations at the post-transcriptional level. The expression levels of Dicer or Drosha are reported to be altered in different malignancies [78, 89, 90]. Drosha upregulation occurs owing to the gain in copy number at chr5p which is observed in majority of cervical SCC (squamous cell carcinoma) cases [90]. Further, hierarchal clustering of miRNA expression data led to classification of cervical SCC cases into two different cohorts based on overexpression of Drosha. It was a significant observation that certain miRNAs were impaired due to overexpression of Drosha, demonstrating that diverse miRNAs react differently to an increase in the miRNA processing mechanism. Remarkably, Drosha has been observed to interact with a tumour-associated fusion protein as a result of chromosomal translocation in certain types of blood cancers [91]. Further, this communication affects pri-miRNA assortment of Drosha resulting in an impaired miRNA expression pattern [2].

9.4 MicroRNA-Associated Regulation of Important Cancer-Related Signalling Pathways

Studies have reported that miRNAs control different functions of cellular senescence and cell cycle along with DNA damage response, and they possess great influence of these on various signalling cascades in different tumours. A detailed list of miRNAs along with its various targets in different tumours have been reported in Table 9.1, and the miRNA-miRNA interaction has been given in Fig. 9.2.

9.4.1 Regulation of Cell Cycle Mechanism and Proliferation

Previous reports have observed the role of miRNAs in cell cycle and proliferation and their contribution to cancer progression by disturbing the crucial cell cycle modulatory signalling pathways. Fundamental to cell cycle control event, the retinoblastoma (pRb) signalling cascade is frequently impaired in various types of tumours [137, 138]. The pRb gene is a significant repressor of the transcription regulators of the E2F family, which control the transcription of genes essential for the advancement and maintenance of cell cycle [139]. This suppression is facilitated by pRb phosphorylation via cyclin-dependent kinases (CDKs),

Table 9.1 List of microRNAs and target genes involved in various malignancies

Malignancy	MicroRNAs	Differential gene expression	Target genes	Reference
Breast cancer	let-7	Downregulated	E2F2, c-Myc, KRAS	[30]
	miR-27a	Upregulated	FOXO1	[92]
	miR-31	Downregulated	RhoA	[93]
	miR-96	Upregulated	FOXO1	[92]
	miR-98	Downregulated	E2F2, c-Myc	[94]
	miR-182	Upregulated	FOXO1, FOXO3	[92]
	miR-205	Downregulated	HER3	[95]
	miR-9-3	Downregulated	p53	[96]
	miR-375	Upregulated	SHOX2	[97]
Lung cancer	miR-21, miR-155	Upregulated	SOCS1, SOCS6, PTEN	[98]
	miR-205	Upregulated	SMAD4	[99]
	miR-16	Upregulated	Bcl-2, HGF	[27, 100]
	miR-17	Downregulated	Bcl-2	[101]
	miR-126-3p	Downregulated	PLXNB2, TSC1	[102]
	let-7a	Downregulated	Cyclin D1	[103]
Colon cancer	miR-21	Downregulated	SPRY2	[104]
	miR-23a	Downregulated	MTSS1	[105]
	miR-31	Upregulated	SATB2, β-catenin, TCF-LEF	[106]
	miR-135b	Upregulated	APC, PTEN/PI3K, SRC	[107]
	miR-193a	Downregulated	KRAS, BRAF	[108]
	mir-338-5p	Downregulated	PIK3C3	[109]
Gastric cancer	miR-25	Upregulated	p57	[110]
	miR-106b	Upregulated	p21, p73	[111]
	miR-93, miR-221	Upregulated	p21, p27, p57	[112, 113]
	miR-512	Downregulated	Mcl-1	[114]
	miR-10b	Upregulated	RhoC	[115]
Glioma	miR-221	Downregulated	PTEN/AKT	[116]
	miR-324-5	Downregulated	GLI1	[117]
Pancreatic cancer	miR-21	Upregulated	MMP2, MPP9, PI3K, AKT	[118]
	miR-192-5p	Upregulated	SERPINE1	[119]
	miR-200c	Downregulated	E-cadherin (CDH1)	[120]
Hepatocellular carcinoma	miR-195	Downregulated	Cyclin D1, E2F3	[121]
	miR-16	Downregulated	Bcl-2	[122]
	miR-18a	Upregulated	ERα, ESR1	[123]
	miR-26a	Downregulated	Cyclin D2, cyclin E2	[124]
	miR-101	Downregulated	Mcl-1	[125]
	miR-145	Downregulated	EGFR, IGF-1R	[126]

(continued)

Table 9.1 (continued)

Malignancy	MicroRNAs	Differential gene expression	Target genes	Reference
Prostate cancer	miR-331	Downregulated	HER2/neu	[127]
	miR-200, miR-200b	Downregulated	ZEB1, ZEB2	[128]
Oral cancer	miR-21	Upregulated	EGFR, APC	[129]
	miR-31	Upregulated	ACOX1, PGE2	[129, 130]
	miR-29b	Upregulated	PTEN	[131]
	miR-144	Upregulated	PTEN	[132]
	miR-187	Upregulated	BARX2	[133]
	miR-143	Downregulated	BCL2, AKT1, MDM2, HRAS, KRAS	[134, 135]
	let-7a	Downregulated	NRAS, HMGA2, KRAS, HRAS, MYC	[136]

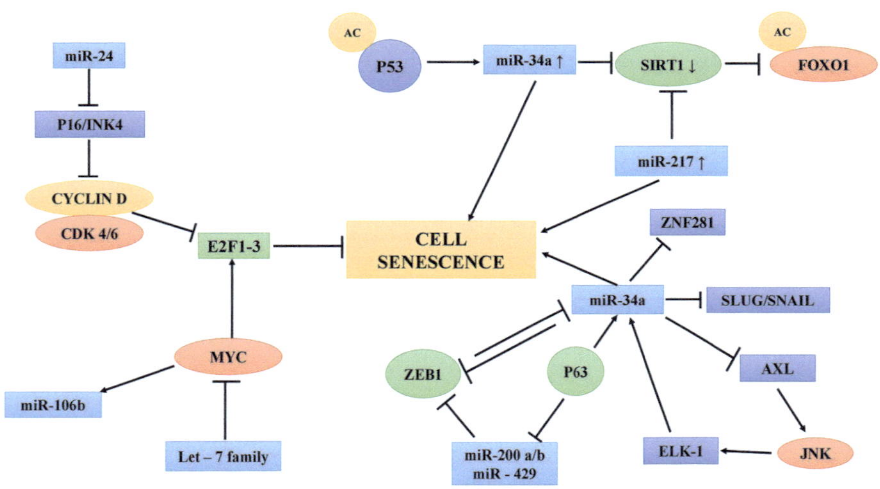

Fig. 9.2 miRNA—Gene interaction network related to different tumours. The microRNA-target gene network was constructed using the predicted interactions and the gene expression data in the miRNET software. The mRNA summary was obtained from earlier published literature. miRNA-mRNA components obtained via population-based probabilistic method was used to establish the different network interactions. In the figure the circles signify genes, and squares signify miRNAs; their interaction is characterized by one edge. The degree is denoted by the centre of the network (i.e. the interaction of one miRNA with the target genes throughout and vice versa)

permitting E2Fs to stimulate gene transcription, such as cyclins and CDKs, which are essential for cell cycle advancement [138]. Explicit cyclin and kinase allies form active CDK complexes, for instance, cyclin D with CDK4/6 where this CDK activity successively activates cell cycle advancement through progressive phases [140].

In addition, cyclins and cyclin-dependent kinases (CDKs) are fundamental growth-suppressing miRNA targets. They control the growth-governing cascades like mitogenic pathways including the MAPK/RAS/RAF axis as well as the p53 pathway which is a growth-inhibiting pathway [140, 141]. Initial reports suggested that the miR-15a-16-1 cluster is absent in various tumours and thus motivated additional exploration in finding the gene targets associated with this miRNA family [13]. The vital positive modulators of the cell cycle, like CDK1/2/6 and cyclins D1/D3/E1, are some of the known targets that assist G1 arrest through these miRNAs [142]. However among these other promoters such as the cyclins [143] and the cell division cycle phosphatases like CDC25A [144] are also the targets of different miRNAs that are downregulated in tumours and aid in inhibiting the cell cycle event [143, 145]. Similar to the miR-17-92 cluster, miR-20a and miR-125b, the E2F transcription factors have been themselves designated as miRNAs targets with tumour suppressor roles [146].

To the contrary, the expression of different negative modulators of the cell cycle are suppressed by various miRNAs. pRb along with p130 and p107 are essential miRNA targets, known to be overexpressed in different tumours [147]. The negative modulators of CDKs signify an essential class of cell cycle inhibitors, which necessitate extensive miRNA-mediated control. For example, Cip1 (p21), a recognized gene target of p53 and an effective activator of G1 arrest, is directed by miR-106b and miR-17-92 clusters, illustrating increased level in several malignancies [144]. Remarkably, although several genes are frequently predicted to be targeted by various miRNAs using in silico analysis, limited genes-miRNA interactions are also validated experimentally in vitro [148]. For instance, in p21 it was confirmed by luciferase reporter assay that among 28 different miRNAs, some are overexpressed in tumours and can possibly target the 3′UTR region of p21 mRNA [16].

Also, the expression of Kip1 (p27) is mainly governed by various post-transcriptional mechanisms [149] and is known to be a target for various miRNAs, one of which is the miR221/222 cluster [150]. This holds significance in glioblastomas and prostate tumours where Kip1 expression levels demonstrate an inverse correlation with miR221 and miR-222 [149, 151]. Additionally, growth-promoting signalling networks have also caused decrease in expression of anti-proliferative miRNAs. The phosphorylation of TRBP reported to be linked with the Dicer complex [152] is also to be influenced by mitogen-activated protein kinase (MAPK) ERK. Levels of the miRNA family of the let-7 tumour suppressor were repressed as a result of repression by ERK following the TRBP phosphorylation, while those of growth-promoting miRNAs including miR-17, miR-20a and miR-92a were stimulated [153].

9.4.2 MicroRNA-Associated Control of Cell Senescence

Senescence is an inevitable withdrawal of the cells from the cell cycle event and grouped into two major subdivisions, namely, premature/stress-induced senescence and replicative senescence. Replicative senescence results when cells achieve a pivotal 'age' as a consequence of telomere shortening, whereas stress-induced senescence may result due to oncogene expression, oxidative stress and stimulation of the DNA damage pathway [154]. However, an important fact is that senescence acts as a blockage for cancer progression.

Furthermore, miRNAs are known to control the different signalling cascades involved in the senescence event (Fig. 9.3). However, several miRNAs negatively regulate cell cycle advancement but possess crucial roles in the stimulation of cell senescence. p16 is an important repressor of CDK4/6 and is inhibited by miR-24, which gets further decreased throughout the replicative senescence event [155, 156]. Also, the p53 gene that is controlled by mainly miR-34a is implicated as a vital senescence regulator through inhibition of multiple targets [53]. The main target of miR-34a—silent information regulator 1 (SIRT1)—is a deacetylase and principal senescence regulator [53, 157]. Expression of miR-34a and SIRT1 inhibition leads to a complex feedback mechanism where SIRT1 deacetylates p53 and further inhibits its activity along with miR-34a transcription [53, 158]. Significantly, miR-34a can also be regulated by one of the members of the ETS family of transcription factors, called ELK1 independently of p53, throughout the oncogene-activated senescence [159].

Moreover, miRNA cluster consisting of hsa-let-7i, hsa-let-7a-d, mir-15b-16-2 and mir-106b-25 is further activated throughout the G1-S shift by E2F1, and E2F3 factor consequently retracts primary fibroblast from quiescence state. These miRNAs essentially hinder the E2F-dependent entry in S-phase by directing numerous target genes and induce cell cycle advancement [160]. Therefore, E2F-induced miRNAs restrain the cellular effects of E2F stimulation leading to prevention of replicative stress. Furthermore, because the expression of these miRNAs are not essentially modified by successive DNA damage, they are more likely to stimulate senescence.

9.4.3 MicroRNAs and DNA Damage Response

Any recognition of an impaired DNA lesion and/or alterations in the chromatin structure causes the initiation of the DNA damage response and further directs the impaired signals to regulatory measures like the DNA-repair mechanism as well as checkpoints of the cell cycle. The damage sensor kinases called ATM, ATR and also CHK1 and CHK2 are triggered, further phosphorylating several protein targets such as the p53 subsequently initiating cellular reactions. Various DNA repair mechanisms prevail as numerous types of DNA lesions may occur. The cells counteract to DNA damage either by stopping the cell cycle advancement or through enduring apoptosis along with repairing DNA adducts or breaks critically connecting DNA damage and cell cycle regulation [141]. In addition, one of the significant roles of miRNA is to regulate the DNA damage and further the transcription and processing of these miRNAs during the damage by distinct components (Fig. 9.4). Thus, the miRNAs inhibit their targets and modulate the DNA damage response mechanism.

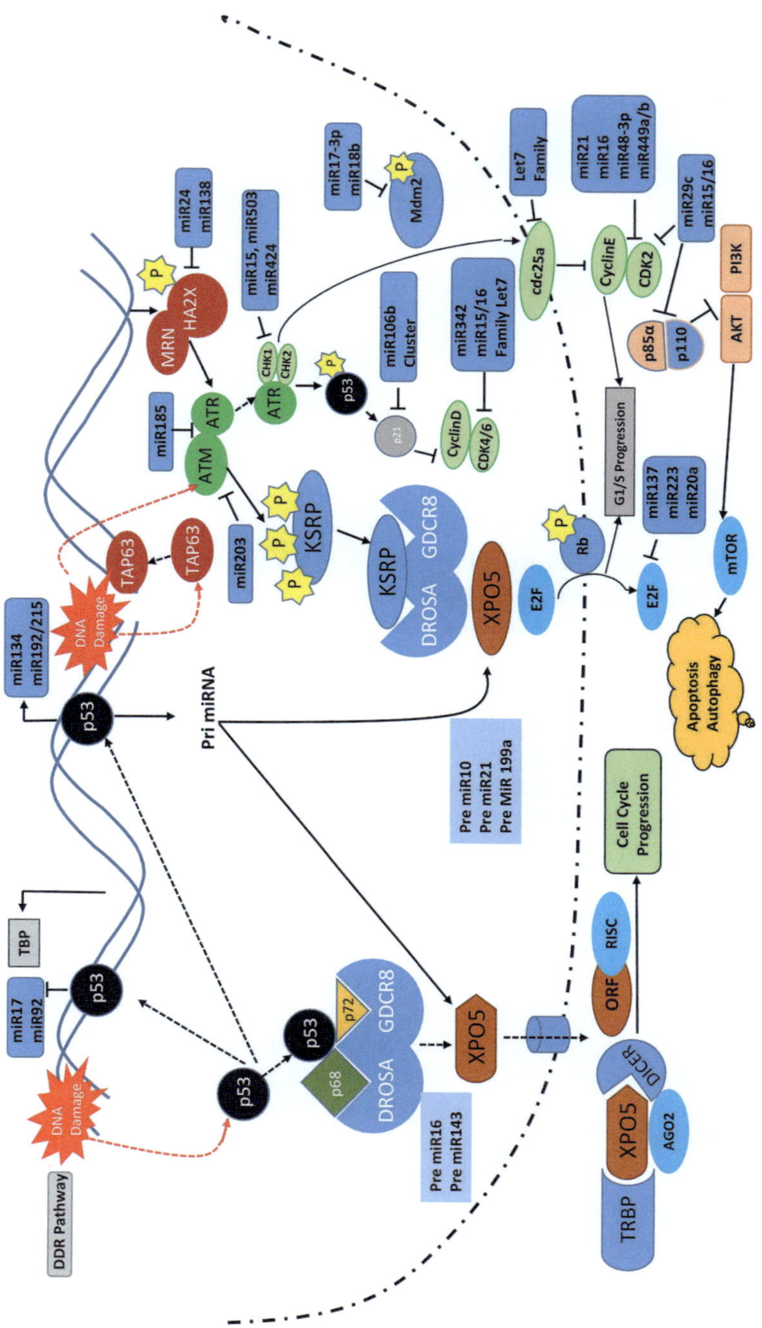

Fig. 9.3 Diagrammatic representation of signalling pathways modulated by microRNAs and their effect on cell senescence

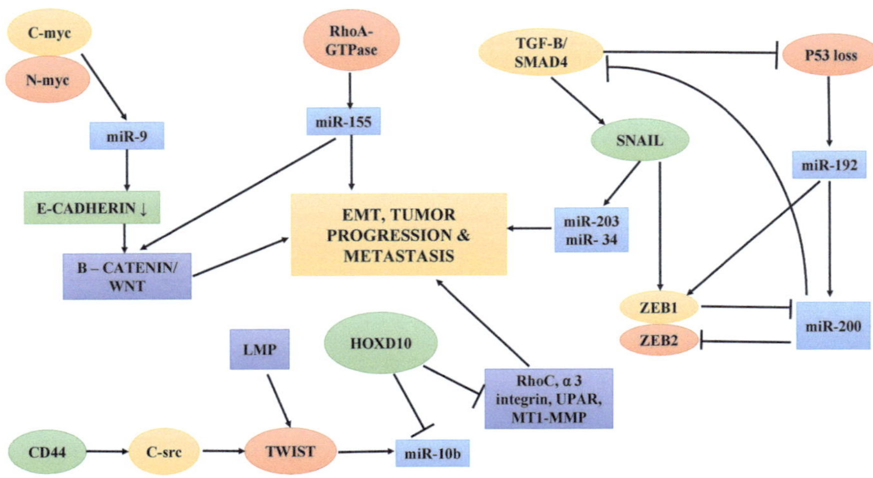

Fig. 9.4 Transcriptional and post-transcriptional control of microRNAs on DNA damage and cell cycle progression

9.4.3.1 Transcriptional Control of miRNA Expression Throughout DNA Damage Event

miRNAs are transcriptionally controlled by transcription factors analogous to that of the protein-coding genes throughout the DNA damage response pathway. Initially, it was identified that p53 was the direct transcriptional target of the miR-34 family [51]. Moreover, various targets of the miR-34 family comprised of the negative modulators of cell cycle progression and apoptosis governing anti-proliferative functions [161]. Nowadays, numerous research studies have reported the miR-34 family to be an important class of tumour suppressors along with its varied functions [52].

MDM2 protein, the crucial negative regulator of p53, is often reported to be amplified in different malignancies. p53 stimulates MDM2 expression that ultimately targets p53 for degradation, thereby contributing to the negative feedback loop. During cellular stress events, the capacity of MDM2 to regulate p53 negatively is decreased, mainly because of MDM2 phosphorylation by the DNA damage kinases, facilitating aggregation of p53 protein and activating its anti-proliferative property [162]. Numerous miRNAs, such as miR-192, miR-194, miR-215, miR-605, miR-143 and miR-145, are transcriptionally stimulated by p53 and participate in controlling p53-MDM2 feedback loop by directly targeting MDM2 [54]. miR-192, miR-194 and miR-215 expression assists in stimulating p53 target gene such as p21 leading to cell cycle arrest, through repression of MDM2. Repression of other cell cycle activating targets additionally leads to the growth inhibitory role of different miRNAs [163]. Also, the same were reported to have downregulated expression in multiple myeloma specimens, whereas inhibition of miRs-143/145 has been reported in the development of epithelial cancers. Additionally, activation of miR-145 by p53 has an important function in p53-mediated inhibition of MYC [164].

Intriguingly, transcriptional suppression of pro-oncogene-associated miRNAs owing to the miR-17-92 polycistronic cluster has been demonstrated to be transcriptionally repressed by p53, and further binding of p53 to the promoter region obstructs binding of the TATA-binding protein [165, 166].

9.4.3.2 Post-transcriptional Control of miRNAs Throughout DNA Damage

Studies have reported that post-transcriptional regulation of miRNA in response to DNA damage arose to be of corresponding significance in comparison to the transcriptional control of miRNA expression level regulation. It is observed that DNA damage causes increase in certain pre-miRNAs along with mature miRNAs but shows no substantial variation in primary miRNA transcript expression. This implies an association among miRNA processing, maturation mechanism and DNA damage response suggesting that the post-transcriptional machineries are possibly causing the initiation of specific miRNAs throughout the DNA damage stress-response process [167]. A study has reported that post-transcriptional miRNA processing also impacts the cellular reaction to UV-stimulated DNA damage causing the cells to become hypersensitive to this UV damage as a result of Ago2 or Dicer silencing. Furthermore, this UV-induced damage-initiated Ago2 re-localization in the stress granules (intracellular RNA—protein aggregates that are formed in stress conditions) is solely a cell cycle-dependent process along with alterations in the miRNA expression levels. However, it is still a matter of debate if involvement of stress granules directly linked to miRNA processing and mRNA suppression or not. Interestingly, it has been observed that alteration in Ago2 and re-localization of CDK and not ATM/ATR activity has known to be of significance. However, for the initiation of DNA damage-inducible miRNA expression, ATM/ATR activity has been reported to be of utmost importance. An important observation was that the modifications in miRNA expression level and stress-granule development occur very promptly, within the initial hours after damage treatment, indicating that miRNA control of the DNA damage response appears initially compared to other transcriptional responses [168]. Therefore, miRNAs play a crucial function in directing the earlier phases of the cellular response to DNA damage.

Following the DNA damage, p53 along with p68 augments the post-transcriptional maturation of numerous miRNAs including miR-145, miR-16-1 and miR-143 that possess the growth-suppressive function. Furthermore, transcriptionally altered p53 mutants restrict the arrangement of Drosha complex and p68, decreasing the rate of miRNA processing machinery [169]. The mutations in p53 gene seen in different malignancies affect both domains essential for DNA binding and control of miRNA processing, making it challenging to segregate. The plausible underlying mechanism may be associated with loss of p53-mediated miRNA functioning that might be directly related with the loss of transcriptional activity facilitating tumour progression. Besides, important proteins encompassed in miRNA biogenesis and regulation consists of binding elements for p53, p63 and p73 proteins, indicating the transcriptional control by the members of this tumour suppressor family. Moreover, the p53-modulated miRNAs target the miRNA biogenesis factors further facilitating a feedback outcome in strongly regulating the expressions of damage-responsive miRNAs [170]. Lately, it has been depicted that following DNA damage, nearly 25% miRNAs are activated through an ATM-dependent pathway [167]. This outcome may be facilitated partly through KH-type splicing regulatory protein (KSRP), an element of Drosha and Dicer miRNA processing units [171]. However, ATM was observed to phosphorylate KSRP, causing an enrichment in the interface between KSRP and pri-miRNAs along with elevated KSRP action in miRNA processing resulting in an overexpression of particular cohort of miRNAs [167]. Furthermore, downstream molecules of ATM/ATR—CHK1 and CHK2 in the DNA damage pathway are activated leading to regulation of miRNA processing mechanism.

9.4.3.3 miRNAs Target Genes that Participate in DNA Damage Control

Several reports have demonstrated that specific miRNAs control vital genes that are important for the DNA damage response event. However, it was observed that the damage sensor kinase ATM is a critical target of miR-421. Moreover, in patients suffering from ataxia-telangiectasia (A-T), disorder caused by impaired ATM levels, it was observed that miR-421 was overexpressed leading to binding blockage of miR-421 to ATM [172]. ATM phosphorylates an enormous number of target genes, such as the histone variant H2AX (vital function in response to DNA double-strand breaks (DDSBs)) [173, 174]. It is a major target of miR-24, causing tumour cells to become hypersensitive to reprivatized drugs and ionizing radiation. In general, miR-24 is overexpressed in differentiated cells, showing a decreased ability to repair the DDSBs [175]. However, in tumours decreased knockdown of miR-24 might impart resistance to different genomic changes. Undeniably, it has been observed that miR-24 expression is repressed by MYC [48]. The other targets for miR-24 are MYC, E2F1 and CDK4/6 that negatively impact the cell cycle progression and contribute to its anti-carcinogenic consequences [176].

In human neuroblastoma and lung fibroblasts, miR-125b mediates the downregulation of the p53 causing inhibition in apoptosis [177]. It has also been observed that miR-504 inhibits p53-modulated programmed cell death and cell cycle arrest via targeting p53 mRNA leading to in vivo carcinogenesis [178]. Additionally, in neuroblastomas miR-380-5p is upregulated owing to amplification of MYCN that has been related with poor patient survival, causing reduction in p53 levels [179]. However, it has been demonstrated that miR-30 family members and miR-25 negatively regulate p53 in certain cancer cell lines [180].

Proficient miRNAs competent of targeting negative controllers of p53 are able to cause an increase in p53-dependent anti-proliferative outcomes demonstrated by miRNAs targeting MDM2. Additionally, miR-29 family members have been reported to target p85-alpha, the controlling subunit of phosphatidylinositol-3 kinase (PI3K) and CDC42, completely influencing the p53-modulated programmed cell death [181]. Moreover, miR-29 shows tumour suppressor property by targeting different DNA methyltransferases [68]. Besides, miR-29b is downregulated in malignant cells and regulates Mcl-1—an anti-apoptotic protein that is simultaneously overexpressed

[86]. Also, miR-122 has been observed to possess an important function in p53 activation by diverse other mechanisms [182].

9.4.4 MicroRNAs Triggering Tumour Progression, Invasion, Migration and Metastasis

Metastasis is a multistep, intricate biological cascade that is characterized by different stages. Epithelial-mesenchymal transition (EMT) is a known important event in the metastatic process, illustrated via loss of cell adhesion by suppression of E-cadherin and stimulation of genes related to invasion and migration. EMT is known to be controlled by different biological signalling cascades with transforming growth factor (TGF)-β having a predominant role on the ZEB, SNAIL and TWIST transcription factors [183]. Cutting-edge facts report that miRNAs have a crucial function in the pathogenesis EMT and tumour metastasis as demonstrated in Fig. 9.5. TGF-β-controlled miRNAs stimulate EMT and facilitate tumour progression, aggressiveness and metastasis. MiR-155 is upregulated in different tumours

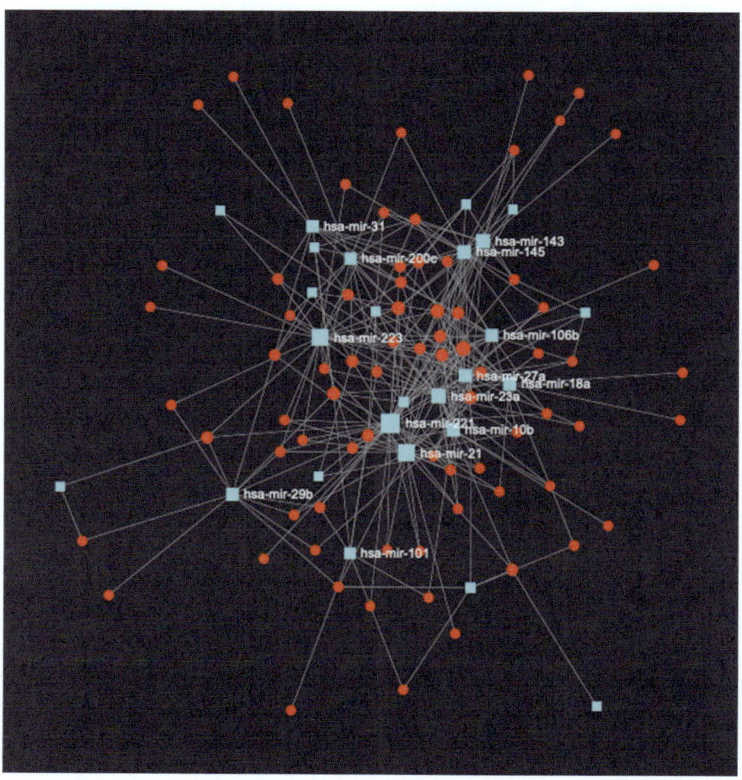

Fig. 9.5 Diagrammatic representation of regulatory effect of microRNAs on tumour progression, epithelial mesenchymal transitions and tumour metastasis

and is activated transcriptionally by TGF-β/SMAD4 signalling network. Recent research depicted that miR-155 stimulates EMT process by targeting RhoA GTPase, a crucial factor of tight junction formation, stability and cellular polarity. Moreover, the silencing of miR-155 represses TGF-β-mediated EMT and tight junction termination, along with cell progression, migration and invasion [184]. Contradictorily, TGF-β suppresses miR-200 and miR-203. However, the miR-200 family is known to influence EMT via hindering the expression of ZEB1 and ZEB2—the E-cadherin associated transcriptional suppressors [185]. As a result, ZEB1 and ZEB2 further suppress the miRNA-200 primary transcript that creates a double negative feedback loop between miR-200 family and the transcription factors. Additionally, the loop was propositioned to elucidate a hypothesis in decoding the underlying mechanism of the metastatic cascade: invasive breast tumour cells having elevated metastatic potential which carry a mesenchymal phenotype have considerably reduced miR-200 expression. Consequently, administered overexpression of miR-200c in the mesenchymal cells escalates E-cadherin leading to an epithelial phenotype by provoking MET [186–188]. Additionally, miR-192 and miR-200 are imperative modulators of p53-regulated EMT, and these miRNAs are trans-activated by p53 that further modulates EMT event through supressing ZEB1/2 expression [185]. Other significant transcription factors are TWIST and SNAIL that stimulate epithelial cell motility, tumour invasiveness migration capacity and metastasis by controlling certain miRNA expressions. In metastatic breast tumour cells, upregulation of miR-10b positively modulates cell invasion and migration that is stimulated by uninterrupted binding of TWIST to miR-10b promoter region. Besides, in primary human breast cancer cell lines—SUM149 and SUM159—an abnormal expression of miR-10b is capable of inducing assertive penetration and micro-metastasis development in (SCID) severe combined immunodeficiency mouse models, stipulating evidence stating that upregulation of discrete miRNAs may be contributing to in vivo metastasis development [189]. Additionally, miRNAs that regulate the gene expression levels of these EMT factors are vital for metastasis development. For example, in aggressive metastatic breast tumour, miR-203 is considerably downregulated owing to hyper-methylation of its promoter. The reestablishment of miR-203 expression in breast tumour cells suppresses in vitro cancer cell invasion and colonization of lung metastatic cells in vivo by inhibiting SNAI2, indicating that the miR-203 and the SNAI2 regulatory circuit is central for EMT and tumour metastasis formation [190, 191].

miR-9 and miR-212 are additional critical miRNAs that contribute in controlling cancer metastasis. C-Myc and n-Myc activate miR-9 expression by directly binding to the miR-9-3 locus. In neuroblastoma tumours, the miR-9 expression level diligently associates with amplification of MYCN, tumour stage, differentiation and metastasis status. miR-9 expression in metastatic breast tumours is much elevated than in primary breast cancer, implying that miR-9 is an impending metastatic cascade regulator. Moreover, it has been identified in breast tumour cells that miR-9 reduces the E-cadherin expression by directly binding to its 3′-untranslated region [189]. This E-cadherin downregulation by miR-9 triggers the β-catenin signalling which further stimulates the downstream oncogenic molecules, leading to elevated cell migration, invasiveness and tumour progression. Moreover, the repression of miR-9 through a miRNA 'sponge' decreases the metastasis development in vivo, suggesting that miR-9 silencing might open newer therapeutic avenues in advanced breast tumours for preventing the development of cancer metastasis [192, 193]. Furthermore, another microRNA, miR-212, is remarkably underexpressed in human colorectal carcinoma owing to promoter hyper-methylation and loss of heterozygosity. The upregulation of miR-212 supresses in vitro CRC cell motility and invasion and in vivo formation of pulmonary metastasis by targeting MnSOD, essential for downregulation of epithelial markers and upregulation of mesenchymal markers in these colorectal carcinoma cells. Hence, miR-212 can be a prognostic marker for CRC patients to predict their overall survival, and both miR-212 and MnSOD can also be explored as therapeutic tools for metastasis therapy [194].

9.4.5 MicroRNAs Modulating Angiogenesis

The process of angiogenesis is an extremely coordinated event that develops new blood vessels from pre-established vessels to provide nutrients and oxygen for tumour growth and cancer metastasis [195]. However, tumour tissues have significantly lower oxygen levels as compared to their proximate normal tissues; thus hypoxia has an essential function in the tumour microenvironment leading to tumour formation and tumour cell maintenance. Hypoxia-inducible factor (HIF) is an important transcription regulator of hypoxia and impacts various miRNA expressions along with its targets. In addition, vascular endothelial growth factor (VEGF) is a focal angiogenic factor that directs the endothelial cells in building new blood vessels on binding to its receptors [196]. This indicates that miRNAs that target HIF or VEGF signalling paths significantly influence the angiogenesis process. Moreover, miR-210 is the most reliable and considerably stimulated miRNA reported throughout the hypoxia process [197]. Different studies have depicted that miR-210 upregulation in human normoxic umbilical vein endothelial cells activates the development of capillary-like structures and VEGF-dependent cellular motility; however, contradictory to this miR-210 blockade alienates these processes [198]. Additionally, miR-210 positively influences angiogenesis by enhancing VEGF and VEGF receptor-2 (VEGFR2) expression as well as by targeting an antiangiogenic factor receptor tyrosine kinase ligand ephrin-A3 [199].

Moreover, miR-424 is another microRNA that is activated during hypoxic conditions in endothelial cells and promotes angiogenesis in vivo and in vitro through directing a scaffolding protein to ubiquitin ligase called cullin 2. This reaction causes the stabilization of HIF1α and permits transcriptional activation of VEGF gene expression [200]. Furthermore, miR-21, another miRNA that stimulates angiogenesis and targets PTEN to trigger Akt/ERK signalling pathway, causes increased HIF1α and VEGF expression levels. Contradictorily, miR-20b and miR-519c target VEGF and/or HIF1α and negatively regulate angiogenesis [201]. miR-107 inhibits the expression of HIF1β besides regulating HIF1α, and so decreased expression of miR-107 causes tumour angiogenesis formation under hypoxic states [55].

Recently, various reports have indicated that exosomal miRNA from tumour cells aids in the development of pre-metastatic niche and modulates the tumour microenvironment. Furthermore, it has been demonstrated that miR-135b, upregulated in exosomes, acquired from hypoxia-resistant multiple myeloma cells, reduces the expression of the factor-inhibiting HIF1 (FIH-1) in endothelial cells and thus influences the development of endothelial tubes through the HIF-FIH signalling cascade. Thus, miR-135b exosomal expression might act as a target for regulating angiogenesis in multiple myeloma and curbing tumour invasiveness and progression [202].

9.5 Clinical Applications of MicroRNAs: From Diagnostics to Therapeutics

9.5.1 MicroRNAs as Diagnostic Markers

The past decade has reported numerous studies on tumour profiling for identification of probable miRNAs and their target genes that are govern by the underlying mechanism involved in carcinogenesis. Different miRNA signatures have been recognized, which may prove to be helpful for differentiating tumours in different organs by further screening resected tumours, biopsy or blood specimens [203]. Moreover, a 4-miRNA signature in leukaemia has been identified that is capable of differentiating acute lymphoblastic leukaemia (ALL) from acute myeloid leukaemia (AML) having a 100% sensitivity as well as specificity [204]. Furthermore, a 97-gene expression panel in breast tumours is capable of classifying the tumour based on the histological grade as compared with lymph-node status, tumour stage and/or size [205]. In pancreatic ductal adenocarcinomas, a panel comprising of seven differentially expressed miRNAs might contribute in more accurate diagnosis as compared to the conventional cytology assessments [206].

9.5.2 MicroRNAs as Prognostic Indicators

Numerous studies have stated that miRNA expression patterns can predict the outcome and prognosis in various tumours. In breast tumours, 31 miRNAs were predominantly attributed to clinical features, whereas the upregulation of 17 different miRNAs was linked with ER-positive stage I/II breast tumours, which showed noticeable clinical outcome [207]. Likewise, the upregulation of miR-210 is related to an elevated recurrence risk and a decreased possibility of relapse-free survival in cancer patients [208]. Moreover, miR-155 overexpression is reported to be linked with poor postoperative survival in B-cell lymphoma and lung cancer patients [209, 210]. Also, miR-96, miR-182 and miR-183 expression have been found to associate with the development of non-small-cell lung carcinoma [211]. Similarly, the expression of miR-200c is associated with overall survival following surgery in CRC patients, and 13 other miRNAs have been revealed to illustrate alterable expression in CLL [212].

9.5.3 MicroRNAs in Cancer Treatment

miRNAs have the property to target numerous genes concurrently. They possess a significant role in carcinogenesis as vital regulators of different cellular pathways by modulating the target gene expression by either mRNA degradation and/or translation repression. Therefore, these miRNAs are interesting candidates that can be used as prognostic indicators as well as therapeutic targets in different malignancies. The characterization of various miRNAs along with its target genes is crucial for treating tumour progression, invasion and metastasis, consequently providing novel therapeutic prospects. There are several methods that can be incorporated for miRNA targeting that include the AMOs (anti-miRNA oligonucleotides) which are single-stranded molecules and cause direct complementarity, therefore inhibiting particular miRNAs. AMOs have been extensively used in vitro and in vivo for targeting mRNAs and assessing their gene functions [213, 214]. Further, the chemical alteration of the AMOs might aid in improving the hybridization affinity of mRNA target in vitro [215] making it defiant to nuclease degradation along with activating RNase or additional proteins and target genes [216]. For in vivo transport, modifying the protein-binding functions of AMOs is crucial to intrusion of plasma clearance and stimulates proper uptake in the cells and tissues [217]. Antago-miRs are single-stranded molecules that are capable of forming complementarity to miRNAs; however, for maintaining the stability along with minimizing degradation, and might additionally be altered with a cholesterol conjugated 20-*O*-methyl [218]. Locked nucleic acids (LNAs) possess a methylene bridge to functionally lock ribose conformation, which ultimately causes increased binding affinity and stability [219]. The function of miRNA sponges is to use multiple additional 3′UTR mRNA sites for a specific miRNA and to bind competitively to miRNA, thus interfering with the normal direction of a single miRNA by targeting it with an antisense oligonucleotide [220]. Additionally, the formation of stable sponges may contribute in reiterating the effects of downregulation of aberrantly expressed miRNAs and structured nanoparticles, the formulations of which may primarily be used for in vitro transfer of miRNAs [221, 222]. Lately, certain research studies have used this miRNA delivery technology into the host cell and/or tissue [223]. The outcomes of earlier studies indicated that by using liposome polycation-hyaluronic acid particles as miRNA carrier for modifications with a tumour targeting monoclonal antibody known as the golgin candidate 4 single-chain variable fragment, they were successful in targeting lung metastasis in a mouse model developed for metastatic melanoma [16, 224–226].

9.6 Concluding Notes

Uninterrupted research into the field of miRNAs lead to the initial discovery of a vital cluster of modulators in all multicellular organisms to a later phase where miRNA-based events are promptly entering the clinics as significant diagnostic/prognostic as well as promising therapeutic tools. Although certain mechanisms such as the post-transcriptional gene expression and its modulation in different cell types are not clearly understood, tremendous research studies associate uncontrolled miRNA expression to the different tumour aetiologies. Evolving research suggests that miRNAs are important participants in the carcinogenesis event as they have crucial roles in governing gene expression and uplifting cellular differentiation processes, are involved in cell fate decisions and cellular maintenance and stabilize the plasticity and de-differentiation processes. Besides, they intensely govern the central nodes in cell cycle regulation, apoptosis, genome integrity, stress responses, tumour development, aggressiveness and metastasis. Additionally, genetic representations have substantiated that different miRNAs pose as oncogenes and that cancers may become predisposed to oncogenic miRNA upregulation, which might have a potential for the use of miRNA inhibitors in therapeutics. However, there is still much scope of identifying important miRNAs that might have clinical significance in different tumours, but the rapid development in this field is plausibly aiding in the advancement of many preclinical endeavours for the near future. A prospective stipulation is that because the presently used drug varieties have broad outcomes and may affect several signalling cascades, miRNAs are fundamentally associated with regulating groups of targets frequently resulting in pleiotropic outcomes. Moreover, only a few in vitro studies have shed light on understanding the role of miRNAs, and thus there is a clear need to discover their dependency on cellular framework and study their interaction in different tumour lesions.

Competing Interests Statement The authors declare no competing interests.

References

1. Lee RC, Ambros V (2001) An extensive class of small RNAs in Caenorhabditis elegans. Science 294(5543):862–864. https://doi.org/10.1126/science.1065329
2. Lee YS, Dutta A (2009) MicroRNAs in cancer. Annu Rev Pathol 4:199–227. https://doi.org/10.1146/annurev.pathol.4.110807.092222
3. Fire A, Xu S, Montgomery MK, Kostas SA, Driver SE, Mello CC (1998) Potent and specific genetic interference by double-stranded RNA in Caenorhabditis elegans. Nature 391(6669):806–811. https://doi.org/10.1038/35888
4. Lee RC, Feinbaum RL, Ambros V (1993) The C. elegans heterochronic gene lin-4 encodes small RNAs with antisense complementarity to lin-14. Cell 75(5):843–854
5. Wightman B, Ha I, Ruvkun G (1993) Posttranscriptional regulation of the heterochronic gene lin-14 by lin-4 mediates temporal pattern formation in C. elegans. Cell 75(5):855–862
6. Calin GA, Cimmino A, Fabbri M, Ferracin M, Wojcik SE, Shimizu M, Taccioli C, Zanesi N, Garzon R, Aqeilan RI, Alder H, Volinia S, Rassenti L, Liu X, Liu CG, Kipps TJ, Negrini M, Croce CM (2008) MiR-15a and miR-16-1 cluster functions in human leukemia. Proc Natl Acad Sci U S A 105(13):5166–5171. https://doi.org/10.1073/pnas.0800121105
7. Klein U, Lia M, Crespo M, Siegel R, Shen Q, Mo T, Ambesi-Impiombato A, Califano A, Migliazza A, Bhagat G, Dalla-Favera R (2010) The DLEU2/miR-15a/16-1 cluster controls B cell proliferation and its deletion leads to chronic lymphocytic leukemia. Cancer Cell 17(1):28–40. https://doi.org/10.1016/j.ccr.2009.11.019

8. Peng Y, Croce CM (2016) The role of MicroRNAs in human cancer. Signal Transduct Target Ther 1:15004. https://doi.org/10.1038/sigtrans.2015.4
9. Lee Y, Kim M, Han J, Yeom KH, Lee S, Baek SH, Kim VN (2004) MicroRNA genes are transcribed by RNA polymerase II. EMBO J 23(20):4051–4060. https://doi.org/10.1038/sj.emboj.7600385
10. Macfarlane LA, Murphy PR (2010) MicroRNA: biogenesis, function and role in cancer. Curr Genomics 11(7):537–561. https://doi.org/10.2174/138920210793175895
11. Bartel DP (2009) MicroRNAs: target recognition and regulatory functions. Cell 136(2):215–233. https://doi.org/10.1016/j.cell.2009.01.002
12. Zhang B, Pan X, Cobb GP, Anderson TA (2007) microRNAs as oncogenes and tumor suppressors. Dev Biol 302(1):1–12. https://doi.org/10.1016/j.ydbio.2006.08.028
13. Calin GA, Dumitru CD, Shimizu M, Bichi R, Zupo S, Noch E, Aldler H, Rattan S, Keating M, Rai K, Rassenti L, Kipps T, Negrini M, Bullrich F, Croce CM (2002) Frequent deletions and down-regulation of micro-RNA genes miR15 and miR16 at 13q14 in chronic lymphocytic leukemia. Proc Natl Acad Sci U S A 99(24):15524–15529. https://doi.org/10.1073/pnas.242606799
14. Ding XM (2014) MicroRNAs: regulators of cancer metastasis and epithelial-mesenchymal transition (EMT). Chin J Cancer 33(3):140–147. https://doi.org/10.5732/cjc.013.10094
15. Carthew RW, Sontheimer EJ (2009) Origins and mechanisms of miRNAs and siRNAs. Cell 136(4):642–655. https://doi.org/10.1016/j.cell.2009.01.035
16. Tan W, Liu B, Qu S, Liang G, Luo W, Gong C (2018) MicroRNAs and cancer: key paradigms in molecular therapy. Oncol Lett 15(3):2735–2742. https://doi.org/10.3892/ol.2017.7638
17. Yi R, Qin Y, Macara IG, Cullen BR (2003) Exportin-5 mediates the nuclear export of pre-microRNAs and short hairpin RNAs. Genes Dev 17(24):3011–3016. https://doi.org/10.1101/gad.1158803
18. Lund E, Guttinger S, Calado A, Dahlberg JE, Kutay U (2004) Nuclear export of microRNA precursors. Science 303(5654):95–98. https://doi.org/10.1126/science.1090599
19. Hutvagner G, McLachlan J, Pasquinelli AE, Balint E, Tuschl T, Zamore PD (2001) A cellular function for the RNA-interference enzyme Dicer in the maturation of the let-7 small temporal RNA. Science 293(5531):834–838. https://doi.org/10.1126/science.1062961
20. Fukuda T, Yamagata K, Fujiyama S, Matsumoto T, Koshida I, Yoshimura K, Mihara M, Naitou M, Endoh H, Nakamura T, Akimoto C, Yamamoto Y, Katagiri T, Foulds C, Takezawa S, Kitagawa H, Takeyama K, O'Malley BW, Kato S (2007) DEAD-box RNA helicase subunits of the Drosha complex are required for processing of rRNA and a subset of microRNAs. Nat Cell Biol 9(5):604–611. https://doi.org/10.1038/ncb1577
21. Davis BN, Hilyard AC, Lagna G, Hata A (2008) SMAD proteins control DROSHA-mediated microRNA maturation. Nature 454(7200):56–61. https://doi.org/10.1038/nature07086
22. Alarcon CR, Lee H, Goodarzi H, Halberg N, Tavazoie SF (2015) N6-methyladenosine marks primary microRNAs for processing. Nature 519(7544):482–485. https://doi.org/10.1038/nature14281
23. Lim LP, Lau NC, Garrett-Engele P, Grimson A, Schelter JM, Castle J, Bartel DP, Linsley PS, Johnson JM (2005) Microarray analysis shows that some microRNAs downregulate large numbers of target mRNAs. Nature 433(7027):769–773. https://doi.org/10.1038/nature03315
24. Liu J, Valencia-Sanchez MA, Hannon GJ, Parker R (2005) MicroRNA-dependent localization of targeted mRNAs to mammalian P-bodies. Nat Cell Biol 7(7):719–723. https://doi.org/10.1038/ncb1274
25. Eulalio A, Behm-Ansmant I, Schweizer D, Izaurralde E (2007) P-body formation is a consequence, not the cause, of RNA-mediated gene silencing. Mol Cell Biol 27(11):3970–3981. https://doi.org/10.1128/MCB.00128-07
26. Chu CY, Rana TM (2006) Translation repression in human cells by microRNA-induced gene silencing requires RCK/p54. PLoS Biol 4(7):e210. pii: 06-PLBI-RA-0036R3
27. Cimmino A, Calin GA, Fabbri M, Iorio MV, Ferracin M, Shimizu M, Wojcik SE, Aqeilan RI, Zupo S, Dono M, Rassenti L, Alder H, Volinia S, Liu CG, Kipps TJ, Negrini M, Croce CM

(2005) miR-15 and miR-16 induce apoptosis by targeting BCL2. Proc Natl Acad Sci U S A 102(39):13944–13949. pii: 0506654102

28. Boyerinas B, Park SM, Hau A, Murmann AE, Peter ME (2010) The role of let-7 in cell differentiation and cancer. Endocr Relat Cancer 17(1):F19–F36. https://doi.org/10.1677/ERC-09-0184
29. He XY, Chen JX, Ou-Yang X, Zhang Z, Peng HM (2010) Construction of let-7a expression plasmid and its inhibitory effect on k-Ras protein in A549 lung cancer cells. Nan Fang Yi Ke Da Xue Xue Bao 30(11):2427–2431
30. Wang YY, Ren T, Cai YY, He XY (2013) MicroRNA let-7a inhibits the proliferation and invasion of nonsmall cell lung cancer cell line 95D by regulating K-Ras and HMGA2 gene expression. Cancer Biother Radiopharm 28(2):131–137. https://doi.org/10.1089/cbr.2012.1307
31. Xia XM, Jin WY, Shi RZ, Zhang YF, Chen J (2010) Clinical significance and the correlation of expression between Let-7 and K-ras in non-small cell lung cancer. Oncol Lett 1(6):1045–1047. https://doi.org/10.3892/ol.2010.164
32. Cheng CY, Hwang CI, Corney DC, Flesken-Nikitin A, Jiang L, Oner GM, Munroe RJ, Schimenti JC, Hermeking H, Nikitin AY (2014) miR-34 cooperates with p53 in suppression of prostate cancer by joint regulation of stem cell compartment. Cell Rep 6(6):1000–1007. pii: S2211-1247(14)00123-5
33. Ji Q, Hao X, Zhang M, Tang W, Yang M, Li L, Xiang D, Desano JT, Bommer GT, Fan D, Fearon ER, Lawrence TS, Xu L (2009) MicroRNA miR-34 inhibits human pancreatic cancer tumor-initiating cells. PLoS One 4(8):e6816. https://doi.org/10.1371/journal.pone.0006816
34. Okada N, Lin CP, Ribeiro MC, Biton A, Lai G, He X, Bu P, Vogel H, Jablons DM, Keller AC, Wilkinson JE, He B, Speed TP, He L (2014) A positive feedback between p53 and miR-34 miRNAs mediates tumor suppression. Genes Dev 28(5):438–450. https://doi.org/10.1101/gad.233585.113
35. Cannell IG, Bushell M (2010) Regulation of Myc by miR-34c: a mechanism to prevent genomic instability? Cell Cycle 9(14):2726–2730. pii: 12182
36. Selcuklu SD, Donoghue MT, Spillane C (2009) miR-21 as a key regulator of oncogenic processes. Biochem Soc Trans 37(Pt 4):918–925. https://doi.org/10.1042/BST0370918
37. Zhang ZW, An Y, Teng CB (2009) [The roles of miR-17-92 cluster in mammal development and tumorigenesis]. Yi Chuan 31(11):1094–1100. pii: 0253-9772(2009)11-1094-7
38. Osada H, Takahashi T (2011) let-7 and miR-17-92: small-sized major players in lung cancer development. Cancer Sci 102(1):9–17. https://doi.org/10.1111/j.1349-7006.2010.01707.x
39. Rinaldi A, Poretti G, Kwee I, Zucca E, Catapano CV, Tibiletti MG, Bertoni F (2007) Concomitant MYC and microRNA cluster miR-17-92 (C13orf25) amplification in human mantle cell lymphoma. Leuk Lymphoma 48(2):410–412. https://doi.org/10.1080/10428190601059738
40. Shuang T, Shi C, Chang S, Wang M, Bai CH (2013) Downregulation of miR-17~92 expression increase paclitaxel sensitivity in human ovarian carcinoma SKOV3-TR30 cells via BIM instead of PTEN. Int J Mol Sci 14(2):3802–3816. https://doi.org/10.3390/ijms14023802
41. Sevignani C, Calin GA, Nnadi SC, Shimizu M, Davuluri RV, Hyslop T, Demant P, Croce CM, Siracusa LD (2007) MicroRNA genes are frequently located near mouse cancer susceptibility loci. Proc Natl Acad Sci U S A 104(19):8017–8022. https://doi.org/10.1073/pnas.0702177104
42. Hayashita Y, Osada H, Tatematsu Y, Yamada H, Yanagisawa K, Tomida S, Yatabe Y, Kawahara K, Sekido Y, Takahashi T (2005) A polycistronic microRNA cluster, miR-17-92, is overexpressed in human lung cancers and enhances cell proliferation. Cancer Res 65(21):9628–9632. https://doi.org/10.1158/0008-5472.CAN-05-2352
43. Tagawa H, Seto M (2005) A microRNA cluster as a target of genomic amplification in malignant lymphoma. Leukemia 19(11):2013–2016. https://doi.org/10.1038/sj.leu.2403942
44. Calin GA, Croce CM (2006) MicroRNAs and chromosomal abnormalities in cancer cells. Oncogene 25(46):6202–6210. https://doi.org/10.1038/sj.onc.1209910
45. Zhang L, Huang J, Yang N, Greshock J, Megraw MS, Giannakakis A, Liang S, Naylor TL, Barchetti A, Ward MR, Yao G, Medina A, O'Brien-Jenkins A, Katsaros D, Hatzigeorgiou A, Gimotty PA, Weber BL, Coukos G (2006) microRNAs exhibit high frequency genomic

alterations in human cancer. Proc Natl Acad Sci U S A 103(24):9136–9141. https://doi.org/10.1073/pnas.0508889103

46. Calin GA, Sevignani C, Dumitru CD, Hyslop T, Noch E, Yendamuri S, Shimizu M, Rattan S, Bullrich F, Negrini M, Croce CM (2004) Human microRNA genes are frequently located at fragile sites and genomic regions involved in cancers. Proc Natl Acad Sci U S A 101(9):2999–3004. https://doi.org/10.1073/pnas.0307323101
47. O'Donnell KA, Wentzel EA, Zeller KI, Dang CV, Mendell JT (2005) c-Myc-regulated microRNAs modulate E2F1 expression. Nature 435(7043):839–843. https://doi.org/10.1038/nature03677
48. Chang TC, Yu D, Lee YS, Wentzel EA, Arking DE, West KM, Dang CV, Thomas-Tikhonenko A, Mendell JT (2008) Widespread microRNA repression by Myc contributes to tumorigenesis. Nat Genet 40(1):43–50. pii: ng.2007.30
49. Wang B, Hsu SH, Wang X, Kutay H, Bid HK, Yu J, Ganju RK, Jacob ST, Yuneva M, Ghoshal K (2014) Reciprocal regulation of microRNA-122 and c-Myc in hepatocellular cancer: role of E2F1 and transcription factor dimerization partner 2. Hepatology 59(2):555–566. https://doi.org/10.1002/hep.26712
50. Han H, Sun D, Li W, Shen H, Zhu Y, Li C, Chen Y, Lu L, Zhang J, Tian Y, Li Y (2013) A c-Myc-MicroRNA functional feedback loop affects hepatocarcinogenesis. Hepatology 57(6):2378–2389. https://doi.org/10.1002/hep.26302
51. He L, He X, Lim LP, de Stanchina E, Xuan Z, Liang Y, Xue W, Zender L, Magnus J, Ridzon D, Jackson AL, Linsley PS, Chen C, Lowe SW, Cleary MA, Hannon GJ (2007) A microRNA component of the p53 tumour suppressor network. Nature 447(7148):1130–1134. pii: nature 05939
52. Hermeking H (2010) The miR-34 family in cancer and apoptosis. Cell Death Differ 17(2):193–199. https://doi.org/10.1038/cdd.2009.56
53. Yamakuchi M, Lowenstein CJ (2009) MiR-34, SIRT1 and p53: the feedback loop. Cell Cycle 8(5):712–715. pii: 7753
54. Xiao J, Lin H, Luo X, Wang Z (2011) miR-605 joins p53 network to form a p53:miR-605:Mdm2 positive feedback loop in response to stress. EMBO J 30(3):524–532. https://doi.org/10.1038/emboj.2010.347
55. Yamakuchi M, Lotterman CD, Bao C, Hruban RH, Karim B, Mendell JT, Huso D, Lowenstein CJ (2010) P53-induced microRNA-107 inhibits HIF-1 and tumor angiogenesis. Proc Natl Acad Sci U S A 107(14):6334–6339. https://doi.org/10.1073/pnas.0911082107
56. Zhang Y, Liao JM, Zeng SX, Lu H (2011) p53 downregulates Down syndrome-associated DYRK1A through miR-1246. EMBO Rep 12(8):811–817. https://doi.org/10.1038/embor.2011.98
57. Eyholzer M, Schmid S, Schardt JA, Haefliger S, Mueller BU, Pabst T (2010) Complexity of miR-223 regulation by CEBPA in human AML. Leuk Res 34(5):672–676. https://doi.org/10.1016/j.leukres.2009.11.019
58. Johnnidis JB, Harris MH, Wheeler RT, Stehling-Sun S, Lam MH, Kirak O, Brummelkamp TR, Fleming MD, Camargo FD (2008) Regulation of progenitor cell proliferation and granulocyte function by microRNA-223. Nature 451(7182):1125–1129. https://doi.org/10.1038/nature06607
59. Stamatopoulos B, Meuleman N, Haibe-Kains B, Saussoy P, Van Den Neste E, Michaux L, Heimann P, Martiat P, Bron D, Lagneaux L (2009) microRNA-29c and microRNA-223 down-regulation has in vivo significance in chronic lymphocytic leukemia and improves disease risk stratification. Blood 113(21):5237–5245. https://doi.org/10.1182/blood-2008-11-189407
60. Wong QW, Lung RW, Law PT, Lai PB, Chan KY, To KF, Wong N (2008) MicroRNA-223 is commonly repressed in hepatocellular carcinoma and potentiates expression of Stathmin1. Gastroenterology 135(1):257–269. https://doi.org/10.1053/j.gastro.2008.04.003
61. Fukao T, Fukuda Y, Kiga K, Sharif J, Hino K, Enomoto Y, Kawamura A, Nakamura K, Takeuchi T, Tanabe M (2007) An evolutionarily conserved mechanism for microRNA-223 expression revealed by microRNA gene profiling. Cell 129(3):617–631. pii: S0092-8674(07)00394-7

62. Fazi F, Rosa A, Fatica A, Gelmetti V, De Marchis ML, Nervi C, Bozzoni I (2005) A minicircuitry comprised of microRNA-223 and transcription factors NFI-A and C/EBPalpha regulates human granulopoiesis. Cell 123(5):819–831. pii: S0092-8674(05)00977-3
63. Han L, Witmer PD, Casey E, Valle D, Sukumar S (2007) DNA methylation regulates microRNA expression. Cancer Biol Ther 6(8):1284–1288. pii: 4486
64. Saito Y, Jones PA (2006) Epigenetic activation of tumor suppressor microRNAs in human cancer cells. Cell Cycle 5(19):2220–2222. pii: 3340
65. Lehmann U, Hasemeier B, Christgen M, Muller M, Romermann D, Langer F, Kreipe H (2008) Epigenetic inactivation of microRNA gene hsa-mir-9-1 in human breast cancer. J Pathol 214(1):17–24. https://doi.org/10.1002/path.2251
66. Lujambio A, Ropero S, Ballestar E, Fraga MF, Cerrato C, Setien F, Casado S, Suarez-Gauthier A, Sanchez-Cespedes M, Git A, Spiteri I, Das PP, Caldas C, Miska E, Esteller M (2007) Genetic unmasking of an epigenetically silenced microRNA in human cancer cells. Cancer Res 67(4):1424–1429. pii: 67/4/1424
67. Scott GK, Mattie MD, Berger CE, Benz SC, Benz CC (2006) Rapid alteration of microRNA levels by histone deacetylase inhibition. Cancer Res 66(3):1277–1281. pii: 66/3/1277
68. Fabbri M, Garzon R, Cimmino A, Liu Z, Zanesi N, Callegari E, Liu S, Alder H, Costinean S, Fernandez-Cymering C, Volinia S, Guler G, Morrison CD, Chan KK, Marcucci G, Calin GA, Huebner K, Croce CM (2007) MicroRNA-29 family reverts aberrant methylation in lung cancer by targeting DNA methyltransferases 3A and 3B. Proc Natl Acad Sci U S A 104(40):15805–15810. pii: 0707628104
69. Fazi F, Racanicchi S, Zardo G, Starnes LM, Mancini M, Travaglini L, Diverio D, Ammatuna E, Cimino G, Lo-Coco F, Grignani F, Nervi C (2007) Epigenetic silencing of the myelopoiesis regulator microRNA-223 by the AML1/ETO oncoprotein. Cancer Cell 12(5):457–466. pii: S1535-6108(07)00268-1
70. Saito Y, Liang G, Egger G, Friedman JM, Chuang JC, Coetzee GA, Jones PA (2006) Specific activation of microRNA-127 with downregulation of the proto-oncogene BCL6 by chromatin-modifying drugs in human cancer cells. Cancer Cell 9(6):435–443. pii: S1535-6108(06)00143-7
71. Lujambio A, Calin GA, Villanueva A, Ropero S, Sanchez-Cespedes M, Blanco D, Montuenga LM, Rossi S, Nicoloso MS, Faller WJ, Gallagher WM, Eccles SA, Croce CM, Esteller M (2008) A microRNA DNA methylation signature for human cancer metastasis. Proc Natl Acad Sci U S A 105(36):13556–13561. https://doi.org/10.1073/pnas.0803055105
72. Donzelli S, Mori F, Bellissimo T, Sacconi A, Casini B, Frixa T, Roscilli G, Aurisicchio L, Facciolo F, Pompili A, Carosi MA, Pescarmona E, Segatto O, Pond G, Muti P, Telera S, Strano S, Yarden Y, Blandino G (2015) Epigenetic silencing of miR-145-5p contributes to brain metastasis. Oncotarget 6(34):35183–35201. https://doi.org/10.18632/oncotarget.5930
73. Lujambio A, Esteller M (2007) CpG island hypermethylation of tumor suppressor microRNAs in human cancer. Cell Cycle 6(12):1455–1459. pii: 4408
74. Thomson JM, Newman M, Parker JS, Morin-Kensicki EM, Wright T, Hammond SM (2006) Extensive post-transcriptional regulation of microRNAs and its implications for cancer. Genes Dev 20(16):2202–2207. pii: gad.1444406
75. Walz AL, Ooms A, Gadd S, Gerhard DS, Smith MA, Guidry Auvil JM, Meerzaman D, Chen QR, Hsu CH, Yan C, Nguyen C, Hu Y, Bowlby R, Brooks D, Ma Y, Mungall AJ, Moore RA, Schein J, Marra MA, Huff V, Dome JS, Chi YY, Mullighan CG, Ma J, Wheeler DA, Hampton OA, Jafari N, Ross N, Gastier-Foster JM, Perlman EJ (2015) Recurrent DGCR8, DROSHA, and SIX homeodomain mutations in favorable histology Wilms tumors. Cancer Cell 27(2):286–297. https://doi.org/10.1016/j.ccell.2015.01.003
76. Iliou MS, da Silva-Diz V, Carmona FJ, Ramalho-Carvalho J, Heyn H, Villanueva A, Munoz P, Esteller M (2014) Impaired DICER1 function promotes stemness and metastasis in colon cancer. Oncogene 33(30):4003–4015. https://doi.org/10.1038/onc.2013.398
77. Faggad A, Budczies J, Tchernitsa O, Darb-Esfahani S, Sehouli J, Muller BM, Wirtz R, Chekerov R, Weichert W, Sinn B, Mucha C, Elwali NE, Schafer R, Dietel M, Denkert C (2010) Prognostic significance of Dicer expression in ovarian cancer-link to global

microRNA changes and oestrogen receptor expression. J Pathol 220(3):382–391. https://doi.org/10.1002/path.2658
78. Karube Y, Tanaka H, Osada H, Tomida S, Tatematsu Y, Yanagisawa K, Yatabe Y, Takamizawa J, Miyoshi S, Mitsudomi T, Takahashi T (2005) Reduced expression of Dicer associated with poor prognosis in lung cancer patients. Cancer Sci 96(2):111–115. pii: CAS015
79. Merritt WM, Lin YG, Han LY, Kamat AA, Spannuth WA, Schmandt R, Urbauer D, Pennacchio LA, Cheng JF, Nick AM, Deavers MT, Mourad-Zeidan A, Wang H, Mueller P, Lenburg ME, Gray JW, Mok S, Birrer MJ, Lopez-Berestein G, Coleman RL, Bar-Eli M, Sood AK (2008) Dicer, Drosha, and outcomes in patients with ovarian cancer. N Engl J Med 359(25):2641–2650. https://doi.org/10.1056/NEJMoa0803785
80. Pampalakis G, Diamandis EP, Katsaros D, Sotiropoulou G (2010) Down-regulation of dicer expression in ovarian cancer tissues. Clin Biochem 43(3):324–327. https://doi.org/10.1016/j.clinbiochem.2009.09.014
81. Dome JS, Coppes MJ (2002) Recent advances in Wilms tumor genetics. Curr Opin Pediatr 14(1):5–11
82. Voller D, Reinders J, Meister G, Bosserhoff AK (2013) Strong reduction of AGO2 expression in melanoma and cellular consequences. Br J Cancer 109(12):3116–3124. https://doi.org/10.1038/bjc.2013.646
83. Zhang J, Fan XS, Wang CX, Liu B, Li Q, Zhou XJ (2013) Up-regulation of Ago2 expression in gastric carcinoma. Med Oncol 30(3):628. https://doi.org/10.1007/s12032-013-0628-2
84. Melo SA, Moutinho C, Ropero S, Calin GA, Rossi S, Spizzo R, Fernandez AF, Davalos V, Villanueva A, Montoya G, Yamamoto H, Schwartz S Jr, Esteller M (2010) A genetic defect in exportin-5 traps precursor microRNAs in the nucleus of cancer cells. Cancer Cell 18(4):303–315. https://doi.org/10.1016/j.ccr.2010.09.007
85. Kluiver J, van den Berg A, de Jong D, Blokzijl T, Harms G, Bouwman E, Jacobs S, Poppema S, Kroesen BJ (2007) Regulation of pri-microRNA BIC transcription and processing in Burkitt lymphoma. Oncogene 26(26):3769–3776. pii: 1210147
86. Mott JL, Kobayashi S, Bronk SF, Gores GJ (2007) mir-29 regulates Mcl-1 protein expression and apoptosis. Oncogene 26(42):6133–6140. pii: 1210436
87. Mineno J, Okamoto S, Ando T, Sato M, Chono H, Izu H, Takayama M, Asada K, Mirochnitchenko O, Inouye M, Kato I (2006) The expression profile of microRNAs in mouse embryos. Nucleic Acids Res 34(6):1765–1771. pii: 34/6/1765
88. Loffler D, Brocke-Heidrich K, Pfeifer G, Stocsits C, Hackermuller J, Kretzschmar AK, Burger R, Gramatzki M, Blumert C, Bauer K, Cvijic H, Ullmann AK, Stadler PF, Horn F (2007) Interleukin-6 dependent survival of multiple myeloma cells involves the Stat3-mediated induction of microRNA-21 through a highly conserved enhancer. Blood 110(4):1330–1333. pii: blood-2007-03-081133
89. Kumar MS, Lu J, Mercer KL, Golub TR, Jacks T (2007) Impaired microRNA processing enhances cellular transformation and tumorigenesis. Nat Genet 39(5):673–677. pii: ng2003
90. Muralidhar B, Goldstein LD, Ng G, Winder DM, Palmer RD, Gooding EL, Barbosa-Morais NL, Mukherjee G, Thorne NP, Roberts I, Pett MR, Coleman N (2007) Global microRNA profiles in cervical squamous cell carcinoma depend on Drosha expression levels. J Pathol 212(4):368–377. https://doi.org/10.1002/path.2179
91. Nakamura T, Canaani E, Croce CM (2007) Oncogenic All1 fusion proteins target Drosha-mediated microRNA processing. Proc Natl Acad Sci U S A 104(26):10980–10985. pii: 0704559104
92. Guttilla IK, White BA (2009) Coordinate regulation of FOXO1 by miR-27a, miR-96, and miR-182 in breast cancer cells. J Biol Chem 284(35):23204–23216. https://doi.org/10.1074/jbc.M109.031427
93. Vire E, Curtis C, Davalos V, Git A, Robson S, Villanueva A, Vidal A, Barbieri I, Aparicio S, Esteller M, Caldas C, Kouzarides T (2014) The breast cancer oncogene EMSY represses transcription of antimetastatic microRNA miR-31. Mol Cell 54(1):203. pii: S1097-2765(14)00274-3

94. Deng ZQ, Yin JY, Tang Q, Liu FQ, Qian J, Lin J, Shao R, Zhang M, He L (2014) Overexpression of miR-98 in FFPE tissues might serve as a valuable source for biomarker discovery in breast cancer patients. Int J Clin Exp Pathol 7(3):1166–1171
95. Wu H, Mo YY (2009) Targeting miR-205 in breast cancer. Expert Opin Ther Targets 13(12):1439–1448. https://doi.org/10.1517/14728220903338777
96. Li X, Xie W, Xie C, Huang C, Zhu J, Liang Z, Deng F, Zhu M, Zhu W, Wu R, Wu J, Geng S, Zhong C (2014) Curcumin modulates miR-19/PTEN/AKT/p53 axis to suppress bisphenol A-induced MCF-7 breast cancer cell proliferation. Phytother Res 28(10):1553–1560. https://doi.org/10.1002/ptr.5167
97. Hong S, Noh H, Teng Y, Shao J, Rehmani H, Ding HF, Dong Z, Su SB, Shi H, Kim J, Huang S (2014) SHOX2 is a direct miR-375 target and a novel epithelial-to-mesenchymal transition inducer in breast cancer cells. Neoplasia 16(4):279–290 e271–275. https://doi.org/10.1016/j.neo.2014.03.010
98. Xue X, Liu Y, Wang Y, Meng M, Wang K, Zang X, Zhao S, Sun X, Cui L, Pan L, Liu S (2016) MiR-21 and MiR-155 promote non-small cell lung cancer progression by downregulating SOCS1, SOCS6, and PTEN. Oncotarget 7(51):84508–84519. https://doi.org/10.18632/oncotarget.13022
99. Zeng Y, Zhu J, Shen D, Qin H, Lei Z, Li W, Liu Z, Huang JA (2017) MicroRNA-205 targets SMAD4 in non-small cell lung cancer and promotes lung cancer cell growth in vitro and in vivo. Oncotarget 8(19):30817–30829. https://doi.org/10.18632/oncotarget.10339
100. Andriani F, Majorini MT, Mano M, Landoni E, Miceli R, Facchinetti F, Mensah M, Fontanella E, Dugo M, Giacca M, Pastorino U, Sozzi G, Delia D, Roz L, Lecis D (2018) MiR-16 regulates the pro-tumorigenic potential of lung fibroblasts through the inhibition of HGF production in an FGFR-1- and MEK1-dependent manner. J Hematol Oncol 11(1):45. https://doi.org/10.1186/s13045-018-0594-4
101. Othman N, Nagoor NH (2014) The role of microRNAs in the regulation of apoptosis in lung cancer and its application in cancer treatment. Biomed Res Int 2014:318030. https://doi.org/10.1155/2014/318030
102. Chen Q, Hu H, Jiao D, Yan J, Xu W, Tang X, Chen J, Wang J (2016) miR-126-3p and miR-451a correlate with clinicopathological features of lung adenocarcinoma: the underlying molecular mechanisms. Oncol Rep 36(2):909–917. https://doi.org/10.3892/or.2016.4854
103. Zhao W, Hu JX, Hao RM, Zhang Q, Guo JQ, Li YJ, Xie N, Liu LY, Wang PY, Zhang C, Xie SY (2018) Induction of microRNAlet7a inhibits lung adenocarcinoma cell growth by regulating cyclin D1. Oncol Rep 40(4):1843–1854. https://doi.org/10.3892/or.2018.6593
104. Sayed D, Rane S, Lypowy J, He M, Chen IY, Vashistha H, Yan L, Malhotra A, Vatner D, Abdellatif M (2008) MicroRNA-21 targets Sprouty2 and promotes cellular outgrowths. Mol Biol Cell 19(8):3272–3282. https://doi.org/10.1091/mbc.E08-02-0159
105. Wang Z, Wei W, Sarkar FH (2012) miR-23a, a critical regulator of "migR"ation and metastasis in colorectal cancer. Cancer Discov 2(6):489–491. https://doi.org/10.1158/2159-8290.CD-12-0177
106. Yu W, Ma Y, Shankar S, Srivastava RK (2017) SATB2/beta-catenin/TCF-LEF pathway induces cellular transformation by generating cancer stem cells in colorectal cancer. Sci Rep 7(1):10939. https://doi.org/10.1038/s41598-017-05458-y
107. Valeri N, Braconi C, Gasparini P, Murgia C, Lampis A, Paulus-Hock V, Hart JR, Ueno L, Grivennikov SI, Lovat F, Paone A, Cascione L, Sumani KM, Veronese A, Fabbri M, Carasi S, Alder H, Lanza G, Gafa R, Moyer MP, Ridgway RA, Cordero J, Nuovo GJ, Frankel WL, Rugge M, Fassan M, Groden J, Vogt PK, Karin M, Sansom OJ, Croce CM (2014) MicroRNA-135b promotes cancer progression by acting as a downstream effector of oncogenic pathways in colon cancer. Cancer Cell 25(4):469–483. https://doi.org/10.1016/j.ccr.2014.03.006
108. Takahashi H, Takahashi M, Ohnuma S, Unno M, Yoshino Y, Ouchi K, Takahashi S, Yamada Y, Shimodaira H, Ishioka C (2017) microRNA-193a-3p is specifically down-regulated and acts as a tumor suppressor in BRAF-mutated colorectal cancer. BMC Cancer 17(1):723. https://doi.org/10.1186/s12885-017-3739-x

109. Chu CA, Lee CT, Lee JC, Wang YW, Huang CT, Lan SH, Lin PC, Lin BW, Tian YF, Liu HS, Chow NH (2019) MiR-338-5p promotes metastasis of colorectal cancer by inhibition of phosphatidylinositol 3-kinase, catalytic subunit type 3-mediated autophagy pathway. EBioMedicine 43:270–281. pii: S2352-3964(19)30244-0
110. Zhao H, Wang Y, Yang L, Jiang R, Li W (2014) MiR-25 promotes gastric cancer cells growth and motility by targeting RECK. Mol Cell Biochem 385(1–2):207–213. https://doi.org/10.1007/s11010-013-1829-x
111. Ivanovska I, Ball AS, Diaz RL, Magnus JF, Kibukawa M, Schelter JM, Kobayashi SV, Lim L, Burchard J, Jackson AL, Linsley PS, Cleary MA (2008) MicroRNAs in the miR-106b family regulate p21/CDKN1A and promote cell cycle progression. Mol Cell Biol 28(7):2167–2174. https://doi.org/10.1128/MCB.01977-07
112. Choi OR, Lim IK (2011) Loss of p21(Sdi1) expression in senescent cells after DNA damage accompanied with increase of miR-93 expression and reduced p53 interaction with p21(Sdi1) gene promoter. Biochem Biophys Res Commun 407(2):406–411. https://doi.org/10.1016/j.bbrc.2011.03.038
113. Sarkar S, Dubaybo H, Ali S, Goncalves P, Kollepara SL, Sethi S, Philip PA, Li Y (2013) Down-regulation of miR-221 inhibits proliferation of pancreatic cancer cells through up-regulation of PTEN, p27(kip1), p57(kip2) and PUMA. Am J Cancer Res 3(5):465–477
114. Kurashina R, Kikuchi K, Iwaki J, Yoshitake H, Takeshita T, Takizawa T (2014) Placenta-specific miRNA (miR-512-3p) targets PPP3R1 encoding the calcineurin B regulatory subunit in BeWo cells. J Obstet Gynaecol Res 40(3):650–660. https://doi.org/10.1111/jog.12217
115. Liu Z, Zhu J, Cao H, Ren H, Fang X (2012) miR-10b promotes cell invasion through RhoC-AKT signaling pathway by targeting HOXD10 in gastric cancer. Int J Oncol 40(5):1553–1560. https://doi.org/10.3892/ijo.2012.1342
116. Papagiannakopoulos T, Friedmann-Morvinski D, Neveu P, Dugas JC, Gill RM, Huillard E, Liu C, Zong H, Rowitch DH, Barres BA, Verma IM, Kosik KS (2012) Pro-neural miR-128 is a glioma tumor suppressor that targets mitogenic kinases. Oncogene 31(15):1884–1895. https://doi.org/10.1038/onc.2011.380
117. Xu HS, Zong HL, Shang M, Ming X, Zhao JP, Ma C, Cao L (2014) MiR-324-5p inhibits proliferation of glioma by target regulation of GLI1. Eur Rev Med Pharmacol Sci 18(6):828–832. pii: 7143
118. Giovannetti E, Funel N, Peters GJ, Del Chiaro M, Erozenci LA, Vasile E, Leon LG, Pollina LE, Groen A, Falcone A, Danesi R, Campani D, Verheul HM, Boggi U (2010) MicroRNA-21 in pancreatic cancer: correlation with clinical outcome and pharmacologic aspects underlying its role in the modulation of gemcitabine activity. Cancer Res 70(11):4528–4538. https://doi.org/10.1158/0008-5472.CAN-09-4467
119. Botla SK, Savant S, Jandaghi P, Bauer AS, Mucke O, Moskalev EA, Neoptolemos JP, Costello E, Greenhalf W, Scarpa A, Gaida MM, Buchler MW, Strobel O, Hackert T, Giese NA, Augustin HG, Hoheisel JD (2016) Early epigenetic downregulation of microRNA-192 expression promotes pancreatic cancer progression. Cancer Res 76(14):4149–4159. https://doi.org/10.1158/0008-5472.CAN-15-0390
120. Yu J, Ohuchida K, Mizumoto K, Sato N, Kayashima T, Fujita H, Nakata K, Tanaka M (2010) MicroRNA, hsa-miR-200c, is an independent prognostic factor in pancreatic cancer and its upregulation inhibits pancreatic cancer invasion but increases cell proliferation. Mol Cancer 9:169. https://doi.org/10.1186/1476-4598-9-169
121. Yang X, Yu J, Yin J, Xiang Q, Tang H, Lei X (2012) MiR-195 regulates cell apoptosis of human hepatocellular carcinoma cells by targeting LATS2. Pharmazie 67(7):645–651
122. Tsang TY, Tang WY, Chan JY, Co NN, Au Yeung CL, Yau PL, Kong SK, Fung KP, Kwok TT (2011) P-glycoprotein enhances radiation-induced apoptotic cell death through the regulation of miR-16 and Bcl-2 expressions in hepatocellular carcinoma cells. Apoptosis 16(5):524–535. https://doi.org/10.1007/s10495-011-0581-5
123. Li L, Guo Z, Wang J, Mao Y, Gao Q (2012) Serum miR-18a: a potential marker for hepatitis B virus-related hepatocellular carcinoma screening. Dig Dis Sci 57(11):2910–2916. https://doi.org/10.1007/s10620-012-2317-y

124. Zhang Y, Zhang B, Zhang A, Li X, Liu J, Zhao J, Zhao Y, Gao J, Fang D, Rao Z (2013) IL-6 upregulation contributes to the reduction of miR-26a expression in hepatocellular carcinoma cells. Braz J Med Biol Res 46(1):32–38. pii: S0100-879X2012007500155
125. Sheng Y, Li J, Zou C, Wang S, Cao Y, Zhang J, Huang A, Tang H (2014) Downregulation of miR-101-3p by hepatitis B virus promotes proliferation and migration of hepatocellular carcinoma cells by targeting Rab5a. Arch Virol 159(9):2397–2410. https://doi.org/10.1007/s00705-014-2084-5
126. Law PT, Ching AK, Chan AW, Wong QW, Wong CK, To KF, Wong N (2012) MiR-145 modulates multiple components of the insulin-like growth factor pathway in hepatocellular carcinoma. Carcinogenesis 33(6):1134–1141. https://doi.org/10.1093/carcin/bgs130
127. Epis MR, Giles KM, Barker A, Kendrick TS, Leedman PJ (2009) miR-331-3p regulates ERBB-2 expression and androgen receptor signaling in prostate cancer. J Biol Chem 284(37):24696–24704. https://doi.org/10.1074/jbc.M109.030098
128. Liu YN, Yin JJ, Abou-Kheir W, Hynes PG, Casey OM, Fang L, Yi M, Stephens RM, Seng V, Sheppard-Tillman H, Martin P, Kelly K (2013) MiR-1 and miR-200 inhibit EMT via Slug-dependent and tumorigenesis via Slug-independent mechanisms. Oncogene 32(3):296–306. https://doi.org/10.1038/onc.2012.58
129. Zeljic K, Jovanovic I, Jovanovic J, Magic Z, Stankovic A, Supic G (2018) MicroRNA meta-signature of oral cancer: evidence from a meta-analysis. Ups J Med Sci 123(1):43–49. https://doi.org/10.1080/03009734.2018.1439551
130. Lai YH, Liu H, Chiang WF, Chen TW, Chu LJ, Yu JS, Chen SJ, Chen HC, Tan BC (2018) MiR-31-5p-ACOX1 axis enhances tumorigenic fitness in oral squamous cell carcinoma via the promigratory prostaglandin E2. Theranostics 8(2):486–504. https://doi.org/10.7150/thno.22059
131. Jia LF, Huang YP, Zheng YF, Lyu MY, Wei SB, Meng Z, Gan YH (2014) miR-29b suppresses proliferation, migration, and invasion of tongue squamous cell carcinoma through PTEN-AKT signaling pathway by targeting Sp1. Oral Oncol 50(11):1062–1071. https://doi.org/10.1016/j.oraloncology.2014.07.010
132. Manikandan M, Deva Magendhra Rao AK, Arunkumar G, Manickavasagam M, Rajkumar KS, Rajaraman R, Munirajan AK (2016) Oral squamous cell carcinoma: microRNA expression profiling and integrative analyses for elucidation of tumourigenesis mechanism. Mol Cancer 15:28. https://doi.org/10.1186/s12943-016-0512-8
133. Lin SC, Kao SY, Chang JC, Liu YC, Yu EH, Tseng SH, Liu CJ, Chang KW (2016) Up-regulation of miR-187 modulates the advances of oral carcinoma by targeting BARX2 tumor suppressor. Oncotarget 7(38):61355–61365. https://doi.org/10.18632/oncotarget.11349
134. Manikandan M, Deva Magendhra Rao AK, Arunkumar G, Rajkumar KS, Rajaraman R, Munirajan AK (2015) Down regulation of miR-34a and miR-143 may indirectly inhibit p53 in oral squamous cell carcinoma: a pilot study. Asian Pac J Cancer Prev 16(17):7619–7625. https://doi.org/10.7314/apjcp.2015.16.17.7619
135. Siriwardena S, Tsunematsu T, Qi G, Ishimaru N, Kudo Y (2018) Invasion-related factors as potential diagnostic and therapeutic targets in oral squamous cell carcinoma-a review. Int J Mol Sci 19(5). https://doi.org/10.3390/ijms19051462
136. Hilly O, Pillar N, Stern S, Strenov Y, Bachar G, Shomron N, Shpitzer T (2016) Distinctive pattern of let-7 family microRNAs in aggressive carcinoma of the oral tongue in young patients. Oncol Lett 12(3):1729–1736. https://doi.org/10.3892/ol.2016.4892
137. Frankel LB, Lund AH (2012) MicroRNA regulation of autophagy. Carcinogenesis 33(11):2018–2025. https://doi.org/10.1093/carcin/bgs266
138. Henley SA, Dick FA (2012) The retinoblastoma family of proteins and their regulatory functions in the mammalian cell division cycle. Cell Div 7(1):10. https://doi.org/10.1186/1747-1028-7-10
139. Polager S, Ginsberg D (2009) p53 and E2f: partners in life and death. Nat Rev Cancer 9(10):738–748. https://doi.org/10.1038/nrc2718
140. Murray AW (2004) Recycling the cell cycle: cyclins revisited. Cell 116(2):221–234. pii: S0092867403010808

141. Kastan MB, Bartek J (2004) Cell-cycle checkpoints and cancer. Nature 432(7015):316–323. pii: nature03097
142. Liu Q, Fu H, Sun F, Zhang H, Tie Y, Zhu J, Xing R, Sun Z, Zheng X (2008) miR-16 family induces cell cycle arrest by regulating multiple cell cycle genes. Nucleic Acids Res 36(16):5391–5404. https://doi.org/10.1093/nar/gkn522
143. Yu Z, Wang C, Wang M, Li Z, Casimiro MC, Liu M, Wu K, Whittle J, Ju X, Hyslop T, McCue P, Pestell RG (2008) A cyclin D1/microRNA 17/20 regulatory feedback loop in control of breast cancer cell proliferation. J Cell Biol 182(3):509–517. https://doi.org/10.1083/jcb.200801079
144. Sarkar S, Dey BK, Dutta A (2010) MiR-322/424 and -503 are induced during muscle differentiation and promote cell cycle quiescence and differentiation by down-regulation of Cdc25A. Mol Biol Cell 21(13):2138–2149. https://doi.org/10.1091/mbc.E10-01-0062
145. Bueno MJ, Malumbres M (2011) MicroRNAs and the cell cycle. Biochim Biophys Acta 1812(5):592–601. https://doi.org/10.1016/j.bbadis.2011.02.002
146. Huang L, Luo J, Cai Q, Pan Q, Zeng H, Guo Z, Dong W, Huang J, Lin T (2011) MicroRNA-125b suppresses the development of bladder cancer by targeting E2F3. Int J Cancer 128(8):1758–1769. https://doi.org/10.1002/ijc.25509
147. Benetti R, Gonzalo S, Jaco I, Munoz P, Gonzalez S, Schoeftner S, Murchison E, Andl T, Chen T, Klatt P, Li E, Serrano M, Millar S, Hannon G, Blasco MA (2008) A mammalian microRNA cluster controls DNA methylation and telomere recombination via Rbl2-dependent regulation of DNA methyltransferases. Nat Struct Mol Biol 15(9):998. pii: nsmb0908-998b
148. Krek A, Grun D, Poy MN, Wolf R, Rosenberg L, Epstein EJ, MacMenamin P, da Piedade I, Gunsalus KC, Stoffel M, Rajewsky N (2005) Combinatorial microRNA target predictions. Nat Genet 37(5):495–500. pii: ng1536
149. le Sage C, Nagel R, Egan DA, Schrier M, Mesman E, Mangiola A, Anile C, Maira G, Mercatelli N, Ciafre SA, Farace MG, Agami R (2007) Regulation of the p27(Kip1) tumor suppressor by miR-221 and miR-222 promotes cancer cell proliferation. EMBO J 26(15):3699–3708. pii: 7601790
150. Kim YK, Yu J, Han TS, Park SY, Namkoong B, Kim DH, Hur K, Yoo MW, Lee HJ, Yang HK, Kim VN (2009) Functional links between clustered microRNAs: suppression of cell-cycle inhibitors by microRNA clusters in gastric cancer. Nucleic Acids Res 37(5):1672–1681. https://doi.org/10.1093/nar/gkp002
151. Galardi S, Mercatelli N, Giorda E, Massalini S, Frajese GV, Ciafre SA, Farace MG (2007) miR-221 and miR-222 expression affects the proliferation potential of human prostate carcinoma cell lines by targeting p27Kip1. J Biol Chem 282(32):23716–23724. pii: M701805200
152. Chendrimada TP, Gregory RI, Kumaraswamy E, Norman J, Cooch N, Nishikura K, Shiekhattar R (2005) TRBP recruits the Dicer complex to Ago2 for microRNA processing and gene silencing. Nature 436(7051):740–744. pii: nature03868
153. Paroo Z, Ye X, Chen S, Liu Q (2009) Phosphorylation of the human microRNA-generating complex mediates MAPK/Erk signaling. Cell 139(1):112–122. https://doi.org/10.1016/j.cell.2009.06.044
154. Kuilman T, Michaloglou C, Mooi WJ, Peeper DS (2010) The essence of senescence. Genes Dev 24(22):2463–2479. https://doi.org/10.1101/gad.1971610
155. Nishino J, Kim I, Chada K, Morrison SJ (2008) Hmga2 promotes neural stem cell self-renewal in young but not old mice by reducing p16Ink4a and p19Arf expression. Cell 135(2):227–239. https://doi.org/10.1016/j.cell.2008.09.017
156. Lal A, Kim HH, Abdelmohsen K, Kuwano Y, Pullmann R Jr, Srikantan S, Subrahmanyam R, Martindale JL, Yang X, Ahmed F, Navarro F, Dykxhoorn D, Lieberman J, Gorospe M (2008) p16(INK4a) translation suppressed by miR-24. PLoS One 3(3):e1864. https://doi.org/10.1371/journal.pone.0001864
157. Brooks CL, Gu W (2009) How does SIRT1 affect metabolism, senescence and cancer? Nat Rev Cancer 9(2):123–128. https://doi.org/10.1038/nrc2562

158. Langley E, Pearson M, Faretta M, Bauer UM, Frye RA, Minucci S, Pelicci PG, Kouzarides T (2002) Human SIR2 deacetylates p53 and antagonizes PML/p53-induced cellular senescence. EMBO J 21(10):2383–2396. https://doi.org/10.1093/emboj/21.10.2383
159. Christoffersen NR, Shalgi R, Frankel LB, Leucci E, Lees M, Klausen M, Pilpel Y, Nielsen FC, Oren M, Lund AH (2010) p53-independent upregulation of miR-34a during oncogene-induced senescence represses MYC. Cell Death Differ 17(2):236–245. https://doi.org/10.1038/cdd.2009.109
160. Bueno MJ, Gomez de Cedron M, Laresgoiti U, Fernandez-Piqueras J, Zubiaga AM, Malumbres M (2010) Multiple E2F-induced microRNAs prevent replicative stress in response to mitogenic signaling. Mol Cell Biol 30(12):2983–2995. https://doi.org/10.1128/MCB.01372-09
161. Chang TC, Wentzel EA, Kent OA, Ramachandran K, Mullendore M, Lee KH, Feldmann G, Yamakuchi M, Ferlito M, Lowenstein CJ, Arking DE, Beer MA, Maitra A, Mendell JT (2007) Transactivation of miR-34a by p53 broadly influences gene expression and promotes apoptosis. Mol Cell 26(5):745–752. pii: S1097-2765(07)00310-3
162. Wade M, Wang YV, Wahl GM (2010) The p53 orchestra: Mdm2 and Mdmx set the tone. Trends Cell Biol 20(5):299–309. https://doi.org/10.1016/j.tcb.2010.01.009
163. Georges SA, Biery MC, Kim SY, Schelter JM, Guo J, Chang AN, Jackson AL, Carleton MO, Linsley PS, Cleary MA, Chau BN (2008) Coordinated regulation of cell cycle transcripts by p53-inducible microRNAs, miR-192 and miR-215. Cancer Res 68(24):10105–10112. https://doi.org/10.1158/0008-5472.CAN-08-1846
164. Sachdeva M, Zhu S, Wu F, Wu H, Walia V, Kumar S, Elble R, Watabe K, Mo YY (2009) p53 represses c-Myc through induction of the tumor suppressor miR-145. Proc Natl Acad Sci U S A 106(9):3207–3212. https://doi.org/10.1073/pnas.0808042106
165. Concepcion CP, Bonetti C, Ventura A (2012) The microRNA-17-92 family of microRNA clusters in development and disease. Cancer J 18(3):262–267. https://doi.org/10.1097/PPO.0b013e318258b60a
166. Yan HL, Xue G, Mei Q, Wang YZ, Ding FX, Liu MF, Lu MH, Tang Y, Yu HY, Sun SH (2009) Repression of the miR-17-92 cluster by p53 has an important function in hypoxia-induced apoptosis. EMBO J 28(18):2719–2732. https://doi.org/10.1038/emboj.2009.214
167. Zhang X, Wan G, Berger FG, He X, Lu X (2011) The ATM kinase induces microRNA biogenesis in the DNA damage response. Mol Cell 41(4):371–383. https://doi.org/10.1016/j.molcel.2011.01.020
168. Pothof J, Verkaik NS, van IW, Wiemer EA, Ta VT, van der Horst GT, Jaspers NG, van Gent DC, Hoeijmakers JH, Persengiev SP (2009) MicroRNA-mediated gene silencing modulates the UV-induced DNA-damage response. EMBO J 28(14):2090–2099. https://doi.org/10.1038/emboj.2009.156
169. Suzuki HI, Yamagata K, Sugimoto K, Iwamoto T, Kato S, Miyazono K (2009) Modulation of microRNA processing by p53. Nature 460(7254):529–533. https://doi.org/10.1038/nature08199
170. Boominathan L (2010) The tumor suppressors p53, p63, and p73 are regulators of microRNA processing complex. PLoS One 5(5):e10615. https://doi.org/10.1371/journal.pone.0010615
171. Trabucchi M, Briata P, Garcia-Mayoral M, Haase AD, Filipowicz W, Ramos A, Gherzi R, Rosenfeld MG (2009) The RNA-binding protein KSRP promotes the biogenesis of a subset of microRNAs. Nature 459(7249):1010–1014. https://doi.org/10.1038/nature08025
172. Hu H, Du L, Nagabayashi G, Seeger RC, Gatti RA (2010) ATM is down-regulated by N-Myc-regulated microRNA-421. Proc Natl Acad Sci U S A 107(4):1506–1511. https://doi.org/10.1073/pnas.0907763107
173. Matsuoka S, Ballif BA, Smogorzewska A, McDonald ER, 3rd, Hurov KE, Luo J, Bakalarski CE, Zhao Z, Solimini N, Lerenthal Y, Shiloh Y, Gygi SP, Elledge SJ (2007) ATM and ATR substrate analysis reveals extensive protein networks responsive to DNA damage. Science 316(5828):1160–1166. pii: 316/5828/1160

174. Stucki M, Clapperton JA, Mohammad D, Yaffe MB, Smerdon SJ, Jackson SP (2005) MDC1 directly binds phosphorylated histone H2AX to regulate cellular responses to DNA double-strand breaks. Cell 123(7):1213–1226. pii: S0092-8674(05)01165-7
175. Lal A, Pan Y, Navarro F, Dykxhoorn DM, Moreau L, Meire E, Bentwich Z, Lieberman J, Chowdhury D (2009) miR-24-mediated downregulation of H2AX suppresses DNA repair in terminally differentiated blood cells. Nat Struct Mol Biol 16(5):492–498. https://doi.org/10.1038/nsmb.1589
176. Lal A, Navarro F, Maher CA, Maliszewski LE, Yan N, O'Day E, Chowdhury D, Dykxhoorn DM, Tsai P, Hofmann O, Becker KG, Gorospe M, Hide W, Lieberman J (2009) miR-24 inhibits cell proliferation by targeting E2F2, MYC, and other cell-cycle genes via binding to "seedless" 3′UTR microRNA recognition elements. Mol Cell 35(5):610–625. https://doi.org/10.1016/j.molcel.2009.08.020
177. Le MT, Teh C, Shyh-Chang N, Xie H, Zhou B, Korzh V, Lodish HF, Lim B (2009) MicroRNA-125b is a novel negative regulator of p53. Genes Dev 23(7):862–876. https://doi.org/10.1101/gad.1767609
178. Hu W, Chan CS, Wu R, Zhang C, Sun Y, Song JS, Tang LH, Levine AJ, Feng Z (2010) Negative regulation of tumor suppressor p53 by microRNA miR-504. Mol Cell 38(5):689–699. https://doi.org/10.1016/j.molcel.2010.05.027
179. Swarbrick A, Woods SL, Shaw A, Balakrishnan A, Phua Y, Nguyen A, Chanthery Y, Lim L, Ashton LJ, Judson RL, Huskey N, Blelloch R, Haber M, Norris MD, Lengyel P, Hackett CS, Preiss T, Chetcuti A, Sullivan CS, Marcusson EG, Weiss W, L'Etoile N, Goga A (2010) miR-380-5p represses p53 to control cellular survival and is associated with poor outcome in MYCN-amplified neuroblastoma. Nat Med 16(10):1134–1140. https://doi.org/10.1038/nm.2227
180. Kumar M, Lu Z, Takwi AA, Chen W, Callander NS, Ramos KS, Young KH, Li Y (2011) Negative regulation of the tumor suppressor p53 gene by microRNAs. Oncogene 30(7):843–853. https://doi.org/10.1038/onc.2010.457
181. Park SY, Lee JH, Ha M, Nam JW, Kim VN (2009) miR-29 miRNAs activate p53 by targeting p85 alpha and CDC42. Nat Struct Mol Biol 16(1):23–29. https://doi.org/10.1038/nsmb.1533
182. Jansson MD, Lund AH (2012) MicroRNA and cancer. Mol Oncol 6(6):590–610. https://doi.org/10.1016/j.molonc.2012.09.006
183. Kalluri R, Weinberg RA (2009) The basics of epithelial-mesenchymal transition. J Clin Invest 119(6):1420–1428. https://doi.org/10.1172/JCI39104
184. Kong W, Yang H, He L, Zhao JJ, Coppola D, Dalton WS, Cheng JQ (2008) MicroRNA-155 is regulated by the transforming growth factor beta/Smad pathway and contributes to epithelial cell plasticity by targeting RhoA. Mol Cell Biol 28(22):6773–6784. https://doi.org/10.1128/MCB.00941-08
185. Gregory PA, Bert AG, Paterson EL, Barry SC, Tsykin A, Farshid G, Vadas MA, Khew-Goodall Y, Goodall GJ (2008) The miR-200 family and miR-205 regulate epithelial to mesenchymal transition by targeting ZEB1 and SIP1. Nat Cell Biol 10(5):593–601. https://doi.org/10.1038/ncb1722
186. Bracken CP, Gregory PA, Kolesnikoff N, Bert AG, Wang J, Shannon MF, Goodall GJ (2008) A double-negative feedback loop between ZEB1-SIP1 and the microRNA-200 family regulates epithelial-mesenchymal transition. Cancer Res 68(19):7846–7854. https://doi.org/10.1158/0008-5472.CAN-08-1942
187. Hurteau GJ, Carlson JA, Spivack SD, Brock GJ (2007) Overexpression of the microRNA hsa-miR-200c leads to reduced expression of transcription factor 8 and increased expression of E-cadherin. Cancer Res 67(17):7972–7976. pii: 67/17/7972
188. Korpal M, Lee ES, Hu G, Kang Y (2008) The miR-200 family inhibits epithelial-mesenchymal transition and cancer cell migration by direct targeting of E-cadherin transcriptional repressors ZEB1 and ZEB2. J Biol Chem 283(22):14910–14914. https://doi.org/10.1074/jbc.C800074200
189. Ma L, Teruya-Feldstein J, Weinberg RA (2007) Tumour invasion and metastasis initiated by microRNA-10b in breast cancer. Nature 449(7163):682–688. pii: nature06174

190. Ding X, Park SI, McCauley LK, Wang CY (2013) Signaling between transforming growth factor beta (TGF-beta) and transcription factor SNAI2 represses expression of microRNA miR-203 to promote epithelial-mesenchymal transition and tumor metastasis. J Biol Chem 288(15):10241–10253. https://doi.org/10.1074/jbc.M112.443655
191. Zhang Z, Zhang B, Li W, Fu L, Zhu Z, Dong JT (2011) Epigenetic silencing of miR-203 upregulates SNAI2 and contributes to the invasiveness of malignant breast cancer cells. Genes Cancer 2(8):782–791. https://doi.org/10.1177/1947601911429743
192. Almeida MI, Reis RM, Calin GA (2010) MYC-microRNA-9-metastasis connection in breast cancer. Cell Res 20(6):603–604. https://doi.org/10.1038/cr.2010.70
193. Ma L, Young J, Prabhala H, Pan E, Mestdagh P, Muth D, Teruya-Feldstein J, Reinhardt F, Onder TT, Valastyan S, Westermann F, Speleman F, Vandesompele J, Weinberg RA (2010) miR-9, a MYC/MYCN-activated microRNA, regulates E-cadherin and cancer metastasis. Nat Cell Biol 12(3):247–256. https://doi.org/10.1038/ncb2024
194. Meng X, Wu J, Pan C, Wang H, Ying X, Zhou Y, Yu H, Zuo Y, Pan Z, Liu RY, Huang W (2013) Genetic and epigenetic down-regulation of microRNA-212 promotes colorectal tumor metastasis via dysregulation of MnSOD. Gastroenterology 145(2):426–436 e421–426. https://doi.org/10.1053/j.gastro.2013.04.004
195. Carmeliet P (2000) Mechanisms of angiogenesis and arteriogenesis. Nat Med 6(4):389–395. https://doi.org/10.1038/74651
196. Ferrara N (2002) VEGF and the quest for tumour angiogenesis factors. Nat Rev Cancer 2(10):795–803. https://doi.org/10.1038/nrc909
197. Camps C, Buffa FM, Colella S, Moore J, Sotiriou C, Sheldon H, Harris AL, Gleadle JM, Ragoussis J (2008) hsa-miR-210 is induced by hypoxia and is an independent prognostic factor in breast cancer. Clin Cancer Res 14(5):1340–1348. https://doi.org/10.1158/1078-0432.CCR-07-1755
198. Lou YL, Guo F, Liu F, Gao FL, Zhang PQ, Niu X, Guo SC, Yin JH, Wang Y, Deng ZF (2012) miR-210 activates notch signaling pathway in angiogenesis induced by cerebral ischemia. Mol Cell Biochem 370(1–2):45–51. https://doi.org/10.1007/s11010-012-1396-6
199. Liu F, Lou YL, Wu J, Ruan QF, Xie A, Guo F, Cui SP, Deng ZF, Wang Y (2012) Upregulation of microRNA-210 regulates renal angiogenesis mediated by activation of VEGF signaling pathway under ischemia/perfusion injury in vivo and in vitro. Kidney Blood Press Res 35(3):182–191. https://doi.org/10.1159/000331054
200. Ghosh G, Subramanian IV, Adhikari N, Zhang X, Joshi HP, Basi D, Chandrashekhar YS, Hall JL, Roy S, Zeng Y, Ramakrishnan S (2010) Hypoxia-induced microRNA-424 expression in human endothelial cells regulates HIF-alpha isoforms and promotes angiogenesis. J Clin Invest 120(11):4141–4154. https://doi.org/10.1172/JCI42980
201. Liu LZ, Li C, Chen Q, Jing Y, Carpenter R, Jiang Y, Kung HF, Lai L, Jiang BH (2011) MiR-21 induced angiogenesis through AKT and ERK activation and HIF-1alpha expression. PLoS One 6(4):e19139. https://doi.org/10.1371/journal.pone.0019139
202. Umezu T, Tadokoro H, Azuma K, Yoshizawa S, Ohyashiki K, Ohyashiki JH (2014) Exosomal miR-135b shed from hypoxic multiple myeloma cells enhances angiogenesis by targeting factor-inhibiting HIF-1. Blood 124(25):3748–3757. https://doi.org/10.1182/blood-2014-05-576116
203. Stahlhut C, Slack FJ (2013) MicroRNAs and the cancer phenotype: profiling, signatures and clinical implications. Genome Med 5(12):111. https://doi.org/10.1186/gm516
204. de Leeuw DC, van den Ancker W, Denkers F, de Menezes RX, Westers TM, Ossenkoppele GJ, van de Loosdrecht AA, Smit L (2013) MicroRNA profiling can classify acute leukemias of ambiguous lineage as either acute myeloid leukemia or acute lymphoid leukemia. Clin Cancer Res 19(8):2187–2196. https://doi.org/10.1158/1078-0432.CCR-12-3657
205. Sun YF, Leu JD, Chen SM, Lin IF, Lee YJ (2009) Results based on 124 cases of breast cancer and 97 controls from Taiwan suggest that the single nucleotide polymorphism (SNP309) in the MDM2 gene promoter is associated with earlier onset and increased risk of breast cancer. BMC Cancer 9:13. https://doi.org/10.1186/1471-2407-9-13

206. Bolmeson C, Esguerra JL, Salehi A, Speidel D, Eliasson L, Cilio CM (2011) Differences in islet-enriched miRNAs in healthy and glucose intolerant human subjects. Biochem Biophys Res Commun 404(1):16–22. https://doi.org/10.1016/j.bbrc.2010.11.024
207. Wee EJ, Peters K, Nair SS, Hulf T, Stein S, Wagner S, Bailey P, Lee SY, Qu WJ, Brewster B, French JD, Dobrovic A, Francis GD, Clark SJ, Brown MA (2012) Mapping the regulatory sequences controlling 93 breast cancer-associated miRNA genes leads to the identification of two functional promoters of the Hsa-mir-200b cluster, methylation of which is associated with metastasis or hormone receptor status in advanced breast cancer. Oncogene 31(38):4182–4195. https://doi.org/10.1038/onc.2011.584
208. Rothe F, Ignatiadis M, Chaboteaux C, Haibe-Kains B, Kheddoumi N, Majjaj S, Badran B, Fayyad-Kazan H, Desmedt C, Harris AL, Piccart M, Sotiriou C (2011) Global microRNA expression profiling identifies MiR-210 associated with tumor proliferation, invasion and poor clinical outcome in breast cancer. PLoS One 6(6):e20980. https://doi.org/10.1371/journal.pone.0020980
209. Eis PS, Tam W, Sun L, Chadburn A, Li Z, Gomez MF, Lund E, Dahlberg JE (2005) Accumulation of miR-155 and BIC RNA in human B cell lymphomas. Proc Natl Acad Sci U S A 102(10):3627–3632. pii: 0500613102
210. Yang M, Shen H, Qiu C, Ni Y, Wang L, Dong W, Liao Y, Du J (2013) High expression of miR-21 and miR-155 predicts recurrence and unfavourable survival in non-small cell lung cancer. Eur J Cancer 49(3):604–615. https://doi.org/10.1016/j.ejca.2012.09.031
211. Zhu J, Feng Y, Ke Z, Yang Z, Zhou J, Huang X, Wang L (2012) Down-regulation of miR-183 promotes migration and invasion of osteosarcoma by targeting Ezrin. Am J Pathol 180(6):2440–2451. https://doi.org/10.1016/j.ajpath.2012.02.023
212. Toiyama Y, Hur K, Tanaka K, Inoue Y, Kusunoki M, Boland CR, Goel A (2014) Serum miR-200c is a novel prognostic and metastasis-predictive biomarker in patients with colorectal cancer. Ann Surg 259(4):735–743. https://doi.org/10.1097/SLA.0b013e3182a6909d
213. Baigude H, Rana TM (2014) Strategies to antagonize miRNA functions in vitro and in vivo. Nanomedicine (Lond) 9(16):2545–2555. https://doi.org/10.2217/nnm.14.162
214. Weiler J, Hunziker J, Hall J (2006) Anti-miRNA oligonucleotides (AMOs): ammunition to target miRNAs implicated in human disease? Gene Ther 13(6):496–502. pii: 3302654
215. Lennox KA, Behlke MA (2011) Chemical modification and design of anti-miRNA oligonucleotides. Gene Ther 18(12):1111–1120. https://doi.org/10.1038/gt.2011.100
216. Gaglione M, Milano G, Chambery A, Moggio L, Romanelli A, Messere A (2011) PNA-based artificial nucleases as antisense and anti-miRNA oligonucleotide agents. Mol BioSyst 7(8):2490–2499. https://doi.org/10.1039/c1mb05131h
217. Kim JH, Yeom JH, Ko JJ, Han MS, Lee K, Na SY, Bae J (2011) Effective delivery of anti-miRNA DNA oligonucleotides by functionalized gold nanoparticles. J Biotechnol 155(3):287–292. https://doi.org/10.1016/j.jbiotec.2011.07.014
218. Ziegler S, Eberle ME, Wolfle SJ, Heeg K, Bekeredjian-Ding I (2013) Bifunctional oligodeoxynucleotide/antagomiR constructs: evaluation of a new tool for microRNA silencing. Nucleic Acid Ther 23(6):427–434. https://doi.org/10.1089/nat.2013.0447
219. Chabot S, Orio J, Castanier R, Bellard E, Nielsen SJ, Golzio M, Teissie J (2012) LNA-based oligonucleotide electrotransfer for miRNA inhibition. Mol Ther 20(8):1590–1598. https://doi.org/10.1038/mt.2012.95
220. Kluiver J, Slezak-Prochazka I, Smigielska-Czepiel K, Halsema N, Kroesen BJ, van den Berg A (2012) Generation of miRNA sponge constructs. Methods 58(2):113–117. https://doi.org/10.1016/j.ymeth.2012.07.019
221. de Melo Maia B, Ling H, Monroig P, Ciccone M, Soares FA, Calin GA, Rocha RM (2015) Design of a miRNA sponge for the miR-17 miRNA family as a therapeutic strategy against vulvar carcinoma. Mol Cell Probes 29(6):420–426. pii: S0890-8508(15)30028-1
222. Qureshi AT, Monroe WT, Dasa V, Gimble JM, Hayes DJ (2013) miR-148b-nanoparticle conjugates for light mediated osteogenesis of human adipose stromal/stem cells. Biomaterials 34(31):7799–7810. https://doi.org/10.1016/j.biomaterials.2013.07.004

223. Chen Y, Zhu X, Zhang X, Liu B, Huang L (2010) Nanoparticles modified with tumor-targeting scFv deliver siRNA and miRNA for cancer therapy. Mol Ther 18(9):1650–1656. https://doi.org/10.1038/mt.2010.136
224. Gu J, Chen X, Xin H, Fang X, Sha X (2014) Serum-resistant complex nanoparticles functionalized with imidazole-rich polypeptide for gene delivery to pulmonary metastatic melanoma. Int J Pharm 461(1–2):559–569. https://doi.org/10.1016/j.ijpharm.2013.12.029
225. Hayes J, Peruzzi PP, Lawler S (2014) MicroRNAs in cancer: biomarkers, functions and therapy. Trends Mol Med 20(8):460–469. https://doi.org/10.1016/j.molmed.2014.06.005
226. Treiber T, Treiber N, Meister G (2019) Publisher correction: regulation of microRNA biogenesis and its crosstalk with other cellular pathways. Nat Rev Mol Cell Biol 20(5):321. https://doi.org/10.1038/s41580-019-0106-6

Metabolic and Enzyme Engineering for the Microbial Production of Anticancer Terpenoids

10

Suresh Chandra Phulara, Vikrant Singh Rajput, Bidyut Mazumdar, and Ashish Runthala

10.1 Terpenoids

Isoprenoids (terpenoids or terpenes) are the largest class of secondary metabolites produced by almost all living organisms that are comprised of over 55,000 known compounds [1]. Several traditional systems utilize terpenoid-rich extracts for fragrance, flavor, and medicinal purpose. This is due to the tremendous diversity in the structure and functions of terpenoids [2, 3]. Despite their function as secondary metabolites, members of terpenoid family also perform fundamental functions in plants and animals, e.g., as components of electron transport system (quinines, ubiquinone, and plastoquinone), as pigments (carotenoids and side chains of chlorophyll), as hormones (gibberellins, ecdysteroids, dafachronic acids, abscisic acid, etc.), and as sterols (ergosterol, cholesterol, brassinosteroids, etc.) [4]. This is their diverse nature that provides these remarkable biomolecules several other biological activities including protective effects against tumor proliferation [5, 6] and several cancers [7, 8].

S. C. Phulara · A. Runthala (✉)
Department of Biotechnology, Koneru Lakshmaiah Education Foundation, Guntur, Andhra Pradesh, India

V. S. Rajput
School of Biotechnology, JNU, New Delhi, India

B. Mazumdar
Department of Chemical Engineering, National Institute of Technology Raipur, Raipur, Chhattisgarh, India

N. Masood, S. Shakil Malik (eds.), *'Essentials of Cancer Genomic, Computational Approaches and Precision Medicine*, https://doi.org/10.1007/978-981-15-1067-0_10

10.2 Terpenoid Biosynthesis

All the members of terpenoid family are produced from two universal precursors, namely, dimethylallyl pyrophosphate (DMAPP) and isopentenyl pyrophosphate (IPP). There are two pathways responsible for the synthesis of these common precursors in living organisms. The mevalonate (MVA) pathway is the first identified pathway [9, 10] and present in almost all eukaryotic cells and in few prokaryotic cells. For decades, MVA pathway has been thought to be responsible for the production of terpenoids in living organisms. In late 1990s and early 2000s, with the advancement of molecular biology tools and extensive genomic work on prokaryotes, scientists have discovered a MVA-independent pathway in prokaryotes. This pathway utilizes glyceraldehyde-3-phosphate (G3P) and pyruvate to produce IPP and DMAPP [11, 12] and is recognized as 1-deoxy-D-xylulose-5-phosphate (DXP) pathway. It exists in several eubacteria and plant organelles including chloroplast. Together the MVA and DXP pathways are responsible for the synthesis of the largest class of secondary metabolites, i.e., terpenoids.

10.2.1 The MVA Pathway

The MVA pathway takes six enzymatic steps to synthesize IPP and DMAPP from acetyl-CoA [13]. The first three steps are dedicated toward the synthesis of MVA by consuming three molecules of acetyl-CoA. The first enzyme, acetoacetyl-CoA thiolase, catalyzes the condensation of two acetyl-CoA to synthesize acetoacetyl-CoA. HMG-CoA synthase (HMGS) then converts acetoacetyl-CoA into hydroxymethylglutaryl-CoA (HMG-CoA) [14], which is further converted to MVA via reaction catalyzed by HMG-CoA reductase (HMGR) [15]. In the later three steps, MVA is converted to IPP. First, mevalonate kinase (MK) phosphorylates MVA to mevalonate-5-phosphate (MVAP) [16], which is then re-phosphorylated by phosphomevalonate kinase (PMK) to form mevalonate-5-diphosphate (MVAPP) [17]. Lastly, in an ATP-dependent decarboxylation step, phosphomevalonate decarboxylase (PMD) converts MVAPP to IPP [18], and IPP isomerase (IDI) catalyzes the conversion of IPP into DMAPP [19] (Fig. 10.1).

10.2.2 The DXP Pathway

The DXP pathway takes seven enzymatic steps to synthesize IPP and DMAPP in a ratio 5:1 [20, 21]. It starts with the synthesis of DXP via condensation of G3P and pyruvate by DXP synthase (DXS) enzyme [22]. In the later step, DXP is reduced to 2*C*-methyl-D-erythritol-4-phosphate (MEP) by DXP reductoisomerase (DXR or IspC) [23]. MEP-cytidyltransferase (IspD) then catalyzes MEP to 4-diphosphocytidyl-2*C*-methyl-D-erythritol (CDP-ME) [24] which is further converted to 4-diphosphocytidyl-2*C*-methyl-D-erythritol-2-phosphate (CDP-MEP) by the action of CDP-ME kinase (IspE) [25]. MEcP synthase (IspF) subsequently converts CDP-MEP to

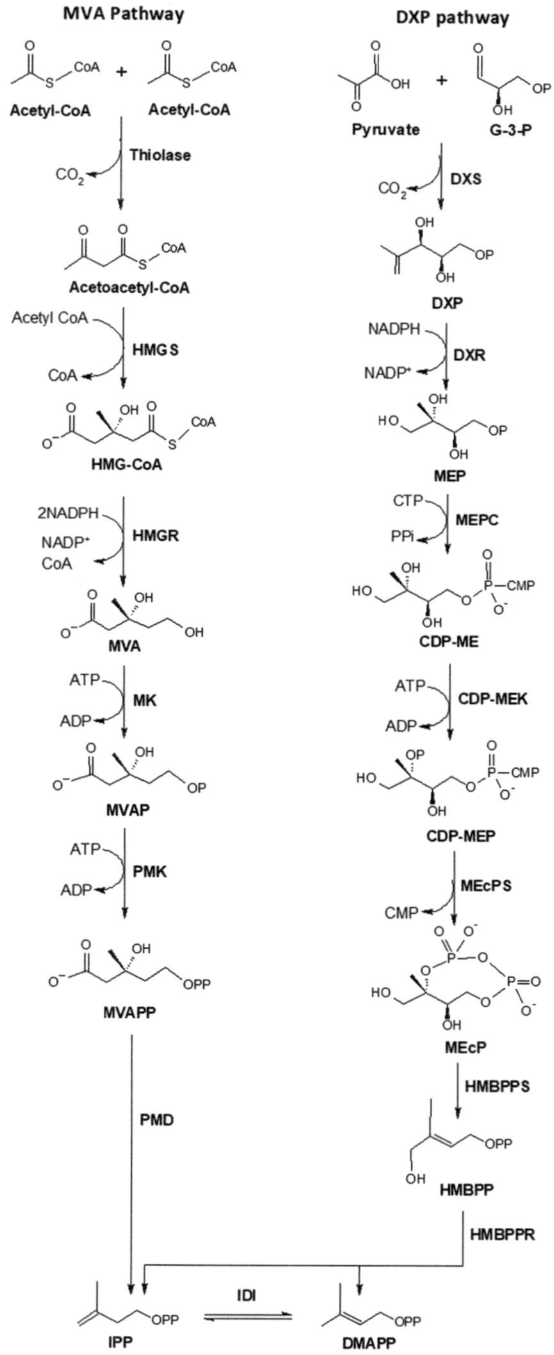

Fig. 10.1 Terpenoid biosynthesis pathways. HMG-CoA 3-hydroxy-3-methylglutaryl-CoA, HMGS 3-hydroxy-3-methylglutaryl-CoAsynthase, HMGR 3-hydroxy-3-methylglutaryl-CoAreductase, MVA mevalonate, MK mevalonate kinase, MVAP mevalonate-5-phosphate, PMK phosphomevalonate kinase, MVAPP mevalonate-5-pyrophosphate, PMD phosphomevalonate decarboxylase, G3P glyceraldehyde-3-phosphate, DXP deoxyxylulose-5-phosphate, DXS DXP synthase, DXR DXP reductase, MEP 2*C*-methyl-D-erythritol-4-phosphate, MEPC MEP cytidyltransferase, CDP-ME diphosphocytidyl-2*C*-methyl-D-erythritol, CDP-MEK CDP-ME kinase, MEcP 2-*C*-methyl-D-erythritol-2,4-cyclopyrophosphate, MECPS MECP synthase, HMBPP 1-hydroxy-2-methyl-2-(*E*)-butenyl-4-diphosphate, HMBPPS HMBPP synthase, HMBPPR HMBPP reductase, IPP isopentenyl pyrophosphate, DMAPP dimethylallyl pyrophosphate, IDI isopentenyl pyrophosphate isomerase

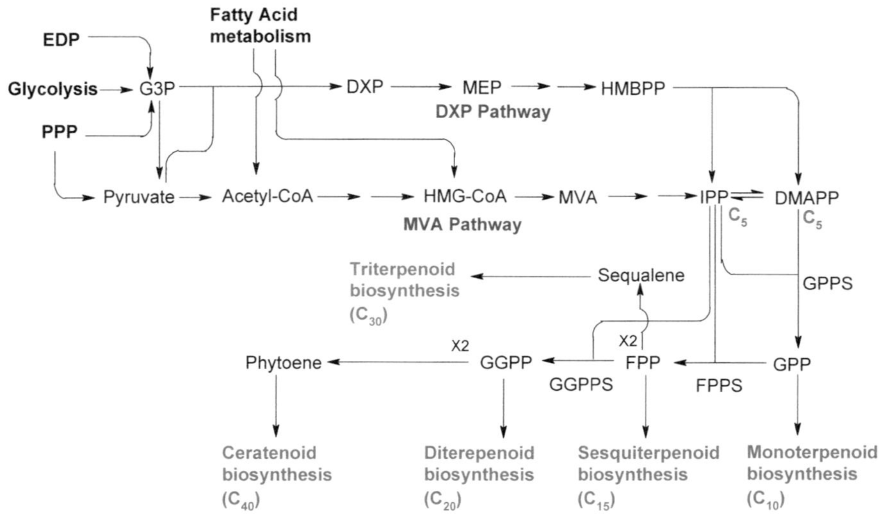

Fig. 10.2 Metabolic routes for the isoprenoids biosynthesis and their precursor supply. PPP pentose phosphate pathway, EDP Entner–Doudoroff pathway, G3P glyceraldehyde-3-phosphate, DXP deoxyxylulose-5-phosphate, MEP 2*C*-methyl-D-erythritol-4-phosphate, HMBPP 1-hydroxy-2-methyl-2-(*E*)-butenyl-4-diphosphate, HMG-CoA 3-hydroxy-3-methylglutaryl-CoA, MVA mevalonate, IPP isopentenyl pyrophosphate, DMAPP dimethylallyl pyrophosphate, GPP geranyl pyrophosphate, GPPS GPP synthase, FPP farnesyl pyrophosphate, FPPS FPP synthase, GGPP geranylgeranyl pyrophosphate, GGPPS GGPP synthase. The PPP and EDP along with glycolysis supply precursors (G3P and pyruvate) to DXP pathway for the biosynthesis of isoprenoids, whereas fatty acid metabolism provides precursors (acetyl-CoA and HMG) for MVA pathway

2-*C*-methyl-D-erythritol-2,4-cyclopyrophosphate (MEcP) [26], which is then converted to prenyl precursors by the action of 1-hydroxy-2-methyl-2-(*E*)-butenyl-4-diphosphate synthase (HMBPP synthase or IspG) and HMBPP reductase (IspH) through two successive reduction and elimination steps [21] (Fig. 10.1).

The IPP and DMAPP are utilized by several downstream enzymes such as geranyl pyrophosphate synthase (GPPS), fernesyl pyrophosphate synthase (FPPS or IspA), and geranylgeranyl pyrophosphate synthase (GGPPS) to synthesize the precursors (such as GPP, FPP, GGPP, etc.) for higher terpenoids molecules including Taxol, bisabolene, pinene, and limonene. The wide range of terpenoid compounds, viz., hemiterpenes (C_5), monoterpenes (C_{10}), sesquiterpenes (C_{15}), diterpenes (C_{20}), triterpenes (C_{30}), and carotenoids (C_{40}), is conventionally classified as per the number of encoded carbon atoms (Fig. 10.2).

10.3 Anticancer Terpenoids

Various forms of terpenoids differently act against the cancer cells, viz., through necrosis or induction of apoptosis, inhibition of angiogenesis, production of oxidative stress on cancer cells, activation of apoptosis via caspases, or inactivation of PI3K/Akt/NF-κB pathway, or they may act in synergistic way with other chemotherapeutic options available [27]. Various anticancer compounds falling in different terpenoid subclasses are hereby summarized.

10.3.1 Monoterpenoids

1. Limonene: It is a chief constituent of many citrus fruits, usually deployed for the industrial manufacturing of cleaning products and flavoring additives. The monocyclic monoterpene and D-limonene are well-known for their chemopreventive property. It is known to enhance the levels of hepatic enzymes, thereby preventing liver cancer. It is also thought that it averts mammary cancer induced by carcinogen at the initiation as well as progression phases [28]. The compound has shown promise in animal models whereby it represses the growth of colon, pancreas, stomach, liver and skin cancers. Antiangiogenesis, antioxidant, and pro-apoptotic properties are responsible for the inhibition of tumor growth and metastasis. The compound is known to hamper with the enzyme 3-hydroxy-3-methylglutanyl coenzyme A (HMGCoA) reductase [29] which in turn suppresses small G proteins like p21 and its membrane localization by protein isoprenylation [30]. Besides inducing the expression of cytochrome C and leading to the cleavage of caspase 3 and 9, it also up-regulates the expression of Bax protein to subsequently induce apoptosis [31].
2. Cantharidin: Being a non-plant origin terpenoid, it has been traditionally used as a Chinese medicine for many years. Almost 1500 species of blister beetles produce the natural defensive toxin which is used against hepatoma and esophageal carcinoma [7, 32]. It also exhibit anticancer effects against colorectal carcinoma, leukemia, breast cancer, and bladder carcinoma [33–35]. However, owing to its extreme side effects and toxicity, the clinical employment of cantharidin is limited. Mechanistically, the molecular targets are serine/threonine protein phosphatase 1 (PP1) and 2A (PP2A), which function to sway apoptosis, cell cycle, and cell-fate determination. The PP2A inhibition is responsible for IKKa/IkBa/p65 NF-κB pathway-dependent cancer cell apoptosis which subsequently activates extrinsic apoptotic signaling molecules such as TRAILR1, TRAILR2, and TNF-a [36]. Additionally, the mitogen-activated protein kinases (MAPKs)/ERK/JNK/p38 signaling is reported in cantharidin-activated apoptosis in cancer cells [37].

10.3.2 Sesquiterpenoid

1. Artemisinin and its derivatives: *Artemisia annua* L. is the origin of artemisinin, a bioactive molecule typically used as a Chinese medicine since many years against malaria. Artemisinin and its derivatives are known to inhibit breast cancer leukemia, ovarian cancer, colon cancer, prostate cancer, gastric cancer, hepatoma, melanoma, and lung cancer [7]. The in vivo anticancer potency has also been proven using xenograft animal models. The application of artemisinin and

its derivatives in combination with gemcitabine or carboplatin is also promising in xenograft tumor models [38, 39]. These molecules lead to G1 cell cycle arrest through cyclin D, cyclin E, CDK2, CDK4, p21, p27, NF-κB, etc. [7] and activate apoptosis in many cancer cell types by triggering p38 MAPK, increasing Fas expression, and inducing caspases [7]. They also suppress angiogenesis, metastasis, and invasion by regulating the amount of matrix metalloproteinases MMP2, MMP7, and MMP9, avb3 integrins, urokinase plasminogen activator (u-PA), and vascular endothelial growth factor (VEGF) [40, 41].

10.3.3 Diterpenoids

1. Tanshinone IIA: *Salvia miltiorrhiza* Bunge, the source of tanshinones, is routinely used in China to treat cardiovascular ailments [42]. Tanshinone IIA is reported to demonstrate in vitro and in vivo anticancer effects against breast cancer, leukemia, hepatocellular carcinoma, and colon cancer [7]. Apart from that, it also demonstrates combinatorial activity with cisplatin and doxorubicin [43–45]. It binds to the minor groove of DNA, thereby damaging the DNA structure to further prevent RNAPII binding. The obstruction within transcription in turn results in ROS generation, downregulation of erythroblastosis oncogene B, upregulation of TNF-a, activation of calcium-dependent signaling pathway, inhibition of the PI3K/AKT pathway, and increase of Bax/Bcl-2 protein ratio which further accounts for the anticancer characteristics of tanshinone IIA [7].
2. Triptolide: It is a triepoxide derived from *Tripterygium wilfordii* Hook.f, and its anti-inflammatory, immunosuppressive, and anti-proliferatory activities are well-known. The xenograft animal models in multiple clinical studies confirm its in vivo activity. The compound majorly attacks the transcriptional apparatus of the cell. It modulates the activity of several transcriptional factors, such as p53, NF-κB, HSF-1, and NF-AT [7]. It inhibits RNAPI and RNAPII to prevent de novo RNA synthesis. Additionally, the induction of proteasome-dependent degradation of the largest subunit of RNAPII (Rpb1) in cancer cells leads to global transcription inhibition. Specific targets include calcium channel polycystin-2 [46], an unknown 90-kDa nuclear protein [47], and a subunit of the transcription factor TFIIH called as the human XPB [48]. The XPB ATPase inhibition accounts for the cellular and physiological effects of the compound. Moreover, factors like impaired nucleotide excision and hypoxia-inducible factor-1a (HIF-1a) accumulation are also responsible for anticancer properties of triptolide.
3. Pseudolaric acid B: It is derived from the extracts of the root bark of *Pseudolarix kaempferi*, a plant found in eastern China. Pseudolaric acids A and B (PAA and PAB) are the major constituents accounting for antifungal and anti-angiogenic properties [7, 47]. PAB is known to inhibit colon, lung, breast, brain, and renal origin cancers [49] by targeting and destabilizing microtubules leading to the tumor cytostatic and anti-angiogenic outcome [47, 50]. It also antagonizes VEGF-stimulated cellular events and inhibits endothelial cell growth and thereby demonstrates a dual anti-angiogenic effect. Apart from microtubule blockage, it

also induces apoptosis through JNK and ERK pathways along with autophagy via Bcl-2 proteins [7].

4. Andrographolide: It is the chief pharmacologically active ingredient of *Andrographis paniculata*, a Chinese medicinal plant widely applied for colds, fever, laryngitis, and diarrhea [7, 51]. It also displays anti-inflammatory and anti-cancer activities [51]. The primary target for its therapeutic effect is NF-κB signaling. The compound binds to p50, a transcription factor of NF-κB, and thereby inhibits the signaling to decrease the amount of chemokines, cytokines, nitric oxide, adhesion molecules, and lipid mediators via suppression of the NF-κB signaling pathway [51]. Apart from NF-κB signaling, it also inhibits the cancer cell proliferation, survival, metastasis, and angiogenesis by affecting the other pathways such as JAK-STAT and PI3K, repression of cyclins, HSP90, cyclin-dependent kinases, metalloproteinases, growth factors, and activation of tumor suppressor proteins p53 and p2 [52].
5. Oridonin: It is extracted from *Rabdosia rubescens*, a Chinese herb known to inhibit many solid tumors, such as osteoma, liver cancer, colorectal cancer, and skin carcinoma along with acute lymphoblastic leukemia, primary adult T-cell leukemia, non-Hodgkin's lymphoma, chronic lymphocytic leukemia, and multiple myeloma cells as well [7, 53]. The in vivo activity has also been established using a colorectal cancer colostomy implantation model [54]. The cancer cells treated with oridonin die from apoptosis caused by the suppression of NF-κB DNA binding. Apoptosis is also induced due to the expression of forkhead box class O (FOXO) transcription factor and glycogen synthase kinase 3 (GSK3) and downregulation of PI3K/Akt signaling. Moreover, the tumor growth is inhibited by downregulation activator protein 1, NF-κB, and p38 pathways [7].
6. Paclitaxel: Paclitaxel is a taxane class therapeutic molecule extracted from the bark of *Taxus brevifolia*, the Pacific yew tree which is well-known to possess broad-spectrum anticancer potential [55]. It is reported to be active against breast cancer, endometrial cancer, non-small cell lung cancer, bladder cancer, and cervical carcinoma [56]. Its application as radio sensitizer against head and neck carcinoma is also reported [57]. Combinatorial therapy with doxorubicin and with anthracycline against breast cancer and with carboplatin and cisplatin for lung cancer has been useful [55, 58]. It acts on rapidly dividing cells by suppressing the microtubule spindle dynamics which leads to obstruction to metaphase-anaphase transitions and an eventual repression of mitosis followed by apoptosis [59]. Paclitaxel prevents tubulin disassembly by associating with polymeric tubulin molecules to stabilize microtubules, and, therefore, its treatment results in G2/M phase-arrested cancer cells [55].

10.3.4 Triterpenoids

1. Celastrol: It is isolated from *Tripterygium wilfordii* Hook.f known for its anticancer, anti-inflammatory properties and antioxidant characteristics [60]. The compound hampers many signaling pathways and suppresses IKKA and β-kinases,

inhibits proteasomes, and inactivates co-chaperones of HSP90 such as Cdc37 and p23 proteins. In addition, it activates HSF1 to trigger the heat shock response and represses AKT/mTOR/P70S6K signaling to inhibit the growth of tumor [7].
2. Cucurbitacins: The oxidized cucurbitane-type tetracyclic triterpenoid, extensively found in plants, exhibits potent anticancer, hepatoprotective, and anti-inflammatory effects [7, 44, 45, 61]. These compounds are known to induce cell cycle arrest, majorly at G2/M and differentiation in several tumor cell lines. They also inhibit tumor cell invasion and migration, both in vivo and in vitro [7]. Cucurbitacins have also shown synergistic effects in combination with cisplatin, doxorubicin, 5-flouroracil, paclitaxel [62], gemcitabine [63, 64], and docetaxel [65] in both in vitro and in vivo models.
3. Pachymic acid: It is isolated from *Poriacocos* and is reported to possess anti-inflammatory and anticancer properties. It demonstrates activity against human prostate cancer DU145 cells, human lung cancer A549 cells, and colon carcinoma HT29 cells and is known to induce apoptosis in LNCaP prostate cancer cells, DU145 and A549 cells [7, 66, 67]. At molecular level, it triggers PARP, caspase 3 and caspase 9. Apart for inhibiting DNA topoisomerase I and II, it represses MDA-MB-231 and MCF-7 breast carcinoma cells invasion and also decreases the PMA-induced transcriptional activity of NF-κB [68].

10.4 Strategies and Concerns for the Production of Anticancer Terpenoids

As discussed, paclitaxel (Taxol) is a commercially important anticancer diterpenoid present in *Taxux* sp. (Yew) plants. It is widely used as a chemotherapeutic agent for the treatment of variety of cancers [69]. The leaves and bark of Yew tree are the major natural source of paclitaxel or similar chemicals, where it is found in very small quantities ranging from 0.01% to 0.05% [70]. In addition, *Taxus* species grow at very slow growth rates, and the efficiency of traditional extraction methods of Taxol from its sources is very less. It has been found that ~10 tons of bark or 300 trees are required to extract 1 kg of Taxol, which can be utilized to treat just few hundred patients [70]. Due to the medicinal and commercial importance of Taxol, the yew species are being heavily exploited for the extraction of Taxol and become endangered. The International Union for Conservation of Nature (IUCN) has also reported an alarming decline (90%) in the population of *Taxus wallichiana* (Himalayan yew) across the Indo-Nepal Himalayan region [71]. Thus, the traditional extraction process of Taxol is environmentally and economically costly.

Due to the environmental concerns and limitations associated with the extraction of Taxol from Yew plants, researchers throughout the globe are now exploring other ways to produce commercially important terpenoid from chemical and/or from microbial route. Taxol is having structural complexities like other counterparts that impart limitations on its production through synthetic routes. Moreover, multiple steps are required for the production of Taxol by chemical route, and at every step, there is a subsequent loss in yield [72], which complicates its economic production. The current process of

Taxol production relies on plant-based semisynthetic routes [73]. Although semisynthetic route has gained some success in the commercial production of Taxol, reliance of this process on plants exerts some limitation on the scale of production and cost [73]. Another limitation that restrains production of such compounds through chemical routes is use of hazardous solvents [74, 75]. Together, the environmental and health concerns associated with the current production methods of terpenoids have led researchers to explore sustainable routes for the production of terpene-based anticancer compounds. Cell cultures of Yew have shown some hope in this regard. This approach has contributed notably to manage the Taxol supply; however, some drawbacks such as the lengthy culture duration, sensitivity of culture to shear stress, poor yield, and high production and extraction cost limit the application of cell culture [76]. To date, several microbial hosts have also been explored for the nonnatural production of terpene-based pharmaceuticals [69, 75] through computer-aided enzyme-design strategies [77].

10.5 Microbial Advances for the Production of Anticancer Terpenoids

Microbes have shown several advantages over plants that include (1) ease in culture and handling in lesser space, (2) higher growth rates, (3) lesser growth medium requirements, and (4) genetic traceability and tractability [78, 79]. Despite these advantages, microbes have also shown great success rates in genetic modifications. Utilization of modern high-throughput synthetic biology tools makes introduction or silencing of an entire pathway in microbial hosts easier than ever [80]. Recent years have seen nonnatural production of terpenoids from microbes either by fine-tuning host's pathways or by introducing foreign pathways/genes or by both [3, 75, 81]. Genetically tractable hosts such as *E. coli* and *S. cerevisiae* are the most widely utilized microbes for the heterologous production of complex terpenoids such as taxadiene and taxadiene-5α-ol [69, 82].

There are several challenges that arise while manipulating a host's genetic code. These include competition for substrate between the foreign and host enzymes, feedback inhibition by pathway intermediates or by end-product itself, and agglomeration of unwanted or toxic byproducts [74]. However, there are always opportunities to prevail over such constraints while working with microbial system rather than plant system. Therefore, past decades have seen several breakthroughs in the field of microbial terpenoid production by utilizing computational, rational, and combinatorial approaches [3, 75]. Alternate endogenous pathways have also been tuned in microbial host for enhancing precursor or cofactor supply for complex terpenoids [83, 84]. To surpass feedback regulation of pathway enzymes by intermediates, protein fusion products have been used [85, 86].

Among vast range of anticancer terpenes, Taxol, a complex diterpene-based natural antineoplastic drug, has gained a considerable interest due to its high efficiency, less toxicity, and broad spectrum. It has been used effectively to treat several types of cancers, such as breast, uterine, colon, ovarian, and other cancers [70, 72]. It is having one of the fast paced and rapidly growing (~9% average growth rate) international markets with a global revenue of US$90 million and is expected to reach US$140 million by 2024 (https://www.reportsweb.com/reports/global-paclitaxel-market-growth-2019-2024). The research for microbial Taxol production is focused on either exploring endophytic fungi capable of Taxol production [72, 76] or genetic modulation of microbes like *E. coli* or *S. cerevisiae* [69, 82].

Taxol-producing endophytic fungi can easily be isolated from explants as roots, stems, leaves, and fruits [70] and can be easily cultured in standard laboratory conditions. The first step in the Taxol production from endophytic fungi is screening of endophytic fungi having natively higher Taxol yield. The functional improvement of the isolated strains is subsequently done by mutagenesis and/or modern biotechnological tools. Finally, production is achieved via advanced fermentation methods [70]. In fungi, production of primeval metabolites can be improved by modulating their mycelium structure via mutations. Both the chemical [ethyl methyl sulfomar (EMS), nitrosoguanidine (NTG), etc.] and physical (ultraviolet, χ-ray, γ-rays, fast neutron, laser, microwave, etc.) mutagens have been used to induce genetic variation in endophytic fungi. It has been found that mutation is able to improve Taxol production over 2.5-folds in the proficient endophytic fungi from *Taxus cuspidate* [87]. It is also observed that treatments, such as UV, NTG, and UV + NTG, could increase bioactive production in the endophytic fungi. Mutation induction via treatment of UV + NTG to a Taxol-producing endophytic fungi has shown ~1.4-fold increase in Taxol yield in mutant strain over the wild type [70].

Taxol biosynthesis is a complex process and has not been determine fully. It is a 19-step process that deploys 8 cytochrome P450-mediated oxygenations [88]. Huang et al. [89] have laid the foundation of microbial Taxol production and achieved taxadiene, a key intermediate of Taxol biosynthesis, from an engineered *E. coli* by the overexpression of downstream terpenoid pathways genes such as IDI, GGPPS, and taxadiene synthase (TS). Later, precursors of Taxol and associated taxoids have been obtained from the recombinant *S. cerevisiae* by the expression of eight taxoid biosynthetic genes [90]. Biosynthetic pathway of Taxol precursors, taxadiene, and taxadiene-5α-ol is shown in Fig. 10.3.

There are three main aspects on which current research is focused for the microbial Taxol production: (1) to enhance GGPP supply, (2) to overexpress TS to convert GGPP into taxadiene [82], and (3) to engineer cytochrome P450-mediated oxygenations for the production of taxadien-5α-ol from taxadiene [69]. To produce taxadiene from recombinant *S. cerevisiae*, a GGPP synthase from *Sulfolobus acidocaldarius* has been overexpressed along with a codon-optimized taxadiene synthase from *Taxus chinensis* [82]. A truncated version of HMG-CoA reductase (tHmg1) has been overexpressed to surpass the steroid-based negative feedback. Further, to facilitate steroid uptake under aerobic environment, mutant *upc2-1* gene of the transcriptional sterol regulator is expressed, and the engineered strain is found to produce ~8.7 mg/L taxadiene after 48 h incubation [82] (Table 10.1). Later, Ajikumar et al. [69] have improved taxadiene titers through the engineered *E. coli* by using the "multivariate-modular pathway engineering (MMPE)" approach. The overall DXP pathway is partitioned into smaller modules, "upper module," and "lower module," and the components of each module are separately fine-tuned to investigate a correct balance

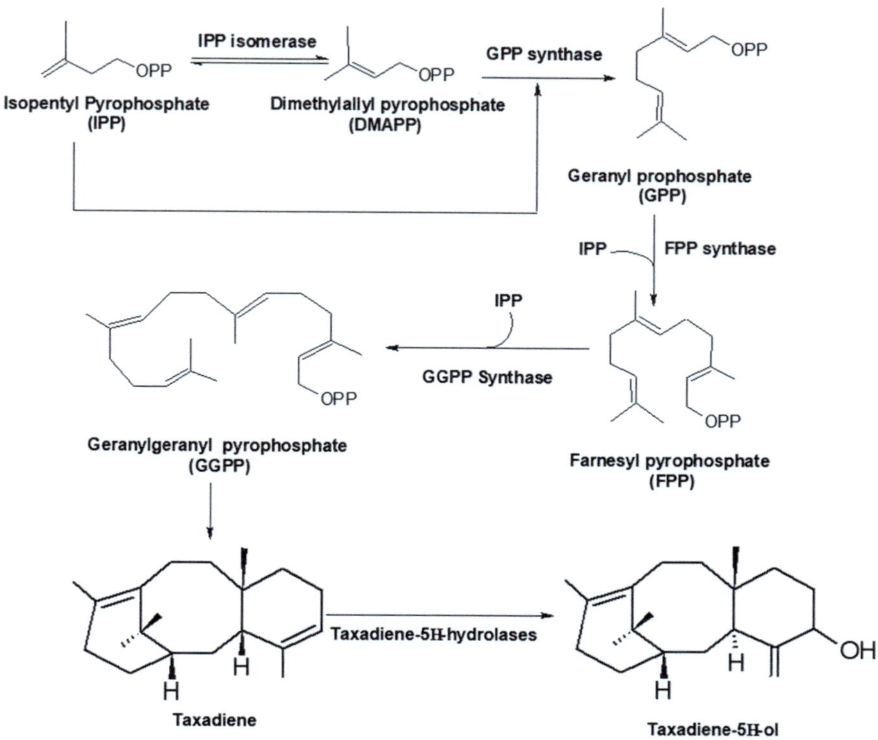

Fig. 10.3 Taxadiene and taxadiene-5α-ol biosynthesis

Table 10.1 Summary of titer, engineered microbe, and production time of Taxol production from engineered microbes

Isoprenoid	Engineered microbes	Titer	Time	References
Taxadiene	*E. coli*	1.3 mg/L	N.A.	[89]
		1 g/L	120 h	[69]
		26.77 mg/L	120 h	[91]
	S. cerevisiae	1 mg/L	65 h	[90]
		8.7 mg/L	N.A.	[82]
Taxadiene-5α-ol	*E. coli*	58 mg/L	100 h	[69]
	S. cerevisiae	~25 μg/L	65 h	[90]

between the upper and lower DXP pathway modules. Identifying the best combination, an engineered *E. coli* is expressed to build a yield of 1.0 g/L taxadiene [69] (Table 10.1). To convert taxadiene into Taxol, a chimeric fusion protein product of CYP450, taxadiene-5α-hydroxylase from *Taxus cuspidate* with its CYP450 reductase (CPR) counterpart, could be expressed in taxadiene-producing strains. A ~58 mg/L taxadiene-5α-ol titer is obtained from resultant strain [69], which is ~2400-fold higher than the previously reported titers in *S. cerevisiae* [90] (Table 10.1). Later, Boghigian et al. [91] have applied a computational approach to increase taxadiene production in *E. coli* [91] by utilizing a variation of minimization of metabolic adjustment (MoMA) algorithm. Though the study has been unable to surpass the taxadiene levels beyond the previously achieved titers [69]; it has identified four targets (outside of the native DXP pathway), which could be utilized together with MMPE for improved cofactor supply for an improved taxadiene accumulation.

10.5.1 *B. subtilis:* A Potential Host for Terpenoid-Based Anticancer Pharmaceuticals

Although, *E. coli* is the most suitable host to achieve higher titers of isoprenoid-based metabolites due to advanced genetic tools available for fine-tuning multiple gene expression, its non-GRAS (generally regarded as safe) status is a major barrier for the commercial production of isoprenoid-based flavors, pharmaceuticals, and their precursors. The rapid expansion of genomics tools provides opportunities to exploit GRAS status microorganisms for the production of desired metabolites [92]. Several alternate microbes such as *B. subtilis*, *Corynebacterium glutamicum*, and *S. cerevisiae* have been explored for the nonnatural production of isoprenoid-based metabolites (such as amorphadiene, pinene, and bisabolene) [92, 93]. This enables researchers to grasp advantages of their desirable properties with simultaneous overexpression of isoprenoid-based metabolites [92, 94–96]. Among the infinite treasure of microbes, nature has gifted a few with the capability of decomposing complex sugars into simple ones, while some others have been endowed with the ability to convert sugars into desired metabolites. The plenteous genetic modifications not only improve product titers but also extend the variety of isoprenoid-based metabolites from alternate microbial hosts [92, 96–99]. Extracting the data regarding the terpenoid biosynthesis pathways of microorganisms in Pubmed, *Bacillales* is found to encode more number of genes and proteins related to terpenoid biosynthesis [97]. However, studies devoted to isoprenoid-based metabolites production from *Bacillales* are a few [99–101].

B. subtilis is a spore-forming gram-positive bacterium and is the member of *Bacillales*. It could be a potential alternate for the isopentenol production due to its GRAS status and rapid growth rate. In addition, it has an innate ability to produce desired metabolites by utilizing a vast array of substrate ranging from glucose to economical carbon feed stocks [100]. Besides these, it has competence to withstand the harsh pH and temperature stress conditions of fermentation process. Most importantly, it yields ~18-fold higher isoprene than *E. coli* and is reported as one among the highest isoprene-producing bacteria [102, 103]. Recently, we have engineered *B. subtilis* strain for the production of hemiterpene alcohols, isopentenol (isoprenol and prenol) by overexpressing endogenous *DXS* and *nudF* genes [104]. Production of higher-carbon number isoprenoid has also been limitedly studied in *B. subtilis* [99, 101]. Yoshida's group has reported the production of C30 carotenoids by incorporating carotenoid synthetic genes *crtM* and *crtN* of *S. aureus* into *B. subtilis* [101]. Production of C30 carotenoids has been further improved by systematic overexpression of DXP pathway genes [99].

10.5.2 IspA: A Key Enzyme for Precursor Supply

As discussed earlier, enzyme engineering of the host's pathway has improved production of a wide range of terpenoids from microbes. It has also been shown that DXP pathway is stoichiometrically more competent than the MVA pathway [105]; however, the titers achieved to date by optimizing DXP pathway [83, 92] do not surpass the level that has been achieved by the expression of heterologous MVA pathway [85, 106]. To produce terpenoid for pharmaceutical application, a GRAS status microbe such as *B. subtilis* is required, and as it is a poor host for heterologous gene expressions, there is always a need to fine-tune the endogenous terpenoid pathway. It is discussed earlier that the primary focuses for Taxol production is to enhance the supply of GGPP. Since microbes do not possess GGPPS, the enzyme needs to be incorporated from other organisms. The GGPPS enzyme catalyzes the condensation reaction between IPP and FPP to form GGPP (Fig. 10.4). Microbes synthesize FPP directly from IPP and DMAPP by an enzyme known as IspA, which is also responsible for GPP synthesis in prokaryotes and simultaneously uptake of GPP to form FPP [107]. Engineering upstream terpenoid pathways in microbial host improves IPP and DMAPP supply for downstream enzymes. In this way, IspA becomes a key enzyme for the supply of FPP to heterologous GPPS.

To increase precursor flux toward higher terpenoid production, IspA enzyme has been overexpressed in microbial hosts [86, 108, 109]. Overexpression of endogenous IspA could utilize the excess IPP and DMAPP to increase FPP flux. There can be two possible stereospecific configurations (E and Z) in an elongating chain of terpenoid. Thus, FPPS can catalyze the formation FPP in four different potential configurations (E,E, E,Z, Z,E, and Z,Z) [110]. It has been found that the endogenous IspA catalyzes the formation of all E configurations of FPP [107], which can be utilized by endogenous enzymes to form other essential terpenoids. However, the Z,E-isoform of FPP cannot be metabolized by microbial host for the synthesis of its essential isoprenoids [111]. Utilization of such isomers of FPP could reduce precursors' flux toward unwanted terpenoid products and minimize metabolic wastes during the desired terpenoid production. To synthesize Z,E-FPP, a heterologous Z,E-FPP synthase (Rv1086) from *Mycobacterium tuberculosis* have been introduced in engineered *E. coli*. Expression of Rv1086 has produced Z,E-isoform of the final product (farnesol); but the production is found to be lower than the E,E-isoform that has been achieved from overexpression of endogenous IspA enzyme. Although the coexpression of Rv1086 with endogenous IspA is found to improve the total

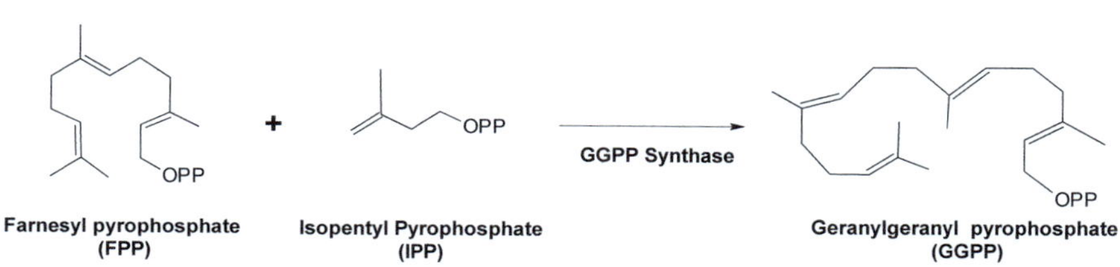

Fig. 10.4 Reaction catalyzed by GGPP synthase

FPP flux in the engineered strain, it reduces Z,E-isoform of the product and it might be due to the consumption of GPP by IspA. Fusion protein expression of Rv1086 with endogenous IspA has been shown to improve the Z,E-FPP flux by increasing GPP availability to Rv1068 [111]. IspA is thus found to be an important enzyme toward the precursor supply for higher terpenoid production in microbial hosts. Fusion protein product of IspA with other terpenoid-specific enzymes such as farnesene synthase has resulted in an improved yield of the final product [86]. Fusion protein expression of IspA with heterologous GGPPS could also be an attractive target to improve GGPP flux toward Taxol/taxadiene production. Even when the experimental structures of these vital proteins are unavailable, the protein structure prediction methodologies should be appropriately deployed to construct their biologically correct model for their detailed functional excavation [112, 113].

10.5.3 In Silico Functional Analysis of IspA

As discussed, FPPS or IspA, catalyzing the formation of farnesyl diphosphate (FPP), is used as precursor for many essential metabolites. As *Bacillus subtilis* is the majorly deployed microbial host industrially. Therefore, in this section in silico functional analysis of *B. Subtilis* IspA protein (NP_390308.2; 296-residues) is considered from the subspecies str. 168. For excavating the detailed structural and functional roles of this protein, the sequence is firstly screened against the conserved signatures of the protein families by InterProScan5 [114]. On basis of homology, the sequence is found to be the member of isoprenoid synthase domain superfamily (IPR008949), and 7-276 residue segment is found to encode the terpenoid synthase domain. Moreover, the PFAM search [115] shows that the 32-268 segment is found to be the member of polyprenyl synthetase (PF00348).

The important physicochemical properties, viz., atomic and residue composition, molecular weight, estimated half-life, extinction coefficient, aliphatic index, theoretical isoelectric point (pI), and instability index, are important properties of every protein to allow its easy experimental discrimination. These properties are estimated by ProtParam from the ExPASY server [116]. The results show that molecular weight of this protein is 32.503 kDa. Theoretical isoelectric point (pI) is found to be 5.28, which indicates that this protein should be a bit acidic in nature. It refers to the pH where the overall net charge of the FPPS protein becomes 0, and hence the pI of 5.28 depicts a bit acidic nature. Within this 296-residue protein, the negatively and positively charged residues are orderly found to be 49 and 37, and logically impart an overall negative charge for the protein. The extinction coefficient value is estimated to be 9190 which refers to the quantity of light that might be possibly absorbed by the FPPS at 280 nm. The instability index value is found to be 37.23, and it shows that the protein is quite stable to indicate that it is a great choice for the enhanced production of the anticancer compound.

For the lack of FPPS structure in the protein data bank, it is predicted through the template-based modeling strategy. Deploying its HMM-based sequence profile by the HHpred algorithm [117], the best functionally similar template 5AYP_B (Length: 297) is considered on basis of the template-ranking strategy [118]. This farnesyl diphosphate synthase (E.C.2.5.1.10) from *Geobacillus stearothermophilus* shows an *E*-value cutoff of 3.4E^{-46}, and it is found to show a coverage span and sequence identity of 100% and 57.24%, respectively. The homology model of the complete FPPS protein is constructed using MODELLER9.19 [119] through its HMM-profile alignment. To remove the nonphysical localized atomic clashes, the predicted model is iteratively sampled by effectively sampling its energetic landscape [120]. The predicted model and not simply its domain topology is subsequently assessed through ERRAT (http://servicesn.mbi.ucla.edu/ERRAT/) and MolProbity [121], and it orderly shows the scores of 94.0559 and 2.67. While the ERRAT analyzes the statistics of non-bonded interactions among different atom types through the error value computed for the 9-residue sliding window, the MolProbity score assesses atomic clashes, non-favored Ramachandran map, and bad side-chain rotamers with a log-weighted measure and indicates the estimated crystallographic resolution for obtaining such scores. As these protein structures have been found to be functionally active as homodimers, the functional active state of the constructed protein model is also constructed on basis of the 5AYP structure along with a subsequent refinement. The monomeric and dimeric states are shown in Fig. 10.5. Further, the Ramachandran map of this protein is evaluated by RAMPAGE server [122], and 97.9% of residues are found to be within the most-favored and allowed regions, and it also indicates a substantial stability of this protein.

10.6 Evolutionary Conservation Analysis

As the functionally important residues are usually conserved throughout evolution, the evolutionary conservation of the FPPS protein is estimated on basis of the constructed structure of the FPPS protein. ConSurf server [123] is deployed through the

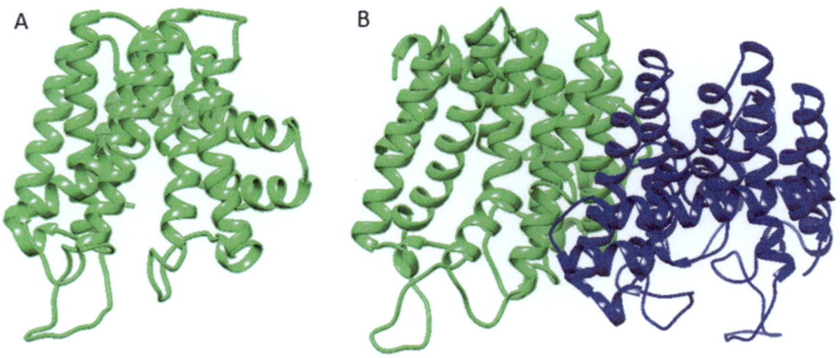

Fig. 10.5 Predicted near-native conformation of the (**a**) monomeric (**b**) dimeric FPPS protein

following set of parameters. For finding the functionally most relevant sites, HMMER is deployed to construct the HMM profile on basis of three iterative rounds and *E*-value cutoff of 0.0001, and the UniRef90 sequence dataset is screened to find the most reliable sequence homologues. The top 100 evolutionarily closest sequences, mutually sharing a sequence identity of 35–95%, are subsequently aligned through MAFFT-L-INS-I. Bayesian method is used to calculate the conservation scores by considering the best model as the evolutionary substitution model.

Through ConSurf, the evolutionary conservation of FPPS protein is analyzed through their resultant conservation score computed on basis of statistical inference methods and machine learning. Conservation scores are mapped onto the protein's surface with a coloring scheme (Fig. 10.6). While the average conservation is marked white, the most conserved and variable loci are respectively marked as maroon and turquoise.

Analyzing the conservation scores across the constructed MSA profile, it is found that the average pairwise distance among the sequence is 1.50966, with the lower and upper bound being 0.209714 and 2.62774, respectively. It defines the average number of residue replacements among any two sequences in the alignment, and thus 0.01 distance indicates that 1 substitution is expected for every 100 positions on an average. Moreover, it is found that the residues D85, D86, D91, R96, K182, and D224 are completely conserved in this class, and the loci L27, D132, E153, and S248 are least conserved. These residue sets are orderly marked blue and red in Fig. 10.7 to show their structural positions.

To date, several microorganisms, including *B. subtilis*, have been modified for the nonnatural production of therapeutic terpenoids, and significant improvements in terms of titers have also been achieved from them. Nonetheless, there is far to go for their commercialization, as the current modern industrial policies are volume dependent. To achieve successful commercialization of terpenoid-based therapeutic, various modern approaches including MMPE, MoME, and saturation mutagenesis can be explored in coordination with fluxomics, metabolomics, and bioprocess techniques.

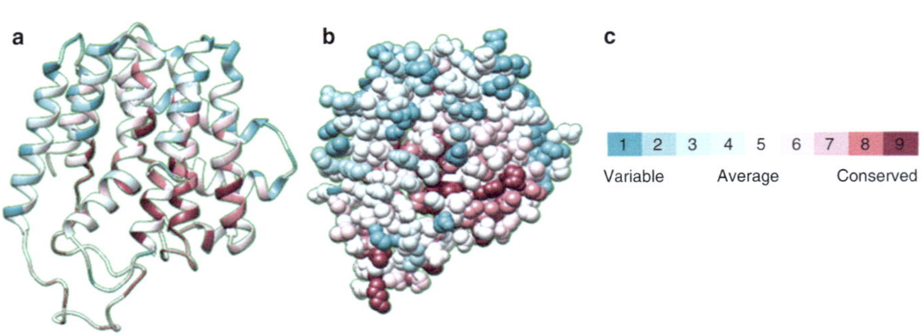

Fig. 10.6 The evolutionary conservation profile of (**a**) FPPS protein (**b**) space-filling model are represented as per the conservation score on basis of (**c**) coloring scheme shown as color-coding bar

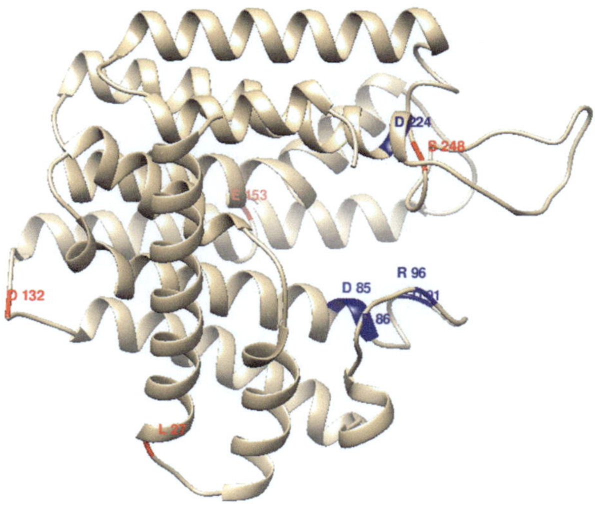

Fig. 10.7 Most conserved (blue) and the least conserved (red) residue sets in the FPPS protein

References

1. Ajikumar PK, Tyo K, Carlsen S, Mucha O, Phon TH, Stephanopoulos G (2008) Terpenoids: opportunities for biosynthesis of natural product drugs using engineered microorganisms. Mol Pharm 5:167–190
2. Breitmaier E (2006) Terpenes: flavors, fragrances, pharmaca, pheromones. Wiley, Weinheim
3. George KW, Alonso-Gutierrez J, Keasling JD, Lee TS (2015) Isoprenoid drugs, biofuels, and chemicals-artemisinin, farnesene, and beyond. Adv Biochem Eng Biotechnol:355–389. https://doi.org/10.1007/10_2014_288
4. Hillier SG, Lathe R (2019) Terpenes, hormones, and life: isoprene rule revisited. J Endocrinol 242:R9–R22. https://doi.org/10.1530/joe-19-0084
5. Burke YD, Stark MJ, Roach SL, Sen SE, Crowell PL (1997) Inhibition of pancreatic cancer growth by the dietary isoprenoids farnesol and geraniol. Lipids 32:151–156
6. He L, Mo H, Hadisusilo S, Qureshi AA, Elson CE (1997) Isoprenoids suppress the growth of murine B16 melanomas in vitro and in vivo. J Nutr 127:668–674
7. Huang M, Lu JJ, Huang MQ, Bao JL, Chen XP, Wang YT (2012) Terpenoids: natural products for cancer therapy. Expert Opin Investig Drugs 21(12):1801–1818
8. Ludwiczuk A, Skalicka-Woźniak K, Georgiev MI (2017) Terpenoids. In: Badal S, Delgoda R (eds) Pharmacognosy. Elsevier, pp 233–266. https://doi.org/10.1016/B978-0-12-802104-0.00011-1
9. Katsuki H, Bloch K (1967) Studies on the biosynthesis of ergosterol in yeast: formation of methylated intermediates. J Biol Chem 242:222–227
10. Lynen F (1967) Biosynthetic pathways from acetate to natural products. Pure Appl Chem 14:137–168
11. Eisenreich W, Menhard B, Hylands PJ, Zenk MH, Bacher A (1996) Studies on the biosynthesis of Taxol: the taxane carbon skeleton is not of mevalonoid origin. Proc Natl Acad Sci U S A 93:6431–6436
12. Rohdich F, Zepeck F, Adam P, Hecht S, Kaiser J, Laupitz R, Grawert T, Amslinger S, Eisenreich W, Bacher A, Arigoni D (2002) The deoxyxylulose phosphate pathway of iso-

prenoid biosynthesis: studies on the mechanisms of the reactions catalyzed by IspG and IspH protein. Proc Natl Acad Sci U S A 100:1586–1591

13. Miziorko HM (2011) Enzymes of the mevalonate pathway of isoprenoid biosynthesis. Arch Biochem Biophys 505:131–143. https://doi.org/10.1016/j.abb.2010.09.028
14. Ferguson JJ, Rudney H (1959) The biosynthesis of β-hydroxy-β-methylglutaryl coenzyme A in yeast: I. Identification and purification of the hydroxymethylglutaryl coenzyme-condensing enzyme. J Biol Chem 234:1072–1075
15. Durr IF, Rudney H (1960) The reduction of β-hydroxy-β-methylglutaryl coenzyme A to mevalonic acid. J Biol Chem 235:2572–2578
16. Tchen TT (1958) Mevalonic kinase: purification and purification. J Biol Chem 233:1100–1103
17. Helling H, Popjak G (1961) Studies on the biosynthesis of cholesterol: XIII. Phosphomevalonic kinase from liver. J. Lipid Res 2:235–243
18. Bloch K, Chaykin S, Phillips AH, De Waard A (1959) Mevalonic acid pyrophosphate and isopentenyl pyrophosphate. J Biol Chem 234:2595–2604
19. Wilding EI, Brown JR, Bryant AP, Chalker AF, Holmes DJ, Ingraham KA, Iordanescu S, So CY, Rosenberg M, Gwynn MN (2000) Identification, evolution, and essentiality of the mevalonate pathway for isopentenyl diphosphate biosynthesis in gram-positive cocci. J Bacteriol 182:4319–4327
20. Hunter WN (2007) The non-mevalonate pathway of isoprenoid precursor biosynthesis. J Biol Chem 282:21573–21577. https://doi.org/10.1074/jbc.R700005200
21. Rohdich F, Hecht S, Gärtner K, Adam P, Krieger C, Amslinger S, Arigoni D, Bacher A, Eisenreich W (2002) Studies on the nonmevalonate terpene biosynthetic pathway: metabolic role of IspH (LytB) protein. Proc Natl Acad Sci U S A 99:1158–1163. https://doi.org/10.1073/pnas.032658999
22. Lange BM, Wildung MR, McCaskill D, Croteau R (1998) A family of transketolases that directs isoprenoid biosynthesis via a mevalonate-independent pathway. Proc Natl Acad Sci U S A 95:2100–2104. https://doi.org/10.1073/pnas.95.5.2100
23. Lange BM, Croteau R (1999) Isoprenoid biosynthesis via a mevalonate-independent pathway in plants: cloning and heterologous expression of 1-deoxy-D-xylulose-5-phosphate reductoisomerase from peppermint. Arch Biochem Biophys 365:170–174
24. Rohdich F, Wungsintaweekul J, Fellermeier M, Sagner S, Herz S, Kis K, Eisenreich W, Bacher A, Zenk MH (1999) Cytidine 5′-triphosphate-dependent biosynthesis of isoprenoids: YgbP protein of *Escherichia coli* catalyzes the formation of 4-diphosphocytidyl-2-C-methylerythritol. Proc Natl Acad Sci U S A 96:11758–11763
25. Lüttgen H, Rohdich F, Herz S, Wungsintaweekul J, Hecht S, Schuhr CA, Fellermeier M, Sagner S, Zenk MH, Bacher A, Eisenreich W (2000) Biosynthesis of terpenoids: YchB protein of *Escherichia coli* phosphorylates the 2-hydroxy group of 4-diphosphocytidyl-2C-methyl-D-erythritol. Proc Natl Acad Sci U S A 97:1062–1067
26. Herz S, Wungsintaweekul J, Schuhr CA, Hecht S, Lüttgen H, Sagner S, Fellermeier M, Eisenreich W, Zenk MH, Bacher A, Rohdich F (2000) Biosynthesis of terpenoids: YgbB protein converts 4-diphosphocytidyl-2C-methyl-D-erythritol 2-phosphate to 2C-methyl-D-erythritol 2,4-cyclodiphosphate. Proc Natl Acad Sci U S A 97:2486–2490
27. Lesgards JF, Baldovini N, Vidal N, Pietri S (2014) Anticancer activities of essential oils constituents and synergy with conventional therapies: a review. Phytother Res 28(10):1423–1446
28. Sun J (2007) D-limonene: safety and clinical applications. Altern Med Rev 12(3):259
29. Clegg RJ, Middleton B, Bell GD, White DA (1982) The mechanism of cyclic monoterpene inhibition of hepatic 3-hydroxy-3-methylglutaryl coenzyme A reductase in vivo in the rat. J Biol Chem 257(5):2294–2299
30. Kawata S, Nagase T, Yamasaki E, Ishiguro H, Matsuzawa Y (1994) Modulation of the mevalonate pathway and cell growth by pravastatin and d-limonene in a human hepatoma cell line (Hep G2). Br J Cancer 69(6):1015

31. Ji J, Zhang L, Wu YY, Zhu XY, Lv SQ, Sun XZ (2006) Induction of apoptosis by d-limonene is mediated by a caspase-dependent mitochondrial death pathway in human leukemia cells. Leuk Lymphoma 47(12):2617–2624
32. Liu D, Chen Z (2009) The effects of cantharidin and cantharidin derivates on tumour cells. Anticancer Agents Med Chem 9(4):392–396
33. Chen YN, Chen JC, Yin SC, Wang GS, Tsauer W, Hsu SF, Hsu SL (2002) Effector mechanisms of norcantharidin-induced mitotic arrest and apoptosis in human hepatoma cells. Int J Cancer 100(2):158–165
34. Huan SKH, Lee HH, Liu DZ, Wu CC, Wang CC (2006) Cantharidin-induced cytotoxicity and cyclooxygenase 2 expression in human bladder carcinoma cell line. Toxicology 223(1-2):136–143
35. Huh JE, Kang KS, Chae C, Kim HM, Ahn KS, Kim SH (2004) Roles of p38 and JNK mitogen-activated protein kinase pathways during cantharidin-induced apoptosis in U937 cells. Biochem Pharmacol 67(10):1811–1818
36. Li W, Chen Z, Zong Y, Gong F, Zhu Y, Zhu Y, Lv J, Zhang J, Xie L, Sun Y, Miao Y, Tao M, Han X, Xu Z (2011) PP2A inhibitors induce apoptosis in pancreatic cancer cell line PANC-1 through persistent phosphorylation of IKKα and sustained activation of the NF-κB pathway. Cancer Lett 304(2):117–127
37. Li W, Xie L, Chen Z, Zhu Y, Sun Y, Miao Y, Xu Z, Han X (2010) Cantharidin, a potent and selective PP2A inhibitor, induces an oxidative stress-independent growth inhibition of pancreatic cancer cells through G2/M cell-cycle arrest and apoptosis. Cancer Sci 101(5):1226–1233
38. Chen T, Li M, Zhang R, Wang H (2009) Dihydroartemisinin induces apoptosis and sensitizes human ovarian cancer cells to carboplatin therapy. J Cell Mol Med 13(7):1358–1370
39. Hou J, Wang D, Zhang R, Wang H (2008) Experimental therapy of hepatoma with artemisinin and its derivatives: in vitro and in vivo activity, chemosensitization, and mechanisms of action. Clin Cancer Res 14(17):5519–5530
40. Buommino E, Baroni A, Canozo N, Petrazzuolo M, Nicoletti R, Vozza A, Tufano MA (2009) Artemisinin reduces human melanoma cell migration by down-regulating αvβ3 integrin and reducing metalloproteinase 2 production. Investig New Drugs 27(5):412–418
41. Rasheed SAK, Efferth T, Asangani IA, Allgayer H (2010) First evidence that the antimalarial drug artesunate inhibits invasion and in vivo metastasis in lung cancer by targeting essential extracellular proteases. Int J Cancer 127(6):1475–1485
42. Zhou L, Zuo Z, Chow MSS (2005) Danshen: an overview of its chemistry, pharmacology, pharmacokinetics, and clinical use. J Clin Pharmacol 45(12):1345–1359
43. Jiao JW, Wen F (2011) Tanshinone IIA acts via p38 MAPK to induce apoptosis and the down-regulation of ERCC1 and lung-resistance protein in cisplatin-resistant ovarian cancer cells. Oncol Rep 25(3):781–788
44. Lee DH, Iwanski GB, Thoennissen NH (2010) Cucurbitacin: ancient compound shedding new light on cancer treatment. Sci World J 10:413–418
45. Lee WY, Cheung CC, Liu KW, Fung KP, Wong J, Lai PB, Yeung JH (2010) Cytotoxic effects of tanshinones from Salvia miltiorrhiza on doxorubicin-resistant human liver cancer cells. J Nat Prod 73(5):854–859
46. Leuenroth SJ, Okuhara D, Shotwell JD, Markowitz GS, Yu Z, Somlo S, Crews CM (2007) Triptolide is a traditional Chinese medicine-derived inhibitor of polycystic kidney disease. Proc Natl Acad Sci 104(11):4389–4394
47. McCallum C, Kwon S, Leavitt P, Shen DM, Liu W, Gurnett A (2007) Triptolide binds covalently to a 90 kDa nuclear protein. Role of epoxides in binding and activity. Immunobiology 212(7):549–556
48. Titov DV, Gilman B, He QL, Bhat S, Low WK, Dang Y, Smeaton M, Demain AL, Miller PS, Kugel JF, Goodrich JA (2011) XPB, a subunit of TFIIH, is a target of the natural product triptolide. Nat Chem Biol 7(3):182

49. Pan DJ, Li ZL, Hu CQ, Chen K, Chang JJ, Lee KH (1990) The cytotoxic principles of Pseudolarix kaempferi: pseudolaric acid-A and-B and related derivatives1. Plantamedica 56(04):383–385
50. Aparicio LMA, Pulido EG, Gallego GA (2012) Vinflunine: a new vision that may translate into antiangiogenic and antimetastatic activity. Anti-Cancer Drugs 23(1):1–11
51. Lim JCW, Chan TK, Ng DS, Sagineedu SR, Stanslas J, Wong WF (2012) Andrographolide and its analogues: versatile bioactive molecules for combating inflammation and cancer. Clin Exp Pharmacol Physiol 39(3):300–310
52. Kuttan G, Pratheeshkumar P, Manu KA, Kuttan R (2011) Inhibition of tumor progression by naturally occurring terpenoids. Pharm Biol 49(10):995–1007
53. Ikezoe T, Yang Y, Bandobashi K, Saito T, Takemoto S, Machida H, Togitani K, Koeffler HP, Taguchi H (2005) Oridonin, a diterpenoid purified from Rabdosiarubescens, inhibits the proliferation of cells from lymphoid malignancies in association with blockade of the NF-κB signal pathways. Mol Cancer Ther 4(4):578–586
54. Jin H, Tan X, Liu X, Ding Y (2011) Downregulation of AP-1 gene expression is an initial event in the oridonin-mediated inhibition of colorectal cancer: studies in vitro and in vivo. J Gastroenterol Hepatol 26(4):706–715
55. Khanna C, Rosenberg M, Vail DM (2015) A review of paclitaxel and novel formulations including those suitable for use in dogs. J Vet Intern Med 29(4):1006–1012
56. Hajek R, Vorlicek J, Slavik M (1996) Paclitaxel (Taxol): a review of its antitumor activity in clinical studies Minireview. Neoplasma 43(3):141–154
57. Zhao Y, Wang SM, Zhang J (2002) Combination chemotherapy with Taxol and cisplatin for 57 patients with non-small cell lung cancer by intraartery and intravenous infusion. Chinese J Cancer 21(12):1365–1367
58. deMagalhaes-Silverman M, Hammert L, Lembersky B, Lister J, Rybka W, Ball E (1998) High-dose chemotherapy and autologous stem cell support followed by post-transplant doxorubicin and Taxol as initial therapy for metastatic breast cancer: hematopoietic tolerance and efficacy. Bone Marrow Transplant 21(12):1207
59. Manfredi JJ, Horwitz SB (1984) Taxol: an antimitotic agent with a new mechanism of action. Pharmacol Ther 25(1):83–125
60. Calixto JB, Campos MM, Otuki MF, Santos AR (2004) Anti-inflammatory compounds of plant origin. Part II. Modulation of pro-inflammatory cytokines, chemokines and adhesion molecules. Plantamedica 70(02):93–103
61. Miro M (1995) Cucurbitacins and their pharmacological effects. Phytother Res 9(3):159–168
62. Hsu HS, Huang PI, Chang YL, Tzao C, Chen YW, Shih HC, Hung SC, Chen YC, Tseng LM, Chiou SH (2011) Cucurbitacin I inhibits tumorigenic ability and enhances radiochemosensitivity in non-small cell lung cancer-derived CD133-positive cells. Cancer 117(13):2970–2985
63. Iwanski GB, Lee DH, En-Gal S, Doan NB, Castor B, Vogt M, Toh M, Bokemeyer C, Said JW, Thoennissen NH, Koeffler HP (2010) Cucurbitacin B, a novel in vivo potentiator of gemcitabine with low toxicity in the treatment of pancreatic cancer. Br J Pharmacol 160(4):998–1007
64. Thoennissen NH, Iwanski GB, Doan NB, Okamoto R, Lin P, Abbassi S, Song JH, Yin D, Toh M, Xie WD, Said JW (2009) Cucurbitacin B induces apoptosis by inhibition of the JAK/STAT pathway and potentiates antiproliferative effects of gemcitabine on pancreatic cancer cells. Cancer Res 69(14):5876–5884
65. Liu T, Zhang M, Zhang H, Sun C, Yang X, Deng Y, Ji W (2008) Combined antitumor activity of cucurbitacin B and docetaxel in laryngeal cancer. Eur J Pharmacol 587(1-3):78–84
66. Giner EM, Máñez S, Recio MC, Giner RM, Cerdá-Nicolás M, Ríos JL (2000) In vivo studies on the anti-inflammatory activity of pachymic and dehydrotumulosic acids. Plantamedica 66(03):221–227
67. Prieto JM, Recio MC, Giner RM, Manez S, Giner-Larza EM, Rios JL (2003) Influence of traditional Chinese anti-inflammatory medicinal plants on leukocyte and platelet functions. J Pharm Pharmacol 55(9):1275–1282

68. Ling H, Zhang Y, Ng KY, Chew EH (2011) Pachymic acid impairs breast cancer cell invasion by suppressing nuclear factor-κB-dependent matrix metalloproteinase-9 expression. Breast Cancer Res Treat 126(3):609–620
69. Ajikumar PK, Xiao W-H, Tyo KEJ, Wang Y, Simeon F, Leonard E, Mucha O, Phon TH, Pfeifer B, Stephanopoulos G (2010) Isoprenoid pathway optimization for Taxol precursor overproduction in *Escherichia coli*. Science 330:70–74. https://doi.org/10.1126/science.1191652
70. Zhou X, Zhu H, Liu L, Lin J, Tang K (2010) A review: recent advances and future prospects of Taxol-producing endophytic fungi. Appl Microbiol Biotechnol 86:1707–1717. https://doi.org/10.1007/s00253-010-2546-y
71. Thomas P, Farjon A (2011) Taxus wallichiana. IUCN Red List Threat. Species. https://doi.org/10.2305/IUCN.UK.2011-2.RLTS.T46171879A9730085.en
72. Li Y, Zhang G, Pfeifer BA (2009) Current and emerging options for Taxol production. In: Schrader J, Bohlmann J (eds) Biotechnology of isoprenoids. Advances in biochemical engineering/biotechnology. Springer, pp 1–35
73. Chandran SS, Kealey JT, Reeves CD (2011) Microbial production of isoprenoids. Process Biochem 46:1703–1710. https://doi.org/10.1016/j.procbio.2011.05.012
74. Gupta P, Phulara SC (2015) Metabolic engineering for isoprenoid-based biofuel production. J Appl Microbiol 119:605–619. https://doi.org/10.1111/jam.12871
75. Tippmann S, Chen Y, Siewers V, Nielsen J (2013) From flavors and pharmaceuticals to advanced biofuels: production of isoprenoids in *Saccharomyces cerevisiae*. Biotechnol J 8:1435–1444. https://doi.org/10.1002/biot.201300028
76. Kusari S, Singh S, Jayabaskaran C (2014) Rethinking production of Taxol W (paclitaxel) using endophyte. Trends Biotechnol 32:304–311
77. Amrein BA, Runthala A, Kamerlin SCL (2019) In silico-directed evolution using CADEE. Methods Mol Biol 1851:381–415
78. Keasling JD (2008) Synthetic biology for synthetic chemistry. ACS Chem Biol 3:64–76
79. Phulara SC, Chaturvedi P, Gupta P (2016) Isoprenoid-based biofuels: homologous expression and heterologous expression in prokaryotes. Appl Environ Microbiol 82:5730–5740. https://doi.org/10.1128/AEM.01192-16
80. Li Y, Pfeifer BA (2014) Heterologous production of plant-derived isoprenoid products in microbes and the application of metabolic engineering and synthetic biology. Curr Opin Plant Biol 19:8–13. https://doi.org/10.1016/j.pbi.2014.02.005
81. Wong J, Rios-solis L, Keasling JD (2017) Microbial production of isoprenoids. In: Lee S (ed) Consequences of microbial interactions with hydrocarbons, oils, and lipids: production of fuels and chemicals, Handbook of hydrocarbon and lipid microbiology. Springer, pp 1–24. https://doi.org/10.1007/978-3-319-31421-1
82. Engels B, Dahm P, Jennewein S (2008) Metabolic engineering of taxadiene biosynthesis in yeast as a first step towards Taxol (paclitaxel) production. Metab Eng 10:201–206. https://doi.org/10.1016/J.YMBEN.2008.03.001
83. Liu H, Wang Y, Tang Q, Kong W, Chung W-J, Lu T (2014) MEP pathway-mediated isopentenol production in metabolically engineered *Escherichia coli*. Microb Cell Factories 13:135. https://doi.org/10.1186/s12934-014-0135-y
84. Zhao J, Li Q, Sun T, Zhu X, Xu H, Tang J, Zhang X, Ma Y (2013) Engineering central metabolic modules of *Escherichia coli* for improving beta-carotene production. Metab Eng 17:42–50. https://doi.org/10.1016/j.ymben.2013.02.002
85. Sarria S, Wong B, Martín HG, Keasling JD, Peralta-Yahya P (2014) Microbial synthesis of pinene. ACS Synth Biol 3:466–475. https://doi.org/10.1021/sb4001382
86. Wang C, Yoon SH, Jang HJ, Chung YR, Kim JY, Choi ES, Kim SW (2011) Metabolic engineering of *Escherichia coli* for α-farnesene production. Metab Eng 13:648–655. https://doi.org/10.1016/j.ymben.2011.08.001
87. Zhou D, Sun J, Yu H, Ping W, Zheng X (2001) *Nodulisporium*, a genus new to China. Mycosystema 20:277–278

88. Croteau R, Ketchum REB, Long RM, Kaspera R, Wildung MR (2006) Taxol biosynthesis and molecular genetics. Phytochem Rev 5:75–97. https://doi.org/10.1007/s11101-005-3748-2
89. Huang Q, Roessner CA, Croteau R, Scott AI (2001) Engineering *Escherichia coli* for the synthesis of taxadiene, a key intermediate in the biosynthesis of Taxol. Bioorg Med Chem 9:2237–2242. https://doi.org/10.1016/S0968-0896(01)00072-4
90. DeJong JHM, Liu Y, Bollon AP, Long RM, Jennewein S, Williams D, Croteau RB (2006) Genetic engineering of Taxol biosynthetic genes in *Saccharomyces cerevisiae*. Biotechnol Bioeng 93:212–224. https://doi.org/10.1002/bit.20694
91. Boghigian BA, Armando J, Salas D, Pfeifer BA (2012) Computational identification of gene over-expression targets for metabolic engineering of taxadiene production. Appl Microbiol Biotechnol 93:2063–2073. https://doi.org/10.1007/s00253-011-3725-1
92. Kang M-K, Eom J-H, Kim Y, Um Y, Woo HM (2014) Biosynthesis of pinene from glucose using metabolically-engineered *Corynebacterium glutamicum*. Biotechnol Lett 36:2069–2077. https://doi.org/10.1007/s10529-014-1578-2
93. Peralta-Yahya PP, Ouellet M, Chan R, Mukhopadhyay A, Keasling JD, Lee TS (2011) Identification and microbial production of a terpene-based advanced biofuel. Nat Commun 2:483. https://doi.org/10.1038/ncomms1494
94. Davies FK, Work VH, Beliaev AS, Posewitz MC (2014) Engineering limonene and bisabolene production in wild type and a glycogen-deficient mutant of *Synechococcus* sp. PCC 7002. Front Bioeng Biotechnol 2:21. https://doi.org/10.3389/fbioe.2014.00021
95. Halfmann C, Gu L, Gibbons W, Zhou R (2014) Genetically engineering cyanobacteria to convert CO2, water, and light into the long-chain hydrocarbon farnesene. Appl Microbiol Biotechnol 98:9869–9877. https://doi.org/10.1007/s00253-014-6118-4
96. Phelan RM, Sekurova ON, Keasling JD, Zotchev SB (2014) Engineering terpene biosynthesis in *Streptomyces* for production of the advanced biofuel precursor bisabolene. ACS Synth Biol 4:393–399. https://doi.org/10.1021/sb5002517
97. Guan Z, Xue D, Abdallah II, Dijkshoorn L, Setroikromo R, Lv G, Quax WJ (2015) Metabolic engineering of *Bacillus subtilis* for terpenoid production. Appl Microbiol Biotechnol 99:9395–9406. https://doi.org/10.1007/s00253-015-6950-1
98. Halfmann C, Gu L, Zhou R (2014) Engineering cyanobacteria for the production of a cyclic hydrocarbon fuel from CO2 and H2O. Green Chem 16:3175–3185. https://doi.org/10.1039/c3gc42591f
99. Xue D, Abdallah II, de Haan IEM, Sibbald MJJB, Quax WJ (2015) Enhanced C30 carotenoid production in *Bacillus subtilis* by systematic overexpression of MEP pathway genes. Appl Microbiol Biotechnol 99:5907–5915. https://doi.org/10.1007/s00253-015-6531-3
100. Xue J, Ahring BK (2011) Enhancing isoprene production by genetic modification of the 1-deoxy-d-xylulose-5-phosphate pathway in *Bacillus subtilis*. Appl Environ Microbiol 77:2399–2405. https://doi.org/10.1128/AEM.02341-10
101. Yoshida K, Ueda S, Maeda I (2009) Carotenoid production in *Bacillus subtilis* achieved by metabolic engineering. Biotechnol Lett 31:1789–1793. https://doi.org/10.1007/s10529-009-0082-6
102. Fall R, Copley SD (2000) Bacterial sources and sinks of isoprene, a reactive atmospheric hydrocarbon. Environ Microbiol 2:123–130
103. Kuzma J, Nemecek-Marshall M, Pollock WH, Fall R (1995) Bacteria produce the volatile hydrocarbon isoprene. Curr Microbiol 30:97–103. https://doi.org/10.1007/BF00294190
104. Phulara SC, Chaurasia D, Diwan B, Chaturvedi P, Gupta P (2018) *In-situ* isopentenol production from *Bacillus subtilis* through genetic and culture condition modulation. Process Biochem 72:47–54
105. Dugar D, Stephanopoulos G (2011) Relative potential of biosynthetic pathways for biofuels and bio-based products. Nat Biotechnol 29:1074–1078. https://doi.org/10.1038/nbt.2055
106. George KW, Thompson MG, Kang A, Baidoo E, Wang G, Chan LJG, Adams PD, Petzold CJ, Keasling JD, Lee TS (2015) Metabolic engineering for the high-yield production of isoprenoid-based C 5 alcohols in *E. coli*. Sci Rep 5:11128. https://doi.org/10.1038/srep11128

107. Fujisaki S, Hara H, Nishimura Y, Horiuchi K, Nishino T (1990) Cloning and nucleotide sequence of the ispA gene responsible for farnesyl diphosphate synthase activity in *Escherichia coli*. J Biochem 108:995–1000
108. Henke NA, Wichmann J, Baier T, Frohwitter J, Lauersen KJ, Risse JM, Peters-Wendisch P, Kruse O, Wendisch VF (2018) Patchoulol production with metabolically engineered *Corynebacterium glutamicum*. Genes (Basel). https://doi.org/10.3390/genes9040219
109. Wang C, Kim JY, Choi ES, Kim SW (2011) Microbial production of farnesol (FOH): current states and beyond. Process Biochem 46:1221–1229. https://doi.org/10.1016/j.procbio.2011.02.020
110. Thulasiram HV, Erickson HK, Poulter CD (2007) Chimeras of two isoprenoid synthases catalyze all four coupling reactions in isoprenoid biosynthesis. Science 316:73–76. https://doi.org/10.1126/science.1137786
111. Wang C, Zhou J, Jang H, Yoon S, Kim J, Lee G, Choi E, Kim S (2013) Engineered heterologous FPP synthases-mediated Z,E-FPP synthesis in *E coli*. Metab Eng 18:53–59. https://doi.org/10.1016/j.ymben.2013.04.002
112. Runthala A (2012) Protein structure prediction: challenging targets for CASP10. J Biomol Struct Dyn 30(5):607–615
113. Runthala A, Chowdhury S (2016) Unsolved problems of ambient computationally intelligent TBM algorithms. In: Hybrid soft computing approaches: research and applications, pp 75-105
114. Madeira F, Park YM, Lee J, Buso N, Gur T, Madhusoodanan N, Basutkar P, Tivey ARN, Potter SC, Finn RD, Lopez R (2019) The EMBL-EBI search and sequence analysis tools APIs in 2019. Nucleic Acids Res 47(W1):W636–W641
115. El-Gebali S, Mistry J, Bateman A, Eddy SR, Luciani A, Potter SC, Qureshi M, Richardson LJ, Salazar GA, Smart A, Sonnhammer ELL, Hirsh L, Paladin L, Piovesan D, Tosatto SCE, Finn RD (2019) The Pfam protein families database in 2019. Nucleic Acids Res 47(D1):D427–D432
116. Artimo P, Jonnalagedda M, Arnold K, Baratin D, Csardi G, de Castro E, Duvaud S, Flegel V, Fortier A, Gasteiger E, Grosdidier A, Hernandez C, Ioannidis V, Kuznetsov D, Liechti R, Moretti S, Mostaguir K, Redaschi N, Rossier G, Xenarios I, Stockinger H (2012) ExPASy: SIB bioinformatics resource portal. Nucleic Acids Res 40(W1):W597–W603
117. Zimmermann L, Stephens A, Nam SZ, Rau D, Kübler J, Lozajic M, Gabler F, Söding J, Lupas AN, Alva V (2018) A completely reimplemented MPI bioinformatics toolkit with a new HHpred server at its core. J Mol Biol 430(15):2237–2243
118. Runthala A, Chowdhury S (2019) Refined template selection and combination algorithm significantly improves template-based modeling accuracy. J Bioinforma Comput Biol 17(2):1950006–1950006
119. Webb B, Sali A (2016) Comparative protein structure modeling using MODELLER. Curr Protoc Bioinformatics 54:5.6.1–5.6.37
120. Runthala A, Chowdhury S (2014) Iterative optimal TM_Score and Z_Score guided sampling significantly improves model topology, lecture notes in engineering and computer science: proceedings of the international multiconference of engineers and computer scientists, Hong Kong, 2014, pp 123–128
121. Chen VB, Arendall WB 3rd, Headd JJ, Keedy DA, Immormino RM, Kapral GJ, Murray LW, Richardson JS, Richardson DC (2010) MolProbity: all-atom structure validation for macromolecular crystallography. Acta Crystallogr D Biol Crystallogr 66(1):12–21
122. Lovell SC, Davis IW, Arendall WB III, De Bakker PI, Word JM, Prisant MG, Richardson DC (2003) Structure validation by Cα geometry: ϕ, ψ and Cβdeviation. Proteins 50(3):437–450
123. Ashkenazy H, Abadi S, Martz E, Chay O, Mayrose I, Pupko T, Ben-Tal N (2016) ConSurf 2016: an improved methodology to estimate and visualize evolutionary conservation inmacromolecules. Nucleic Acids Res 44:344–350

Translational Research in Oncology

11

Asma Saleem Qazi, Samina Akbar, Rida Fatima Saeed,
and Muhammad Zeeshan Bhatti

11.1 Cancer Biomarker Identification and Risk Assessment

11.1.1 Introduction

During the last decades, there has been a tremendous increase in knowledge and molecular technologies to study cancer biomarkers. Understanding and developing biomarkers are important for patients' usage, which can be accepted in routine medical practice. Biomarker is defined by the National Cancer Institute (NCI) as "a biological molecule found in blood, other bodily fluids, or tissues that is a sign of a normal or abnormal process, or of a condition or diseases" (https://www.cancer.gov/publications/dictionaries/cancer-terms/def/biomarker?redirect=true) in the case of cancer. This definition has been expanded and involved the characteristics of biological molecules that can be accurately measured and evaluated as an indicator of normal and pathological mechanisms, molecular interactions, or pharmacological responses to a therapeutic intervention [1]. There are two main classifications of biomarkers: biomarkers of exposure (applied in risk prediction) and biomarkers of disease such as screening, monitoring, and diagnosis of disease [2]. Biomarkers present an important tool for detecting and monitoring disease state from normal state. During the progression of disease, biomarkers act as the hallmark of the physical state of cell at a given time [3]. They can be found in circulation (blood plasma), excretion/secretions (stool, saliva, nipple discharge, or urine) and are noninvasive or minimally invasive compared to biopsy or screening evaluation of cancer.

A. S. Qazi (✉) · S. Akbar · R. F. Saeed · M. Z. Bhatti (✉)
Department of Biological Sciences, National University of Medical Sciences, Rawalpindi, Pakistan
e-mail: asma.qazi@numspak.edu.pk; samina.akbar@numspak.edu.pk; rida.saeed@numspak.edu.pk; zeeshan.bhatti@numspak.edu.pk

N. Masood, S. Shakil Malik (eds.), *'Essentials of Cancer Genomic, Computational Approaches and Precision Medicine*,
https://doi.org/10.1007/978-981-15-1067-0_11

There is a diverse range of available biomarkers, including proteins (enzymes), nucleic acids (microRNA), DNA sequence (germline or somatic), miRNA antibodies, peptides, or metabolic products [4, 5]. High-throughput proteomic technologies, for example, mass spectrometry and microarrays, have been applied with other techniques to identify candidate markers in cancer biology, tumor microenvironment, or molecular pathway. With these techniques, a lot of data is generated which highlights the need to monitor study design and analyses, in order to reduce the false-positive results [5]. However, there are some limitations such as insensitivity toward low-quantity biomarkers, and therefore, the reduced biological heterogeneity found in cancer is important to achieve the best outcome of cancer proteome mining [6]. These issues may often be hindered by the use of the ultraviolet laser microscope system with pressure catapulting for cell populations, or flow cytometry, which is another powerful technique employed for cell sorting, counting, and biomarker detection [7, 8]. Methods for sample processing are helpful to analyze proteins and are essential to capture critical biomarker information for detection and risk assessment [9].

Biomarkers are also beneficial in risk assessment, monitoring, or detecting cancer. Hereditary and environmental exposures (i.e., infectious agents or carcinogens) play an important role to modulate cancer risk over a period of time. Various tumor-suppressor genes, oncogenes, and microRNA genes in malignant cells either develop or alter during cancer progressions [10]. Hence, it is important to know the risk biomarkers or non-cancer biomarkers for early detection and risk assessment of cancer [11]. In high risk early breast cancer patient, the serum samples from 81 patients indicated 83% of patients for metastatic relapse and might be an important prognostic factor in high risk early breast cancer [12]. It can be concluded that proteomic technologies identify new cancer biomarkers not only for risk assessment but also for therapeutic interventions and early detection. In advance epithelial malignancies, there is an accumulation of a large number of genomic abnormalities that is not present in normal cells, such as mutations, loss of heterozygosity, and aneuploidy [13–15]. This provides significant insights for understanding the evolution of cell changes from normal to cancerous state, and therefore the suitable biomarkers are necessary for cancer risk predictions and early cancer diagnosis.

11.1.2 Cancer Heterogeneity and Diagnosis at Early Stage

It is well-known that cancer is not developed from only one type of cell; rather different types of cancer cells are developed and usually consist of multiple distinct subtypes. Cell-to-cell variability has introduced a different progression level of cancers, such as drug resistance, early-stage diagnosis, and evolution of the disease. Yet it is difficult to access and detect cancer heterogeneity [16].

Some scientists of the field consider cancer heterogeneity as one of the crucial points in understanding the disease process and designing the treatment especially the personalized medicine approach for patients' treatment. Proteomic techniques revealed that most of the biomarkers do not show heterogeneity, but it mostly depends upon the cell type [17]. It is suggested that combining techniques such as MALDI with imaging mass spectroscopy (MALDI-IMS) allow both cancer- and patient-specific information for specific tissue classification in terms of heterogeneity, cell morphology, and biomarker discovery [18, 19]. These techniques also allow creating peptide reference datasets that can help in identifying the specific cancer types linked with peptides, yet the limitation of this technique is low signal-to-noise ratio and mass accuracy [19]. A biopsy-related simulation procedure was discovered by Shipitsin and his coworkers for identifying cancer cell aggregates through biomarker identification irrespective of different types of cancer [20].

Cancer survival rate depends on its early diagnosis, i.e., if the cancer is diagnosed between Stage 0 to Stage I, the survival rate reaches to 90%, whereas it decreases about 10% at Stage IV diagnosis. The high mortality rate of the disease is due to the absence of major symptoms especially at an early stage [21]. These findings clearly indicate the importance of biomarker research in the field whether it is of biomarkers associated at different stages of cancers as diagnostic biomarker, assessing clinical prognosis and disease recurrence as prognostic biomarkers, disease monitoring and treatment response as surveillance biomarkers, or relative to treatment and patient response to treatment as predictive biomarkers [22]. Clear understanding of cancer heterogeneity and its effect on the disease progression may serve as a way forward for early-stage diagnosis and development of drug system in cancer treatment in the future.

11.1.3 Determining Factors of Tumor Spread and Risk Assessment

Cancer is the leading cause of death with 18.1 million new cases and 9.6 million cancer-associated deaths reported in 2018 [23]. Overall, 90% of human malignancies are derived from epithelial cells. In addition, due to the heterogeneity associated with the biological and clinical aspects of most tumors, an increased understanding about their development and progression may improve diagnostic and therapeutic strategies [24]. In general, cancer cells escape the normal regulatory mechanisms that control cell division. This multistep process of tumorigenesis involves in the mutations and other genetic changes that result in the expression of dominantly acting proto-oncogenes or a downregulation of tumor suppressor genes [25]. Moreover, an accumulation of mutations leads to the deregulation of cell cycle, inhibition of apoptosis, and an enhanced ability of cells to invade in surrounding tissues and metastasize to distant sites [26]. The oncogenes are amended form of normal genes known as proto-oncogenes, which regulate the normal growth and differentiation of cells. Proton products of proto-oncogenes are in many cases involved in signaling processes in the cell. Among the products of the proto-oncogenes are growth factors and their receptors (s-sis, cerbB, c-Met), small G-proteins (c-Ras), nuclear transcription factors (c-Fos, c-Jun), and protein kinases (c-Raf) [27]. Alterations in proto-oncogenes such as deletions, translocations, mutations, and amplifications lead to an uncontrolled cellular signaling. The tumor suppressor genes, such as p53, are frequently involved in the inhibition of cellular proliferation in various types of human cancers [28]. Proteomic technologies are recently used for the identification and quantification of protein biomarkers to meet the challenges in cancer biology. Cancer cells like normal cells are complex and have a wide range of protein abundance, due to an altered regulation at both transcriptional and posttranslational levels, which are the main factors behind their increased growth and motility [29]. Cancer biomarkers function as the main players in the disease risk assessment in tissue for diagnosis and/or in blood, saliva, and urine to evaluate healthy individuals [30].

Besides this, cancer risk assessment models collect information about the family history including genetic mutations that may be associated with cancer [31, 32]. The genetic risk assessment is critical to identify the individual's higher disease susceptibility that helps the detection at an early stage in order to develop preventive strategies. In this way, the individuals with a genetic disorder may be subjected to genetic testing and counseling in order to help them understand the complications associated with predisposition to cancer. Moreover, newer risk assessment models are also considering the environmental and behavioral factors (smoke, alcohol consumption, lifestyle, exposure to radiation, chemicals, etc.) which are potentially modifiable and contribute in the development of around 90–95% of all cancers [33]. These risk assessment tools include the US NCI colorectal cancer risk detection tool [34]; the NCI breast cancer risk detection tool, which uses the breast cancer risk prediction [35]; and MelaPRO for detecting risk of melanoma [36]. However, due to the limited effectiveness of these tools in cancer screening, the involvement of clinical and the healthcare bodies with appropriate screening procedures must be assured to increase the assessment reliability.

11.1.4 Proteomic Analyses in Different Cancer Types

During the past two decades, there has been enormous development in molecular biology that led us to a better understanding of the molecular, cellular, and genetic bases of various diseases including cancer. The alterations in gene expression can be studied using functional genomics [37]. However, there are some limitations using the genomic analysis, such as the inability to identify the proteins' role at cellular levels [38, 39]. Other limiting factors, including the posttranslational modification events, can add different functional groups to proteins (i.e., sugars) and result in changed protein products. There is variation in the rate of protein synthesis and functions which gives rise to inconsistencies in their correlation [38]. Hence, proteomic techniques have advantages over genomic assays, as it involves direct analysis of cell physiology such as posttranslational modification and hence plays an important role to study cancer pathogenesis.

There is a huge amount of proteins present in a living organism, and it appears that proteomics contributes greatly in understanding various biological mechanisms such as genetic codes, RNA processing (alternative splicing), and many others. For example, neurexins that belong to cell surface protein family are specific for the brain and have more than 1000 isoforms, which are formed due to alternative splicing [40]. To understand the levels of proteins using proteomics is very important, i.e., some messenger RNAs are non-coding, and as a result there is no formation of protein products; sequence data are limited to give information about pseudogenes, protein modifications, protein stability, and degradation rate [38, 39, 41]. The early progress in DNA microarray technology has encouraged the development of a wide range of arrays, which contributes greatly to the detailed study of protein fields of modern proteomic analysis [42]. Though the two-dimensional gel electrophoresis (2DE) technique with MS has provided valuable information about various proteins, the clinical benefits of this technique in proteomic studies are limited. The technical challenges associated with this technique include difficulties in the reproducibility of 2D gels and in identifying the lower abundance of target proteins [43].

Modern proteomic technologies such as MS-based profiling of serum pattern and protein microarray have proved to be useful in revealing new molecular markers and therapeutic targets in various types of human cancers [44]. Additionally, the analysis of serum proteomic pattern has suggested important diagnostic signatures for various cancers including ovarian [45], breast [46], prostate [47], and liver cancer [48].

11.1.4.1 Lung Cancer

Lung cancer holds a high mortality rate (27% of all cancer deaths per year) due to late stage diagnosis and lack of effective treatments [49]. The advances in proteomic techniques have played a key role in understanding the molecular biology of lung cancer, especially in the identification of biomarkers, since the DNA-based biomarkers show lack of sensitivity, specificity, and repeated sampling [50]. Therefore, it is very crucial to identify better biomarkers for lung cancer diagnosis, and prognosis was reviewed in detail [51]. A proteomic approach (2D-PAGE with Western blot analysis) has led to the discovery of the circulating autoantibodies against annexins I and/or II in sera from lung cancer patients, which were associated with high circulating levels of an inflammatory cytokine, IL-6 [52]. This study has described an approach for the development of serum-based assay and to diagnose lung cancer.

In lung cancer, noninvasive biomarkers, including blood, sputum, exhaled breath condensate, and urine, have been utilized [53]. To identify a marker which can be measured in pre-diagnostic sera is an important objective, as it carries the potential for screening strategies or blood-based early detection of lung cancer, besides the potential usage for monitoring of cancer [54]. Further, identification and circulation of plasma-based biomarkers such as EGFR, SFTPB, and WFDC2 were significantly altered in different cases of lung cancer compared to control [54]. In addition, serum proteins (including alpha-1 antitrypsin, carcinoembryonic antigen, retinol-binding protein, and squamous cell carcinoma antigen) can also be useful for diagnosis of lung cancer [55]. This approach has utility of developing serum-based assays for cancer diagnosis. Current technologies contributing in proteomics and imaging tools are being used as stated in the previous section, with favorable results, thus increasing our understanding of lung cancer pathogenesis at the molecular levels

[56]. Cancer cells shed various forms of secreted proteins in blood, serum, and tissues, and their levels may rise in early stages of cancer and hence correlate with proliferation of cancer cells [57, 58]. Therefore, secreted proteins can be employed as promising serum biomarkers of cancer, for example, secreted proteins in non-small cell lung cancer cell line (A549) have been identified using MS and database search by Huang and his colleagues [59]. They identified 14 proteins, and dihydrodiol dehydrogenase was selected as a novel serological marker of NSCLC [59]. The identification of secreted protein is an effective and practical approach for discovering the potential cancer biomarkers in serum.

Another form of noninvasive biomarker is exhaled breath condensate (EBC), which is a simple and new technique involving fluid from lower respiratory tract for sampling. EBC has been a wide interest due to presence of biomarkers for lung cancer detection and progression [60]. In this section, the identification of new potential diagnostic and prognostic biomarkers for lung cancer, using proteomics methodologies, has been discussed here.

11.1.4.2 Breast Cancer

There has been a promising progress in both therapeutic and diagnostic applications of breast cancer, the most common type of invasive cancer and the major cause of cancer-related deaths in females [23]. FDA has approved the biomarker named as CA15.3 (sensitivity 58.2% and specificity 96.0%, respectively) to detect breast cancer, but its specificity and sensitivity are not high enough for early cancer detection [61].

Development of high-throughput proteomic approaches (as stated in Sect. 11.2.4) has been applied in studying and discovering the biomarkers that are involved in the molecular mechanisms of breast cancer and yield a promising role in therapeutic and diagnostic applications [62]. A combination of in vitro and in vivo technology in a two-step approach has been applied to culture cells that were taken from tumors of defined breast cancer stages. Human breast cancer tissues were also taken and validated by MS and immunohistochemistry on tissue microarrays [63]. In transformed cells, the proteomic signatures showed loss of tissue architecture and metabolic changes, suggesting that proteomic analysis gives information related to tumor progression and protein changes in breast cancer [63]. In this study, they identified 8750 proteins, from which the higher levels of IDH2 and CRABP2 and low levels of SEC14L2 could be used as prognostic markers for breast cancer, suggesting that proteomic analysis gives information related to protein changes specifically for tumor progression [63].

Tissue samples and biological fluids (such as saliva, plasma, nipple aspirate, and cerebrospinal fluid) have been used in proteome research to identify diagnostic and predictive biomarkers [51]. Fascinatingly, the plasma proteome in breast cancer also shows the proteins derived from the microenvironment involved in various physiological processes such as wound repair, tissue modeling, metabolic homeostasis, and immune response [64]. Moreover, proteome technology was used to identify a serum protein, named nuclear matrix protein (designated NMP66; 28.3 kD) which can differentiate the malignant disease state from benign and normal control conditions [65]. This potential biomarker is now being evaluated in large-scale clinical trials for early detection of breast cancer as it is involved in malignant transformation [65].

11.1.4.3 Colorectal Cancer

Colorectal cancer (CRC) is one of the most leading causes of cancer deaths. Although early-stage detection is an effective tool for cancer treatment and genomic studies provided information related to cancer prognosis, mutations, and treatment system, it has given the static picture of the model. To add more in the molecular studies, proteomics was introduced in the field of cancer research [66]. Research related to biomarkers has shown a great impact on the risk assessment analysis, early-stage diagnosis and prognosis, cancer therapeutics, and concept of personalized medicine. Mass spectrometry is one of basic applications to identify the potential biomarkers in colorectal cancer. Then LC-MS/MS-based shotgun proteomic assays can identify various subtypes of colorectal cancer through clustering method [67]. It is reported that five subtypes of colorectal cancer have identified genes, clinical signatures, biomarkers, and proteins as a targeted site for cancer treatments using this proteomic approach [68]. This study has also identified the importance of an integrated field of genomic and proteomic for colorectal cancer. Another study has reported 95 samples of colorectal cancer using these techniques and has developed a panel for colorectal cancer highlighting considerable heterogeneity of CRC subtypes [69].

Targeted therapies also become non-responders to specific therapeutic agent due to mutations, e.g., in patients with advanced colorectal cancer, specific mutation in 12 and 13 codon of KARS gene changes targeted therapies to cetuximab and panitumumab [70, 71] by enhancing proliferative effect of cancer cell treatment. Similarly, a mutation in gene UGT1A1 changes the drug irinotecan effect on cancer cell, making the drug ineffective [72].

However, studying proteome and its modification for understanding biomarkers is crucially important to identify signature biomarkers for clinical practice and to promote personalized medicine [73]. Proteomic approach can be used while studying CRC and can be administered to shotgun proteomics, which is a promising technique for screening effect of cancer biomarkers and then analyzing the CRC samples through mass spectrometry [74]. Protein quantification can be performed as label-free quantification (LFQ), stable isotope labeling by amino acid in cell cultures (SILAC), tandem mass tag (TMT), isobaric tags for relative and absolute quantification (iTRAQ), etc. These techniques may be helpful for the multiplexing of samples and analyzing these samples in many conditions through LC-MS/MS [75]. These techniques strengthen the validation step clinically.

11.1.4.4 Prostate Cancer

Prostate cancer is the second common cause of cancer deaths in male. There is a need for screening the malignancy at an early stage and detection of prostate cancer antigen (PSA) [76]. The first proteomic study was done in 2000 by analyzing prostate cancer through laser capture microdissection (LCM) followed by 2D-PAGE [77]. This study has also provided the comparative analysis of normal and malignant cell progression in prostate cancer cell lines [78]. Commonly used treatment for prostate cancer is androgen-dependent therapy, to which most of the patients do respond, yet some patients show differential expression of PSA and some other proteins. Such expression pattern may lead to the identification of new biomarkers [79]. Diagnosis using serum proteins may be useful in deciding patient biopsy with an elevated PSA level. It is also shown that mass spectral analysis of benign hyperplasia and prostate malignancy leads to identification of novel biomarkers [80]. In vitro analyses have shown increased expression of HMGCL, BDH1, OXCT1, and ACAT1 proteins and are useful biomarkers for early detection of prostate cancer.

11.1.4.5 Gastric Cancer

Gastric cancers are considered the fifth most common type of cancer that develops very fast and are fetal, if remained uncured. It has a survival rate of less than 20% due to late diagnosis, and the most common type of this cancer is adenocarcinoma [81]. These cancers are usually diffusing and undifferentiated, while intestinal cancers are very well differentiated. Other types are neuroendocrine tumors, gastrointestinal tumors, and gastric lymphomas [82]. *Helicobacter pylori* is one of the best carcinogens for adenocarcinomas. It is mentioned in previous studies that gastrokine family has an explicit role in gastric cancer. Among this family gastrokine 3 and 1 are considered the most putative biomarkers. Their expression decreases at the onset of disease [83]. Pepsinogen C is also considered one of the vital biomarkers and plays a role in cancer prognosis. Its expression diminishes in gastritis and completely lost in gastric ulcers [84].

High-throughput molecular proteomic determination methods characterize the differential expression of proteins well and are associated with thermal resistance in human cell lines [85]. To check the expression levels of proteins Cathepsin B, HSP 27 (heat shock protein), protein isomerase A3, NSP3, and transgelin and prohibitin expression were found higher in gastric cancer using proteomic approaches (2D-PAGE and mass spectrometry) and associated with lesser survival rate [86]. Using histo-proteomic analysis, keratin, calcyclin, lipoprotein A1 precursor, 14-3-3 zeta, IPO-38, nucleoside-diphosphate kinase, nicotinamide *N*-methyltransferase, pyridoxal kinase, and pepsinogen C were identified as potential biomarkers in gastric cancers. Techniques used for identification were chip array and SELDI-TOF MS [87, 88].

11.1.4.6 Liver Cancer

Liver cancer, particularly hepatocellular carcinoma (HCC), is a major cause of cancer mortality and morbidity with continuously increasing incidence. Earlier and accurate diagnosis through biomarkers can provide an effective therapy to the patients. α-Fetoprotein (AFP) and des-γ-carboxy prothrombin are widely used biomarkers for histopathological diagnosis [89, 90], whereas glypican-3, heat shock protein 70, and glutamine synthetase help in the diagnosis through immunohistochemistry. Still for accurate diagnosis, there is a need to identify novel biomarkers in liver cancer [91]. Proteomics has also provided a versatile platform for these studies as they not only provide data related to biomarker discovery but also are helpful in understanding cancer progression, metastasis, and reoccurrence.

In proteomic analysis, experiments are designed with sample isolation either from the patient or through cell lines and animal models. Usually top-down and bottom-up approaches are used for the analysis. In the top-down approach, protein is separated through 2D-DIGE and then analyzed using mass spectrometry [92]. In the bottom-up strategy, proteins are digested into peptides and then analyzed through liquid chromatography and tandem mass spectrometry (LC-MS/MS). Then finally, proteins are identified via protein databases or de novo sequencing [93]. For proteomic studies, biomarkers need to be highly specific and sensitive for excellent diagnosis and should be validated across a broad range of populations.

Cell culture models are helpful in designing these studies, as they are homogenous irrespective of cancer cells that are heterogeneous. Yokoo et al. have analyzed 9 AFP-positive cell lines and 7 AFP-negative cell lines through 2D-DIGE, and MALDI-TOF MS have identified 11 proteins out of 2000 proteins that are involved in metabolism, apoptosis, and posttranslational modification [94]. Cell lines also help in monitoring chemical (exogenous and endogenous) effects in protein expression and metabolic pathways and provide informative data about variable enzyme expression in cells. LC-MS/MS analysis of human hepatocyte cells, HepG2, and Hep3B has identified an overlap in expressing proteins and demonstrated these proteins as HCC-specific biomarkers [95, 96]. Other than a cell culture, animals, body fluids, and specific tissues are also used as a model for proteomic analysis. Animal models are characterized well and provide an in vivo analysis, implementing appropriate diagnosis and therapeutics. However, limitation includes faster development of liver cancer in animals as compared to humans leading to incomplete understanding of metastasis [97]. Among body fluids, serum proteins may reflect the pathological state of the cell for tissue leakage and aberrant secretions and can serve as the dynamic range for developing potential biomarker panels.

11.1.4.7 Leukemia

Numerous proteomic technologies have been applied to characterize potential biomarkers associated with prognosis, diagnosis, and targeted therapy in leukemia patients. Nowadays, leukemia is subclassified by proteomic application since the cytogenetic analysis is laborious and expensive [98]. Novel protein biomarkers in acute lymphoblastic leukemia (ALL) (APOA4, CLUS, GELS, CERU, APOE, APOA1, AMBP, S10A9, CATA, ACTB, and AFAM) were identified using 2DE and MALDI-TOF-MS for protein identification, playing a significant role in the diagnosis and prognosis of leukemia [99]. Current developments in proteomic technologies are expected to improve efficacy and diminish the toxicity of current treatment of leukemia.

Acute myeloid leukemia (AML) is the most common in adults and has a low survival rate despite huge development in therapeutic strategies [100]. Proteomic techniques such as protein analysis play a promising role, not only in the diagnosis of myeloid leukemia at a molecular level but also in monitoring the therapy response

[101]. The subclassification of AML using 2DE and MALDI-TOF PMF analysis identified protein biomarkers (alpha-enolase, annexin A10, RhoGD12, and catalase), which are known to play an important role in glycolysis, apoptosis, tumor suppression, and metastasis. These biomarkers can be used to monitor the prognosis, hence proving new potential therapeutic targets for AML [102]. In a pilot study, 2D electrophoresis was used to compare the protein expression patterns in human B-cell chronic lymphocytic leukemia. In this study, protein expression profiles of 24 patients were correlated with their chromosomal features or clinical data such as survival time. The shorter survival time in patients was, in turn, associated with a changed pattern of different proteins and enzymes, providing better insight to understand the molecular aspects of leukemia [103].

The clinical trial results strongly compelled minimal residual disease (MRD) as a potential biomarker for treating and prognosis of patients with ALL and AML. Jongen-Lavrencic and his colleagues found that MRD is highly correlated with relapse and overall survival for AML patients [104]. In this study, they used bone marrow samples from 482 patients and detected mutations using multiparameter flow cytometry and targeted next-generation sequencing (NGS). Nearly 54 mutations in genes were detected that can be used as a potential marker of MRD [104]. Furthermore, five serum peptides named as glutathione S-transferase P1, isoform 1 of fibrinogen alpha chain precursor, fibrinogen alpha chain, platelet factor 4, and connective tissue active peptide III were identified in adult ALL for MRD monitoring and assessing therapeutic response in clinical practice [105].

11.1.4.8 Brain Tumors

These tumors are classified based on the cell morphology and stage of cancers. Primary tumors arise from glial cells and are called gliomas. Their subtypes are astrocytoma, oligodendroglioma, and ependymoma. Proteomic studies reveal that cellular response to the surrounding environment is important to understand the process of disease spread [106]. For better understanding of protein expression by genome and their successors is very important to investigate the disease progression as expression level of a particular protein, structural modifications, mutations, understanding of analytical methods may lead to discovery of novel biomarkers [107]. 2D analysis in proteomics is considered almost accurate for protein quantification. HSP27, brain-specific transglutaminase, major vault protein, G-proteins, and cystatin B are involved in glioma malignancies [108]. Moreover, Peroxiredoxins transcription factor BTF3 and α-B-crystallin were also found with increased level of expression in astrocytomas. In vivo analysis of expression levels is still a challenge due to structural and functional complexities. LC-MS/MS can detect and compare the protein expression range to confirm the predicted amino acid [109]. After the data collection, the identified proteins are matched using software (SEQUEST and Mascot, etc.) and by isotope labeling approaches such as ICAT and iTRAQ [110]. Still, we need to design proper study method and statistical analysis of protein aberrations.

11.1.4.9 Ovarian Cancer

Ovarian cancer is the fifth most common cause of cancer-related death in women worldwide. The 5-year survival rate of the disease would significantly increase in the early detection of Stage I [111]. Disastrously, the diagnosis of the disease is possible once it has spread to Stage III or beyond Stage IV in about 80% of women [112]. Moreover, women with Stage III or IV ovarian cancer show a 5-year survival rate of 15–20%, while ovarian cancer patients at Stage I show a 5-year survival rate of about 95% with surgical intervention [113]. The MS coupled with a computer algorithm developed a system for the profiling of low molecular weight serum proteins and identified a specific protein pattern associated with asymptomatic women with a high risk of developing ovarian cancer [42]. Proteomic analysis in ovarian cancer diagnosis consists of proteomic pattern diagnostic or serum proteome profiling, which includes the complex mass spectrometric differences between proteomic patterns of normal vs cancer samples, determined through bioinformatic tools [114]. The discovery of new biomarkers in proteomic patterns diagnostic by MS as well as the pattern of several biomarkers could hold a prominent level of discriminatory information than a single biomarker alone across the patient population with variable characteristics [115]. Numerous studies showed that proteomic pattern analysis on ovarian cancer appears to be a novel and highly sensitive diagnostic tool for an early stage assessment [116]. However, despite the auspicious results in terms of sensitivity and specificity for the detection of ovarian cancer, few concerns have been raised with respect to standard operating procedures, reproducibility, quality control, sample collection, shipping, and handling [117].

11.1.4.10 Skin Cancer

Skin cancer has varying degrees of malignancies depending upon skin layer penetration. Basal cell carcinoma was found one of the most common types of skin cancer [118]. It is mentioned in previous investigations that mutations in skin cancer alter the specific gene that also affect regulators of cell proliferation and viability through NF-B and ARF/p53 pathways [119]. Since 2000 proteomic techniques have provided a wide variety of biomarkers of the skin, comprehensive profiling is yet to complete [120]. Transplantation antigen of HSP90 family specific to skin tumors was identified that further determine six chaperones: HSP27, 60, 70, and 84, ER 60, and GRP 78. This study has compared epidermal stem cell with their differentiated transit amplifying cells [121]. Arbutin was found a potent biomarker using A37 cell line. MALDI-Q-TOF MS and MS/MS have identified 7 upregulated and 19 downregulated proteins that have anticancer effect [122]. It was also found that 14 differentially expressed proteins of p53 tumor suppressor regulate cell apoptosis and have a significant role in the suppression of cancer proliferation [123].

11.2 Proteomic Approaches for Cancer Treatments

11.2.1 Introduction

Proteomics is globally used to determine the gene expression at protein level, which provides the quantitative analysis of cell's response to the surrounding environments [124]. Proteomic deals with the different protein-based techniques, including posttranslational modifications, isotope-coded affinity, and protein arrays [113]. Proteome in cell undergoes modifications, such as posttranslational, regulatory, and degradative processes which have impact on the structure, location, and function of the gene products [114]. Therefore, proteomics-based analysis provides platform to better understand the biology of cancer via identification of protein expression that causes structural changes and protein-protein interaction in cell or fluid. Proteomic technologies are critical for the identification of biomarkers related to cancer diagnosis, progression, and investigation of therapeutic targets [125]. The physiological state of cancer cells is usually determined by ELISA, Western blot, and immunohistochemistry-based tools for the identification and quantification of specific proteins. However, these methodologies are difficult, costly and none of them characterizes the absolute abundance of the biomarkers in biological samples [126]. Thus, adoption of proteomic approaches plays an important role in the processes of cancer. Cancer proteomics includes the identification and quantitative analysis of protein expression from preneoplasia to neoplasia at various stages of disease [127]. The identification of these changes occurs during transformation of healthy cells into neoplastic cells with altered protein expression and protein modification, thereby affecting cellular functions that lie under the theme of cancer proteomics [128].

Moreover, two-dimensional gel electrophoresis (2DE) analysis was carried out in the early detection of tumor progression and metastasis of mammary adenocarcinoma in rat model [129]. 2DE-based identification of ubiquinol-cytochrome c reductase is potential biomarker in renal cell carcinoma [130]. Furthermore, 2DE method was used in the identification of protein expression for molecular diagnosis of ovarian and breast cancer [131, 132]. In addition, mass spectrometry (MS)-based analysis in human glioblastoma showed increased protein expression as compared to control (healthy tissue). Moreover, tandem MS (MS/MS) and liquid chromatography-MS (LC-MS) were used to identify thymosin beta-4 protein in tumor tissues [133]. Besides, matrix-assisted laser desorption/ionization (MALDI)-MS system showed increased expression of redox, nuclear metric, and cytoskeletal proteins in breast carcinoma, elevated retinoic acid-binding protein and carbohydrate-binding proteins in ovarian carcinomas, and increased cathepsin D protein in lung adenocarcinoma [134]. Next, surface-enhanced laser desorption-ionization (SELDI)-MS is used to identify the down- or upregulation of potential markers in prostate cancer cells and body fluids [135]. The SELDI protein profiles of lung, ovarian, and prostate cancer may provide insights into the protein expression changes from normal to benign and from premalignant to malignant lesions [136]. For the functional proteomics, protein arrays generate large set of well-characterized antibodies and expression profiles for cancer monitoring. Protein arrays containing immobilized proteins of microdissected cells have been used to identify the cancer progression. In this review, we have focused on the proteomic technologies that reveal the advantages, limitations, and perspectives of cancer treatments.

11.2.2 Mechanisms of Proteomic Alterations in Cancer

Cancer is a multifaceted disease associated with the alteration in genetic and epigenetic mechanisms, including mutations and chromosomal abnormalities at the cellular or tissue levels, leading to the human malignancies development [137]. Globally, the rate of cancer incidence and mortality is rapidly increasing, and hence it becomes the main focus of biomedical scientists to prevent the spread of this disease.

"Onco-proteomics" involves studying proteins and protein-protein interactions in cancer cells using proteomic applications, which can be applied to diagnose cancer. There has been increasing development of proteomics in cancer research with the widespread involvement of mass spectrometry [138]. As we know, current cancer screening tests lack sensitivity and specificity, posing a huge clinical challenge to identify malignant cancer [41]. During the last decades, there have been huge rise and fall in the development and understanding of cancer biology using proteomics and have shed light on the underlying mechanism of factors causing cancer formation. Hence, there is a strong interest in using proteomics to ameliorate understanding of cancer pathogenesis, which could lead to the identification of new cancer biomarkers for cancer early detection and therapeutic efficiency [138].

Onco-proteomics involves the identification of various overexpressed proteins in cancer relative to healthy tissues, as proteomic technologies have been broadly applied to identify cancer diagnostic biomarkers, monitoring disease progression and discovering therapeutic interventions [9]. Nearly 200 proteins that are post-translationally modified affect various cellular mechanisms including protein-protein interaction, half-life, degradation, stability, targeting, etc., since one gene may result in a huge amount of protein products [9]. However, the exact mechanism causing different types of cancers is still undefined. But one possible reason for the proteomic variation in cancer is the dysregulations of posttranslational modifications (includes protein acetylation, glycosylation, and phosphorylation), which have been shown to be associated in a wide spectrum of human diseases. Hence, understanding which pathway triggers the tumor cascade is important for therapeutic strategies [139].

The improvements in mass spectrometry technique have led to an increased sensitivity, accuracy, and rapidity of analyses to identify several thousand proteins per experiments, especially in the event of large-scale analysis of posttranslational modifications (i.e., phosphorylation and ubiquitination conducted by functional proteomics) [140]. Proteomics has shown vast applications in the identification of different protein markers involved in cancer signaling pathway.

A study performed by Mellinghoff in 2005 on glioblastoma showed that epidermal growth factor receptor (EGFR) and phosphatase and tensin homologue deleted on chromosome 10 tumor-suppressor protein (PTEN) co-expression were associated with an increased response to tyrosine kinase inhibitors (i.e., erlotinib), whereas the cells expressing EGFR but not PTEN did not respond to the drug therapy [141]. Posttranslational modifications are most studied using proteomic approaches as it regulates many biological mechanisms, including signal transduction [142]. But it still remains a challenge as the sensitivity and selectivity of purification methods still need to be defined [143].

Another possible mechanism is the alteration in protein structure and functions, and the main cause involves the mutations affecting cancer-related genes, resulting in the formation of defective protein structure, and altering protein interactions and degradation [62, 144]. Hence, the structural description of proteins, their complexity, and interactions have become the center of attention while using proteomic techniques [145]. Henceforth, the onco-proteomics holds promise as a biological indicator of discovering novel biomarkers for monitoring cancer progression, early diagnosis, and drug efficacy of therapeutic agents [138]. Consequently, cellular pathways that are involved in cell functions, proliferation, and survival are potential therapeutic targets of cancer [41, 146].

11.2.3 Need for Proteomic Approaches in Cancer

Current goals of proteomics aim at the development and establishment of new methodologies for analyzing protein expression and function in various physiological and pathological conditions [147]. Proteomics gives an insight of cell response to changes, and hence, scientists take the advantages of current high-throughput techniques to understand the protein profiles in various diseases including cancer. For example, prostate cancer has been studied using different proteomic techniques (including difference gel electrophoresis (DIGE), MS profiling, 2D-PAGE, shotgun proteomics with label-based (ICAT, iTRAQ) and label-free (SWATH) quantification, MudPIT) to search for the diagnostic biomarkers and their clinical applications [148]. A synergistic combination of powerful technologies (stated in Sect. 11.2.4) will provide further knowledge to identify novel drug targets and biomarkers for human cancers.

Over the years, proteomic tools have been progressively used to study the cancer biomarkers [149]. Initially, the proteome analysis in cancer was based on 2DE in which selected spots for proteins were identified by matrix-assisted laser desorption-ionization MS. Overall, 11 proteins were identified in human melanoma cell lysates (A375) [150]. Notably, gel-based proteomics has contributed significantly in cancer research, particularly on colorectal [151], breast [152], and pancreatic cancer [153]. Due to some advantages, gel-based proteomic experiments have been moderately substituted by MS-based proteomic techniques. Nonetheless, 2DE-based perspectives are still widely used due to some specific advantages in cancer research [154]. New strategies are required for designing the process, labeling, fractionation, and analysis via bioinformatic tools, which will increase the sensitivity and development of next-generation MS proteomic fields of study [155]. These techniques significantly boost the quantification, identification, and monitoring of huge data related to the expression of protein biomarkers, modifications at posttranslational level, and other regulatory as well as molecular aspects of cancer that may be important from clinical perspectives. These kinds of studies have been found to be the most beneficial for the development of novel diagnostic and therapeutic strategies while also allowing a better understanding of the mechanisms involved during cancer progression [149].

11.2.4 Molecular Diagnostic Tools for Cancer

Cancer is a heterogeneous disease which involves multiple pathways resulting from a combination of tumorigenesis and metastasis. Diagnosis of cancer, especially at an early stage, is highly significant for improving the patient's outcome. For a long time, proteins in cancer cells are mainly identified using Western blotting, ELISA, and immunohistochemistry. But these methodologies are costly and laborious [149]. Proteomic tools have significantly developed from 2D to MALDI-MS and have played a momentous role in pancreatic and breast cancers [153, 156]. The designing of new experimental strategies for sample labeling, processing, fractionation, and bioinformatic analyses combined with proteomic technologies enables us to identify, monitor, and quantify the data related to biomarkers, posttranslational modifications, and other molecular mechanisms [149]. These outcomes are important for the development of novel diagnostic and therapeutic tools, leading to a better understanding of the mechanism involved in cancer.

Research on the protein alteration in cancer studies have been carried out more than 70 years ago [157]. However, recent proteomic technologies are utilized in deciphering the differential expression of proteins in human cancers. Numerous metabolic diseases and genetic abnormalities are associated with the cellular transcription and translation status by creating variations in the proteome [158]. The proteomic approaches for the discovery and assessment of proteins have been developed during the last 12 years. Identification and validation of biomarkers are accomplished by various proteomics-based methods, such as protein profiling/activity profiling, protein linkage maps, protein microarrays, phosphorylation analysis, 2DE, DIGE, MS, shotgun/bottom-up proteomics, selected reaction monitoring protein arrays, and bioinformatic analysis (Fig. 11.1).

11.2.4.1 Two-Dimensional Gel Electrophoresis

Two-dimensional gel electrophoresis (2DE) was first introduced in 1975 and became a method of choice for protein separation and expression analysis [159]. 2DE is one of the most important tools in the field of proteomics that can identify hundreds or thousands of proteins in a single gel sample and the possibility to directly detect the posttranslational modifications of proteome [160]. Proteins are separated on the basis of charge (isoelectric focusing) and mass on the

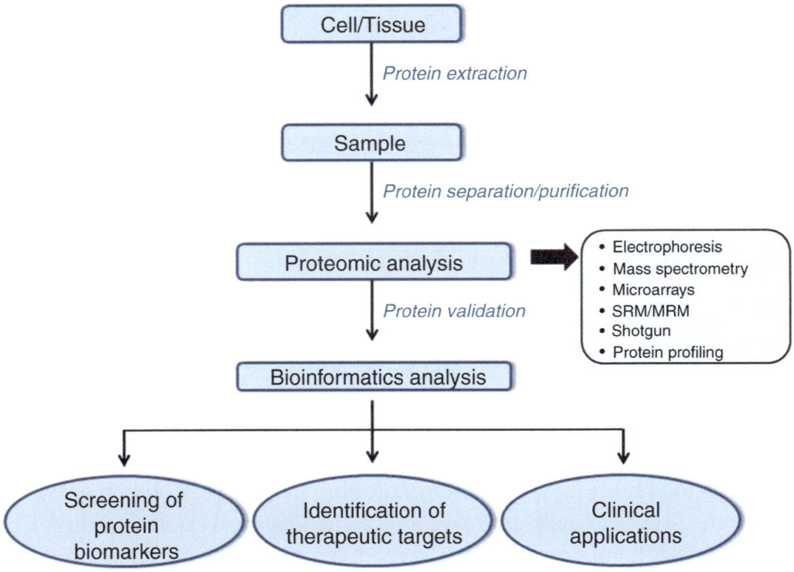

Fig. 11.1 A typical method describing the diagnostic tools using proteomic approaches. *SRM* selected reaction monitoring, *MRM* multiple reaction monitoring

polyacrylamide gel. Approximately 3000 proteins can be visualized on a single gel using silver staining and by PDQuest™ software [134]. The information obtained on the mass-to-charge ratio identifies the protein, whereas the protein database also determines the type and location of protein modifications. Several studies have reported that 2DE proteomic analysis can detect the protein spots between normal and cancer samples [161]. The proteomic analysis by 2DE methodology of bladder tumors exhibited downregulation of cytokeratins, galectin 7, psoriasin, and statifin in tumor with low degree of differentiation, and psoriasin in urine was observed in squamous cell carcinoma patients [162]. The changes in calgranulin B protein expression in dysplastic polyps from colon carcinoma and ulcerative colitis patients were analyzed by 2DE [163]. Furthermore, 2DE combined with MS technology leads to the identification of discriminating protein spots for discovery of proteins associated with disease [164]. Though 2DE is widely used for the protein detection, this technique has some restrictions, including reduced dynamic range and visualization of proteins in proteomic methods. Moreover, 2DE demonstrates hydrophobic relevance in regulatory or signaling proteins, which causes difficulty in the detection of very basic proteins.

11.2.4.2 Difference Gel Electrophoresis (DIGE)

DIGE was first discovered by Unlu in 1997 [165]; this technique is used to overcome the limitation of 2DE by recognizing the correct quantitation, reproducibility, and separation of proteins [166]. The main advantage of DIGE analysis includes the independent labeling of two or more protein samples with cyanine-based fluorescent dyes (Cy3 and Cy5), followed by the separation and visualization on a single gel and measurement of the relative ratio of separated protein fluorescence detected by ImageMaster 2D Platinum (GE Healthcare, Uppsala, Sweden) [167]. Thus, the reproducibility and reliability of protein expression analysis for normal and cancer tissues have been improved by DIGE method. The overexpression of receptor tyrosine kinase 2 (ErbB-2) in breast cancer cells [168] and the analysis of different bacterial growth conditions have been detected by DIGE analysis [169]. The main limitation of DIGE analysis is the hydrophobic nature of cyanine dyes, which causes reduction in the solubility of labeled proteins that may lead to protein precipitation before gel electrophoresis [170].

11.2.4.3 Mass Spectrometry

Proteomic studies were based on 2DE and sequential mass spectrometry approach which facilitates the identification of peptide sequences in proteins that were present in differential abundance on gel [171]. MS techniques identify and measure the molecules on the basis of mass-to-charge ratio by high-energy laser detector. It mainly consists of three basic components, such as ion source, mass analyzer, and detector [172]. MS has played important role in cancer research and other disease models through discovery of protein biomarkers. MS-based bioinformatic analysis enabled researchers and clinicians to distinguish between cancer and healthy patients through mass spectra and pattern identification. This technique is highly sensitive (picomole to femtomole) for the detection of cancer biomarkers, such as small polar molecules, oligonucleotides, phosphoproteins, and glycoproteins [173]. Recently, MS technique has been improved and modified to analyze biomolecules, proteins, and peptides. Two MS-based approaches, developed for the investigation of new biomarker discovery in proteomic, are matrix-assisted laser desorption-ionization time-of-flight (MALDI-TOF) and surface-enhanced laser desorption-ionization time-of-flight (SELDI-TOF). MALDI-TOF-MS analysis can detect nanomolar to picomolar protein and separates the proteins based on mass, whereas SELDI-TOF-MS separation is dependent on charge, where the hydrophobic proteins are characterized by protein chips, chromatography, and MS-based detection [166]. Moreover, liquid chromatography coupled with mass spectrometry (LC-MS) is used to identify and separate thousands of proteins in biological samples, such as serum, plasma, tissue, cells, etc. [174]. However, MS analysis has limitations for the detection of high molecular weight and heavily glycosylated proteins.

11.2.4.4 Protein Microarrays

Protein microarray technique has the ability to analyze the modifications in protein phosphorylation at high-throughput level of proteins. This technique is based on the antigen-antibody interaction of cell population for profiling the proteome [175]. There are two major types of protein microarrays, i.e., forward-phase arrays (FPAs) and reverse-phase arrays (RPAs). In FPAs, antibodies are arrayed and probed with cell lysates, while in RPAs, the cell lysates are arrayed and then probed with the specific antibodies. RPAs provide labeling-free cellular protein lysates, which represent high-throughput platform for investigation of therapeutics and screening of biomarkers in the pathophysiological studies [176]. During the clinical trials, RPAs have the exclusive ability to analyze signaling pathways of small number of cells or cells isolated from the human tissues by laser capture microdissection [177]. Studies have revealed the use of RPAs for the identification and discovery of therapeutic targets in cancer. However, the main restriction of RPAs includes the need for specific antibodies to conduct proteomic profile [178]. Protein arrays are essential tool in tumor research for the identification and characterization of biomarkers in different biological samples, including tumor biopsies and tissue culture lysates and serum [179]. Therefore, proteomics-based protein microarray approach is widely used for the discovery of novel antigens for cancer diagnosis [180].

11.2.4.5 Selected Reaction Monitoring Protein Arrays

Selected reaction monitoring (SRM) is an ideal tool for the accurate quantification of the proteins, which is very helpful in biomarker development with excellent specificity and sensitivity. SRM has its extension called multiple reaction monitoring (MRM), which has the capacity to quantify small molecules [181]. They can also perform protein/peptide analysis and can monitor the intensity of the parent/daughter ion (m/z ions) with great specificity. This quantification can be achieved by isobaric labeling (iTRAQ) of the target proteins or by spiking isotopic peptides into sample proteins and controls [182, 183]. Limitation of these techniques includes high costs, and sometimes isotopic labeling remains incomplete during large-scale validation of data.

11.2.4.6 Shotgun/Bottom-Up Proteomics

Shotgun proteomics or bottom-up protein analysis was introduced in 1998 by Yates [184]. Shotgun protein analysis refers to proteolytic digestion of proteins into short peptides that can be resolved by different fractionation strategies; normally, fractionated peptide mixtures are subjected to LC-MS analysis [185]. Shotgun proteomic analysis has achieved a relatively high-throughput analysis of proteome and provides a snapshot of the major protein constituents [186]. The applications of shotgun analysis include protein-protein interaction, protein quantification, proteome profiling, and protein modification [187]. Shotgun proteomics has been used for the advanced biological discoveries, and it is divided into two types, i.e., label-free MS-based proteomic and label-based technologies (isotopic or isobaric tags). The main advantage of shotgun method is its efficiency in terms of sorting out thousands of proteins involved in biological conditions [188]. Shotgun proteomic analysis can identify thousands of proteins with high accuracy and resolution in a single experiment. However, digested and fragmented peptides usually occur in abundance in each protein sample and are more likely to overlook less abundant proteins which is the main limitation of shotgun analysis in proteomics [127].

11.2.4.7 Protein Profiling/Activity Profiling and Protein Linkage Maps

Protein profiling is a diagnostic tool that is more sensitive and specific than biomarker detection. Surface-enhanced laser desorption-ionization time-of-flight mass spectrometry (SELDI-TOF MS) is the major tool in protein profiling or activity profiling. However, the standardization and reproducibility present the major limitation of this tool [45]. A protein chip system of this technique is the fastest and more reliable to discover and identify the biomarkers. To avoid errors in sample collection method, material type and time for the ionization need to be very accurate and standardized. In SELDI-TOF MS, calibration step is important for calculating the exact mass of sample protein. This step is also necessary for desorption and ionization of the sample in the chip reader [189]. Proteomic profiling of platelet extracts using SELDI-TOF MS method to analyze protein mixtures displays the increased amounts of angiogenesis regulatory proteins (i.e., VEGF) [98]. This selective process detects tiny size of platelets in cancer, which is not possible with the available methods. SELDI-TOF MS and protein chip have also been used for detection of new biomarkers and building diagnostic models of breast cancer, suggesting that SELDI is relatively highly sensitive and specific tool for screening and discovering novel cancer biomarkers [190].

For activity profiling, usually specific probes with fluorescent, radioactive compounds and affinity tags are used [191] to identify markers and enzymatic inhibitors by comparative analysis of protein expression levels in healthy and diseased tissues [192]. Other known applications of these techniques include the development of therapeutic agents and interaction proteins for better understanding of regulatory proteins [193]. This technique may also provide quantitative analysis of binding proteins and can facilitate the therapeutic response of a patient to the particular therapeutic agent. It may also provide the opportunity of developing noninvasive imaging technologies for diagnosis. Nanoelectrospray (nanoES) is also used in addition to this technique if the full-length sequence is not available. It can also generate a partial sequence as a peptide sequence tag to complete the mass information [194].

Protein linkage mapping provides the quantitative study and highlights any mutational changes in protein expression whether in a cell or tissue. It can determine proteins in abundance and detect posttranslational modification that can characterize protein of interest. These protein maps also enable the comparative analysis of protein expression and modifications [195].

11.2.4.8 Phosphorylation Analysis

Protein phosphorylation is a critical posttranslational modification and key regulatory factor of the tumor growth and progression. It is well-known that initiation of cellular signaling through tyrosine receptors promotes protein-protein interaction and phosphorylation by involving signaling proteins like MAP kinases [196]. Moreover, protein phosphorylation can induce changes in gene expression and protein synthesis modifications that affect the cell proliferation, cell migration, and molecular mechanisms of cancer cell progression and inhibition. In this regard, EGFR is one of the best examples in different kinds of cancers [197]. To better understand the signaling mechanisms of cancer development, various techniques are applied for the detection of phosphopeptides. Immunoaffinity-based strategy has been developed to characterize and identify tyrosine phosphorylation by phosphoproteome [198]. Moreover, phosphotyrosine-specific antibodies are extracted from protease-digested cancer cells by MS/MS analysis. Similarly, phosphotyrosine immunoprecipitation with immobilized metal affinity chromatography-tandem MS, SILAC, and tandem MS is used for the study of phosphoproteome in cancer cells [199]. The identification and characterization of phosphorylation sites in posttranslational modifications reveal potential signaling mechanisms in cancer biology.

11.2.4.9 Bioinformatic Analysis

For any disease, bioinformatics can play a vital role in identifying disease-associated genetic variants in which single nucleotide polymorphisms (SNPs) and copy number variations (CNVs) can be identified. These two also play crucial roles in developing personalized medicine. Bioinformatic and biological approaches can identify or discover functional variants using the system-level approach, gene expression data, epigenetic data, and regulatory and pathway data [200]. The analysis is usually based on the most susceptible loci besides evaluating disease risk. Bioinformatics also provides knowledge of computational methodologies, developing algorithms to process genomic data with accuracy. It also provides the systematical methods to eliminate noises from collected data and to normalize the data type. They can also help in maintaining electronic health record in case of developing personalized medicine data; this field has to face the challenge of heterogeneous data obtained from different patients [201]. Yet bioinformatic infrastructure can store, manage, and analyze data according to disease environment, mutations in genes, and sometimes individual's living style. Bioinformatic tools need speed for analyzing the progression of disease and taking clinical decisions as cancer, and some of the acute diseases have faster progression [202]. Some examples of standard tools are DAVID, BINGO, GoMiner and Cytoscape that provide flexibility in analysis.

11.2.5 Importance of Cancer Diagnostics

Early detection of cancer is the main challenge in treating cancer. Even though there is a wide range of current techniques that can be used to identify cancer, i.e., mammography for breast cancer in addition to the prostate serum antigen for prostate cancer, their reliability for early cancer detection is uncertain due to the lack of specificity and sensitivity [203]. For that reason, cancer detection, especially at the early stage, is very important and is possible through proteomic technique, which encompasses analysis of differentially expressed proteins in molecular pathway of cancer [9]. Proteomic approaches have appeared as an addition to genomics and antibody-based techniques to identify tumor biomarkers, to study protein patterns, and to identify therapeutic targets of cancer [98]. It is important that these tumor markers can be validated and identify tumor. The molecular changes in cancer are responsible for altering protein expression, posttranslational modifications, as well as cellular signaling pathway which can be studied using proteomic approaches [203]. This leads to a better understanding of the pathological and molecular basis of cancer, but the exact cause is still not clearly defined. In the past decades, a huge development in high-throughput technologies, such as DNA microarrays, has resulted in their wide implications in classifying cancers at molecular level.

In proteome analysis, serum or other body fluids can be used for the identifications of biomarkers that may lead to the cancer diagnosis at an early stage. Biomarkers have gained so much interest, as the tumor-derived secretary products can be identified in serum or other fluids [204]. In addition, it may also be used to detect different protein levels in the serum of cancer patients. These changes in the serum proteome caused by cancer-specific metabolic or cancer-associated pathways, somewhat independent of mass or tumor size, assist in the early detection of cancer [204]. A practical technique for serum protein profiling was developed by Miller et al. (2003), in which they used antibody microarrays to identify promising biomarkers in prostate cancer sera. They compared protein abundance of prostate cancer and control serum samples using two-color fluorescence assay. They recognized five proteins (villin, von Willebrand factor, immunoglobulin G, alpha1-antichymotrypsin, and immunoglobulin M) using a set of reliable microarray measurements that differ in prostate cancer samples compared to the control samples. These advances allow the direct use of protein microarrays and high-density antibody in biomarker discovery studies [205].

11.2.6 Study Design Guidelines for Biomarker Development

A biomarker can indicate and quantify a health or disease state of the body and can indicate the body response to therapeutic treatment [206]. More specifically, a biomarker shows clinical applications by evaluating the risk assessment, disease progression, and potential therapeutic responses, thereby being useful in clinical decision-making. Biomarker development is a complicated process that involves multiple steps with the objective to attain useful clinical outcomes [68, 207]

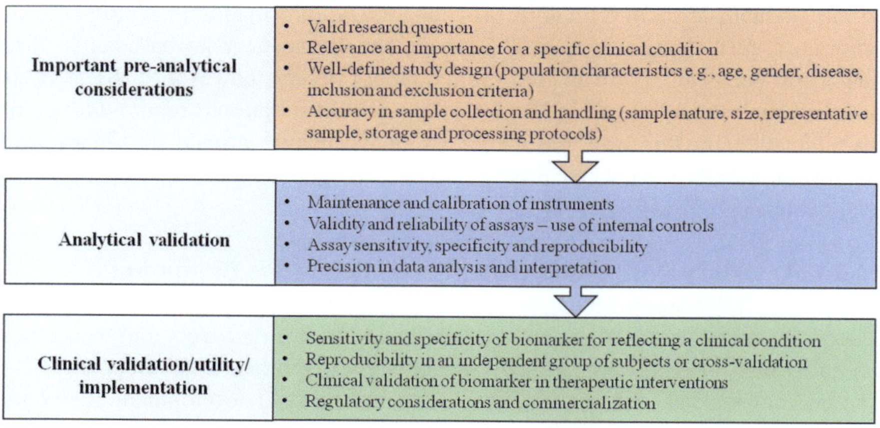

Fig. 11.2 Guidelines for biomarker development

(Fig. 11.2). The process is typically based upon a clear and concise research hypothesis in order to identify the promising biomarkers that are relevant, highly specific, sensitive, and important to monitor a clinical condition.

11.2.6.1 Pre-analytical Considerations (Sample Collection and Handling)

This step takes into considerations the important criteria for sample selection. It is also important for a biomarker to be easily detectable in samples taken in a noninvasive or minimally invasive manner, such as the liquid biopsies (urine, saliva, or blood). The details about the sample's nature, size, collection, and storage procedures should be clearly mentioned [5]. As in cancer research, the sample collection is a critical step due to the heterogeneity of samples, and therefore, the sample size and the selection of a representative sample acquire much importance [208]. Furthermore, the characteristics of the samples obtained from a study design (subjects' age, gender, health status, etc.) should be well-defined, because of their importance in guiding the clinical applications and implementations of the candidate biomarkers for a target population (Fig. 11.2).

11.2.6.2 Analytical Validation (Assay Reliability and Accuracy)

This step mainly focuses on the accuracy and reliability of the analytical procedures employed to detect a biomarker. It is important to validate the robustness, sensitivity, specificity, and reproducibility of an assay with quality control measures in order to avoid the detection of false positives due to experimental errors [209, 210]. The precision and calibrations of the instruments used to perform these assays must also be given equal importance [62] (Fig. 11.2).

11.2.6.3 Clinical Validation and Utility

Clinical validity refers to the ability of a biomarker to precisely identify the subjects more or less likely to suffer a clinical condition [68]. Clinical utility corresponds to the effectiveness of a biomarker in improving the clinical outcome of patients and defining benefit-to-harm ratio, thus providing useful information to avoid the inappropriate clinical decisions [5, 68, 70]. Finally, the diagnostic assay based on in vitro diagnostic needs an approval from the regulatory bodies; however, if the assay is based on a laboratory-developed test, only analytical validation is required for commercialization. In this way, the regulatory bodies play a crucial role in making healthcare decisions about the effectiveness of a diagnostic tool and its therapeutic applications [70, 73] (Fig. 11.2).

11.2.6.4 Study Design and Other Issues Related to Biomarker Development

Indeed, there is an increasing gap between the biomarker discovery and their clinical utility due to several limitations and challenges in biomarker development [62]. The bias can arise at each phase of biomarker research and development, including sample collection and handling procedures, study design, validity and verification of analytical assays, data analysis, interpretation, and reproducibility in an independent group of individuals [211, 212]. Nevertheless, the study design presents the main source of bias in biomarker research and development, partly due to the sample acquisition. The sample collection should be based on well-designed prospective clinical trials with specified inclusion and exclusion criteria in order to minimize the potential biases [212]. The characteristics of the target population and the information related to patients' follow-up are crucial factors in defining the molecular traits that evolve with time. Most often, the subject selection is based on incidentally available specimens, rather than a pre-defined study protocol for biomarker discovery. This retrospective study design raises huge bias due to the confounding factors that could lead to false-positive discoveries and thus shows limited clinical validity and utility. While the prospective setting for sample collection and follow-up is considered an ideal option, the biomarker detection is costly and lengthy method, which presents a big hurdle in their deployment [213]. In order to ameliorate the study design of a clinical trial and to overcome biases in biomarker research, a "prospective-retrospective" strategy was proposed, which utilizes the samples obtained from previously conducted prospective trials [214, 215].

Moreover, adequate funding along with the development of good-quality and large integrated biobanks with optimal sample handling would also contribute greatly toward biomarker discovery research [216, 217]. In addition, the implementation of biomarkers and their use in clinical practice requires regulatory and legislative procedures, which further hampers the pace of biomarker development [73, 211].

Although, with advancements in omics technology, a wide array of biomarkers has been discovered, only few novel biomarkers have shown clinical implementations due to the contradictory results obtained from trials with methodological limitations [218]. For instance, despite the discovery of several tumor biomarkers reported in literature, only few of them have been approved by FDA [211]. Different signature-based assays have been designed to measure the gene expression profiles in breast cancer prediction. These include MammaPrint which measures 70 genes [219] and Oncotype Dx Breast Cancer Assay which measures 21-gene prognostic profile [220]. Similar assays have also been developed to measure gene expression profiles in prostate and colon cancer tissues [221, 222]. In the future, biomarker discovery research needs more rigorous study designs and protocols to avoid biases. Careful consideration of clinical applications and implementations together with accompanying biomarker performance characteristics in study designs will lead to meaningful translational outcomes.

11.2.7 Importance of Biomarkers in Therapy Designs

In recent years, biomarkers have gained substantial importance in defining the layouts of a therapy design, due to their wide range of applications in risk assessment, disease diagnosis, drug discovery, and patient stratification according to drug response [223–225]. Biomarkers make major contribution by providing insight into the disease evolution and therapy responses, as prognostic (disease evolution, risk assessment), diagnostic (recurrence risk detection), predictive (responsiveness to a particular therapy), or pharmacodynamic biomarkers (optimization of pharmacological doses) as well as surrogate endpoints (measurement of the clinical outcome of a treatment, as a substitute for a clinical endpoint) [68, 226–229] (Fig. 11.3).

In cancer research, the main challenge is to deal with the heterogeneity among different cancers that presents a main hurdle in the identification and development of candidate biomarkers. However, the precise evaluation, monitoring, and management of cancer largely depend upon the use of biomarkers at different stages of the disease. The most widely used established biomarkers include PSA, for screening and monitoring of prostate cancer [230]; HE4 and CA-125 in diagnosis and therapy monitoring of ovarian cancer [231, 232]; and CEA to detect the recurrence of patients diagnosed with colorectal cancer [233, 234].

The efficacy of various anticancer therapies has been found to be reduced due to the absence of predictive biomarkers, which show the ability to identify the molecular mechanisms of action or resistance of a particular drug. Hence, it is recommended that all drugs should ideally have such biomarkers. The identification of these biomarkers will be greatly helpful in understanding the mechanisms of drug resistance and to devise strategies to manage these issues. As in the case of melanoma, a combination therapy of *MEK* and *BRAF* inhibitors is employed to get effective outcomes [235], whereas a new generation of EGFR inhibitors has been designed for non-small cell lung cancer [236]. Nevertheless, a careful consideration is required for the selection of biomarkers used in various cancer types, the standardization of study designs, as well as the validation strategies. Together, this reveals that appropriate approaches should be necessarily implemented in order to develop better therapy designs and identify important biomarkers in different types of tumors.

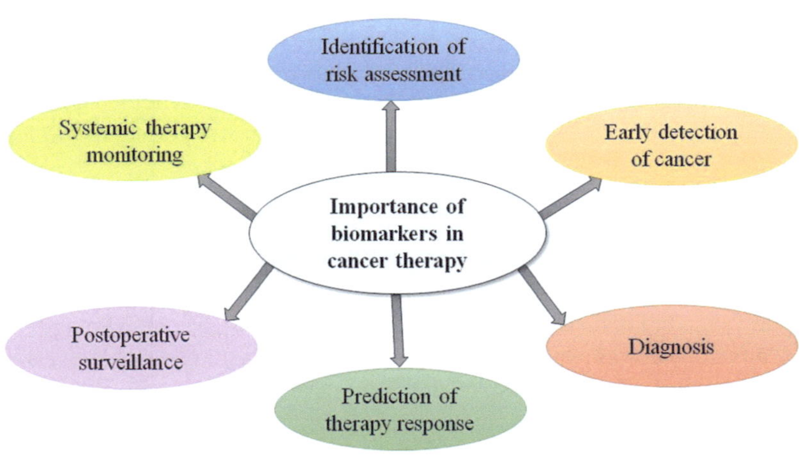

Fig. 11.3 Role of biomarker in cancer therapy design

11.3 Concept of Personalized Medicine Based on Proteomics

11.3.1 Introduction

A great body of evidence over the last few decades has revealed that a significant number of variations in drug response are associated with an individual's genetic profile as well as some interrelated factors including age, diet, environment, health status, and therapeutic interventions. Moreover, in order to achieve an effective drug response, the variations among the individuals due to their geographic locations and ethnical differences should also be taken into consideration.

11.3.1.1 Historical Background

Various events in the early 1950s have highlighted the importance of evaluating the genetic basis underlying the variations in drug response in different clinical conditions. Adverse events, such as the hemolytic anemia, were reported with the use of antimalarial drugs (e.g., primaquine) in patients with glucose-6-phosphate dehydrogenase deficiency [237]. Furthermore, a respiratory arrest was observed upon the administration of a muscle relaxant, succinylcholine, due to a genetic defect in succinylcholine esterase enzyme that converts succinylcholine into an inactive form [238]. Similarly, peripheral neuropathy was reported in individuals who received isoniazid for tuberculosis treatment, due to the inherited defect in *N*-acetyl transferase enzyme [239]. In addition, during the 1970s, the adverse response to an antihypertensive drug, debrisoquine, was reported in individuals with a polymorphism of CYP2D6, a drug-metabolizing enzyme [240, 241].

All these findings of individualized drug responses gave rise to the field of pharmacogenetics [242], which falsified the paradigm of "one size fits all." Pharmacogenetics aims to identify DNA sequence variations to characterize the molecular mechanisms underlying an individual's drug response. In 1990s, the advent of the human genome sequencing and genotyping facilities evolved the field of pharmacogenetics into pharmacogenomics, which seeks to explore the differential gene expression profiles in relation to drug response at individual or population level [243]. The increasing technological developments and advancements in the field of genomics and molecular diagnostics have allowed a vast understanding of translational aspects, a personalized approach to clinical care.

11.3.1.2 Perception of Personalized Medicine Approach

Personalized medicine refers to the prediction of disease susceptibility, prevention, diagnosis, and treatment response based on inter-individual variations in genetic and lifestyle factors [244]. The emerging field of personalized medicine aims at ensuring an early risk assessment and improved patient healthcare while considering that an individual's genetic profile determines the individual's particular response to a pharmacological intervention as well as dietary and lifestyle modifications [245]. Therefore, the main concept of personalized medicine is perceived as "the right treatment for the right person at the right time" [246]. Inter-individual variations may arise due to the differences in their genetic profiles that may render a drug less efficient or allow it to stay in the plasma for a longer time than normal, causing toxicity. Personalized medicine approach focuses on identifying and reporting all these genetic variations associated with a drug response for patient's stratifications [247]. Personalized medicine relies on developing the therapies that are aimed to target the groups of patients that are unable to respond to a specific treatment and thereby are deprived of appropriate healthcare. Personalized medicine, therefore, promises to improve the healthcare system with lowering costs, by providing each individual with the opportunity for earlier diagnosis, risk predictions, and well-suited treatments (Fig. 11.4).

11.3.1.3 Omics Technologies in Personalized Medicine

The improvement in omics technologies has contributed a great deal to facilitate the stratification of individuals by enabling omics profiling including whole genomics, epigenomics, glycomics, lipidomics, transcriptomics, proteomics, metabolomics, and pharmacogenomics [248]. These high-throughput analyses performed on different biomolecules can detect the variation in an individual's genetic and metabolic profiles related to certain disorders, thus affecting their response to a specific therapy. These omics facilities have wide applications throughout the life span in the prediction of disease risk factor, diagnosis, and progression as well as the targeted therapeutic approaches [249]. This also provides a better understanding of molecular and cellular mechanisms involved in human health and disease. The integrated omics approach in clinical practice as well as the availability of different biomarkers has greatly facilitated the stratification of patient based on their responses to specific treatment, in order to decide the best-suitable therapeutic regimens [250, 251].

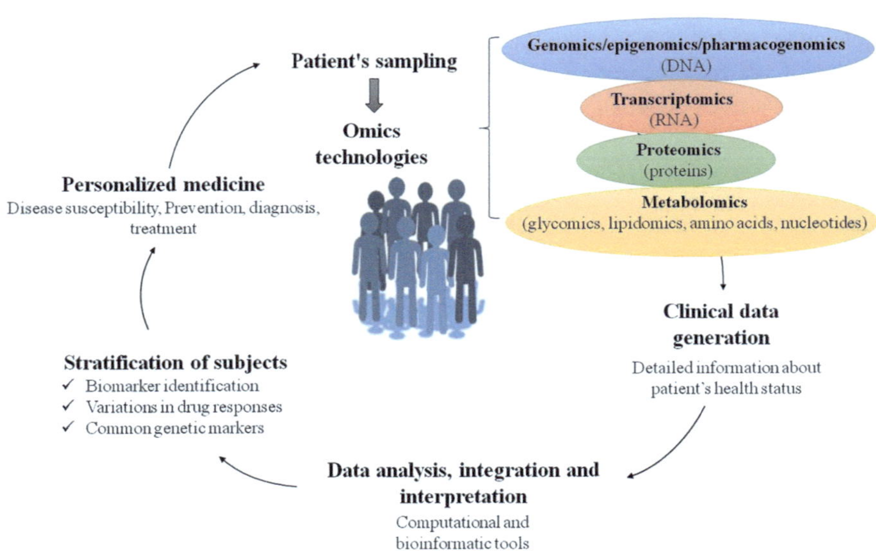

Fig. 11.4 Concept of personalized medicine

11.3.1.4 Ethical Aspects of Personalized Medicine

Providing a personalized care within a clinical setting is a complex process that requires related issues of social legal and ethical aspects to be addressed properly while designing a study [252]. Apart from these elements, there are many major obstacles for the development in the field of personalized medicine [245, 253, 254]. Maintenance of privacy with individual patient's dignity is very important so that the sensitive data may not become the cause of embarrassment for patients. Taking informed consent of individual patient or in specific cases with the guardian protects the patient and physician relationship and helps in avoiding discrimination. However, efforts should be made including the improved comprehension and clarity in acquiring patient's informed consent, protection from violating confidentiality of information as well as keeping a balance between individual/social benefits and scientific progress and development. Together, this may be helpful in solving ethical challenges associated with personalized medicine.

11.3.2 Driving Factors in Personalized Medicine

Personalized medicine can be regarded as a continuously evolving approach to define treatments based on an individual's genetic profile and physiological parameters [255]. During the past few years, however, increasing technological developments and the availability of a vast scientific knowledge have diversified the field of personalized medicine with an overall improvement in personalized healthcare. The promising advances in the fields of pharmacogenetics and pharmacogenomics are considered as crucial driving factors for personalized medicine [256]. Recent advances in high-throughput approaches for genetic analyses (genotyping, next-generation sequencing, etc.) combined with the emergence of computational and bioinformatics tools have revolutionized the area of molecular medicine with the objective to attain precise understanding of various complex diseases [250]. This has also resulted in the identification of novel genetic variants and germline mutations involved in various genetic disorders. In the field of cancer, these technologies have facilitated the detection of genetic polymorphisms which predict the patient's response to therapy [257, 258]. Today, the decreased cost of human genome sequencing, accompanying with the availability of genome-wide association studies (GWAS) and the 1000 Genomes Project, has facilitated the identification of genetic variants in different populations [259]. This leads to a better understanding and management of various disorders and contributes to the development of novel diagnostic and therapeutic strategies.

The rapid development of individualized targeted therapies provides investment opportunities as well as diversification of the pharmaceutical industries, which are emerging as another driving factor for personalized medicine. The investment in the development of targeted treatments with regard to personalized medicine allows the pharmaceutical companies to manage the issues including patent expiry or generic competition [260, 261]. This also renders pharmaceutical companies to contribute significantly in the accessibility of personalized treatments to the patients. In short, it suggests that the effective coordination among scientific and regulatory frames as well as pharmaceutical companies will play a key role in driving the progress and evolution in the field of personalized medicine and thus strengthening the integrated healthcare system.

11.3.3 Challenges in Designing the Personalized Medicine

With the passage of time and advancement in knowledge, there is a gradual shift from traditional treatment methods. The most common practice in drug designing and developmental research was to target and study the effect of drug on almost complete population. However, individual patients have inherent different genetic makeup, and thus they respond differently to the same treatment, and thus desirable results were not obtained [262]. With these observations idea of tailoring the treatment to the unique genetic makeup of individual patient was evolved, that is, the idea of tailoring the personalized medicine. Yet it is also obvious that attaining this goal was not an easy task and has many challenges.

Acquiring the individual data for designing the personalized medicine, analysis and maintaining of big omics data, library establishment for biological samples, and obtaining informed consent keeping all involved medical ethics alive especially for major usage in the future for research purposes are some of the challenges that are being faced in this field [263]. Another huge challenge is finding unknown genetic or molecular domains of human genome for personalized medicine development [264]. Basically, the term precision medicine involves multiple omics profile of individual patients including genomics, proteomics, metabolomics, transcriptomics, metagenomics, epigenomics, and pharmacogenomics along with family history and patient lifestyle for designing tailored treatment strategy (as also described in Sect. 11.3.1.3). Complex disease (cancer, diabetes, etc.) also involves patient exposure to the environment and standard of living to assess more individual approach for designing precision medicine especially for most vulnerable patients [265]. It also highlights the shortcomings of healthcare system for diagnostics and therapeutics of more neglected diseases and their pathologies along with their epidemic and endemic.

The most challenging element in designing personalized therapy is related to ethical issues. These include the concerns about the establishment of new biobanks, confidentiality, and handling of data stored in these biobanks [266, 267]. Patient's authorization for genetic testing (informed consent) [268], the appropriate use and interpretation of genetic data [269], genetic discrimination on subject selection based on race or ethnicity [270, 271].

Genomic studies have provided a lot of information about cancer susceptibility gene identification of potential targets for cancer therapeutics and molecular expression profile of the disease and have open many ways for designing drug delivery systems. Still the overview provided through these studies is insufficient for designing personalized medicine therapy and correlating gene transcript with protein expression level in the living system [272]. Moreover, genomic studies may not provide any insight for posttranslational modification such as glycosylation, phosphorylation, lipidation, cleavage, and protein-protein interactions that is important in understanding the disease etiology [145]. Signaling proteins have much more importance in cancer diagnostics and therapeutics as posttranslational modification forms the complex, interrelated signaling cascade that may cause delays in cell apoptosis, cell migration, and division patterns and thus leading to cancer.

In addition, identification of individual gene responsible, related expressed proteins with clinical signatures, biomarkers use as therapeutic or diagnostic candidate for each expressed proteins or its subtype, all these challanges implies for validation and implication of personalized medicine treatment. Another limitation is that there are many potential biomarkers that are identified in published literature, but still research work is required for its proper validation [273]. Their identification in literature does not suffice the criteria for their clinical applications for any treatment and diagnosis or even for categorization according to individual patient treatment for personalized medicine. This has limited the critical element of translational research in the field of cancer. With all these mentioned challenges, still the field of precision or personalized medicine has some initial achievements that can revolutionize general traditional medical practices for patient treatment. Still, it requires the extensive collaboration with a lot of time and money investment. This field is remarkable and can open many pathways to design and provide idealized treatment for patients, but still there is a long way to go.

11.3.4 Proteomic Research Findings and Their Application in Translational Oncology

Proteomics is one of the most important fields in order to understand the actual working of the cell and disease process in this post-genomic era. Cancer proteome involves the study of protein expression of cancer cells and their effects on signaling pathways and other related activities including tumor progression and spread mechanism. Advancement in this field not only provides the information of the protein pathway network, generation of protein repertoire, specific protein interactions and binding, posttranslational modifications, structure, function, characterization, and quantification but also provides the most relevant data for drug development that also helps in the clinical applications of the drug [274]. Every cell has different types of proteome that is unique according to the cell type, but it can be altered according to the tissue microenvironment where it resides. Data based on proteomics are much helpful in cell classification and understanding of protein modification along with cellular mechanism involving the spread of disease [275].

Proteomic research findings are very important to provide the important biological information that is beneficial in designing personalized medicine and early diagnosis especially in the form of biomarkers. This aspect could serve as a major tool in personalized medicine application in translational oncology as it is based on the molecular diagnosis for each patient irrespective of morphological assessment of patients. Type and quality of data that is generated play a vital role in developing genomic and proteomic signatures and biomarker discoveries into anticancer agents for translational oncology [276]. Along with these, monitoring of disease progression and chances of recurrence and therapeutic response of individual patients also play key role in the application of translational oncology. The high accuracy and sensitivity of present-day genomic techniques can characterize more targeted and effective treatments for cancer patients, but current reimbursement and management strategies need to be revised for addition in policies for the introduction of personalized medicine treatment strategies in the routine medical systems. It is also reported previously by Wilhelm et al. through MS-based draft that human proteome expression has high levels of functional proteins of specific cancer [277]. For example, EGFR was found in a very confined expressive manner at high levels in breast cancer [278], and beta-catenin of Wnt signaling pathway was found in colon cancer development [277].

Proteomic research findings on various cancers have shown promising results for detection of novel biomarkers that can be quite useful for cancer diagnosis at initial stage and in designing therapeutics even for individualized patient. Researchers can also design projects that aim to discover novel anticancer agents. This may in turn open many gateways for drug discoveries. Clinical proteomics that is a new subdiscipline of this field deals with molecular technologies for cancer marker discoveries. This discipline can do wonders with more and more research in cancer diagnostics, especially in early stage, and can help not only in saving lives but also reducing the national economic burden.

11.3.5 Personalized Medicine Implications in Healthcare System: Perspective in Oncology

Cancer can be considered as the best study model for the understanding of disease, its functions, and therapeutics, as it can provide the vast research platform for its applications at the bedside. Cancer proteomics covers both basic and clinical elements of proteomics that ultimately lead to cover the translational oncology [41]. Discovery of biomarkers leads to find out the new promising target sites for the treatment and to design patient-specific therapy. The detailed study of cancer proteomics opens new pathways to understand the role of effector protein molecules, their phenotype, and signaling pathways that ultimately leads to the understanding of molecular basis needed to design personalized medicine.

11.3.5.1 Why Personalized Medicine?

At present, personalized medicine approach is higher in demand as it can cover the variability among the individuals resulting in designing of targated therapies. Proteomics plays major role in precision medicine implication as it has an open window for improved therapeutic outcomes [279]. However, for complete treatment understanding and outcomes, the field still requires a lot of advancement.

To date, most of the cancer diagnosis relies on physical examination, imaging, pathological evaluations, and biopsies. However, very limited insight is available in terms of molecular qualities of individual patient profile or morphological assessment of specific tumor tissues/cells that has become the driving factors for developing personalized medicine. The transition of traditional diagnostic and therapeutic methods to personalized real-time molecular approach would be a major drift in cancer treatment. It may also enable high-throughput molecular profiling of individual patient in the future that will be more beneficial than the present-day molecular analysis through PCR for clonal population, in situ hybridization, immunohistochemistry, and chromosomal analysis. Personalized medicine is a hand-in-hand tool for targeted therapies based on the individual patient molecular profile [279].

11.3.5.2 Translational Elements from Bench to Bedside

Translational oncology is the field where the implementation of personalized medicine has enabled scientist to increase their understanding of control of metastasis and some contribution to the improved healthcare system as it provides a better therapeutic approach that is beneficial for the patient as well [280]. While designing a unique treatment plan for an individual patient, the scientist and clinicians closely monitor factors contributing the disease interaction, posttranslational modifications, and their epigenetics and genetics in the diverse presentation of cancer.

Mostly the bench research relies on the molecular assessment of cancer based on cell culture and animal studies. Usually these studies provide an insight of molecular mechanism of disease, signaling pathways, extra- and intracellular matrix, biomarker expression analysis, etc., but it is still difficult to translate these research outcomes for patients' benefit directly due to lack of available knowledge for molecular determinants of specific cancer type and individual patient [281]. Microarray analysis has also confirmed divergence among different cancerous cells and even among same cancer type in different patients [282]. Another limitation of this field is that extracted cell lines are not subject to provide a complete three-dimensional picture of molecular stimuli and tumor microenvironment of complete tissue. Secondly, there are evidences of finding differences between proteomic contents of primary and metastatic tumors [283].

11.4 Biomedical Applications, Challenges, and Future Prospective in Onco-proteomics

Understanding of onco-proteomics is very important for early diagnosis along with cancer management and development of personalized medicine. Knowledge of the pathobiology of cancer leads to the novel diagnostic strategies and improved pharmacological approaches [284]. Discovery of biomarker prognostics, diagnostic and therapeutic site identification, and development of proteomic sequence with the signature posttranslational modification may lead to the properly designed individualized medicine. Still the major components of characterizing the individualized therapy with its complete infrastructure are not discovered yet [274].

11.4.1 Understanding Cancer Pathogenicity

The etiology of diseases is a multifaceted mechanism; several cases of protein malfunctions cause pathogenesis of disease; thus understanding of applied proteomics is a must for understanding the disease [285]. Similarly, cancer pathogenesis is a key factor in order to understand and develop test technologies for personalized medicine design and molecular profiling of individual patients. Furthermore, new tissue collection system for patient specimen must be introduced as generally practiced formalin-based fixation method, which is good enough for morphological/structural assessment and molecular profiling. However, it is insufficient for patient proteomic profiling and related posttranslational modifications, so one requirement is to preserve the morphology of tissue with stabilize RNA and proteins for complete proteomic profiling [140].

Some diseases are also caused by mutation resulting in cystic fibrosis (single-gene mutation) or environmental factors. Furthermore, cancer alters the genome of cells affecting the DNA-repair mechanism and hence modifying the DNA. Biomedical research is very important, especially using the proteomic technologies for shedding light on diseases' pathology, diagnosis, treatment, and prognosis, since it is done using different levels of omics (genomics, transcriptomics, proteomics, and metabolomics) [285]. For example, in order to understand the metastasis, genes need to be analyzed at genomic, proteomic and transcriptomic levels. Biomarker discovery is still a huge challenge posing multiple hurdles in its clinical applications [140]. Existing biomarkers or novel potential biomarkers struggle with proper identification, validation, and reliability along with limited specificity and sensitivity [286].

11.4.2 Onco-proteomic Innovations and Integration with Other Proteomic Tools

Conjunct technologies in proteomics have a larger application in facilitating diagnostics and therapeutics. One of the promising fields is *nano-proteomics* that can help in the understanding of application of nano-biotechnology for the improvement of nano-oncology [287]. This field has shown a promising potential in healthcare system, and in developing personalized medicine approach, yet there is a lot that needs to be worked out along with overcoming technical obstacles for the proper utilization and implication of this emerging field in the healthcare system and translation of cancer research from bench to bedside. *Antibody microarray* is another advancement in proteomics that relies on automation and high-throughput multiplexed analysis of proteins. They can measure even a single sample of different proteins of cancer network, yet one limitation is amplification of sample as done in PCR [288]. Therefore, highly sensitive arrays are required to detect and quantify biomarkers. *Aptamer-based molecular probes* are useful to make ligand with high specificity and affinity due to their 3D structures. These can identify protein signatures of cells, as they have tended to highlight short DNA folding [289]. This technology can also be used with biochips and mass spectrometry for protein monitoring. *Cancer immunomics* can identify autoantibody signatures formed in response of cancer, particularly breast or colorectal cancer [290]. This can also be performed with immunoblotting, immunoaffinity, 2DE, and chromatography to identify isolated antigens. *Tissue microarray* is also used to analyze biomarkers and development of diagnostic tests. It can combine with laser capture microdissection to identify embedded tissue samples [291].

Various technologies have already been developed for protein quantification, functional analysis, posttranslational modification, and biomarker identification. Data generated using these technologies are useful in understanding biological system and cancer. However, the current focus in proteomics understands the nature of proteins with complete analytical capabilities of expression level and mutational changes.

11.4.3 Challenges

Although proteomics is a promising field in cancer studies, it faces many challenges technically in protein separation analysis, genetic mutations, capillary electrophoresis, and cancer repositories, while designing personalized medicine for cancer therapy. Development of biomarker panel and validation of identifying cancer biomarkers are another challenge of the field. Bioinformatics plays a key role in providing initial information and is a powerful tool for analyzing data. Mishandling in this field may result in total shift of obtained results. Careful interpretation of the data may reveal the underlying mechanism of disease spread. Cancer heterogeneity is another challenge that can be minimized by proper study design and developing robust validation assays. Cancer is a complex disease, and in vitro analysis may differ from in vivo analysis in the tumor microenvironment. Studies designed in animal models may differ in humans, as the rate of cancer spread is different. Overall proteomics and related technologies do enable molecular results in clinical validation, but there is still a long way to go.

11.4.4 Future Prospects

Interdisciplinary collaboration among basic scientists, medical professionals like pathologist, radiologist, and oncologist and then bioinformatician, epidemiologists, and bioethicists is necessary for translating bench research to clinical side, developing multicenter clinical trials, managements of big omics data, and a panel of biomarkers to adapt to the personalized medicine paradigm.

To accommodate this fast growing era of personalized medicine, training and education programs for physicians, nurses, residents, and students in the field are a requirement. Disease-related biomarkers need to be evaluated even for low molecular weight serum proteins for the early-stage diagnosis. Cancer diagnosis at early stage is a healthy sign for complete and proper treatment of patients. Other than the abovementioned perspectives, there is need to address some regulatory challenges and policies to be designed by the authorities to cope up with these challenges for the development of the new discipline of personalized medicine, which may provide promising treatment of diseases through the field in the healthcare system.

11.5 Conclusion

Proteomics play an integral role in the different approaches of cancer prognosis, diagnosis, understanding melagnancies, patient monitoring and response to particular therapies and risk assessments. Proteomics data serves as a large-scale analyzer of understanding oncogenes and onco-proteins. It is a promising tool that can enable scientist and clinicians in the field to evaluate and understand cancer at the molecular level and in designing personalized therapies. Furthermore, this field also aids in understanding protein interactions, biomarker role, signaling pathways, tumor heterogeneity, proliferation and spread of disease, mutational changes, and disease pathological and pathophysiological conditions. Still, with such dynamic applications, it also has some pitfalls and there are chances of errors. Therefore, the researchers need to carefully design the study that is also beneficial statistically according to the study question. To fulfill all the aspect of research, a strong and intense collaboration among different cancer field specialists is required to produce quality results that are robust and reliable as well. Discovery along with validation study is a need of the hour to understand the complex and mechanistic changes of cancer. However, it is very hard to lead a uniform impact of cancer research after these highlighted points and recommendations due to diverse and variable challenges.

References

1. Naylor S (2003) Biomarkers: current perspectives and future prospects. Expert Rev Mol Diagn 3(5):525–5299. https://doi.org/10.1586/14737159.3.5.525
2. Mayeux R (2004) Biomarkers: potential uses and limitations. NeuroRx 1(2):182–188. https://doi.org/10.1602/neurorx.1.2.182
3. Wulfkuhle JD, Liotta LA, Petricoin EF (2003) Proteomic applications for the early detection of cancer. Nat Rev Cancer 3(4):267–275. https://doi.org/10.1038/nrc1043

4. Hudler P, Kocevar N, Komel R (2014) Proteomic approaches in biomarker discovery: new perspectives in cancer diagnostics. Sci World J 2014:260348. https://doi.org/10.1155/2014/260348
5. Henry NL, Hayes DF (2012) Cancer biomarkers. Mol Oncol 6(2):140–146. https://doi.org/10.1016/j.molonc.2012.01.010
6. Zhang Z, Chan DW (2005) Cancer proteomics: in pursuit of "true" biomarker discovery. Cancer Epidemiol Biomarkers Prev 14(10):2283–2286. https://doi.org/10.1158/1055-9965.EPI-05-0774
7. Srinivasan R (1986) Ablation of polymers and biological tissue by ultraviolet lasers. Science 234(4776):559–565. https://doi.org/10.1126/science.3764428
8. Han Y, Gu Y, Zhang AC, Lo YH (2016) Review: imaging technologies for flow cytometry. Lab Chip 16(24):4639–4647. https://doi.org/10.1039/c6lc01063f
9. Srinivas PR, Srivastava S, Hanash S, Wright GL Jr (2001) Proteomics in early detection of cancer. Clin Chem 47(10):1901–1911
10. Croce CM (2008) Oncogenes and cancer. N Engl J Med 358(5):502–511. https://doi.org/10.1056/NEJMra072367
11. Li X, Blount PL, Vaughan TL, Reid BJ (2011) Application of biomarkers in cancer risk management: evaluation from stochastic clonal evolutionary and dynamic system optimization points of view. PLoS Comput Biol 7(2):e1001087. https://doi.org/10.1371/journal.pcbi.1001087
12. Goncalves A, Esterni B, Bertucci F, Sauvan R, Chabannon C, Cubizolles M, Bardou VJ, Houvenaegel G, Jacquemier J, Granjeaud S, Meng XY, Fung ET, Birnbaum D, Maraninchi D, Viens P, Borg JP (2006) Postoperative serum proteomic profiles may predict metastatic relapse in high-risk primary breast cancer patients receiving adjuvant chemotherapy. Oncogene 25(7):981–989. https://doi.org/10.1038/sj.onc.1209131
13. Li X, Galipeau PC, Sanchez CA, Blount PL, Maley CC, Arnaudo J, Peiffer DA, Pokholok D, Gunderson KL, Reid BJ (2008) Single nucleotide polymorphism-based genome-wide chromosome copy change, loss of heterozygosity, and aneuploidy in Barrett's esophagus neoplastic progression. Cancer Prev Res (Phila) 1(6):413–423. https://doi.org/10.1158/1940-6207.CAPR-08-0121
14. Greenman C, Stephens P, Smith R, Dalgliesh GL, Hunter C, Bignell G, Davies H, Teague J, Butler A, Stevens C, Edkins S, O'Meara S, Vastrik I, Schmidt EE, Avis T, Barthorpe S, Bhamra G, Buck G, Choudhury B, Clements J, Cole J, Dicks E, Forbes S, Gray K, Halliday K, Harrison R, Hills K, Hinton J, Jenkinson A, Jones D, Menzies A, Mironenko T, Perry J, Raine K, Richardson D, Shepherd R, Small A, Tofts C, Varian J, Webb T, West S, Widaa S, Yates A, Cahill DP, Louis DN, Goldstraw P, Nicholson AG, Brasseur F, Looijenga L, Weber BL, Chiew YE, DeFazio A, Greaves MF, Green AR, Campbell P, Birney E, Easton DF, Chenevix-Trench G, Tan MH, Khoo SK, Teh BT, Yuen ST, Leung SY, Wooster R, Futreal PA, Stratton MR (2007) Patterns of somatic mutation in human cancer genomes. Nature 446(7132):153–158. https://doi.org/10.1038/nature05610
15. Baudis M (2007) Genomic imbalances in 5918 malignant epithelial tumors: an explorative meta-analysis of chromosomal CGH data. BMC Cancer 7:226. https://doi.org/10.1186/1471-2407-7-226
16. Litzenburger UM, Buenrostro JD, Wu B, Shen Y, Sheffield NC, Kathiria A, Greenleaf WJ, Chang HY (2017) Single-cell epigenomic variability reveals functional cancer heterogeneity. Genome Biol 18(1):15. https://doi.org/10.1186/s13059-016-1133-7
17. Wang X, Markowetz F, De Sousa EMF, Medema JP, Vermeulen L (2013) Dissecting cancer heterogeneity--an unsupervised classification approach. Int J Biochem Cell Biol 45(11):2574–2579. https://doi.org/10.1016/j.biocel.2013.08.014
18. Gustafsson OJ, Eddes JS, Meding S, McColl SR, Oehler MK, Hoffmann P (2013) Matrix-assisted laser desorption/ionization imaging protocol for in situ characterization of tryptic peptide identity and distribution in formalin-fixed tissue. Rapid Commun Mass Spectrom 27(6):655–670. https://doi.org/10.1002/rcm.6488

19. Meding S, Martin K, Gustafsson OJ, Eddes JS, Hack S, Oehler MK, Hoffmann P (2013) Tryptic peptide reference data sets for MALDI imaging mass spectrometry on formalin-fixed ovarian cancer tissues. J Proteome Res 12(1):308–315. https://doi.org/10.1021/pr300996x
20. Shipitsin M, Small C, Choudhury S, Giladi E, Friedlander S, Nardone J, Hussain S, Hurley AD, Ernst C, Huang YE, Chang H, Nifong TP, Rimm DL, Dunyak J, Loda M, Berman DM, Blume-Jensen P (2014) Identification of proteomic biomarkers predicting prostate cancer aggressiveness and lethality despite biopsy-sampling error. Br J Cancer 111(6):1201–1212. https://doi.org/10.1038/bjc.2014.396
21. Siegel RL, Miller KD, Jemal A (2018) Cancer statistics, 2018. CA Cancer J Clin 68(1):7–30. https://doi.org/10.3322/caac.21442
22. Corbo C, Cevenini A, Salvatore F (2017) Biomarker discovery by proteomics-based approaches for early detection and personalized medicine in colorectal cancer. Proteomics Clin Appl 11(5–6). https://doi.org/10.1002/prca.201600072
23. Bray F, Ferlay J, Soerjomataram I, Siegel RL, Torre LA, Jemal A (2018) Global cancer statistics 2018: GLOBOCAN estimates of incidence and mortality worldwide for 36 cancers in 185 countries. CA Cancer J Clin 68(6):394–424. https://doi.org/10.3322/caac.21492
24. Lee JY, Yoon JK, Kim B, Kim S, Kim MA, Lim H, Bang D, Song YS (2015) Tumor evolution and intratumor heterogeneity of an epithelial ovarian cancer investigated using next-generation sequencing. BMC Cancer 15:85. https://doi.org/10.1186/s12885-015-1077-4
25. Mabert K, Cojoc M, Peitzsch C, Kurth I, Souchelnytskyi S, Dubrovska A (2014) Cancer biomarker discovery: current status and future perspectives. Int J Radiat Biol 90(8):659–677. https://doi.org/10.3109/09553002.2014.892229
26. Sever R, Brugge JS (2015) Signal transduction in cancer. Cold Spring Harb Perspect Med 5(4). https://doi.org/10.1101/cshperspect.a006098
27. Monica L, Savu L (2013) A different approach for cellular oncogene identification came from Drosophila genetics. In: Oncogene and cancer - from bench to clinic. https://doi.org/10.5772/54150
28. Yan H, Chen X, Li Y, Fan L, Tai Y, Zhou Y, Chen Y, Qi X, Huang R, Ren J (2019) MiR-1205 functions as a tumor suppressor by disconnecting the synergy between KRAS and MDM4/E2F1 in non-small cell lung cancer. Vaccine 9(2):312–329
29. Albertson DG, Collins C, McCormick F, Gray JW (2003) Chromosome aberrations in solid tumors. Nat Genet 34(4):369–376. https://doi.org/10.1038/ng1215
30. Sauter ER (2017) Exosomes in blood and cancer. Transl Cancer Res 6(S8):S1316–S1320. https://doi.org/10.21037/tcr.2017.08.13
31. Aaltonen L, Johns L, Jarvinen H, Mecklin JP, Houlston R (2007) Explaining the familial colorectal cancer risk associated with mismatch repair (MMR)-deficient and MMR-stable tumors. Clin Cancer Res 13(1):356–361. https://doi.org/10.1158/1078-0432.CCR-06-1256
32. Walker JG, Licqurish S, Chiang PP, Pirotta M, Emery JD (2015) Cancer risk assessment tools in primary care: a systematic review of randomized controlled trials. Ann Fam Med 13(5):480–489. https://doi.org/10.1370/afm.1837
33. Yarnall JM, Crouch DJ, Lewis CM (2013) Incorporating non-genetic risk factors and behavioural modifications into risk prediction models for colorectal cancer. Cancer Epidemiol 37(3):324–329. https://doi.org/10.1016/j.canep.2012.12.008
34. Services USDoHaH (2014) The Colorectal Cancer Risk Assessment Tool. National Institutes of Health
35. Gail MH, Brinton LA, Byar DP, Corle DK, Green SB, Schairer C, Mulvihill JJ (1989) Projecting individualized probabilities of developing breast cancer for white females who are being examined annually. J Natl Cancer Inst 81(24):1879–1886. https://doi.org/10.1093/jnci/81.24.1879
36. Wang W, Niendorf KB, Patel D, Blackford A, Marroni F, Sober AJ, Parmigiani G, Tsao H (2010) Estimating CDKN2A carrier probability and personalizing cancer risk assessments in hereditary melanoma using MelaPRO. Cancer Res 70(2):552–559. https://doi.org/10.1158/0008-5472.CAN-09-2653

37. Wilson KE, Ryan MM, Prime JE, Pashby DP, Orange PR, O'Beirne G, Whateley JG, Bahn S, Morris CM (2004) Functional genomics and proteomics: application in neurosciences. J Neurol Neurosurg Psychiatry 75(4):529–538. https://doi.org/10.1136/jnnp.2003.026260
38. Kellner R (2000) Proteomics. Concepts and perspectives. Fresenius J Anal Chem 366:517–524
39. Klein JB, Thongboonkerd V (2004) Overview of proteomics. Contrib Nephrol 141:1–10
40. Ullrich B, Ushkaryov YA, Südhof TC (1995) Cartography of neurexins: more than 1000 isoforms generated by alternative splicing and expressed in distinct subsets of neurons. Neuron 14(3)
41. Shruthi BS, Vinodhkumar P, Selvamani (2016) Proteomics: a new perspective for cancer. Adv Biomed Res 5:67. https://doi.org/10.4103/2277-9175.180636
42. Carr KM, Rosenblatt K, Petricoin EF, Liotta LA (2004) Genomic and proteomic approaches for studying human cancer: prospects for true patient-tailored therapy. Hum Genomics 1(2):134–140
43. Vaezzadeh AR, Steen H, Freeman MR, Lee RS (2009) Proteomics and opportunities for clinical translation in urological disease. J Urol 182(3):835–843. https://doi.org/10.1016/j.juro.2009.05.001
44. Liotta LA, Kohn EC, Petricoin EF (2001) Clinical proteomics. JAMA 286(18). https://doi.org/10.1001/jama.286.18.2211
45. Petricoin EF, Ardekani AM, Hitt BA, Levine PJ, Fusaro VA, Steinberg SM, Mills GB, Simone C, Fishman DA, Kohn EC, Liotta LA (2002) Use of proteomic patterns in serum to identify ovarian cancer. Lancet 359(9306):572–577. https://doi.org/10.1016/s0140-6736(02)07746-2
46. Li J, Zhang Z, Rosenzweig J, Wang YY, Chan DW (2002) Proteomics and bioinformatics approaches for identification of serum biomarkers to detect breast cancer. Clin Chem 48(8):1296–1304
47. Adam BL, Qu Y, Davis JW, Ward MD, Clements MA, Cazares LH, Semmes OJ, Schellhammer PF, Yasui Y, Feng Z, Wright GL Jr (2002) Serum protein fingerprinting coupled with a pattern-matching algorithm distinguishes prostate cancer from benign prostate hyperplasia and healthy men. Cancer Res 62(13):3609–3614
48. Poon TC, Yip TT, Chan AT, Yip C, Yip V, Mok TS, Lee CC, Leung TW, Ho SK, Johnson PJ (2003) Comprehensive proteomic profiling identifies serum proteomic signatures for detection of hepatocellular carcinoma and its subtypes. Clin Chem 49(5):752–760
49. Siegel RL, Miller KD, Jemal A (2016) Cancer statistics, 2016. CA Cancer J Clin 66(1):7–30. https://doi.org/10.3322/caac.21332
50. Sung HJ, Cho JY (2008) Biomarkers for the lung cancer diagnosis and their advances in proteomics. BMB Rep 41(9):615–625. https://doi.org/10.5483/bmbrep.2008.41.9.615
51. Luo L, Dong LY, Yan QG, Cao SJ, Wen XT, Huang Y, Huang XB, Wu R, Ma XP (2014) Research progress in applying proteomics technology to explore early diagnosis biomarkers of breast cancer, lung cancer and ovarian cancer. Asian Pac J Cancer Prev 15(20):8529–8538. https://doi.org/10.7314/apjcp.2014.15.20.8529
52. Brichory FM, Misek DE, Yim AM, Krause MC, Giordano TJ, Beer DG, Hanash SM (2001) An immune response manifested by the common occurrence of annexins I and II autoantibodies and high circulating levels of IL-6 in lung cancer. Proc Natl Acad Sci U S A 98(17):9824–9829. https://doi.org/10.1073/pnas.171320598
53. Zamay TN, Zamay GS, Kolovskaya OS, Zukov RA, Petrova MM, Gargaun A, Berezovski MV, Kichkailo AS (2017) Current and prospective protein biomarkers of lung cancer. Cancers (Basel) 9(11). https://doi.org/10.3390/cancers9110155
54. Taguchi A, Politi K, Pitteri SJ, Lockwood WW, Faca VM, Kelly-Spratt K, Wong CH, Zhang Q, Chin A, Park KS, Goodman G, Gazdar AF, Sage J, Dinulescu DM, Kucherlapati R, Depinho RA, Kemp CJ, Varmus HE, Hanash SM (2011) Lung cancer signatures in plasma based on proteome profiling of mouse tumor models. Cancer Cell 20(3):289–299. https://doi.org/10.1016/j.ccr.2011.08.007
55. Patz EF Jr, Campa MJ, Gottlin EB, Kusmartseva I, Guan XR, Herndon JE 2nd (2007) Panel of serum biomarkers for the diagnosis of lung cancer. J Clin Oncol 25(35):5578–5583. https://doi.org/10.1200/JCO.2007.13.5392

56. Cheung CHY, Juan HF (2017) Quantitative proteomics in lung cancer. J Biomed Sci 24(1):37. https://doi.org/10.1186/s12929-017-0343-y
57. Wu CC, Chien KY, Tsang NM, Chang KP, Hao SP, Tsao CH, Chang YS, Yu JS (2005) Cancer cell-secreted proteomes as a basis for searching potential tumor markers: nasopharyngeal carcinoma as a model. Proteomics 5(12):3173–3182. https://doi.org/10.1002/pmic.200401133
58. Welsh JB, Sapinoso LM, Kern SG, Brown DA, Liu T, Bauskin AR, Ward RL, Hawkins NJ, Quinn DI, Russell PJ, Sutherland RL, Breit SN, Moskaluk CA, Frierson HF Jr, Hampton GM (2003) Large-scale delineation of secreted protein biomarkers overexpressed in cancer tissue and serum. Proc Natl Acad Sci U S A 100(6):3410–3415. https://doi.org/10.1073/pnas.0530278100
59. Huang LJ, Chen SX, Huang Y, Luo WJ, Jiang HH, Hu QH, Zhang PF, Yi H (2006) Proteomics-based identification of secreted protein dihydrodiol dehydrogenase as a novel serum markers of non-small cell lung cancer. Lung Cancer 54(1):87–94. https://doi.org/10.1016/j.lungcan.2006.06.011
60. Conrad DH, Goyette J, Thomas PS (2008) Proteomics as a method for early detection of cancer: a review of proteomics, exhaled breath condensate, and lung cancer screening. J Gen Intern Med 23(Suppl 1):78–84. https://doi.org/10.1007/s11606-007-0411-1
61. Polanski M, Anderson NL (2007) A list of candidate cancer biomarkers for targeted proteomics. Biomark Insights 1:1–48
62. Sallam RM (2015) Proteomics in cancer biomarkers discovery: challenges and applications. Dis Markers 2015:321370. https://doi.org/10.1155/2015/321370
63. Geiger T, Madden SF, Gallagher WM, Cox J, Mann M (2012) Proteomic portrait of human breast cancer progression identifies novel prognostic markers. Cancer Res 72(9):2428–2439. https://doi.org/10.1158/0008-5472.CAN-11-3711
64. Pitteri SJ, Kelly-Spratt KS, Gurley KE, Kennedy J, Buson TB, Chin A, Wang H, Zhang Q, Wong CH, Chodosh LA, Nelson PS, Hanash SM, Kemp CJ (2011) Tumor microenvironment-derived proteins dominate the plasma proteome response during breast cancer induction and progression. Cancer Res 71(15):5090–5100. https://doi.org/10.1158/0008-5472.CAN-11-0568
65. Luftner D, Possinger K (2002) Nuclear matrix proteins as biomarkers for breast cancer. Expert Rev Mol Diagn 2(1):23–31. https://doi.org/10.1586/14737159.2.1.23
66. Samadder NJ, Jasperson K, Burt RW (2015) Hereditary and common familial colorectal cancer: evidence for colorectal screening. Dig Dis Sci 60(3):734–747. https://doi.org/10.1007/s10620-014-3465-z
67. Guinney J, Dienstmann R, Wang X, de Reynies A, Schlicker A, Soneson C, Marisa L, Roepman P, Nyamundanda G, Angelino P, Bot BM, Morris JS, Simon IM, Gerster S, Fessler E, De Sousa EMF, Missiaglia E, Ramay H, Barras D, Homicsko K, Maru D, Manyam GC, Broom B, Boige V, Perez-Villamil B, Laderas T, Salazar R, Gray JW, Hanahan D, Tabernero J, Bernards R, Friend SH, Laurent-Puig P, Medema JP, Sadanandam A, Wessels L, Delorenzi M, Kopetz S, Vermeulen L, Tejpar S (2015) The consensus molecular subtypes of colorectal cancer. Nat Med 21(11):1350–1356. https://doi.org/10.1038/nm.3967
68. Chauvin A, Boisvert FM (2018) Clinical proteomics in colorectal cancer, a promising tool for improving personalised medicine. Proteomes 6(4). https://doi.org/10.3390/proteomes6040049
69. Zhang B, Wang J, Wang X, Zhu J, Liu Q, Shi Z, Chambers MC, Zimmerman LJ, Shaddox KF, Kim S, Davies SR, Wang S, Wang P, Kinsinger CR, Rivers RC, Rodriguez H, Townsend RR, Ellis MJ, Carr SA, Tabb DL, Coffey RJ, Slebos RJ, Liebler DC, Nci C (2014) Proteogenomic characterization of human colon and rectal cancer. Nature 513(7518):382–387. https://doi.org/10.1038/nature13438
70. Dobbin KK, Cesano A, Alvarez J, Hawtin R, Janetzki S, Kirsch I, Masucci GV, Robbins PB, Selvan SR, Streicher HZ, Zhang J, Butterfield LH, Thurin M (2016) Validation of biomarkers to predict response to immunotherapy in cancer: volume II - clinical validation and regulatory considerations. J Immunother Cancer 4:77. https://doi.org/10.1186/s40425-016-0179-0

71. Di Nicolantonio F, Martini M, Molinari F, Sartore-Bianchi A, Arena S, Saletti P, De Dosso S, Mazzucchelli L, Frattini M, Siena S, Bardelli A (2008) Wild-type BRAF is required for response to panitumumab or cetuximab in metastatic colorectal cancer. J Clin Oncol 26(35):5705–5712. https://doi.org/10.1200/JCO.2008.18.0786
72. Takano M, Sugiyama T (2017) UGT1A1 polymorphisms in cancer: impact on irinotecan treatment. Pharmgenomics Pers Med 10:61–68. https://doi.org/10.2147/PGPM.S108656
73. Mischak H, Ioannidis JP, Argiles A, Attwood TK, Bongcam-Rudloff E, Broenstrup M, Charonis A, Chrousos GP, Delles C, Dominiczak A, Dylag T, Ehrich J, Egido J, Findeisen P, Jankowski J, Johnson RW, Julien BA, Lankisch T, Leung HY, Maahs D, Magni F, Manns MP, Manolis E, Mayer G, Navis G, Novak J, Ortiz A, Persson F, Peter K, Riese HH, Rossing P, Sattar N, Spasovski G, Thongboonkerd V, Vanholder R, Schanstra JP, Vlahou A (2012) Implementation of proteomic biomarkers: making it work. Eur J Clin Invest 42(9):1027–1036. https://doi.org/10.1111/j.1365-2362.2012.02674.x
74. Jennings L, Van Deerlin VM, Gulley ML, College of American Pathologists Molecular Pathology Resource C (2009) Recommended principles and practices for validating clinical molecular pathology tests. Arch Pathol Lab Med 133(5):743–755. https://doi.org/10.1043/1543-2165-133.5.743
75. Duffy MJ, O'Donovan N, Crown J (2011) Use of molecular markers for predicting therapy response in cancer patients. Cancer Treat Rev 37(2):151–159. https://doi.org/10.1016/j.ctrv.2010.07.004
76. Hoffman RM (2011) Clinical practice. Screening for prostate cancer. N Engl J Med 365(21):2013–2019. https://doi.org/10.1056/NEJMcp1103642
77. Wang X, Yu J, Sreekumar A, Varambally S, Shen R, Giacherio D, Mehra R, Montie JE, Pienta KJ, Sanda MG, Kantoff PW, Rubin MA, Wei JT, Ghosh D, Chinnaiyan AM (2005) Autoantibody signatures in prostate cancer. N Engl J Med 353(12):1224–1235. https://doi.org/10.1056/NEJMoa051931
78. Ornstein DK, Gillespie JW, Paweletz CP, Duray PH, Herring J, Vocke CD, Topalian SL, Bostwick DG, Linehan WM, Petricoin EF, Emmert-Buck MR (2000) Proteomic analysis of laser capture microdissected human prostate cancer and in vitro prostate cell lines. Electrophoresis 21(11):2235–2242. https://doi.org/10.1002/1522-2683(20000601)21:11<2235::Aid-elps2235>3.0.Co;2-a
79. Hood BL, Darfler MM, Guiel TG, Furusato B, Lucas DA, Ringeisen BR, Sesterhenn IA, Conrads TP, Veenstra TD, Krizman DB (2005) Proteomic analysis of formalin-fixed prostate cancer tissue. Mol Cell Proteomics 4(11):1741–1753. https://doi.org/10.1074/mcp.M500102-MCP200
80. Saraon P, Cretu D, Musrap N, Karagiannis GS, Batruch I, Drabovich AP, van der Kwast T, Mizokami A, Morrissey C, Jarvi K, Diamandis EP (2013) Quantitative proteomics reveals that enzymes of the ketogenic pathway are associated with prostate cancer progression. Mol Cell Proteomics 12(6):1589–1601. https://doi.org/10.1074/mcp.M112.023887
81. Cho WC (2014) Proteomics in translational cancer research: biomarker discovery for clinical applications. Expert Rev Proteomics 11(2):131–133. https://doi.org/10.1586/14789450.2014.899908
82. He QY, Cheung YH, Leung SY, Yuen ST, Chu KM, Chiu JF (2004) Diverse proteomic alterations in gastric adenocarcinoma. Proteomics 4(10):3276–3287. https://doi.org/10.1002/pmic.200300916
83. Altieri F, Di Stadio CS, Severino V, Sandomenico A, Minopoli G, Miselli G, Di Maro A, Ruvo M, Chambery A, Quagliariello V, Masullo M, Rippa E, Arcari P (2014) Anti-amyloidogenic property of human gastrokine 1. Biochimie 106:91–100. https://doi.org/10.1016/j.biochi.2014.08.004
84. Menheniott TR, Peterson AJ, O'Connor L, Lee KS, Kalantzis A, Kondova I, Bontrop RE, Bell KM, Giraud AS (2010) A novel gastrokine, Gkn3, marks gastric atrophy and shows evidence of adaptive gene loss in humans. Gastroenterology 138(5):1823–1835. https://doi.org/10.1053/j.gastro.2010.01.050

85. Lin LL, Huang HC, Juan HF (2012) Discovery of biomarkers for gastric cancer: a proteomics approach. J Proteomics 75(11):3081–3097. https://doi.org/10.1016/j.jprot.2012.03.046
86. Jang JSJ, Cho HY, Lee YJ, Ha WS, Kim HW (2004) The differential proteome profile of stomach cancer: identification of the biomarker candidates. Oncol Res Featuring Preclin Clin Cancer Ther 14(10):491–499. https://doi.org/10.3727/0965040042380441
87. Melle C, Ernst G, Schimmel B, Bleul A, Kaufmann R, Hommann M, Richter KK, Daffner W, Settmacher U, Claussen U, von Eggeling F (2005) Characterization of pepsinogen C as a potential biomarker for gastric cancer using a histo-proteomic approach. J Proteome Res 4(5):1799–1804. https://doi.org/10.1021/pr050123o
88. Hao Y, Yu Y, Wang L, Yan M, Ji J, Qu Y, Zhang J, Liu B, Zhu Z (2008) IPO-38 is identified as a novel serum biomarker of gastric cancer based on clinical proteomics technology. J Proteome Res 7(9):3668–3677. https://doi.org/10.1021/pr700638k
89. Di Bisceglie AM, Sterling RK, Chung RT, Everhart JE, Dienstag JL, Bonkovsky HL, Wright EC, Everson GT, Lindsay KL, Lok ASF, Lee WM, Morgan TR, Ghany MG, Gretch DR, the H-CTG (2005) Serum alpha-fetoprotein levels in patients with advanced hepatitis C: results from the HALT-C Trial. J Hepatol 43(3):434–441. https://doi.org/10.1016/j.jhep.2005.03.019
90. Liebman HA, Furie BC, Tong MJ, Blanchard RA, Lo KJ, Lee SD, Coleman MS, Furie B (1984) Des-gamma-carboxy (abnormal) prothrombin as a serum marker of primary hepatocellular carcinoma. N Engl J Med 310(22):1427–1431. https://doi.org/10.1056/NEJM198405313102204
91. Di Tommaso L, Franchi G, Park YN, Fiamengo B, Destro A, Morenghi E, Montorsi M, Torzilli G, Tommasini M, Terracciano L, Tornillo L, Vecchione R, Roncalli M (2007) Diagnostic value of HSP70, glypican 3, and glutamine synthetase in hepatocellular nodules in cirrhosis. Hepatology 45(3):725–734. https://doi.org/10.1002/hep.21531
92. Wu Z, Pang W, Coghill GM (2015) An integrative top-down and bottom-up qualitative model construction framework for exploration of biochemical systems. Soft Comput 19(6):1595–1610. https://doi.org/10.1007/s00500-014-1467-6
93. Megger DA, Naboulsi W, Meyer HE, Sitek B (2014) Proteome analyses of hepatocellular carcinoma. J Clin Transl Hepatol 2(1):23–30. https://doi.org/10.14218/JCTH.2013.00022
94. Yokoo H, Kondo T, Fujii K, Yamada T, Todo S, Hirohashi S (2004) Proteomic signature corresponding to alpha fetoprotein expression in liver cancer cells. Hepatology 40(3):609–617. https://doi.org/10.1002/hep.20372
95. Fu WM, Zhang JF, Wang H, Tan HS, Wang WM, Chen SC, Zhu X, Chan TM, Tse CM, Leung KS, Lu G, Xu HX, Kung HF (2012) Apoptosis induced by 1,3,6,7-tetrahydroxyxanthone in Hepatocellular carcinoma and proteomic analysis. Apoptosis 17(8):842–851. https://doi.org/10.1007/s10495-012-0729-y
96. Zhang J, Niu D, Sui J, Ching CB, Chen WN (2009) Protein profile in hepatitis B virus replicating rat primary hepatocytes and HepG2 cells by iTRAQ-coupled 2-D LC-MS/MS analysis: insights on liver angiogenesis. Proteomics 9(10):2836–2845. https://doi.org/10.1002/pmic.200800911
97. Albrethsen J, Miller LM, Novikoff PM, Angeletti RH (2011) Gel-based proteomics of liver cancer progression in rat. Biochim Biophys Acta 1814(10):1367–1376. https://doi.org/10.1016/j.bbapap.2011.05.018
98. Jain KK (2008) Innovations, challenges and future prospects of oncoproteomics. Mol Oncol 2(2):153–160. https://doi.org/10.1016/j.molonc.2008.05.003
99. Braoudaki M, Lambrou GI, Vougas K, Karamolegou K, Tsangaris GT, Tzortzatou-Stathopoulou F (2013) Protein biomarkers distinguish between high- and low-risk pediatric acute lymphoblastic leukemia in a tissue specific manner. J Hematol Oncol 6:52. https://doi.org/10.1186/1756-8722-6-52
100. Prada-Arismendy J, Arroyave JC, Rothlisberger S (2017) Molecular biomarkers in acute myeloid leukemia. Blood Rev 31(1):63–76. https://doi.org/10.1016/j.blre.2016.08.005
101. Hjelle SM, Forthun RB, Haaland I, Reikvam H, Sjoholt G, Bruserud O, Gjertsen BT (2010) Clinical proteomics of myeloid leukemia. Genome Med 2(6):41. https://doi.org/10.1186/gm162

102. Lopez-Pedrera C, Villalba JM, Siendones E, Barbarroja N, Gomez-Diaz C, Rodriguez-Ariza A, Buendia P, Torres A, Velasco F (2006) Proteomic analysis of acute myeloid leukemia: identification of potential early biomarkers and therapeutic targets. Proteomics 6(Suppl 1):S293–S299. https://doi.org/10.1002/pmic.200500384
103. Voss T, Ahorn H, Haberl P, Döhner H, Wilgenbus K (2001) Correlation of clinical data with proteomics profiles in 24 patients with B-cell chronic lymphocytic leukemia. Int J Cancer 91(2):180–186. https://doi.org/10.1002/1097-0215(200002)9999:9999 <::Aid-ijc1037>3.0.Co;2-j
104. Jongen-Lavrencic M, Grob T, Hanekamp D, Kavelaars FG, Al Hinai A, Zeilemaker A, Erpelinck-Verschueren CAJ, Gradowska PL, Meijer R, Cloos J, Biemond BJ, Graux C, van Marwijk Kooy M, Manz MG, Pabst T, Passweg JR, Havelange V, Ossenkoppele GJ, Sanders MA, Schuurhuis GJ, Lowenberg B, Valk PJM (2018) Molecular minimal residual disease in acute myeloid leukemia. N Engl J Med 378(13):1189–1199. https://doi.org/10.1056/NEJMoa1716863
105. Bai J, He A, Huang C, Yang J, Zhang W, Wang J, Yang Y, Zhang P, Zhang Y, Zhou F (2014) Serum peptidome based biomarkers searching for monitoring minimal residual disease in adult acute lymphocytic leukemia. Proteome Sci 12(1):49. https://doi.org/10.1186/s12953-014-0049-y
106. Odreman F, Vindigni M, Gonzales ML, Niccolini B, Candiano G, Zanotti B, Skrap M, Pizzolitto S, Stanta G, Vindigni A (2005) Proteomic studies on low- and high-grade human brain astrocytomas. J Proteome Res 4(3):698–708. https://doi.org/10.1021/pr0498180
107. Hu Y, Huang X, Chen GYJ, Yao SQ (2004) Recent advances in gel-based proteome profiling techniques. Mol Biotechnol 28(1):63–76. https://doi.org/10.1385/mb:28:1:63
108. Iwadate Y, Sakaida T, Hiwasa T, Nagai Y, Ishikura H, Takiguchi M, Yamaura A (2004) Molecular classification and survival prediction in human gliomas based on proteome analysis. Cancer Res 64(7):2496–2501. https://doi.org/10.1158/0008-5472.CAN-03-1254
109. Liu H, Sadygov RG, Yates JR 3rd (2004) A model for random sampling and estimation of relative protein abundance in shotgun proteomics. Anal Chem 76(14):4193–4201. https://doi.org/10.1021/ac0498563
110. Ross PL, Huang YN, Marchese JN, Williamson B, Parker K, Hattan S, Khainovski N, Pillai S, Dey S, Daniels S, Purkayastha S, Juhasz P, Martin S, Bartlet-Jones M, He F, Jacobson A, Pappin DJ (2004) Multiplexed protein quantitation in Saccharomyces cerevisiae using amine-reactive isobaric tagging reagents. Mol Cell Proteomics 3(12):1154–1169. https://doi.org/10.1074/mcp.M400129-MCP200
111. Jacobs IJ, Skates SJ, MacDonald N, Menon U, Rosenthal AN, Davies AP, Woolas R, Jeyarajah AR, Sibley K, Lowe DG, Oram DH (1999) Screening for ovarian cancer: a pilot randomised controlled trial. Lancet 353(9160):1207–1210. https://doi.org/10.1016/s0140-6736(98)10261-1
112. Cohen LS, Escobar PF, Scharm C, Glimco B, Fishman DA (2001) Three-dimensional power Doppler ultrasound improves the diagnostic accuracy for ovarian cancer prediction. Gynecol Oncol 82(1):40–48. https://doi.org/10.1006/gyno.2001.6253
113. Conrads TP, Zhou M, Petricoin EF III, Liotta L, Veenstra TD (2003) Cancer diagnosis using proteomic patterns. Expert Rev Mol Diagn 3(4):411–420
114. Plebani M (2005) Proteomics: the next revolution in laboratory medicine? Clin Chim Acta 357(2):113–122. https://doi.org/10.1016/j.cccn.2005.03.017
115. Diamandis EP (2003) Proteomic patterns in biological fluids: do they represent the future of cancer diagnostics? Clin Chem 49(8):1272–1275. https://doi.org/10.1373/49.8.1272
116. Lin YW, Lin CY, Lai HC, Chiou JY, Chang CC, Yu MH, Chu TY (2006) Plasma proteomic pattern as biomarkers for ovarian cancer. Int J Gynecol Cancer 16(Suppl 1):139–146. https://doi.org/10.1111/j.1525-1438.2006.00475.x
117. Petricoin E (2003) The vision for a new diagnostic paradigm. Clin Chem 49(8):1276–1278. https://doi.org/10.1373/49.8.1276
118. Green CL, Khavari PA (2004) Targets for molecular therapy of skin cancer. Semin Cancer Biol 14(1):63–69. https://doi.org/10.1016/j.semcancer.2003.11.007

119. Kasparian NA, McLoone JK, Meiser B (2009) Skin cancer-related prevention and screening behaviors: a review of the literature. J Behav Med 32(5):406–428. https://doi.org/10.1007/s10865-009-9219-2
120. Franssen ME, Zeeuwen PL, Vierwinden G, van de Kerkhof PC, Schalkwijk J, van Erp PE (2005) Phenotypical and functional differences in germinative subpopulations derived from normal and psoriatic epidermis. J Invest Dermatol 124(2):373–383. https://doi.org/10.1111/j.0022-202X.2004.23612.x
121. Huang CM, Foster KW, DeSilva T, Zhang J, Shi Z, Yusuf N, Van Kampen KR, Elmets CA, Tang DC (2003) Comparative proteomic profiling of murine skin. J Invest Dermatol 121(1):51–64. https://doi.org/10.1046/j.1523-1747.2003.12327.x
122. Hamideh MF, Hakimeh Z, Mostafa RT, Parviz T (2010) Roteomic analysis of gene expression in basal cell carcinoma. Iran J Dermatol 13(4):112–117
123. Cheng SL, Liu RH, Sheu JN, Chen ST, Sinchaikul S, Tsay GJ (2007) Toxicogenomics of A375 human malignant melanoma cells treated with arbutin. J Biomed Sci 14(1):87–105. https://doi.org/10.1007/s11373-006-9130-6
124. Penque D (2009) Two-dimensional gel electrophoresis and mass spectrometry for biomarker discovery. Proteomics Clin Appl 3(2):155–172. https://doi.org/10.1002/prca.200800025
125. Rai AJ, Gelfand CA, Haywood BC, Warunek DJ, Yi J, Schuchard MD, Mehigh RJ, Cockrill SL, Scott GB, Tammen H, Schulz-Knappe P, Speicher DW, Vitzthum F, Haab BB, Siest G, Chan DW (2005) HUPO Plasma Proteome Project specimen collection and handling: towards the standardization of parameters for plasma proteome samples. Proteomics 5(13):3262–3277. https://doi.org/10.1002/pmic.200401245
126. Aebersold R, Burlingame AL, Bradshaw RA (2013) Western blots versus selected reaction monitoring assays: time to turn the tables? Mol Cell Proteomics 12(9):2381–2382. https://doi.org/10.1074/mcp.E113.031658
127. Elschenbroich S, Ignatchenko V, Clarke B, Kalloger SE, Boutros PC, Gramolini AO, Shaw P, Jurisica I, Kislinger T (2011) In-depth proteomics of ovarian cancer ascites: combining shotgun proteomics and selected reaction monitoring mass spectrometry. J Proteome Res 10(5):2286–2299. https://doi.org/10.1021/pr1011087
128. Anderson NL, Matheson AD, Steiner S (2000) Proteomics: applications in basic and applied biology. Curr Opin Biotechnol 11(4):408–412. https://doi.org/10.1016/s0958-1669(00)00118-x
129. Welch DR, McClure SA, Aeed PA, Bahner MJ, Adams LD (1990) Tumor progression- and metastasis-associated proteins identified using a model of locally recurrent rat mammary adenocarcinomas. Clin Exp Metastasis 8(6):533–551. https://doi.org/10.1007/bf00135876
130. Sarto C, Marocchi A, Sanchez JC, Giannone D, Frutiger S, Golaz O, Wilkins MR, Doro G, Cappellano F, Hughes G, Hochstrasser DF, Mocarelli P (1997) Renal cell carcinoma and normal kidney protein expression. Electrophoresis 18(3–4):599–604. https://doi.org/10.1002/elps.1150180343
131. Alaiya AA, Franzén B, Fujioka K, Moberger B, Schedvins K, Silfversvärd C, Linder S, Auer G (1997) Phenotypic analysis of ovarian carcinoma: polypeptide expression in benign, borderline and malignant tumors. Int J Cancer 73(5):678–682. https://doi.org/10.1002/(sici)1097-0215(19971127)73:5<678::Aid-ijc11>3.0.Co;2-2
132. Franzen B, Linder S, Uryu K, Alaiya AA, Hirano T, Kato H, Auer G (1996) Expression of tropomyosin isoforms in benign and malignant human breast lesions. Br J Cancer 73(7):909–913. https://doi.org/10.1038/bjc.1996.162
133. Stoeckli M, Chaurand P, Hallahan DE, Caprioli RM (2001) Imaging mass spectrometry: a new technology for the analysis of protein expression in mammalian tissues. Nat Med 7(4):493–496. https://doi.org/10.1038/86573
134. Bergman A-C, Benjamin T, Alaiya A, Waltham M, Sakaguchi K, Franzén B, Linder S, Bergman T, Auer G, Appella E, Wirth PJ, Jörnvall H (2000) Identification of gel-separated tumor marker proteins by mass spectrometry. Electrophoresis 21(3):679–686. https://doi.org/10.1002/(sici)1522-2683(20000201)21:3<679::Aid-elps679>3.0.Co;2-a

135. Wright GL Jr, Cazares LH, Leung SM, Nasim S, Adam BL, Yip TT, Schellhammer PF, Gong L, Vlahou A (1999) Proteinchip(R) surface enhanced laser desorption/ionization (SELDI) mass spectrometry: a novel protein biochip technology for detection of prostate cancer biomarkers in complex protein mixtures. Prostate Cancer Prostatic Dis 2(5-6):264–276. https://doi.org/10.1038/sj.pcan.4500384
136. Paweletz CP, Gillespie JW, Ornstein DK, Simone NL, Brown MR, Cole KA, Wang Q-H, Huang J, Hu N, Yip T-T, Rich WE, Kohn EC, Linehan WM, Weber T, Taylor P, Emmert-Buck MR, Liotta LA, Petricoin EF (2000) Rapid protein display profiling of cancer progression directly from human tissue using a protein biochip. Drug Dev Res 49(1):34–42. https://doi.org/10.1002/(sici)1098-2299(200001)49:1<34::Aid-ddr6>3.0.Co;2-w
137. Sadikovic B, Al-Romaih K, Squire JA, Zielenska M (2008) Cause and consequences of genetic and epigenetic alterations in human cancer. Curr Genomics 9(6):394–408. https://doi.org/10.2174/138920208785699580
138. Cho WC (2007) Contribution of oncoproteomics to cancer biomarker discovery. Mol Cancer 6:25. https://doi.org/10.1186/1476-4598-6-25
139. Krueger KE, Srivastava S (2006) Posttranslational protein modifications: current implications for cancer detection, prevention, and therapeutics. Mol Cell Proteomics 5(10):1799–1810. https://doi.org/10.1074/mcp.R600009-MCP200
140. Kolch W, Pitt A (2010) Functional proteomics to dissect tyrosine kinase signalling pathways in cancer. Nat Rev Cancer 10(9):618–629. https://doi.org/10.1038/nrc2900
141. Mellinghoff IK, Wang MY, Vivanco I, Haas-Kogan DA, Zhu S, Dia EQ, Lu KV, Yoshimoto K, Huang JH, Chute DJ, Riggs BL, Horvath S, Liau LM, Cavenee WK, Rao PN, Beroukhim R, Peck TC, Lee JC, Sellers WR, Stokoe D, Prados M, Cloughesy TF, Sawyers CL, Mischel PS (2005) Molecular determinants of the response of glioblastomas to EGFR kinase inhibitors. N Engl J Med 353(19):2012–2024. https://doi.org/10.1056/NEJMoa051918
142. Darie CC (2013) Mass spectrometry and proteomics: principle, workflow, challenges and perspectives. Mod Chem Appl 01(02). https://doi.org/10.4172/2329-6798.1000e105
143. Swaney DL, Villen J (2016) Proteomic analysis of protein posttranslational modifications by mass spectrometry. Cold Spring Harb Protoc 2016 (3):pdb top077743. https://doi.org/10.1101/pdb.top077743
144. Tainsky MA (2009) Genomic and proteomic biomarkers for cancer: a multitude of opportunities. Biochim Biophys Acta 1796(2):176–193. https://doi.org/10.1016/j.bbcan.2009.04.004
145. Tyers M, Mann M (2003) From genomics to proteomics. Nature 422(6928):193–197. https://doi.org/10.1038/nature01510
146. Gulati S, Cheng TM, Bates PA (2013) Cancer networks and beyond: interpreting mutations using the human interactome and protein structure. Semin Cancer Biol 23(4):219–226. https://doi.org/10.1016/j.semcancer.2013.05.002
147. Aebersold R, Cravatt BF (2002) Proteomics – advances, applications and the challenges that remain. Trends Biotechnol 20(12):s1–s2. https://doi.org/10.1016/s1471-1931(02)00206-9
148. Davalieva K, Polenakovic M (2015) Proteomics in diagnosis of prostate cancer. Pril (Makedon Akad Nauk Umet Odd Med Nauki) 36(1):5–36
149. Faria SS, Morris CF, Silva AR, Fonseca MP, Forget P, Castro MS, Fontes W (2017) A timely shift from shotgun to targeted proteomics and how it can be groundbreaking for cancer research. Front Oncol 7:13. https://doi.org/10.3389/fonc.2017.00013
150. Clauser KR, Hall SC, Smith DM, Webb JW, Andrews LE, Tran HM, Epstein LB, Burlingame AL (1995) Rapid mass spectrometric peptide sequencing and mass matching for characterization of human melanoma proteins isolated by two-dimensional PAGE. Proc Natl Acad Sci U S A 92(11):5072–5076. https://doi.org/10.1073/pnas.92.11.5072
151. Ang CS, Rothacker J, Patsiouras H, Gibbs P, Burgess AW, Nice EC (2011) Use of multiple reaction monitoring for multiplex analysis of colorectal cancer-associated proteins in human feces. Electrophoresis 32(15):1926–1938. https://doi.org/10.1002/elps.201000502
152. Milioli HH, Vimieiro R, Riveros C, Tishchenko I, Berretta R, Moscato P (2015) The discovery of novel biomarkers improves breast cancer intrinsic subtype prediction and reconciles

the labels in the METABRIC data set. PLoS One 10(7):e0129711. https://doi.org/10.1371/journal.pone.0129711
153. Chen J, Wu W, Chen L, Zhou H, Yang R, Hu L, Zhao Y (2013) Profiling the potential tumor markers of pancreatic ductal adenocarcinoma using 2D-DIGE and MALDI-TOF-MS: up-regulation of Complement C3 and alpha-2-HS-glycoprotein. Pancreatology 13(3):290–297. https://doi.org/10.1016/j.pan.2013.03.010
154. Guo L, Zhang C, Zhu J, Yang Y, Lan J, Su G, Xie X (2016) Proteomic identification of predictive tissue biomarkers of sensitive to neoadjuvant chemotherapy in squamous cervical cancer. Life Sci 151:102–108. https://doi.org/10.1016/j.lfs.2016.03.006
155. Mesri M (2014) Advances in proteomic technologies and its contribution to the field of cancer. Adv Med 2014:238045. https://doi.org/10.1155/2014/238045
156. Milioli HH, Santos Sousa K, Kaviski R, Dos Santos Oliveira NC, De Andrade Urban C, De Lima RS, Cavalli IJ, De Souza Fonseca Ribeiro EM (2015) Comparative proteomics of primary breast carcinomas and lymph node metastases outlining markers of tumor invasion. Cancer Genomics Proteomics 12(2):89–101
157. Longsworth LG, Shedlovsky T, Macinnes DA (1939) Electrophoretic patterns of normal and pathological human blood serum and plasma. J Exp Med 70(4):399–413. https://doi.org/10.1084/jem.70.4.399
158. Di Girolamo F, Del Chierico F, Caenaro G, Lante I, Muraca M, Putignani L (2012) Human serum proteome analysis: new source of markers in metabolic disorders. Biomark Med 6(6):759–773. https://doi.org/10.2217/bmm.12.92
159. O'Farrell PH (1975) High resolution two-dimensional electrophoresis of proteins. J Biol Chem 250(10):4007–4021
160. Norbeck J, Blomberg A (1997) Two-dimensional electrophoretic separation of yeast proteins using a non-linear wide range (pH 3–10) immobilized pH gradient in the first dimension; reproducibility and evidence for isoelectric focusing of alkaline (pI >7) proteins. Yeast 13(16):1519–1534. https://doi.org/10.1002/(sici)1097-0061(199712)13:16<1519::Aid-yea211>3.0.Co;2-u
161. Doustjalali SR, Yusof R, Govindasamy GK, Bustam AZ, Pillay B, Hashim OH (2006) Patients with nasopharyngeal carcinoma demonstrate enhanced serum and tissue ceruloplasmin expression. J Med Invest 53(1,2):20–28. https://doi.org/10.2152/jmi.53.20
162. Oestergaard M, Wolf H, Oerntoft TF, Celis JE (1999) Psoriasin (S100A7): a putative urinary marker for the follow-up of patients with bladder squamous cell carcinomas. Electrophoresis 20(2):349–354. https://doi.org/10.1002/(sici)1522-2683(19990201)20:2<349::Aid-elps349>3.0.Co;2-b
163. Jungblut PR, Zimny-Arndt U, Zeindl-Eberhart E, Stulik J, Koupilova K, Pleißner K-P, Otto A, Müller E-C, Sokolowska-Köhler W, Grabher G, Stöffler G (1999) Proteomics in human disease: cancer, heart and infectious diseases. Electrophoresis 20(10):2100–2110. https://doi.org/10.1002/(sici)1522-2683(19990701)20:10<2100::Aid-elps2100>3.0.Co;2-d
164. Chevalier F (2010) Highlights on the capacities of "Gel-based" proteomics. Proteome Sci 8:23. https://doi.org/10.1186/1477-5956-8-23
165. Unlu M, Morgan ME, Minden JS (1997) Difference gel electrophoresis: a single gel method for detecting changes in protein extracts. Electrophoresis 18(11):2071–2077. https://doi.org/10.1002/elps.1150181133
166. Zhang B, Barekati Z, Kohler C, Radpour R, Asadollahi R, Holzgreve W, Zhong XY (2010) Proteomics and biomarkers for ovarian cancer diagnosis. Ann Clin Lab Sci 40(3):218–225
167. Karp NA, Feret R, Rubtsov DV, Lilley KS (2008) Comparison of DIGE and post-stained gel electrophoresis with both traditional and SameSpots analysis for quantitative proteomics. Proteomics 8(5):948–960. https://doi.org/10.1002/pmic.200700812
168. Gharbi S, Gaffney P, Yang A, Zvelebil MJ, Cramer R, Waterfield MD, Timms JF (2002) Evaluation of two-dimensional differential gel electrophoresis for proteomic expression analysis of a model breast cancer cell system. Mol Cell Proteomics 1(2):91–98. https://doi.org/10.1074/mcp.t100007-mcp200

169. Gade D, Thiermann J, Markowsky D, Rabus R (2003) Evaluation of two-dimensional difference gel electrophoresis for protein profiling. Soluble proteins of the marine bacterium Pirellula sp. strain 1. J Mol Microbiol Biotechnol 5(4):240–251. https://doi.org/10.1159/000071076
170. Shaw J, Rowlinson R, Nickson J, Stone T, Sweet A, Williams K, Tonge R (2003) Evaluation of saturation labelling two-dimensional difference gel electrophoresis fluorescent dyes. Proteomics 3(7):1181–1195. https://doi.org/10.1002/pmic.200300439
171. Zhou G, Li H, DeCamp D, Chen S, Shu H, Gong Y, Flaig M, Gillespie JW, Hu N, Taylor PR, Emmert-Buck MR, Liotta LA, Petricoin EF, Zhao Y (2002) 2D differential in-gel electrophoresis for the identification of esophageal scans cell cancer-specific protein markers. Mol Cell Proteomics 1(2):117–123. https://doi.org/10.1074/mcp.M100015-MCP200
172. Govorun VM, Archakov AI (2002) Proteomic technologies in modern biomedical science. Biochemistry (Mosc) 67(10):1109–1123
173. Petricoin EF, Zoon KC, Kohn EC, Barrett JC, Liotta LA (2002) Clinical proteomics: translating benchside promise into bedside reality. Nat Rev Drug Discov 1:683. https://doi.org/10.1038/nrd891
174. Chen EI, Yates JR 3rd (2007) Cancer proteomics by quantitative shotgun proteomics. Mol Oncol 1(2):144–159. https://doi.org/10.1016/j.molonc.2007.05.001
175. Bouwman K, Qiu J, Zhou H, Schotanus M, Mangold LA, Vogt R, Erlandson E, Trenkle J, Partin AW, Misek D, Omenn GS, Haab BB, Hanash S (2003) Microarrays of tumor cell derived proteins uncover a distinct pattern of prostate cancer serum immunoreactivity. Proteomics 3(11):2200–2207. https://doi.org/10.1002/pmic.200300611
176. Charboneau L, Tory H, Chen T, Winters M, Petricoin EF 3rd, Liotta LA, Paweletz CP (2002) Utility of reverse phase protein arrays: applications to signalling pathways and human body arrays. Brief Funct Genomic Proteomic 1(3):305–315
177. Sheehan KM, Calvert VS, Kay EW, Lu Y, Fishman D, Espina V, Aquino J, Speer R, Araujo R, Mills GB, Liotta LA, Petricoin EF 3rd, Wulfkuhle JD (2005) Use of reverse phase protein microarrays and reference standard development for molecular network analysis of metastatic ovarian carcinoma. Mol Cell Proteomics 4(4):346–355. https://doi.org/10.1074/mcp.T500003-MCP200
178. Wulfkuhle JD, Aquino JA, Calvert VS, Fishman DA, Coukos G, Liotta LA, Petricoin EF 3rd (2003) Signal pathway profiling of ovarian cancer from human tissue specimens using reverse-phase protein microarrays. Proteomics 3(11):2085–2090. https://doi.org/10.1002/pmic.200300591
179. Paweletz CP, Charboneau L, Bichsel VE, Simone NL, Chen T, Gillespie JW, Emmert-Buck MR, Roth MJ, Petricoin IE, Liotta LA (2001) Reverse phase protein microarrays which capture disease progression show activation of pro-survival pathways at the cancer invasion front. Oncogene 20(16):1981–1989. https://doi.org/10.1038/sj.onc.1204265
180. Pereira-Faca SR, Kuick R, Puravs E, Zhang Q, Krasnoselsky AL, Phanstiel D, Qiu J, Misek DE, Hinderer R, Tammemagi M, Landi MT, Caporaso N, Pfeiffer R, Edelstein C, Goodman G, Barnett M, Thornquist M, Brenner D, Hanash SM (2007) Identification of 14-3-3 theta as an antigen that induces a humoral response in lung cancer. Cancer Res 67(24):12000–12006. https://doi.org/10.1158/0008-5472.CAN-07-2913
181. Anderson L, Hunter CL (2006) Quantitative mass spectrometric multiple reaction monitoring assays for major plasma proteins. Mol Cell Proteomics 5(4):573–588. https://doi.org/10.1074/mcp.M500331-MCP200
182. Gerber SA, Rush J, Stemman O, Kirschner MW, Gygi SP (2003) Absolute quantification of proteins and phosphoproteins from cell lysates by tandem MS. Proc Natl Acad Sci U S A 100(12):6940–6945. https://doi.org/10.1073/pnas.0832254100
183. Wolf-Yadlin A, Hautaniemi S, Lauffenburger DA, White FM (2007) Multiple reaction monitoring for robust quantitative proteomic analysis of cellular signaling networks. Proc Natl Acad Sci U S A 104(14):5860–5865. https://doi.org/10.1073/pnas.0608638104
184. Yates JR (1998) Mass spectrometry and the age of the proteome. J Mass Spectrom 33(1):1–19. https://doi.org/10.1002/(sici)1096-9888(199801)33:1<1::Aid-jms624>3.0.Co;2-9

185. Timmins-Schiffman E, Nunn BL, Goodlett DR, Roberts SB (2013) Shotgun proteomics as a viable approach for biological discovery in the Pacific oyster. Conserv Physiol 1(1):cot009. https://doi.org/10.1093/conphys/cot009
186. Abdallah C, Dumas-Gaudot E, Renaut J, Sergeant K (2012) Gel-based and gel-free quantitative proteomics approaches at a glance. Int J Plant Genomics 2012:494572. https://doi.org/10.1155/2012/494572
187. Zhang Y, Fonslow BR, Shan B, Baek MC, Yates JR 3rd (2013) Protein analysis by shotgun/bottom-up proteomics. Chem Rev 113(4):2343–2394. https://doi.org/10.1021/cr3003533
188. Nwabo Kamdje AH, Seke Etet PF, Vecchio L, Muller JM, Krampera M, Lukong KE (2014) Signaling pathways in breast cancer: therapeutic targeting of the microenvironment. Cell Signal 26(12):2843–2856. https://doi.org/10.1016/j.cellsig.2014.07.034
189. Wiesner A (2004) Detection of tumor markers with ProteinChip® technology. Curr Pharm Biotechnol 5(1):45–67. https://doi.org/10.2174/1389201043489675
190. Hu Y, Zhang S, Yu J, Liu J, Zheng S (2005) SELDI-TOF-MS: the proteomics and bioinformatics approaches in the diagnosis of breast cancer. Breast 14(4):250–255. https://doi.org/10.1016/j.breast.2005.01.008
191. Nomura DK, Dix MM, Cravatt BF (2010) Activity-based protein profiling for biochemical pathway discovery in cancer. Nat Rev Cancer 10(9):630–638. https://doi.org/10.1038/nrc2901
192. Sadaghiani AM, Verhelst SH, Bogyo M (2007) Tagging and detection strategies for activity-based proteomics. Curr Opin Chem Biol 11(1):20–28. https://doi.org/10.1016/j.cbpa.2006.11.030
193. Fonovic M, Bogyo M (2008) Activity-based probes as a tool for functional proteomic analysis of proteases. Expert Rev Proteomics 5(5):721–730. https://doi.org/10.1586/14789450.5.5.721
194. Karas M, Bahr U, Dülcks T (2000) Nano-electrospray ionization mass spectrometry: addressing analytical problems beyond routine. Fresenius J Anal Chem 366(6-7):669–676. https://doi.org/10.1007/s002160051561
195. Abo M, Li C, Weerapana E (2018) Isotopically-labeled iodoacetamide-alkyne probes for quantitative cysteine-reactivity profiling. Mol Pharm 15(3):743–749. https://doi.org/10.1021/acs.molpharmaceut.7b00832
196. Ardito F, Giuliani M, Perrone D, Troiano G, Lo Muzio L (2017) The crucial role of protein phosphorylation in cell signaling and its use as targeted therapy (Review). Int J Mol Med 40(2):271–280. https://doi.org/10.3892/ijmm.2017.3036
197. Yarden Y (2001) The EGFR family and its ligands in human cancer. Eur J Cancer 37:3–8. https://doi.org/10.1016/s0959-8049(01)00230-1
198. Rush J, Moritz A, Lee KA, Guo A, Goss VL, Spek EJ, Zhang H, Zha XM, Polakiewicz RD, Comb MJ (2005) Immunoaffinity profiling of tyrosine phosphorylation in cancer cells. Nat Biotechnol 23(1):94–101. https://doi.org/10.1038/nbt1046
199. Chi A, Huttenhower C, Geer LY, Coon JJ, Syka JE, Bai DL, Shabanowitz J, Burke DJ, Troyanskaya OG, Hunt DF (2007) Analysis of phosphorylation sites on proteins from Saccharomyces cerevisiae by electron transfer dissociation (ETD) mass spectrometry. Proc Natl Acad Sci U S A 104(7):2193–2198. https://doi.org/10.1073/pnas.0607084104
200. Hagen JB (2000) The origins of bioinformatics. Nat Rev Genet 1(3):231–236. https://doi.org/10.1038/35042090
201. Colinge J, Bennett KL (2007) Introduction to computational proteomics. PLoS Comput Biol 3(7):e114. https://doi.org/10.1371/journal.pcbi.0030114
202. Perez-Iratxeta C, Andrade-Navarro MA, Wren JD (2007) Evolving research trends in bioinformatics. Brief Bioinform 8(2):88–95. https://doi.org/10.1093/bib/bbl035
203. Zamanian-Azodi M, Rezaei-Tavirani M, Mortazavian A, Vafaee R, Rezaei-Tavirani M, Zali H, Soheili-Kashani M (2015) Application of proteomics in cancer study. Am J Cancer Sci 2:1–18
204. Ebert MP, Korc M, Malfertheiner P, Rocken C (2006) Advances, challenges, and limitations in serum-proteome-based cancer diagnosis. J Proteome Res 5(1):19–25. https://doi.org/10.1021/pr050271e

205. Miller JC, Zhou H, Kwekel J, Cavallo R, Burke J, Butler EB, Teh BS, Haab BB (2003) Antibody microarray profiling of human prostate cancer sera: antibody screening and identification of potential biomarkers. Proteomics 3(1):56–63. https://doi.org/10.1002/pmic.200390009
206. FDA-NIH (2016) BEST (Biomarkers, EndpointS, and other Tools) Resource [Internet]. In: (MD) SS (ed) BEST (Biomarkers, EndpointS, and other Tools) Resource. Silver Spring (MD)
207. Pepe MS, Etzioni R, Feng Z, Potter JD, Thompson ML, Thornquist M, Winget M, Yasui Y (2001) Phases of biomarker development for early detection of cancer. J Natl Cancer Inst 93(14):1054–1061. https://doi.org/10.1093/jnci/93.14.1054
208. Cyll K, Ersvaer E, Vlatkovic L, Pradhan M, Kildal W, Avranden Kjaer M, Kleppe A, Hveem TS, Carlsen B, Gill S, Loffeler S, Haug ES, Waehre H, Sooriakumaran P, Danielsen HE (2017) Tumour heterogeneity poses a significant challenge to cancer biomarker research. Br J Cancer 117(3):367–375. https://doi.org/10.1038/bjc.2017.171
209. Baggerly KA, Morris JS, Coombes KR (2004) Reproducibility of SELDI-TOF protein patterns in serum: comparing datasets from different experiments. Bioinformatics 20(5):777–785. https://doi.org/10.1093/bioinformatics/btg484
210. Masucci GV, Cesano A, Hawtin R, Janetzki S, Zhang J, Kirsch I, Dobbin KK, Alvarez J, Robbins PB, Selvan SR, Streicher HZ, Butterfield LH, Thurin M (2016) Validation of biomarkers to predict response to immunotherapy in cancer: volume I - pre-analytical and analytical validation. J Immunother Cancer 4:76. https://doi.org/10.1186/s40425-016-0178-1
211. Goossens N, Nakagawa S, Sun X, Hoshida Y (2015) Cancer biomarker discovery and validation. Transl Cancer Res 4(3):256–269. https://doi.org/10.3978/j.issn.2218-676X.2015.06.04
212. Selleck MJ, Senthil M, Wall NR (2017) Making meaningful clinical use of biomarkers. Biomark Insights 12:1177271917715236. https://doi.org/10.1177/1177271917715236
213. Zheng Y (2018) Study design considerations for cancer biomarker discoveries. J Appl Lab Med 3(2):282–289. https://doi.org/10.1373/jalm.2017.025809
214. Pepe MS, Feng Z, Janes H, Bossuyt PM, Potter JD (2008) Pivotal evaluation of the accuracy of a biomarker used for classification or prediction: standards for study design. J Natl Cancer Inst 100(20):1432–1438. https://doi.org/10.1093/jnci/djn326
215. Simon RM, Paik S, Hayes DF (2009) Use of archived specimens in evaluation of prognostic and predictive biomarkers. J Natl Cancer Inst 101(21):1446–1452. https://doi.org/10.1093/jnci/djp335
216. Watson RW, Kay EW, Smith D (2010) Integrating biobanks: addressing the practical and ethical issues to deliver a valuable tool for cancer research. Nat Rev Cancer 10(9):646–651. https://doi.org/10.1038/nrc2913
217. Pepe MS, Li CI, Feng Z (2015) Improving the quality of biomarker discovery research: the right samples and enough of them. Cancer Epidemiol Biomarkers Prev 24(6):944–950. https://doi.org/10.1158/1055-9965.EPI-14-1227
218. Fraser GA, Meyer RM (2007) Biomarkers and the design of clinical trials in cancer. Biomark Med 1(3):387–397. https://doi.org/10.2217/17520363.1.3.387
219. van de Vijver MJ, He YD, van't Veer LJ, Dai H, Hart AA, Voskuil DW, Schreiber GJ, Peterse JL, Roberts C, Marton MJ, Parrish M, Atsma D, Witteveen A, Glas A, Delahaye L, van der Velde T, Bartelink H, Rodenhuis S, Rutgers ET, Friend SH, Bernards R (2002) A gene-expression signature as a predictor of survival in breast cancer. N Engl J Med 347(25):1999–2009. https://doi.org/10.1056/NEJMoa021967
220. Paik S, Shak S, Tang G, Kim C, Baker J, Cronin M, Baehner FL, Walker MG, Watson D, Park T, Hiller W, Fisher ER, Wickerham DL, Bryant J, Wolmark N (2004) A multigene assay to predict recurrence of tamoxifen-treated, node-negative breast cancer. N Engl J Med 351(27):2817–2826. https://doi.org/10.1056/NEJMoa041588
221. Nguyen HG, Welty CJ, Cooperberg MR (2015) Diagnostic associations of gene expression signatures in prostate cancer tissue. Curr Opin Urol 25(1):65–70. https://doi.org/10.1097/MOU.0000000000000131

222. You YN, Rustin RB, Sullivan JD (2015) Oncotype DX((R)) colon cancer assay for prediction of recurrence risk in patients with stage II and III colon cancer: a review of the evidence. Surg Oncol 24(2):61–66. https://doi.org/10.1016/j.suronc.2015.02.001
223. Colburn WA (2003) Biomarkers in drug discovery and development: from target identification through drug marketing. J Clin Pharmacol 43(4):329–341. https://doi.org/10.1177/0091270003252480
224. Freidlin B, McShane LM, Korn EL (2010) Randomized clinical trials with biomarkers: design issues. J Natl Cancer Inst 102(3):152–160. https://doi.org/10.1093/jnci/djp477
225. Gosho M, Nagashima K, Sato Y (2012) Study designs and statistical analyses for biomarker research. Sensors (Basel) 12(7):8966–8986. https://doi.org/10.3390/s120708966
226. Sargent DJ, Conley BA, Allegra C, Collette L (2005) Clinical trial designs for predictive marker validation in cancer treatment trials. J Clin Oncol 23(9):2020–2027. https://doi.org/10.1200/JCO.2005.01.112
227. Buyse M, Michiels S, Sargent DJ, Grothey A, Matheson A, de Gramont A (2011) Integrating biomarkers in clinical trials. Expert Rev Mol Diagn 11(2):171–182. https://doi.org/10.1586/erm.10.120
228. Chakravarty AG, Rothmann M, Sridhara R (2011) Regulatory issues in use of biomarkers in oncology trials. Stat Biopharm Res 3(4):569–576. https://doi.org/10.1198/sbr.2011.09026
229. Jenkins M, Flynn A, Smart T, Harbron C, Sabin T, Ratnayake J, Delmar P, Herath A, Jarvis P, Matcham J, Group PSIBSI (2011) A statistician's perspective on biomarkers in drug development. Pharm Stat 10(6):494–507. https://doi.org/10.1002/pst.532
230. Kontos CK, Adamopoulos PG, Scorilas A (2015) Prognostic and predictive biomarkers in prostate cancer. Expert Rev Mol Diagn 15(12):1567–1576. https://doi.org/10.1586/14737159.2015.1110022
231. Bast RC Jr, Feeney M, Lazarus H, Nadler LM, Colvin RB, Knapp RC (1981) Reactivity of a monoclonal antibody with human ovarian carcinoma. J Clin Invest 68(5):1331–1337. https://doi.org/10.1172/jci110380
232. Dochez V, Caillon H, Vaucel E, Dimet J, Winer N, Ducarme G (2019) Biomarkers and algorithms for diagnosis of ovarian cancer: CA125, HE4, RMI and ROMA, a review. J Ovarian Res 12(1):28. https://doi.org/10.1186/s13048-019-0503-7
233. Bhatti I, Patel M, Dennison AR, Thomas MW, Garcea G (2015) Utility of postoperative CEA for surveillance of recurrence after resection of primary colorectal cancer. Int J Surg 16:123–128. https://doi.org/10.1016/j.ijsu.2015.03.002
234. Vallam KC, Guruchannabasavaiah B, Agrawal A, Rangarajan V, Ostwal V, Engineer R, Saklani A (2017) Carcinoembryonic antigen directed PET-CECT scanning for postoperative surveillance of colorectal cancer. Colorectal Dis 19(10):907–911. https://doi.org/10.1111/codi.13695
235. Flaherty KT, Infante JR, Daud A, Gonzalez R, Kefford RF, Sosman J, Hamid O, Schuchter L, Cebon J, Ibrahim N, Kudchadkar R, Burris HA 3rd, Falchook G, Algazi A, Lewis K, Long GV, Puzanov I, Lebowitz P, Singh A, Little S, Sun P, Allred A, Ouellet D, Kim KB, Patel K, Weber J (2012) Combined BRAF and MEK inhibition in melanoma with BRAF V600 mutations. N Engl J Med 367(18):1694–1703. https://doi.org/10.1056/NEJMoa1210093
236. Janne PA, Yang JC, Kim DW, Planchard D, Ohe Y, Ramalingam SS, Ahn MJ, Kim SW, Su WC, Horn L, Haggstrom D, Felip E, Kim JH, Frewer P, Cantarini M, Brown KH, Dickinson PA, Ghiorghiu S, Ranson M (2015) AZD9291 in EGFR inhibitor-resistant non-small-cell lung cancer. N Engl J Med 372(18):1689–1699. https://doi.org/10.1056/NEJMoa1411817
237. Carson PE, Flanagan CL, Ickes CE, Alving AS (1956) Enzymatic deficiency in primaquine-sensitive erythrocytes. Science 124(3220):484–485. https://doi.org/10.1126/science.124.3220.484-a
238. Kalow W, Staron N (1957) On distribution and inheritance of atypical forms of human serum cholinesterase, as indicated by dibucaine numbers. Can J Biochem Physiol 35(12):1305–1320
239. Evans DA, Manley KA, Mc KV (1960) Genetic control of isoniazid metabolism in man. Br Med J 2(5197):485–491. https://doi.org/10.1136/bmj.2.5197.485

240. Mahgoub A, Dring LG, Idle JR, Lancaster R, Smith RL (1977) Polymorphic hydroxylation of debrisoquine in man. Lancet 310(8038):584–586. https://doi.org/10.1016/s0140-6736(77)91430-1
241. Bertilsson L, Dengler HJ, Eichelbaum M, Schulz HU (1980) Pharmacogenetic covariation of defective N-oxidation of sparteine and 4-hydroxylation of debrisoquine. Eur J Clin Pharmacol 17(2):153–155. https://doi.org/10.1007/bf00562624
242. Vogel F (1959) Moderne Probleme der Humangenetik. In: Heilmeyer L, Schoen R, de Rudder B (eds) Ergebnisse der Inneren Medizin und Kinderheilkunde, vol 12. Springer, Berlin, Heidelberg. https://doi.org/10.1007/978-3-642-94744-5_2
243. EMEA (2002) Position paper on terminology in pharmacogenetics. Committee for proprietary medicinal products. European Agency for the Evaluation of Medicinal Products
244. Redekop WK, Mladsi D (2013) The faces of personalized medicine: a framework for understanding its meaning and scope. Value Health 16(6 Suppl):S4–S9. https://doi.org/10.1016/j.jval.2013.06.005
245. Salari P, Larijani B (2017) Ethical issues surrounding personalized medicine: a literature review. Acta Med Iran 55(3):209–217
246. Annas GJ (2014) Personalized medicine or public health? Bioethics, human rights, and choice. Revista Portuguesa de Saúde Pública 32(2):158–163. https://doi.org/10.1016/j.rpsp.2014.04.003
247. Vogenberg FR, Isaacson Barash C, Pursel M (2010) Personalized medicine: part 1: evolution and development into theranostics. P T 35(10):560–576
248. Chen R, Snyder M (2013) Promise of personalized omics to precision medicine. Wiley Interdiscip Rev Syst Biol Med 5(1):73–82. https://doi.org/10.1002/wsbm.1198
249. Ginsburg GS, Phillips KA (2018) Precision medicine: from science to value. Health Aff (Millwood) 37(5):694–701. https://doi.org/10.1377/hlthaff.2017.1624
250. Alyass A, Turcotte M, Meyre D (2015) From big data analysis to personalized medicine for all: challenges and opportunities. BMC Med Genomics 8:33. https://doi.org/10.1186/s12920-015-0108-y
251. Popa ML, Albulescu R, Neagu M, Hinescu ME, Tanase C (2019) Multiplex assay for multiomics advances in personalized-precision medicine. J Immunoassay Immunochem 40(1):3–25. https://doi.org/10.1080/15321819.2018.1562940
252. Sharrer GT (2017) Personalized medicine: ethical aspects. Methods Mol Biol 1606:37–50. https://doi.org/10.1007/978-1-4939-6990-6_3
253. Badzek L, Henaghan M, Turner M, Monsen R (2013) Ethical, legal, and social issues in the translation of genomics into health care. J Nurs Scholarsh 45(1):15–24. https://doi.org/10.1111/jnu.12000
254. Joly Y, Saulnier KM, Osien G, Knoppers BM (2014) The ethical framing of personalized medicine. Curr Opin Allergy Clin Immunol 14(5):404–408. https://doi.org/10.1097/ACI.0000000000000091
255. Salari K, Watkins H, Ashley EA (2012) Personalized medicine: hope or hype? Eur Heart J 33(13):1564–1570. https://doi.org/10.1093/eurheartj/ehs112
256. Kurnat-Thoma EL (2011) Genetics and genomics: the scientific drivers of personalized medicine. Annu Rev Nurs Res 29:27–54
257. Martincorena I, Campbell PJ (2015) Somatic mutation in cancer and normal cells. Science 349(6255):1483–1489. https://doi.org/10.1126/science.aab4082
258. Cocca M, Bedognetti D, La Bianca M, Gasparini P, Girotto G (2016) Pharmacogenetics driving personalized medicine: analysis of genetic polymorphisms related to breast cancer medications in Italian isolated populations. J Transl Med 14:22. https://doi.org/10.1186/s12967-016-0778-z
259. Tavares P, Dias L, Palmeiro A, Rendeiro P, Tolias P (2011) Single-test parallel assessment of multiple genetic disorders. Pers Med 8(3):375–379. https://doi.org/10.2217/pme.11.23
260. Roth M, Keeling P, Smart D (2010) Driving personalized medicine: capturing maximum net present value and optimal return on investment. Pers Med 7(1):103–114. https://doi.org/10.2217/pme.09.64

261. Steffen JA, Steffen JS (2013) Driving forces behind the past and future emergence of personalized medicine. J Pers Med 3(1):14–22. https://doi.org/10.3390/jpm3010014
262. Goldberger JJ, Buxton AE (2013) Personalized medicine vs guideline-based medicine. JAMA 309(24):2559–2560. https://doi.org/10.1001/jama.2013.6629
263. Chen R, Snyder M (2012) Systems biology: personalized medicine for the future? Curr Opin Pharmacol 12(5):623–628. https://doi.org/10.1016/j.coph.2012.07.011
264. Zoon CK, Starker EQ, Wilson AM, Emmert-Buck MR, Libutti SK, Tangrea MA (2009) Current molecular diagnostics of breast cancer and the potential incorporation of microRNA. Expert Rev Mol Diagn 9(5):455–467. https://doi.org/10.1586/erm.09.25
265. Pardanani A, Wieben ED, Spelsberg TC, Tefferi A (2002) Primer on medical genomics. Part IV: expression proteomics. Mayo Clin Proc 77(11):1185–1196. https://doi.org/10.4065/77.11.1185
266. Haga SB, Beskow LM (2008) Ethical, legal, and social implications of biobanks for genetics research. Adv Genet 60:505–544. https://doi.org/10.1016/S0065-2660(07)00418-X
267. Chalmers D (2011) Genetic research and biobanks. Methods Mol Biol 675:1–37. https://doi.org/10.1007/978-1-59745-423-0_1
268. Jamal L, Sapp JC, Lewis K, Yanes T, Facio FM, Biesecker LG, Biesecker BB (2014) Research participants' attitudes towards the confidentiality of genomic sequence information. Eur J Hum Genet 22(8):964–968. https://doi.org/10.1038/ejhg.2013.276
269. Caulfield T, McGuire AL, Cho M, Buchanan JA, Burgess MM, Danilczyk U, Diaz CM, Fryer-Edwards K, Green SK, Hodosh MA, Juengst ET, Kaye J, Kedes L, Knoppers BM, Lemmens T, Meslin EM, Murphy J, Nussbaum RL, Otlowski M, Pullman D, Ray PN, Sugarman J, Timmons M (2008) Research ethics recommendations for whole-genome research: consensus statement. PLoS Biol 6(3):e73. https://doi.org/10.1371/journal.pbio.0060073
270. Goh AM, Chiu E, Yastrubetskaya O, Erwin C, Williams JK, Juhl AR, Paulsen JS, Group IR-HIOTHS (2013) Perception, experience, and response to genetic discrimination in Huntington's disease: the Australian results of The International RESPOND-HD study. Genet Test Mol Biomarkers 17(2):115–121. https://doi.org/10.1089/gtmb.2012.0288
271. Matloff ET, Bonadies DC, Moyer A, Brierley KL (2014) Changes in specialists' perspectives on cancer genetic testing, prophylactic surgery and insurance discrimination: then and now. J Genet Couns 23(2):164–171. https://doi.org/10.1007/s10897-013-9625-z
272. Pierce JD, Fakhari M, Works KV, Pierce JT, Clancy RL (2007) Understanding proteomics. Nurs Health Sci 9(1):54–60. https://doi.org/10.1111/j.1442-2018.2007.00295.x
273. Carlson RJ (2009) The disruptive nature of personalized medicine technologies: implications for the health care system. Public Health Genomics 12(3):180–184. https://doi.org/10.1159/000189631
274. Celis JE, Kruhøffer M, Gromova I, Frederiksen C, Østergaard M, Thykjaer T, Gromov P, Yu J, Pálsdóttir H, Magnusson N, Ørntoft TF (2000) Gene expression profiling: monitoring transcription and translation products using DNA microarrays and proteomics. FEBS Lett 480(1):2–16. https://doi.org/10.1016/s0014-5793(00)01771-3
275. Agyeman AA, Ofori-Asenso R (2015) Perspective: does personalized medicine hold the future for medicine? J Pharm Bioallied Sci 7(3):239–244. https://doi.org/10.4103/0975-7406.160040
276. Mosca R, Ceol A, Aloy P (2013) Interactome3D: adding structural details to protein networks. Nat Methods 10(1):47–53. https://doi.org/10.1038/nmeth.2289
277. Wilhelm M, Schlegl J, Hahne H, Gholami AM, Lieberenz M, Savitski MM, Ziegler E, Butzmann L, Gessulat S, Marx H, Mathieson T, Lemeer S, Schnatbaum K, Reimer U, Wenschuh H, Mollenhauer M, Slotta-Huspenina J, Boese JH, Bantscheff M, Gerstmair A, Faerber F, Kuster B (2014) Mass-spectrometry-based draft of the human proteome. Nature 509(7502):582–587. https://doi.org/10.1038/nature13319
278. Hanash S, Taguchi A (2010) The grand challenge to decipher the cancer proteome. Nat Rev Cancer 10(9):652–660. https://doi.org/10.1038/nrc2918

279. Khan SR, Khurshid Z, Akhbar S, Moin FS (2016) Advances of salivary proteomics in Oral Squamous Cell Carcinoma (OSCC) detection: an update. Proteomes 4(4). https://doi.org/10.3390/proteomes4040041
280. Shah FD, Begum R, Vajaria BN, Patel KR, Patel JB, Shukla SN, Patel PS (2011) A review on salivary genomics and proteomics biomarkers in oral cancer. Indian J Clin Biochem 26(4):326–334. https://doi.org/10.1007/s12291-011-0149-8
281. Behjati S, Haniffa M (2017) Genetics: taking single-cell transcriptomics to the bedside. Nat Rev Clin Oncol 14(10):590–592. https://doi.org/10.1038/nrclinonc.2017.117
282. MacBeath G (2002) Protein microarrays and proteomics. Nat Genet 32(Suppl):526–532. https://doi.org/10.1038/ng1037
283. Celis JE, Gromov P (2003) Proteomics in translational cancer research: toward an integrated approach. Cancer Cell 3(1):9–15. https://doi.org/10.1016/s1535-6108(02)00242-8
284. Vaidyanathan G (2012) Redefining clinical trials: the age of personalized medicine. Cell 148(6):1079–1080. https://doi.org/10.1016/j.cell.2012.02.041
285. Sanchez JC, Couté Y, Allard L, Lescuyer P, Hochstrasser DF (2007) Biomedical applications of proteomics. Principles and practice. Springer, Berlin, Heidelberg, Proteome Research. https://doi.org/10.1007/978-3-540-72910-5_9
286. Barbosa EB, Vidotto A, Polachini GM, Henrique T, Marqui AB, Tajara EH (2012) Proteomics: methodologies and applications to the study of human diseases. Rev Assoc Med Bras (1992) 58(3):366–375. https://doi.org/10.1590/S0104-42302012000300019
287. Jain KK (2008) Recent advances in nanooncology. Technol Cancer Res Treat 7(1):1–13. https://doi.org/10.1177/153303460800700101
288. Kopf E, Zharhary D (2007) Antibody arrays--an emerging tool in cancer proteomics. Int J Biochem Cell Biol 39(7–8):1305–1317. https://doi.org/10.1016/j.biocel.2007.04.029
289. Shangguan D, Cao Z, Meng L, Mallikaratchy P, Sefah K, Wang H, Li Y, Tan W (2008) Cell-specific aptamer probes for membrane protein elucidation in cancer cells. J Proteome Res 7(5):2133–2139. https://doi.org/10.1021/pr700894d
290. Hardouin J, Lasserre JP, Sylvius L, Joubert-Caron R, Caron M (2007) Cancer immunomics: from serological proteome analysis to multiple affinity protein profiling. Ann N Y Acad Sci 1107:223–230. https://doi.org/10.1196/annals.1381.024
291. Voduc D, Kenney C, Nielsen TO (2008) Tissue microarrays in clinical oncology. Semin Radiat Oncol 18(2):89–97. https://doi.org/10.1016/j.semradonc.2007.10.006

Molecular Profiling of Breast Cancer in Clinical Trials: A Perspective

12

Saima Shakil Malik, Iqra, Nosheen Akhtar, Iffat Fatima, Zaineb Akram, and Nosheen Masood

12.1 Introduction

Breast cancer is one of the most common malignancies and accounts for more than 30% of cancer diagnosis among women throughout the world [1]. Increased breast cancer incidence rate can be evidenced from the findings that every eighth women in the United States is at risk of developing this brutal disease. Women not only from underdeveloped or developing countries become victim of this disease and struggle for survival, but also women from developed countries are also facing the same issue [2–5]. Breast cancer has heterogeneous nature in histological, pathological, and clinical investigations, and it is always a challenge for surgeons/oncologists to identify suitable treatment for every patient [6, 7]. Conventionally, breast tumors were categorized by using slide-based techniques and histopathological attributes responsible for diagnosing ductal or lobular breast carcinoma and characterizing

Nosheen Akhtar and Iffat Fatima contributed equally with all other contributors.

S. S. Malik (✉)
Fatima Jinnah Women University, Rawalpindi, Pakistan

Armed Forces Institute of Pathology, Rawalpindi, Pakistan
e-mail: saimamalik25@yahoo.com

Iqra · N. Masood
Microbiology and Biotechnology Research Lab, Fatima Jinnah Women University, Rawalpindi, Pakistan

N. Akhtar
National University of Medical Science, Rawalpindi, Pakistan

I. Fatima
Quaid-i-Azam University, Islamabad, Pakistan

Z. Akram
Armed Forces Bone Marrow Transplant Centre, Rawalpindi, Pakistan

N. Masood, S. Shakil Malik (eds.), *'Essentials of Cancer Genomic, Computational Approaches and Precision Medicine*,
https://doi.org/10.1007/978-981-15-1067-0_12

tumor size, grade, and involvement of lymph nodes [8, 9]. With the advancement in molecular biology-related knowledge, different breast cancer molecular subtypes have been recognized based on the status of HR and HER2, which differ in chemotherapeutic responsiveness and disease prognosis [10]. Epithelial carcinoma is the most commonly diagnosed breast cancer type and, therefore, gathers greater attention in this chapter. Basic intrinsic epithelial breast carcinoma types are "luminal A, luminal B, $HER2^+$, and basal-like cancer" [11, 12]. Androgen receptor-based epithelial breast carcinoma types have also been reported [13].

Identifying precise molecular breast carcinoma subtypes could lead to more personalized method for breast cancer treatment via targeted therapies [14]. Furthermore, the clinical advantage experienced with agents targeting HER2/hormone signaling has opened new ways to identify and test more molecular targets [15]. Advancement in the molecular profiling-related knowledge has revealed many novel genetic and epigenetic alterations/modifications as possible drivers of breast carcinoma biology [16]. Some of these genetic alterations that can help in characterizing currently available breast cancer molecular subtypes are shown in Fig. 12.1.

After BRCA1/BRCA2, many other genetically targeted agents were explored in breast cancer and now in progress to become clinically important markers. Most important factor in recognizing some molecular marker is its role in treatment and patient's overall survival. To address the potential of various biomarkers, response to treatment was evaluated with the help of clinical trials as a best source of confirmation and many are still in progress. The current chapter will highlight recent advancements in the molecular profiling of breast cancer leading to better disease diagnosis and treatment.

12.2 Molecular Profiling in Breast Cancer

Breast cancer molecular profiling is capable of monitoring and predicting treatment response in different ways [23] and can be determined with different techniques including RT-PCR [24, 25], immunohistochemistry [26, 27], fluorescence in situ hybridization (FISH) [28], DNA hybridization-based analysis [29], and *next-generation sequencing* (*NGS*) [30].

12.2.1 Genomic Tools for Detection of Breast Cancer

Genomics refers to the analysis of sequence and structural variations in DNA. It also involves investigation of gene expression and functional element annotation at a genomic scale. Genomic tools are used to detect indels, single nucleotide polymorphisms, and epigenetic modifications [31]. Genomic analyses lead to the development of diagnostic tests which provided patients personalized diagnostic information [32]. It also helped for the development of personalized treatment plans, consequently preventing resistance, toxicity, and nonresponsiveness. Due to lack of knowledge involved in carcinogenesis, we are still targeting one drug, one gene, and one organ site model [33].

Characteristics	HR^+ (ER^+ / PR^+)		$HER2^+$	TNBC (HR^- & $HER2^-$)
Typical intrinsic subtypes	Luminal A ($HER2^-$)	Luminal B ($HER2^+$ / $HER2^-$)	HER2	Basal
Frequency among breast cancers	40 – 60%	Approximately 15%	Approximately 10%	10 – 25%
Grade	Lower	Higher	High	High
Prognosis	Good	Intermediate	General	General
Targeted therapy	Endocrine Letrozole, tamoxifen, exemestane, anastrozole, fluvestrant	Endocrine Letrozole, tamoxifen, exemestane, anastrozole, fluvestrant	Anti HER2 Trastuzumab, lapatinib, T-DM1, pertuzumab	DNA repair targeting agents are under investigation like PARP inhibitors
Chemotherapy	Lower response	Intermediate response	Anthracycline based chemotherapy	Platinum based chemotherapy
Genetic profile	Ki-67 low expression GATA-3, XBP1, ESR1 & FOX1 high expression MAP3K1 & MAP2K4 frequent mutation	ER related genes low expression Proliferation genes increased expression CCND1 – frequent amplification	HER2 related & proliferation genes increased expression TP53 mutation High genomic instability	Expression of genes characteristic of normal breast myoepithelial cells (cytokeratins 5, 6, and 17) high expression of DNA repair proteins frequent TP53 mutations

Fig. 12.1 Breast cancer tumor's molecular subtypes [17–22]

12.2.1.1 Oncotype DX

Oncotype DX is RT-PCR-based genomic assay, optimized for FFPE biopsy specimens [34]. The assay was established to predict recurrence score in breast cancer patients of stage I and II, lymph node-negative, hormone receptor-positive, and metastatic cancer, treated with tamoxifen [35]. It utilizes set of important genes customized after data evaluation form 447 patients. During the project, 250 genes were studied, and panel of 21 genes was derived for HR+ breast cancer patients, likely considered to be the prognostic for breast cancer. In this panel, 16 genes are related to cancer and 5 are reference genes as internal control [36]. The cancer-related gene panel is associated with the genes of known functions involved in basic tumorigenesis pathways, i.e., cell proliferation, invasion, hormone response, and other oncogenes. Genes specifically related to breast cancer, incorporated on Oncotype DX, are shown in Fig. 12.2. It stratifies recurrence score between 0 and 100 [37]. Score correlates to disease recurrence possibility among patients successfully treated with chemotherapy within 10 years of diagnosis. The significance of this assay was evaluated and validated by using cohort study from the National Surgical Adjuvant Breast and Bowel Project (NSABP) and trials B-14 and B-20 [38]. Oncotype Dx predicts potential benefit from adjuvant chemotherapy. To date, Oncotype DX is the only multigene assay for breast cancer and incorporated in the guidelines of National Comprehensive Cancer Network (NCCN), highlighting its use and ability to predict the risk of recurrence and benefits from adjuvant chemotherapy [39–41]. According to guidelines, once patients treated with tamoxifen have been classified to lower risk of recurrence by the Oncotype DX assay, they can be spared from adjuvant chemotherapy [42].

Oncotype DX has become the most commonly used clinical assay, but few studies showed that immunohistochemistry (IHC) score provides similar prognostic information which is a less expensive and simpler alternative [36]. Other reports

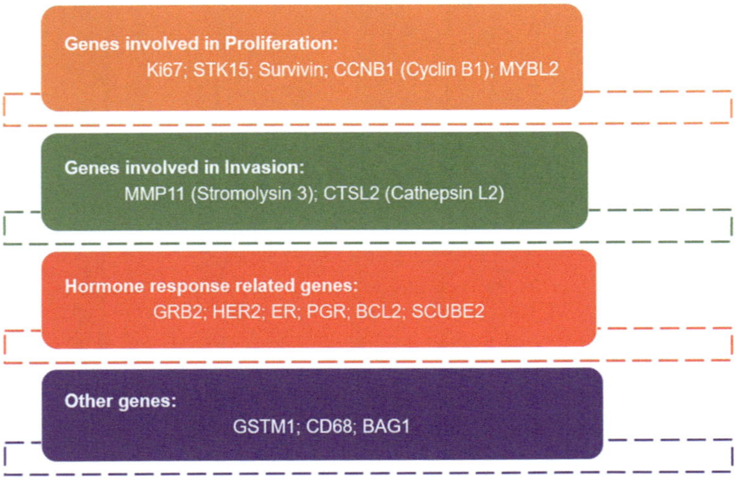

Fig. 12.2 Gene profile of Oncotype DX assay [44–46]

show that Oncotype DX also provides information which can predict benefits from adjuvant chemotherapy [43].

12.2.1.2 MammaPrint

MammaPrint is a molecular diagnostic assay which involves microarray-based approach to predict tumor recurrence in breast cancer patients [44]. It consists of a customized panel of 70 genes that has been displayed sovereign prognostic value for lymph node-negative breast cancer patients and is associated with tumor development and metastasis [47, 48]. These genes are the hallmarks of cancer and play roles in regulation of cell cycle, metastasis, invasion, proliferation, extravasation, adaptation to microenvironment, survival in circulation, and angiogenesis [36]. MammaPrint was initially established from expression arrays of whole genome using a cohort of breast cancer patients who had gone through definitive surgery only, with known clinical outcomes and with no systemic therapy [49].

In MammaPrint gene expression levels are determined by the probe-specific hybridization of complementary DNA [50]. In 2007, US FDA approved MammaPrint for freshly frozen tissue samples. During the process, RNA after extraction from tissues is amplified, co-hybridized is carried out using a standard reference, and 70-gene expression profile is obtained [51]. MammaPrint has been shown as prognostic indicator, independent of clinicopathologic features such as size of tumor, HER2 status, and hormone receptor status [52, 53]. This method has been reported to have significantly higher correlation of prognostic prediction to tumor recurrence [42]. In MammaPrint, patients are classified into low-risk and high-risk groups corresponding to a 10-year distant metastasis-free survival rate.

MammaPrint is a useful diagnostic tool, but there are many limitations that must be considered. The patient recommended for MammaPrint screenings should be of stage I or II lymph node-negative invasive breast cancer with tumor size less than 5 mm^3 [50, 54]. Further, MammaPrint is restricted to patients with less than 65 years of age, and it also needs large amount of specimen. Collection of tissue samples and handling make this assay hard for use in normal clinical practice [55]. Collection is very critical for optimum results and requires regions clear of both stromal and necrotic tissue with at least 30% of malignant cells, which may be impossible to obtain from a biopsy [56]. For these limitations, ASCO required further data and recommendations for usage of MammaPrint in clinical settings. To date, only Agendia laboratory (Amsterdam) performs this assay [57, 58].

12.2.1.3 PAM50 (Prosigna)

PAM50 is also a molecular test for tumor profiling which helps to evaluate chemotherapy benefits in addition to hormone therapy for ER-positive and HER2-negative breast cancers. It investigates the activity of 50 genes to predict the risk of distant recurrence from 5 to 10 years. It is based on qRT-PCR that has been recommended for FFPE tissue specimens of ER-positive, HER2-negative, basal, luminal A- and luminal B-like breast cancers [36]. It estimates the chances of metastasis for postmenopausal women with stage I and II lymph node-negative breast cancers. However, multivariate analyses have revealed this assay also provides information that is independent of clinicopathologic variables [59]. PAM50 provides the detailed quantitative information about luminal gene expression, proliferation, PGR, ESR1, and ERBB2 and, consequently, can be used for opting proper treatment decisions [36]. Different work is in progress to assess the efficacy of this test and has been reported to be superior to IHC and Oncotype DX for predicting the emergence of late relapses following adjuvant endocrine therapy. Prosigna is manufactured by NanoString Technologies, distributed to different pathology labs and is approved for use in the European Union [60].

12.2.1.4 Genomic Grade Index (GGI) (Ipsogen)

The GGI is a microarray-based test which includes 97 genes, created by Sotiriou et al., with the intention of making tumor grading system more precise. It was developed from the data of 189 breast cancer cohort and validated in different subtypes of 597 tumors [61]. GGI grades tumor into high risk and low risk instead of 1, 2, and 3 grades of histopathology. GGI provides valuable information for estimation of breast cancer prognosis in ER-positive breast cancers and is also shown to help in prediction of relapse in endocrine-treated cancers [62] and prognosis in the patients with neoadjuvant therapy. The FDA has authorized the marketing of GGI to ipsogen JAK2 RGQ PCR Kit, manufactured by QIAGEN GmbH [63].

12.2.1.5 Breast Cancer Index (BCI)

Biotheranostics' Breast Cancer Index (BCI) is a quantitative RT-PCR-based prognostic test. For BCI formalin-fixed and FFPE tissue blocks are used. There are two outputs of this assay, based on unique gene signatures, which include BCI predictive and BCI prognostic. BCI prognostic helps for assessment of patient's individualized risk for distant recurrence, while BCI predictive provides possibility of benefit from extended endocrine therapy, possibly more than 5 years. BCI includes two independent biomarkers, IL17BR:HOXB13 and five cell cycle-associated gene index, which helps to assess tumor grade. The test is limited to patients with ER^+ and lymph node-negative cancer. So far, BCI has not added value information to other available prognostic tests limiting its clinical utility [64].

12.2.1.6 Theros H/I^{SM} and MGI^{SM}

These are transcriptomic-based biomarkers. In Theros H/I^{SM} clinical output of breast cancer individuals is determined who were treated with tamoxifen by evaluating the expression of two genes HOXB13 and IL17BR. If the expression ratio of these mentioned genes is high, then it represents no response to tamoxifen and tumor aggressiveness [65]. MGISM is also a molecular diagnostic test. This test is carried out to check the recurrence risk by using five-gene expression index for ER-positive breast cancer individuals [66]. Thus, more data is required for superiority of Theros H/I^{SM} and MGI^{SM} compared with other conventional methods.

To date, many genomic tests have been developed to improve the diagnosis and therapy of breast cancer. The IMPAKT 2012 group assessed the effectiveness of different available tests, i.e., MammaPrint, Oncotype DX, Genomic Grade Index, PAM50, and EndoPredict. They reported that MammaPrint and Oncotype DX have considerable validity and significance for both analytical and clinical aspects, in ER^+ breast cancer patients. Unfortunately, no significant association of other tests with prognosis was observed, and further studies are required for their convincing clinical validity [64].

12.3 Immunohistochemistry in Molecular Profiling of Breast Cancer

12.3.1 Significance of Immunohistochemistry as a Diagnostic Tool

Personalized cancer therapy demands use of several biomarkers during histopathological diagnosis [67]. Surgical pathology heavily relies on immunohistochemistry for diagnosing various malignancies. Protein localization and tumor classification can be done by IHC [68], although molecular profiling assists immunohistochemistry (IHC) which is currently performed with the conventional markers for breast cancer prognosis. However, only ER-positive cancer patients get benefit from this information [69]. Immunohistochemistry is used to measure the expression level of predictive markers including estrogen receptor/progesterone receptor (ER/PR) and human epidermal growth factor receptor 2 (HER2) during clinical assessment of tumors [70]. Treatment approaches with antiestrogen or anti-HER2-based therapies are followed for subgroups of patients selected based on these predictive markers. In addition, this approach also aids in analyzing the recurring risk of cancer in such patients [71].

12.3.2 Advancements and Limitations of IHC Techniques

There are several limiting factors due to which conventional methods of IHC are not well acknowledged recently. These include extra labor, time expenditure, expenses, and the large amount of sample tissue required for the procedure. This can be explained by example of Oncotype Dx test used for identification and prognosis of breast cancer. It demands much time and labor as more than 20 genes need to be examined for their role in breast cancer [72, 73]. Although these issues are assumed to be resolved by using an automated IHC machine, expenditures of both money and time still remain major issues while dealing with a large number of biomarkers and tissue sample, respectively. Additionally, limitations like variations in results, qualitative evaluation, and subjective decision make this technique a less reputable proteomic tool [72].

12.3.2.1 Multicolored-Based Immunohistochemistry

In recent investigations, multiplexing method with molecular dyes and quantum dots (QDs) is used for multicolored-based IHC assays [74, 75]. Multicolor IHC has advantage that it facilitates co-expression of several biomarkers with both direct and indirect sequential staining. However, several drawbacks are associated with multicolor staining [76]. These include increased labor and time expenditure, higher reagent costs, and sensitive procedure of probe conjugation using less stable primary antibodies and non-specific binding of secondary probes. These undesired factors lessen the effectiveness of multicolored immunohistochemistry [77].

12.3.2.2 Microfluidic-Based Multiplexed Immunohistochemistry (MMIHC)

Integration of IHC-based assays with an appropriate multiplexing method can prove an efficient diagnostic method for cancer patients [78]. Immunohistochemistry has been further modified with microfluidic parallel multiplexed design for diagnosing breast cancer quantitatively. This methodology provides an enclosed microenvironment in which fluids can be easily and timely manipulated [79]. Development of MMIHC platform demonstrates the enhanced IHC performance with accurate diagnosis, time, and cost-effectiveness as compared to previous methods which employ analysis of whole sections of breast cancer tissues [80]. Usually microfluidic devices are designed in such a way that glass slide and microchannel are permanently bonded together, and introduction of an interface between a microfluidic device and tissue slide has not been commonly reported by previous studies. Thus, it can be assumed that use of microfluidic design is not frequently practiced in studies with human clinical specimens [80–82].

Structural Design of Microfluidic Devices

Kim et al. had designed a microfluidic device by taking into consideration of solution number, biomarker count, and adequate reaction channel dimensions. Four biomarkers were used including estrogen (ER), Ki-67, progesterone (PR), and human epidermal growth factor 2 (HER2) receptors. The device contained six and four reservoirs for reagents and biomarkers, respectively. In addition, microvalves for both reagent and biomarker reservoirs, four reaction channels, and one outlet were included in the design. Lastly, to maintain constant pressure and creating a temporary seal, a weight was put on the top of the device [80, 83].

Preparation and Assembly of MMIHC Assay

The procedure employed for the preparation of MMIHC device involved two-step soft lithography, poly(dimethylsiloxane) (PDMS; Sylgard 184; Dow Corning, MA) replica molding and aligning processes. To minimize tissue damage, an appropriate interface between MMIHC device and tissue slide was prepared. To assemble, bottom plate of device was loaded with tissue slide. Afterward, tissue was treated with washing buffer, and four reaction channels containing MMIHC device were placed on it. Buffer was filled in microchannels carefully to avoid creation of micro-bubbles. Lastly, upper plate of the device was loaded with a weight so any leakage could be avoided, and tissues would be pressed with walls of microchannels [84, 85].

12.3.2.3 Analysis of Human Breast Cancer Tissue with MMIHC

After initial testing and trials of MMIHC device, Kim et al. used this platform for examination of tumor tissues of patients. This modified technique minimizes need of additional externally connected equipment. A major advantage of using MMIHC platform is that probability of assay failure is reduced under 1%, which is frequently observed in case of clinically rare samples. Immunohistochemical staining can be easily repeated in this setup due to an enclosed microenvironment and semi-automation of the staining process, and antibody consumption is reduced up to 200-fold along with speedy immunological reaction. Additionally, comparison of MMIHC results with those of western blotting revealed that this technique can give better results for semiquantitative analysis of cell blocks. Its effectiveness is exhibited by the fact that more accurate results are obtained during relative quantification due to single site biomarker staining which enables direct comparison and eliminates undesired variation as observed in multistep conventional IHC [80].

Quantification with image analyses needs further advancements and improvements in algorithms for clear scoring. Although MMIHC was considered more advantageous than earlier techniques, reliability of its results was doubted when compared to conventional whole tissue analysis [85]. These concerns are primarily based on scoring discrepancy probably caused by inborn errors of IHC due to variation in laboratory conditions or observer's skills. Other reasons include selection of specimens, processing errors, representation methods of MMIHC results, etc. In conclusion, after required modifications, a more applicable, fast, and easy to quantify MMIHC platform can improve the patient care conditions by facilitating clinical diagnosis of breast cancer [85, 86].

12.4 High-Throughput Sequencing (NGS) Technologies

Human genome consists around 3 billion nucleotides and 22,000 genes comprising on 23 chromosomes. Conventional methods took 10–12 weeks for genetic testing of known genes involved in breast cancer. This turnaround time, along with cost and area of genome studied, improved with the advent of new technologies, i.e., next-generation sequencing [87]. It has also helped to achieve new treatment avenues and make patient's lives better. Next-generation sequencing (NGS) has played very important role for investigations in such a heterogeneous and complex disease like breast cancer [88]. Firstly, it helped to characterize genome and exome of cancer patients. Along with unraveling the mutational processes, large-scale studies have discovered new genes associated with the disease. Advanced tools allow deep investigations of whole genome data and its correlation with disease stage, prognosis, and treatment options [89, 90].

12.4.1 Identification of New Genes

NGS has led to the discovery of new "driver" and "passenger" mutations. It all particularly was at the highest peak in 2012, with exceptional unraveling of mutational landscape. Some of the mutations newly identified in 2012 are shown in Table 12.1.

12.4.2 Delineating the Mutational Steps in Cancer

Many studies illustrated the mutational process underlying the cause and propagation of breast cancer, out of which the study published by Nik-Zainal [95] was the most appealing one of that time. According to this most important driver mutation in case of breast cancer patients occur in genes like TP53, *GATA3*, *PIK3CA*, *MAP2K4*, *SMAD4*, *MLL2*, *MLL3*, etc., duration and strength of each mutation determine the mutational process or pathway to the disease.

12.4.3 Detecting Minimal Residual Disease (MRD)

Generally, circulating tumor cell in blood and bone marrow has impact in development of breast cancer [96]. Nested real-time PCR has been used to detect tumor DNA in serum of relapsed breast cancer patients and to detect MRD. Early diagnosis can also be made by detecting serum DNA using NGS [97].

12.4.4 Drug Response Prediction

Various prognostic markers have been recognized which can not only identify patients with better or worse outcome of disease but can also predict response of patients to a certain treatment. It can not only reduce cost but save time as well. The most important markers studied till today in case of breast cancer are ER and HER2, having both prognostic and predictive roles. Oncotype Dx or recurrence score is used to estimate the expression level of 21 genes for stratifying ER breast cancer

Table 12.1 Mutated genes identified through next-generation sequencing (NGS)

S. No	Study	Mutated genes
1	Stephens et al. [91]	AKT2, TBX3, ARID1B, CDKN1B, NCOR1, MAP3K1, MAP3K13, SMARCD1, CASP8
2	Banerji et al. [92]	RUNX1, CBFB
3	Shah et al. [93]	USH2A, COL6A3, MYO3A, NRC31, PRKCE, PRKCQ, PRKG1, PRPS2, PRKCZ
4	Cancer Genome Atlas [94]	AFF2, OR6A2, PIK3R1, PTPRD, NF1, RPGR, SF3B1, CCND3, CTCF, TBL1XR1, NCOR1, ZFP36L1, GPS2, CLEC19A, RYR2, HIST1H2BC, GPR32, SEPT13, PTPN22, DCAF4L2, OR6A2

into high- and low-risk groups, using microarray analysis [98]. The use of whole genome sequencing techniques has given the insight into intra-tumor heterogeneity. Firstly, it showed the different subtypes of tumor with changed rearrangement patterns and mutations; secondly, metastasis is altered in case of primary tumors. Thirdly, it has been proven that tumor can progress using distinct pathways.

12.5 Biomarkers in Randomized Clinical Trials (RCT)

Biomarkers are naturally occurring molecules, characteristics, or genes used to perform a clinical assessment (prediction, identification, and monitoring the health states of individuals) and planning new therapeutics. In clinical trials of different tumor types, the relationship between drug response to presence, absence, or any kind of change in biomarker was tested. This consists of proof-of-concept trials, which include integral and integrated biomarkers. In integral biomarkers trials, patients with presence or absence of specific biomarkers were included only, while in integrated biomarkers trials, biomarkers effect mainly on drug response was tested [99]. Main goal of biomarkers incorporation into clinical trials was specific selection of patients who were expected to be benefitted from some specific therapies and to give more inclusive sight of how novel therapies function. But, incorporation of biomarkers into clinical trials is still challenging, because there is a need for considering some assays which can act as standards in different countries and clinical practices. A study of phase Ib/randomized phase II trial (double-blind clinical trial of tamoxifen plus taselisib or placebo) for HR+ metastatic breast cancer patients found that clinical outcomes can be improved by combining PI3K-AKT-mTOR pathway inhibitors with prior endocrine therapy. Taselisib is PI3K inhibitor having higher selectivity for mutant (MUT) PI3Kα isoforms than wild type. POSEIDON phase Ib data with tamoxifen (TAM) plus taselisib revealed greater performance in metastatic Ca breast individuals with an acceptable toxicity profile. Patients were grouped based on histology, menopausal status, no prior chemotherapy history, and treatment centers [100]. First randomized double-blind controlled clinical trial MANTICORE (Multidisciplinary Approach to Novel Therapies in Cardiology Oncology Research) was carried out on 100 early breast cancer patients at 2 centers. It was carried out in HER2+ early breast cancer (EBC) patients for evaluation of heart failure pharmacotherapy in the prevention of adjuvant trastuzumab-mediated left ventricular (LV) dysfunction. Adjuvant trastuzumab (TRZ) is mostly done for HER2+ overexpressing EBC patients with survival rates of 5 years. However, it has fivefold increased clinical heart failure rate. For prevention of such negative sequelae, LV remodeling is recognized as an early indicator of heart diseases. One of the methods used for quantifying LV remodeling and function is cardiac magnetic resonance imaging (CMR). So, MANTICORE trial was designed for evaluation of heart failure pharmacotherapy in the prevention of adjuvant trastuzumab-mediated left ventricular (LV) dysfunction. Patients were randomized to receive perindopril, bisoprolol, or placebo prior to initiating TRZ. So, this study has the potential to implement change in clinical practices with TRZ-based adjuvant therapy [101].

Programmed cell death-1 receptor and its ligands (PD-L1) are considered as therapeutic targets in reactivation of immune responses against cancer. Avelumab, an anti-PD-L1 antibody in clinical trials of metastatic breast cancer or locally advanced cancer, is being investigated (a phase Ib JAVELIN solid tumor trial). Immunohistochemistry was used to assess tumor PD-L1 with various cutoff criteria. Total 168 metastatic patients with HER2+, HER2−/ER+ or PR+, triple negative (TNBC = HER2−/ER−/PR−), or unknown biomarker were treated with avelumab. It showed a significant safety profile and had clinical activity in a subgroup of metastatic breast cancer patients. In patients with triple negative breast cancer, clinical response to avelumab is associated with the presence of PD-L1-expressing immune cells within tumor cells [102].

A single-arm clinical trial (phase II) with only one agent platinum was conducted on TNB patients along with correlated biomarkers. In case of metastatic TNBC, with germline BRCA1/BRCA2 mutations, platinum is used as active chemotherapeutic agent. Patients can be identified who could benefit from platinum therapy based on measurement of tumor DNA repair functions. Well-designed potential controlled trials that use diagnostically certified assays and predefined criteria are warranted to assess the clinical utility of DNA repair measurement for analyzing responsiveness to DNA-damaging agents and platinum [103]. These enrichment biomarkers, presently in clinical trials, may become predictive biomarker in the future after being clinically proven. Some examples are *RAS* mutations for both MAPK and PI3K pathway inhibitors, IGF mutations with IGF-1R antibodies and PTEN loss, and *PIK3CA* mutations for PI3K-Akt-mTOR pathway inhibitors. Various biomarker panels have been developed, like TruSeq Amplicon—Cancer Panel (TSACP) to assist identification of significant breast cancer-associated biomarkers for research and for clinical practices [104] (Table 12.2).

12.6 Conclusion

Advancement in molecular profiling of breast tumor types has showed differential molecular features that affect responsiveness, prognosis, and resistance to therapy. In this new era, importance of molecular profiling for breast cancer diagnosis and treatment can be evidenced with the emergence of vast variety of techniques and assays in clinical practice. These technologies have proven to solve various diagnostic issues, increased the information available from clinical trials, and paved toward personalized medicine overcoming the challenges of traditional techniques. Research is still in progress via clinical trials incorporating biomarkers to secure maximum benefits for breast cancer patients.

Table 12.2 Completed and ongoing biomarker-driven clinical trials of breast cancer (mentioned in text)

Trial name/ID	Agents	Phase	Patient population	Status
NCT02530424	Palbociclib, fulvestrant, trastuzumab, and pertuzumab expression of Ki67	Phase II	Triple targeting of ER, HER2, and RB1 in HER2- and ER-positive Ca breast, *n* = 36 patients	Ongoing
NCT02032277	Veliparib plus carboplatin or carboplatin PARP inhibitor, neoadjuvant chemotherapy	Phase III	*n* = 634 patients triple-negative breast cancer, clinical stage II–III	Ongoing
NCT02162719 LOTUS	Ipatasertib plus paclitaxel versus placebo plus paclitaxel, PI3K/AKT pathway inhibitor	Phase II	Metastatic triple-negative breast cancer, *n* = 166 patients	Ongoing
NSABP B-42 Double-blinded, randomized trial	Placebo-controlled trial of extended adjuvant endocrine therapy (tx) with letrozole (*L*) (aromatase inhibitor (AI))	Phase II	Stage I–III, postmenopausal, and hormone receptor (+) Ca breast, *n* = 3966	Completed
Nanoparticle albumin-bound (nab) paclitaxel	ab-paclitaxel followed by FEC (5-FU [fluorouracil], epirubicin, and cyclophosphamide)	Phase II	HER2-negative breast cancer *n* = 25 with no previous chemotherapy	Completed
NCT01889238 MDV3100 open label trial	Enzalutamide	Phase II	Androgen receptor-positive TNBC	Not recruiting anymore
NCT01990209	Orteronel	Phase II	Androgen receptor positive with metastatic breast cancer; *n* = 86	Ongoing
NCT01528345	Dovitinib, dovitinib placebo and fulvestrant	Phase II	Her− and HR+ metastatic postmenopausal individuals having progression after endocrine therapy, *n* = 97	Completed
NCT01791985	AZD4547 activity with either anastrozole or letrozole or both	Phase I/II	ER+ breast cancer patients with disease progression by letrozole and anastrozole, *n* = 56	Ongoing
NCT02437318 Double-blind randomized trial	Placebo controlled study of faslodex and alpelisib in combination	Phase III	HER2−, hormone receptor+, postmenopausal females and men with disease progression after aromatase inhibitor therapy, *n* = 572	Ongoing

(continued)

Table 12.2 (continued)

Trial name/ID	Agents	Phase	Patient population	Status
NCT00773695 Multicenter randomized study	Avastin activity was evaluated in combination with neoadj therapy. (antiangiogenic therapy done in this trial)	Phase II	Effect of this treatment was evaluated in primary tumors of HER2− Ca breast patients, $n = 150$	Completed
NCT01965522	Anti-proliferative effects of vitamin D3 (2000 IU daily) or placebo, and to melatonin (20 mg/day) or placebo in breast cancer (MELO-D) as measured by Ki67	Phase II	144 women with histologically confirmed invasive breast cancer (ductal, lobular, or mixed) Change in microRNA blood serum was studied	Completed
NCT01612871	Anastrozole, tamoxifen, exemestane and letrozole (hormonal therapy)	Phase IV	Metastatic Ca breast $n = 39$, specific circulating microRNAs were detected before and after given treatment	Completed
NCT02656589	Capecitabine, trastuzumab drugs given to patients, microRNAs expression was analyzed		300 participants, microRNA of HER2+ individuals treated with Herceptin having stage IV	Ongoing
NCT01907529	Neoadjuvant docetaxel, epirubicin, cyclophosphamide, and human recombinant endostatin (endostar)	Phase II/III	300 participants with histologically confirmed invasive breast cancer having stage III breast cancer and belonging to age group 18–70. This trial is designed on hypothesis that active angiogenesis agent combined to chemotherapy could enhance the pathological response rate	Completed

References

1. Siegel RL, Miller KD, Jemal A (2019) Cancer statistics. CA Cancer J Clin 69(1):7–34
2. Wadasadawala T, Lewis S, Parmar V, Budrukkar A, Gupta S, Nair N, Shet T, Badwe R, Sarin R (2018) Bilateral breast cancer after multimodality treatment: a report of clinical outcomes in an Asian population. Clin Breast Cancer 18(4):e727–e737
3. Bray F, Ferlay J, Soerjomataram I, Siegel RL, Torre LA, Jemal A (2018) Global cancer statistics 2018: GLOBOCAN estimates of incidence and mortality worldwide for 36 cancers in 185 countries. CA Cancer J Clin 68(6):394–424

4. Adeloye D, Sowunmi OY, Jacobs W, David RA, Adeosun AA, Amuta AO, Misra S, Gadanya M, Auta A, Harhay MO (2018) Estimating the incidence of breast cancer in Africa: a systematic review and meta-analysis. J Glob Health 8(1):010419
5. Malik SS, Mubarik S, Masood N, Khadim MT (2018) An insight into clinical outcome of XPG polymorphisms in breast cancer. Mol Biol Rep 45(6):2369–2375
6. Pang JMB, Gorringe KL, Fox SB (2016) Ductal carcinoma in situ–update on risk assessment and management. Histopathology 68(1):96–109
7. Martínez-Pérez C, Turnbull AK, Ekatah GE, Arthur LM, Sims AH, Thomas JS, Dixon JM (2017) Current treatment trends and the need for better predictive tools in the management of ductal carcinoma in situ of the breast. Cancer Treat Rev 55:163–172
8. Holten-Rossing H, Talman MLM, Jylling AMB, Lænkholm AV, Kristensson M, Vainer B (2017) Application of automated image analysis reduces the workload of manual screening of sentinel lymph node biopsies in breast cancer. Histopathology 71(6):866–873
9. Malik SS, Masood N, Asif M, Ahmed P, Shah ZU, Khan JS (2018) Expressional analysis of MLH1 and MSH2 in breast cancer. Curr Probl Cancer 43(2):97–105
10. Yersal O, Barutca S (2014) Biological subtypes of breast cancer: prognostic and therapeutic implications. World J Clin Oncol 5(3):412
11. Hoadley KA, Yau C, Wolf DM, Cherniack AD, Tamborero D, Ng S, Leiserson MD, Niu B, McLellan MD, Uzunangelov V (2014) Multiplatform analysis of 12 cancer types reveals molecular classification within and across tissues of origin. Cell 158(4):929–944
12. Russnes HG, Lingjaerde OC, Børresen-Dale A-L, Caldas C (2017) Breast cancer molecular stratification: from intrinsic subtypes to integrative clusters. Am J Pathol 187(10):2152–2162
13. Guedj M, Marisa L, De Reynies A, Orsetti B, Schiappa R, Bibeau F, Macgrogan G, Lerebours F, Finetti P, Longy M (2012) A refined molecular taxonomy of breast cancer. Oncogene 31(9):1196
14. Becht E, de Reyniès A, Giraldo NA, Pilati C, Buttard B, Lacroix L, Selves J, Sautès-Fridman C, Laurent-Puig P, Fridman WH (2016) Immune and stromal classification of colorectal cancer is associated with molecular subtypes and relevant for precision immunotherapy. Clin Cancer Res 22(16):4057–4066
15. Bristow RG, Alexander B, Baumann M, Bratman SV, Brown JM, Camphausen K, Choyke P, Citrin D, Contessa JN, Dicker A (2018) Combining precision radiotherapy with molecular targeting and immunomodulatory agents: a guideline by the American Society for Radiation Oncology. Lancet Oncol 19(5):e240–e251
16. Coyle KM, Boudreau JE, Marcato P (2017) Genetic mutations and epigenetic modifications: driving cancer and informing precision medicine. Biomed Res Int 2017:9620870
17. Cadoo KA, Traina TA, King TA (2013) Advances in molecular and clinical subtyping of breast cancer and their implications for therapy. Surg Oncol Clin 22(4):823–840
18. Serrano-Gómez SJ, Fejerman L, Zabaleta J (2018) Breast cancer in Latinas: a focus on intrinsic subtypes distribution. Cancer Epidemiol Prev Biomarkers 27(1):3–10
19. Hernandez-Aya LF, Ma CX (2016) Chemotherapy principles of managing stage IV breast cancer in the United States. Chin Clin Oncol 5(3):42
20. Ong FS, Das K, Wang J, Vakil H, Kuo JZ, Blackwell W-LB, Lim SW, Goodarzi MO, Bernstein KE, Rotter JI (2012) Personalized medicine and pharmacogenetic biomarkers: progress in molecular oncology testing. Expert Rev Mol Diagn 12(6):593–602
21. Matissek KJ, Onozato ML, Sun S, Zheng Z, Schultz A, Lee J, Patel K, Jerevall P-L, Saladi SV, Macleay A (2018) Expressed gene fusions as frequent drivers of poor outcomes in hormone receptor–positive breast cancer. Cancer Discov 8(3):336–353
22. Veeraraghavan J, Tan Y, Cao X-X, Kim JA, Wang X, Chamness GC, Maiti SN, Cooper LJ, Edwards DP, Contreras A (2014) Recurrent ESR1–CCDC170 rearrangements in an aggressive subset of oestrogen receptor-positive breast cancers. Nat Commun 5:4577
23. Nuciforo PG (2016) Quantitative analysis of HER family proteins using mass spectrometry as a predictive tool of response to anti-HER therapies in breast cancer. Department of Surgery, University of Barcelona. ISBN: 9788449065507

24. Mangolini A, Ferracin M, Zanzi MV, Saccenti E, Ebnaof SO, Poma VV, Sanz JM, Passaro A, Pedriali M, Frassoldati A (2015) Diagnostic and prognostic microRNAs in the serum of breast cancer patients measured by droplet digital PCR. Biomarker Res 3(1):12
25. Munson DJ, Egelston CA, Chiotti KE, Parra ZE, Bruno TC, Moore BL, Nakano TA, Simons DL, Jimenez G, Yim JH (2016) Identification of shared TCR sequences from T cells in human breast cancer using emulsion RT-PCR. Proc Natl Acad Sci 113(29):8272–8277
26. Snider J (2014) Overview of immunohistochemistry. Thermo Fisher Scientific Inc. Retrieved 05 Jan 2014 Disponible en http://www.piercenet.com/method
27. Sinn H-P, Schneeweiss A, Keller M, Schlombs K, Laible M, Seitz J, Lakis S, Veltrup E, Altevogt P, Eidt S (2017) Comparison of immunohistochemistry with PCR for assessment of ER, PR, and Ki-67 and prediction of pathological complete response in breast cancer. BMC Cancer 17(1):124
28. Bahreini F, Soltanian AR, Mehdipour P (2015) A meta-analysis on concordance between immunohistochemistry (IHC) and fluorescence in situ hybridization (FISH) to detect HER2 gene overexpression in breast cancer. Breast Cancer 22(6):615–625
29. Wang Y, Cottman M, Schiffman JD (2012) Molecular inversion probes: a novel microarray technology and its application in cancer research. Cancer Genet 205(7-8):341–355
30. Pant S, Weiner R, Marton MJ (2014) Navigating the rapids: the development of regulated next-generation sequencing-based clinical trial assays and companion diagnostics. Front Oncol 4:78
31. Nishizaki SS, Boyle AP (2017) Mining the unknown: assigning function to noncoding single nucleotide polymorphisms. Trends Genet 33(1):34–45
32. Laskin J, Jones S, Aparicio S, Chia S, Ch'ng C, Deyell R, Eirew P, Fok A, Gelmon K, Ho C (2015) Lessons learned from the application of whole-genome analysis to the treatment of patients with advanced cancers. Mol Case Stud 1(1):a000570
33. Moffat JG, Vincent F, Lee JA, Eder J, Prunotto M (2017) Opportunities and challenges in phenotypic drug discovery: an industry perspective. Nat Rev Drug Discov 16(8):531
34. McVeigh TP, Kerin MJ (2017) Clinical use of the Oncotype DX genomic test to guide treatment decisions for patients with invasive breast cancer. Breast Cancer Targets Ther 9:393
35. Roberts MC, Miller DP, Shak S, Petkov VI (2017) Breast cancer-specific survival in patients with lymph node-positive hormone receptor-positive invasive breast cancer and oncotype DX recurrence score results in the SEER database. Breast Cancer Res Treat 163(2):303–310
36. Kittaneh M, Montero AJ, Glück S (2013) Molecular profiling for breast cancer: a comprehensive review. Biomarkers Cancer 5:S9455
37. Cronin M, Sangli C, Liu M-L, Pho M, Dutta D, Nguyen A, Jeong J, Wu J, Langone KC, Watson D (2007) Analytical validation of the Oncotype DX genomic diagnostic test for recurrence prognosis and therapeutic response prediction in node-negative, estrogen receptor–positive breast cancer. Clin Chem 53(6):1084–1091
38. Cronin M, Pho M, Dutta D, Stephans JC, Shak S, Kiefer MC, Esteban JM, Baker JB (2004) Measurement of gene expression in archival paraffin-embedded tissues: development and performance of a 92-gene reverse transcriptase-polymerase chain reaction assay. Am J Pathol 164(1):35–42
39. Senkus E, Kyriakides S, Ohno S, Penault-Llorca F, Poortmans P, Rutgers E, Zackrisson S, Cardoso F (2015) Primary breast cancer: ESMO clinical practice guidelines for diagnosis, treatment and follow-up. Ann Oncol 26(suppl_5):v8–v30
40. Coates AS, Winer EP, Goldhirsch A, Gelber RD, Gnant M, Piccart-Gebhart M, Thürlimann B, Senn H-J, Members P, André F (2015) Tailoring therapies—improving the management of early breast cancer: St Gallen International Expert Consensus on the Primary Therapy of Early Breast Cancer 2015. Ann Oncol 26(8):1533–1546
41. Wood DE (2015) National Comprehensive Cancer Network (NCCN) clinical practice guidelines for lung cancer screening. Thorac Surg Clin 25(2):185–197
42. Duffy M, Harbeck N, Nap M, Molina R, Nicolini A, Senkus E, Cardoso F (2017) Clinical use of biomarkers in breast cancer: updated guidelines from the European Group on Tumor Markers (EGTM). Eur J Cancer 75:284–298

43. Curtit E, Mansi L, Maisonnette-Escot Y, Sautière J-L, Pivot X (2017) Prognostic and predictive indicators in early-stage breast cancer and the role of genomic profiling: focus on the Oncotype DX® Breast Recurrence Score Assay. Eur J Surg Oncol 43(5):921–930
44. Li H, Zhu Y, Burnside ES, Drukker K, Hoadley KA, Fan C, Conzen SD, Whitman GJ, Sutton EJ, Net JM (2016) MR imaging radiomics signatures for predicting the risk of breast cancer recurrence as given by research versions of MammaPrint, Oncotype DX, and PAM50 gene assays. Radiology 281(2):382–391
45. Mariotto A, Jayasekerea J, Petkov V, Schechter CB, Enewold L, Helzlsouer KJ, Feuer EJ, Mandelblatt JS (2019) Expected monetary impact of oncotype DX score-concordant systemic breast cancer therapy based on the TAILORx trial. JNCI: J Natl Cancer Inst. https://doi.org/10.1093/jnci/djz068
46. Chandler Y, Schechter CB, Jayasekera J, Near A, O'Neill SC, Isaacs C, Phelps CE, Ray GT, Lieu TA, Ramsey S (2018) Cost effectiveness of gene expression profile testing in community practice. J Clin Oncol 36(6):554
47. Brandão M, Pondé N, Piccart-Gebhart M (2018) Mammaprint™: a comprehensive review. Future Oncol 15(2):207–224
48. Xin L, Liu Y-H, Martin TA, Jiang WG (2017) The era of multigene panels comes? The clinical utility of Oncotype DX and Mammaprint. World J Oncol 8(2):34
49. Webber VL (2019) Comprehensive gene assessment of estrogen receptor positive breast cancers reveals that HER2 positive status plays an important role in resistance to neoadjuvant letrozole. Cancer Res 73:7683
50. Glas AM, Delahaye L, Krijgsman O (2019) Mammaprint of a multi-marker microarray as a routine diagnostic. In: Molecular diagnostics: the key in personalized cancer medicine. Pan Stanford Publishing, Singapore, p 139
51. Beumer I, Witteveen A, Delahaye L, Wehkamp D, Snel M, Dreezen C, Zheng J, Floore A, Brink G, Chan B (2016) Equivalence of MammaPrint array types in clinical trials and diagnostics. Breast Cancer Res Treat 156(2):279–287
52. Ono M, Tsuda H, Yoshida M, Shimizu C, Kinoshita T, Tamura K (2017) Prognostic significance of progesterone receptor expression in estrogen-receptor positive, HER2-negative, node-negative invasive breast cancer with a low Ki-67 labeling index. Clin Breast Cancer 17(1):41–47
53. Dai X, Li T, Bai Z, Yang Y, Liu X, Zhan J, Shi B (2015) Breast cancer intrinsic subtype classification, clinical use and future trends. Am J Cancer Res 5(10):2929
54. Han HS, Magliocco AM (2016) Molecular testing and the pathologist's role in clinical trials of breast cancer. Clin Breast Cancer 16(3):166–179
55. Barcenas CH, Raghavendra A, Sinha AK, Syed MP, Hsu L, Patangan MG Jr, Chavez-MacGregor M, Shen Y, Hortobagyi GH, Valero V (2017) Outcomes in patients with early-stage breast cancer who underwent a 21-gene expression assay. Cancer 123(13):2422–2431
56. Delahaye LJ, Wehkamp D, Floore AN, Bernards R, van't Veer LJ, Glas AM (2013) Performance characteristics of the MammaPrint® breast cancer diagnostic gene signature. Pers Med 10(8):801–811
57. Bender RA (2009) Company profile: Agendia, Inc. Biomark Med 3(3):225–230
58. Agendia NV (2019) MammaPrint and BluePrint Breast Cancer Recurrence and Molecular Subtyping Kit-Package Insert. available at: https://www.agendia.com/diagnostic-products/_assets/pdfs/M-ROW-133-V2(2018Oct)_NGS_Package_Insert.pdf
59. Chia SK, Bramwell VH, Tu D, Shepherd LE, Jiang S, Vickery T, Mardis E, Leung S, Ung K, Pritchard KI (2012) A 50-gene intrinsic subtype classifier for prognosis and prediction of benefit from adjuvant tamoxifen. Clin Cancer Res 18(16):4465–4472
60. Győrffy B, Hatzis C, Sanft T, Hofstatter E, Aktas B, Pusztai L (2015) Multigene prognostic tests in breast cancer: past, present, future. Breast Cancer Res 17(1):11
61. Sotiriou C, Wirapati P, Loi S, Harris A, Fox S, Smeds J, Nordgren H, Farmer P, Praz V, Haibe-Kains B (2006) Gene expression profiling in breast cancer: understanding the molecular basis of histologic grade to improve prognosis. J Natl Cancer Inst 98(4):262–272

62. Naoi Y, Kishi K, Tanei T, Tsunashima R, Tominaga N, Baba Y, Kim SJ, Taguchi T, Tamaki Y, Noguchi S (2011) High genomic grade index associated with poor prognosis for lymph node-negative and estrogen receptor-positive breast cancers and with good response to chemotherapy. Cancer 117(3):472–479
63. Hsu C-C, Huang C-E, Wu Y-Y, Chen Y-Y, Lung J, Leu Y-W, Li C-P, Tsou H-Y, Chuang W-H, Lu C-H (2018) Quantitative competitive allele-specific TaqMan duplex PCR (qCAST-Duplex PCR) assay: a refined method for highly sensitive and specific detection of JAK2V617F mutant allele burdens. Haematologica 103(10):e450–e454
64. Azim H Jr, Michiels S, Zagouri F, Delaloge S, Filipits M, Namer M, Neven P, Symmans W, Thompson A, Andre F (2013) Utility of prognostic genomic tests in breast cancer practice: the IMPAKT 2012 Working Group Consensus Statement. Ann Oncol 24(3):647–654
65. Zhao L, Zhu S, Gao Y, Wang Y (2014) Two-gene expression ratio as predictor for breast cancer treated with tamoxifen: evidence from meta-analysis. Tumor Biol 35(4):3113–3117
66. Dwivedi S, Purohit P, Misra R, Pareek P, Goel A, Khattri S, Pant KK, Misra S, Sharma P (2017) Diseases and molecular diagnostics: a step closer to precision medicine. Indian J Clin Biochem 32(4):374–398
67. Gonzalez de Castro D, Clarke P, Al-Lazikani B, Workman P (2013) Personalized cancer medicine: molecular diagnostics, predictive biomarkers, and drug resistance. Clin Pharmacol Ther 93(3):252–259
68. Hammond MEH, Hayes DF, Dowsett M, Allred DC, Hagerty KL, Badve S, Fitzgibbons PL, Francis G, Goldstein NS, Hayes M (2010) American Society of Clinical Oncology/College of American Pathologists guideline recommendations for immunohistochemical testing of estrogen and progesterone receptors in breast cancer (unabridged version). Arch Pathol Lab Med 134(7):e48–e72
69. Taylor CR (2018) Introduction to predictive biomarkers: definitions. In: Predictive biomarkers in oncology: applications in precision medicine. Springer, Cham, p 1
70. Gore CR, Gurwale S, Sammi A, Dey I, Deshpande AH (2018) Estrogen, progesterone, and human epidermal growth factor receptor-2 in malignant breast lesions. Med J Dr DY Patil Vidyapeeth 11(1):9
71. Dalerba PD, Clarke MF, Sahoo D, Raab WJ, Salazar LEV (2018) Biomarker for predicting colon cancer responsiveness to anti-tumor treatment. Google Patents
72. Gilbert MTP, Haselkorn T, Bunce M, Sanchez JJ, Lucas SB, Jewell LD, Van Marck E, Worobey M (2007) The isolation of nucleic acids from fixed, paraffin-embedded tissues–which methods are useful when? PLoS One 2(6):e537
73. Bishop DP, Cole N, Zhang T, Doble PA, Hare DJ (2018) A guide to integrating immunohistochemistry and chemical imaging. Chem Soc Rev 47(11):3770–3787
74. Smith AM, Dave S, Nie S, True L, Gao X (2006) Multicolor quantum dots for molecular diagnostics of cancer. Expert Rev Mol Diagn 6(2):231–244
75. Bilan R, Nabiev I, Sukhanova A (2016) Quantum dot-based nanotools for bioimaging, diagnostics, and drug delivery. ChemBioChem 17(22):2103–2114
76. Hofman P, Badoual C, Henderson F, Berland L, Hamila M, Long-Mira E, Lassalle S, Roussel H, Hofman V, Tartour E (2019) Multiplexed immunohistochemistry for molecular and immune profiling in lung cancer—just about ready for prime-time? Cancer 11(3):283
77. Söll I, Hauptmann G (2015) Multicolored visualization of transcript distributions in drosophila embryos. In: In situ hybridization methods. Springer, New York, pp 45–59
78. Lindeman NI, Cagle PT, Aisner DL, Arcila ME, Beasley MB, Bernicker EH, Colasacco C, Dacic S, Hirsch FR, Kerr K (2018) Updated molecular testing guideline for the selection of lung cancer patients for treatment with targeted tyrosine kinase inhibitors: guideline from the College of American Pathologists, the International Association for the Study of Lung Cancer, and the Association for Molecular Pathology. J Thorac Oncol 13(3):323–358
79. Dixit CK, Kadimisetty K, Otieno BA, Tang C, Malla S, Krause CE, Rusling JF (2016) Electrochemistry-based approaches to low cost, high sensitivity, automated, multiplexed protein immunoassays for cancer diagnostics. Analyst 141(2):536–547

80. Kim MS, Kim T, Kong S-Y, Kwon S, Bae CY, Choi J, Kim CH, Lee ES, Park J-K (2010) Breast cancer diagnosis using a microfluidic multiplexed immunohistochemistry platform. PLoS One 5(5):e10441
81. Mitra D (2013) Microfluidic modules for enabling point-of-care biopsy-based cancer diagnostics. UC Berkeley, Berkeley
82. Halldorsson S, Lucumi E, Gómez-Sjöberg R, Fleming RM (2015) Advantages and challenges of microfluidic cell culture in polydimethylsiloxane devices. Biosens Bioelectron 63:218–231
83. Anna SL (2016) Droplets and bubbles in microfluidic devices. Annu Rev Fluid Mech 48:285–309
84. Park J-K (2010) Lab-on-a-chip technology for integrative bioengineering. In: 10th IEEE international conference on nanotechnology. IEEE, Piscataway, pp 156–159
85. Kim MS, Kwon S, Park J-K (2013) Breast cancer diagnostics using microfluidic multiplexed immunohistochemistry. In: Microfluidic diagnostics. Springer, New York, pp 349–364
86. Kwon S, Cho CH, Lee ES, Park J-K (2015) Automated measurement of multiple cancer biomarkers using quantum-dot-based microfluidic immunohistochemistry. Anal Chem 87(8):4177–4183
87. Pitt AR, Kolch W (2018) 24 Genomics, proteomics, and metabolomics. In: Medical Biochemistry E-Book, p. 319
88. Rabbani B, Nakaoka H, Akhondzadeh S, Tekin M, Mahdieh N (2016) Next generation sequencing: implications in personalized medicine and pharmacogenomics. Mol BioSyst 12(6):1818–1830
89. Skol AD, Sasaki MM, Onel K (2016) The genetics of breast cancer risk in the post-genome era: thoughts on study design to move past BRCA and towards clinical relevance. Breast Cancer Res 18(1):99
90. Serratì S, De Summa S, Pilato B, Petriella D, Lacalamita R, Tommasi S, Pinto R (2016) Next-generation sequencing: advances and applications in cancer diagnosis. OncoTargets Ther 9:7355
91. Stephens PJ, Tarpey PS, Davies H, Van Loo P, Greenman C, Wedge DC, Nik-Zainal S, Martin S, Varela I, Bignell GR, Yates LR, Papaemmanuil E, Beare D, Butler A, Cheverton A, Gamble J, Hinton J, Jia M, Jayakumar A, Jones D, Latimer C, Lau KW, McLaren S, McBride DJ, Menzies A, Mudie L, Raine K, Rad R, Chapman MS, Teague J, Easton D, Langerod A, Lee MT, Shen CY, Tee BT, Huimin BW, Broeks A, Vargas AC, Turashvili G, Martens J, Fatima A, Miron P, Chin SF, Thomas G, Boyault S, Mariani O, Lakhani SR, van de Vijver M, van't Veer L, Foekens J, Desmedt C, Sotiriou C, Tutt A, Caldas C, Reis-Filho JS, Aparicio SA, Salomon AV, Borresen-Dale AL, Richardson AL, Campbell PJ, Futreal PA, Stratton MR, Oslo Breast Cancer C (2012) The landscape of cancer genes and mutational processes in breast cancer. Nature 486(7403):400–404. https://doi.org/10.1038/nature11017
92. Banerji S, Cibulskis K, Rangel-Escareno C, Brown KK, Carter SL, Frederick AM, Lawrence MS, Sivachenko AY, Sougnez C, Zou L, Cortes ML, Fernandez-Lopez JC, Peng S, Ardlie KG, Auclair D, Bautista-Pina V, Duke F, Francis J, Jung J, Maffuz-Aziz A, Onofrio RC, Parkin M, Pho NH, Quintanar-Jurado V, Ramos AH, Rebollar-Vega R, Rodriguez-Cuevas S, Romero-Cordoba SL, Schumacher SE, Stransky N, Thompson KM, Uribe-Figueroa L, Baselga J, Beroukhim R, Polyak K, Sgroi DC, Richardson AL, Jimenez-Sanchez G, Lander ES, Gabriel SB, Garraway LA, Golub TR, Melendez-Zajgla J, Toker A, Getz G, Hidalgo-Miranda A, Meyerson M (2012) Sequence analysis of mutations and translocations across breast cancer subtypes. Nature 486(7403):405–409. https://doi.org/10.1038/nature11154
93. Shah SP, Roth A, Goya R, Oloumi A, Ha G, Zhao Y, Turashvili G, Ding J, Tse K, Haffari G, Bashashati A, Prentice LM, Khattra J, Burleigh A, Yap D, Bernard V, McPherson A, Shumansky K, Crisan A, Giuliany R, Heravi-Moussavi A, Rosner J, Lai D, Birol I, Varhol R, Tam A, Dhalla N, Zeng T, Ma K, Chan SK, Griffith M, Moradian A, Cheng SW, Morin GB, Watson P, Gelmon K, Chia S, Chin SF, Curtis C, Rueda OM, Pharoah PD, Damaraju S, Mackey J, Hoon K, Harkins T, Tadigotla V, Sigaroudinia M, Gascard P, Tlsty T, Costello JF, Meyer IM, Eaves CJ, Wasserman WW, Jones S, Huntsman D, Hirst M, Caldas C, Marra MA,

Aparicio S (2012) The clonal and mutational evolution spectrum of primary triple-negative breast cancers. Nature 486(7403):395–399. https://doi.org/10.1038/nature10933
94. Cancer Genome Atlas N (2012) Comprehensive molecular portraits of human breast tumours. Nature 490(7418):61–70. https://doi.org/10.1038/nature11412
95. Nik-Zainal S, Alexandrov LB, Wedge DC, Van Loo P, Greenman CD, Raine K, Jones D, Hinton J, Marshall J, Stebbings LA, Menzies A, Martin S, Leung K, Chen L, Leroy C, Ramakrishna M, Rance R, Lau KW, Mudie LJ, Varela I, DJ MB, Bignell GR, Cooke SL, Shlien A, Gamble J, Whitmore I, Maddison M, Tarpey PS, Davies HR, Papaemmanuil E, Stephens PJ, McLaren S, Butler AP, Teague JW, Jonsson G, Garber JE, Silver D, Miron P, Fatima A, Boyault S, Langerod A, Tutt A, Martens JW, Aparicio SA, Borg A, Salomon AV, Thomas G, Borresen-Dale AL, Richardson AL, Neuberger MS, Futreal PA, Campbell PJ, Stratton MR, Breast Cancer Working Group of the International Cancer Genome C (2012) Mutational processes molding the genomes of 21 breast cancers. Cell 149(5):979–993. https://doi.org/10.1016/j.cell.2012.04.024
96. Naume B, Zhao X, Synnestvedt M, Borgen E, Russnes HG, Lingjaerde OC, Stromberg M, Wiedswang G, Kvalheim G, Karesen R, Nesland JM, Borresen-Dale AL, Sorlie T (2007) Presence of bone marrow micrometastasis is associated with different recurrence risk within molecular subtypes of breast cancer. Mol Oncol 1(2):160–171. https://doi.org/10.1016/j.molonc.2007.03.004
97. Beck J, Urnovitz HB, Mitchell WM, Schutz E (2010) Next generation sequencing of serum circulating nucleic acids from patients with invasive ductal breast cancer reveals differences to healthy and nonmalignant controls. Mol Cancer Res 8(3):335–342. https://doi.org/10.1158/1541-7786.MCR-09-0314
98. Paik S, Shak S, Tang G, Kim C, Baker J, Cronin M, Baehner FL, Walker MG, Watson D, Park T, Hiller W, Fisher ER, Wickerham DL, Bryant J, Wolmark N (2004) A multigene assay to predict recurrence of tamoxifen-treated, node-negative breast cancer. N Engl J Med 351(27):2817–2826. https://doi.org/10.1056/NEJMoa041588
99. Massacesi C, Tomaso E, Fretault N, Hirawat S (2013) Challenges in the clinical development of PI3K inhibitors. Ann N Y Acad Sci 1280(1):19
100. Oliveira M, Baird R, van Rossum A, Beelen K, Garcia-Corbacho J, Mandjes I, Vallier A, van Werkhoven E, Garrigós L, Kumar S (2017) Abstract OT2-01-11: Phase II of POSEIDON: A phase Ib/randomized phase II trial of tamoxifen plus taselisib or placebo in hormone receptor positive, HER2 negative, metastatic breast cancer patients with prior exposure to endocrine treatment. AACR, Philadelphia
101. Pituskin E, Mackey J, Koshman S, Jassal D, Pitz M, Haykowsky M, Thompson R, Oudit G, Ezekowitz J, Paterson I (2016) Abstract PD5-03: Prophylactic beta blockade preserves left ventricular ejection fraction in HER2-overexpresssing breast cancer patients receiving trastuzumab: Primary results of the MANTICORE randomized controlled trial. AACR, Philadelphia
102. Kelly K, Patel MR, Infante JR, Iannotti N, Nikolinakos P, Leach J, Wang D, Chandler JC, Jerusalem GHM, Gurtler JS (2015) Avelumab (MSB0010718C), an anti-PD-L1 antibody, in patients with metastatic or locally advanced solid tumors: assessment of safety and tolerability in a phase I, open-label expansion study. American Society of Clinical Oncology, Alexandria
103. Isakoff SJ, Mayer EL, He L, Traina TA, Carey LA, Krag KJ, Rugo HS, Liu MC, Stearns V, Come SE (2015) TBCRC009: a multicenter phase II clinical trial of platinum monotherapy with biomarker assessment in metastatic triple-negative breast cancer. J Clin Oncol 33(17):1902
104. Chevrier S, Arnould L, Ghiringhelli F, Coudert B, Fumoleau P, Boidot R (2014) Next-generation sequencing analysis of lung and colon carcinomas reveals a variety of genetic alterations. Int J Oncol 45(3):1167–1174

Part IV

Systems Biology and Integrated Computational Methods for Cancer-Associated Mutation Analysis

13

Ayisha Zia and Sajid Rashid

13.1 Systems Biology

Systems biology is the research endeavor that offers the basic scientific groundwork for synthetic biology. It is grounded on the molecular diversity of living systems [1]. It is an integrative system that connects different components in a single biological unit and also links different units like cells and tissues using holistic methods to characterize their functions through computational methods, quantitative approaches, and high-throughput technologies. Cells are made of different constituents that interact and make a network model, for example, metabolic, regulatory, and signaling networks that regulate various cellular functions. Several elaborated and dynamic models are available for signaling pathways [2].

The computational approaches deliver a comprehension to understand the dynamics and interaction within cells, organs, tissues, and organisms. For complex diseases, precision medicine and quantitative methods are influenced by systems biology [3]. The best example of system thinking is the Human Genome Project as it shows different ways to work on the problems in the field of genetics [4]. Its main purpose is to discover the properties of cells, tissues, and organisms working as a whole system whose description is possible only by using systems biology which involves metabolic networks [5]. Interpretation of the systems biology to obtain and investigate complex data sets by interdisciplinary tools and experimental studies generally starts with omics including genomics, transcriptomics, and metabolomics. Other subdisciplines include phosphoproteomics, glycoproteomics, and areas to identify chemically modified proteins, metabolomics-, organismal-, tissue-, or cellular-level measurements of lipids [6].

A. Zia · S. Rashid (✉)
National Centre for Bioinformatics, Functional Informatics Lab, Quaid-i-Azam University, Islamabad, Pakistan
e-mail: azia@bs.qau.edu.pk; sajidrwp@yahoo.co.uk

N. Masood, S. Shakil Malik (eds.), *'Essentials of Cancer Genomic, Computational Approaches and Precision Medicine*,
https://doi.org/10.1007/978-981-15-1067-0_13

13.1.1 Dynamic State Characterization

For complex reaction networks, dynamic analysis involves tracing of time-dependent concentration changes and reaction fluxes over the time period. The three key points of dynamic states are:

- Time constant (the rate of change of a variable is considered by time constant)
- Aggregate variables (the biochemical and physiological events that are involved in unfolding. Basically, we move to the aggregate variables from the original concentration variables that eventually terminate in the overall dynamic features on slower time scales)
- Transitions (intricate networks can transition from one state to another state)

13.1.2 Formulation of Dynamic Network Models

Two different approaches (bottom-up and top-down) are used to formulate dynamic networks. In bottom-up approach, we identify all the events in the network in complexity with the addition of more information from time to time to make the event complete, whereas in top-down approach, all data and information is collected at the same time, and later this data is divided into smaller parts. The bottom-up analysis of any dynamic state of a network is based on the kinetic theory and network topology [2].

13.1.3 Cancer Systems Biology

It comprehends the application of systems biology methods to study the disease with evolving properties at different biological levels. It also helps to analyze how the disturbance in the intracellular pathways and networks of normal cells occurs during carcinogenesis for the development of effective prognostic models. These models can assist scientists in the validations of new treatments and drugs [7]. These perturbations are caused by the instability in tumors that changes the functions of different molecules. It is further convoluted due to the networks in a single cell and by the alterations in the interactions with the environment and whole individual during the tumorigenic process itself. Therefore computational and mathematical methods are used in cancer systems biology to interpret the complexity [8].

Cancer systems biology combines basic and clinical cancer research, and it provides applications of systems biology methods to the cancer research, particularly:

a. The need for improved methods to gain understanding from extensive networks
b. The significance of assimilating multiple types of data in construction of further accurate models
c. Trials in deciphering insights of tumorigenic mechanisms into therapeutic mediations
d. The function of tumor microenvironment at different levels [9]

13.1.4 Analysis of Cells at System Level

The system level provides the information at all the points of cell function. Different technologies are present which are supporting huge data quantity. This data needs to be handled and managed to make it into meaningful knowledge. Hence, organization and scrutinization of all data sets are known as bioinformatics like omics that delivers large amount of information from proteins, metabolites, and mRNA. By utilizing the sequencing technology, one can find genomic sequence and depict its determinants that include single nucleotide polymorphisms (SNPs) and regulatory sites that control particular phenotype or its function in an organism [10]. Epigenomics describes the epigenetic modifications [11], and proteomics measures the proteins and posttranslational modifications [12]. Likewise, transcriptomics measures transcriptome [11], and the study of metabolites in the cells and tissues is metabolomics [13]. These experimental techniques may result in huge data collection that may become a basis for designing novel tools and algorithms to interpret unknown data sets through knowledge-based information and linking the outcome of system-level studies.

13.2 Computational Approaches Used in Systems Biology

The data obtained from omics is organized by various tools of bioinformatics. These data sets are then used to form networks. Topological features can be constructed from these networks of molecular interactions. In these networks, there are network motifs [14] and functional modules that can perform functional tasks and represent dynamical signal properties. Regulatory pathways that include different motifs, feedback loops, and modules could be mined to construct dynamical models [15] which are further used for simulations to understand their promising behavior in time and space. To study the drug actions, they can be combined with PK/PD models [16]. Figure 13.1 shows the computational approaches used in systems biology.

13.2.1 Systems Medicine

Systems medicine is based on systems biology and systems science. It reflects intricate interactions within the human body with respect to the genome, environment, and behavior of the patient [17]. Systems medicine is used in research setups as it uncovers the unique and dynamic network of interactions which are crucial for influencing the progress of medical conditions. It also assists in determining molecular targets against any condition for its therapeutic and diagnostic measures. The relationship between the dry and wet lab is supported by systems medicine as well [18]. The basic dissimilarity among systems biology and systems medicine is that systems biology assumes the data to be useable and correct, while systems medicine ensures to lead with molecular and clinical data sets to produce the pathways that might contribute to medicinal development to the adapted healthcare [19, 20]. The

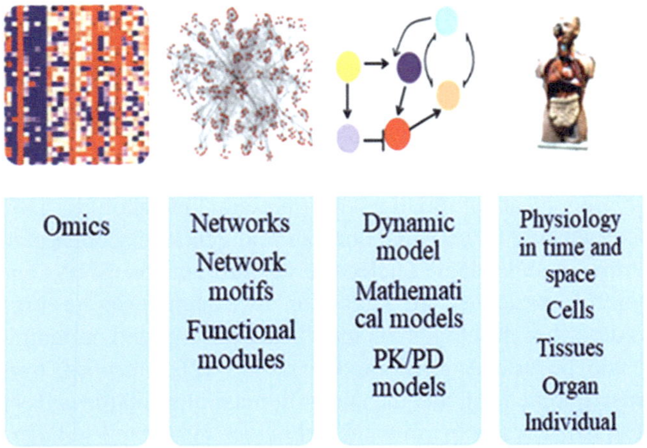

Fig. 13.1 Computational approaches in systems biology. Omics data are arranged using different tools of bioinformatics to construct networks. Regulatory pathways can be extracted from these networks for the formation of dynamic models. From dynamic models, the behavior of the system in time and space can be predicted and combined with PK/PD models for the drug action mechanism

basic difference between systems biology and systems medicine is that systems biology assumes the data to be useable and correct, while systems medicine ensures the validity of molecular and clinical data sets to interpret the pathways that may contribute to therapeutic possibilities to the adapted healthcare [19, 20].

13.2.2 Systems Medicine for Human Diseases and Novel Drugs Research

Systems medicine requires different features to achieve clinical and diagnostic goals [19]. One of the important areas in the systems medicine is the progress of the computational models that help to explain the disease advancement and effects of therapeutic interventions [21]. This is important for the better control of large data sets and also to elucidate wet laboratory in order to develop multifaceted interrelationships among molecular targets.

Systems medicine plays a vital role in drug development whereby drugs are proven to be effective for one condition or ineffective for a different medical condition [22]. Jin et al. performed transcriptome expression analysis before and after the drug administration to observe the off-target effects of drug for signaling pathways. This study recognized a systems-based analytical approach named as Bayesian factor regression model (BFRM) accompanied by cancer signaling bridges (CSB), termed as CSB-BFRM, which is fruitful in the prediction of outcomes of clinical responses arising for Food and Drug Administration (FDA)-approved drugs through validation using three independent cancer models, thereby assuring the accuracy of systems medicine approach [23].

Systems medicine has an impact in recognizing innovative disease networks. The foremost exploration focuses on the connections of models that are influenced by the pathogenesis and are inactive or active in numerous disease conditions. MicroRNA (miRNA) research is one of the typical methodologies to recognize the application of systems medicine. As miRNA controls the transcripts, one miRNA perhaps deregulates the expression of numerous downstream target genes; therefore, it is possible that miRNA can be applied in many clinical conditions probably in a simultaneous manner [24]. Outline of systems medicine is shown in Fig. 13.2.

Systems medicine is paving its way for academics, clinicians, and researchers dealing with experimental research approaches. The probability to investigate an immense data from in silico and experimental approaches offers more understanding into the complex molecular interactions. This assists to the enlightening of unusual dynamic interactions that are vital for medical conditions and therefore serve as clinically significant key molecules for future therapeutics [18, 24].

13.3 Computational Approaches

Extensive measurements of somatic mutations in the tumors are possible through high-throughput DNA sequencing technologies. Cancer genomics purposes to find out all the genes related to cancer and their involvements in cancer development. Cancer-driven mutation and pathways can be detected on the basis of biological networks and different computational approaches. They can be classified into (1)

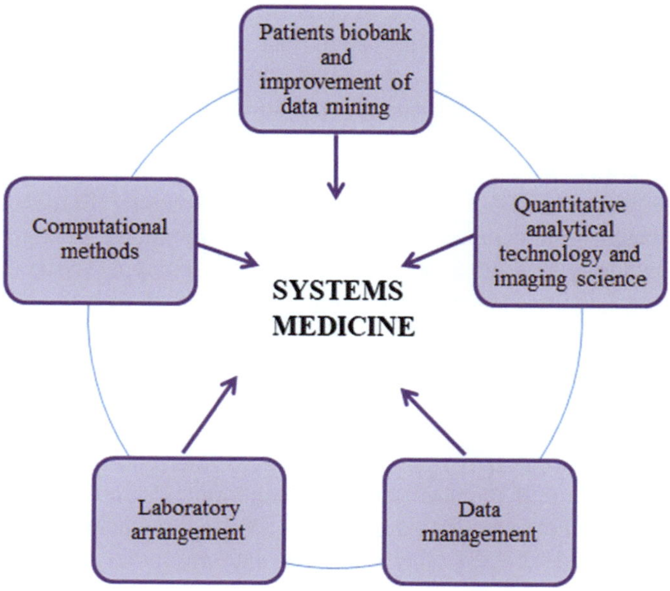

Fig. 13.2 Outline of the mandatory features for execution of systems medicine methods to modern medical research

functional impact-based approach, (2) network- or pathway-based approach, (3) data integration-based approach, (4) mutation frequency-based approach, and (5) structural genomics-based approach [25]. Here, the approaches and the databases used for the identification of cancer genes and pathways will be focused.

13.3.1 Data Resources of Cancer-Related Genes, Networks, and Pathways

Different databases are present that contain information and function about cancer genes. Among them, COSMIC (The Catalogue Of Somatic Mutations In Cancer) is one of the largest databases. It includes mutations from the cancer cell lines and also the whole genome and exome of patients having cancer and hence provides detailed information of somatic mutations [26]. The Cancer Genome Atlas (TCGA) characterizes genomic changes in 33 cancer types which has enhanced the evaluation of genomic changes in cancer genomics. Single base substitutions in TCGA are 2,948,799, among them 1,648,416 are missense variants [27]. The International Cancer Genome Consortium (ICGC) aims to describe the epigenomic, transcriptomic, and genomic profiles of the cancer genomes of 50 different cancer types [28].

cBioportal is a web source of visualizing and investigating cancer genomics data [29]. These annotation databases are helpful to decode the consequences among mutations and protein 3D structures. To identify driver mutations specifically in kinase domain, protein's three-dimensional (3D) structure information is used. In context of the 3D structure, another database is Cancer3D to investigate missense somatic mutations [30]. dSysMap is a resource for mapping the missense mutations through the structurally annotated interactome of human. Recently, for studying function of noncoding somatic mutations, different projects have been initialized as protein-coding human genome is just <2% [31]. These include Encyclopedia of DNA Elements (ENCODE) [32], the functional annotation of the mammalian genome 5 (FANTOM5) [33], and NIH Roadmap Epigenomics [34]. These databases offer comprehensive resources of functional genomics data to describe regulatory role of noncoding mutations. Genotype-Tissue Expression (GTEx) project delivers genetic expression and regulation data for many human tissues. It helps to study the tissue-specific regulatory pathways that are changed by somatic mutations Consortium GT. Human genomics [35]. To study somatic cancer mutation, the Database of Curated Mutations (DoCM) is used. It includes 1276 missense mutations and 1364 variants from 122 cancer subtypes [36]. Another community-edited web source named as Clinical Interpretations of Variants in Cancer (CIViC) is used for discovering different variants in cancer. It includes 1767 variants until February 2018 and enables precision medicine for cancer treatment [37]. Table 13.1 [38] shows all the data resources for cancer-driven mutations.

Table 13.1 Data resources for the assessment of computational tools for somatic mutation genes and driver mutations in cancer

Name	Depiction
COSMIC	Comprehensive resources of somatic mutations
TCGA	Characterize genomic changes in 33 cancer types
ICGC	Describe epigenomic, transcriptomic, and genomic profiles of the cancer genomes
cBioPortal	Visualization and investigation of cancer genomics data
Cancer3D	Functional roles of somatic mutations via protein 3D structure
dSysMap	For mapping the missense mutation on the structurally annotated interactome of human
ENCODE	Comprehensive resources of functional genomics data
NIH Roadmap Epigenomics	Resources of functional genomics data
FANTOM	Regulatory role of noncoding mutations
GTEx	A resource for the tissue-specific regulation and gene expression
DoCM	For somatic cancer mutations
CIViC	For variants in cancer

13.3.2 Data Resources for Networks and Pathways

Detailed analysis based on gene networks has been applied to interpret somatic mutations in the cancer [39]. Protein-protein interaction (PPI) and pathway-related databases have been established such as Reactome [40], WikiPathways [41], Pathway Interaction Database (PID) [42], and Pathway Commons [43]. These databases have been widely used to assess the role of variants and somatic mutations [44].

Some important PPI databases include BioGRID [45], HPRD [46], MINT [47], IntAct [48], STRING [49], PINA [50], PhosphoSitePlus [51], Phospho.ELM [52], PTMcode [53], Interactome3D [54], Instruct [55], and 3did [56].

PPI databases provide a network resource of complementary molecular interactions to decipher the consequences of somatic variations in various cancers as they enlist literature-derived and experimental PPIs, 3D structure PPIs, and kinase-substrate-specific phosphorylation events (Fig. 13.3).

13.4 Computational Approaches and Methods

Computational methods help in the fastest way to characterize the disease. General approaches used for the investigation of somatic mutations are shown in Fig. 13.4. Through whole genome sequencing, list of mutations leading to cancer can be obtained.

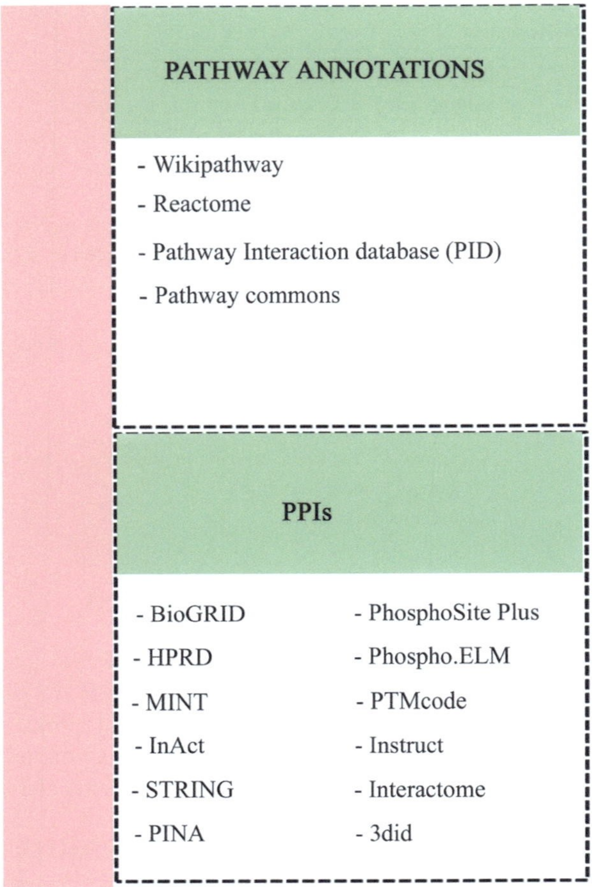

Fig. 13.3 Data resources for prioritizing driver mutations and pathways in cancer

13.4.1 Mutation Frequency-Based Approaches

Significantly mutated genes (SMGs) in the cancer are defined by categorizing the genes that undergo more mutations than those based on the mutation model in a certain cancer type [57]. Table 13.2 [38] summarizes the computational approaches based on the mutation frequency such as Mutational Significant in Cancer (MuSiC). It incorporates the clinical data with sequence-based data to find out the relationship among affected genes, mutations, and pathways [58]. Similarly, ContrastRank compares alleged defective rate of every gene against normal data [59]. As the model with low mutation frequency may lead to false positive results, thus other methods were projected. SMGs based on the gain of function mutation can be identified by OncodriveCLUST [60]. It showed that silent mutations play a vital role in cancer. OncodriveCLUST uses silent mutation as the background. Lawrence et al.

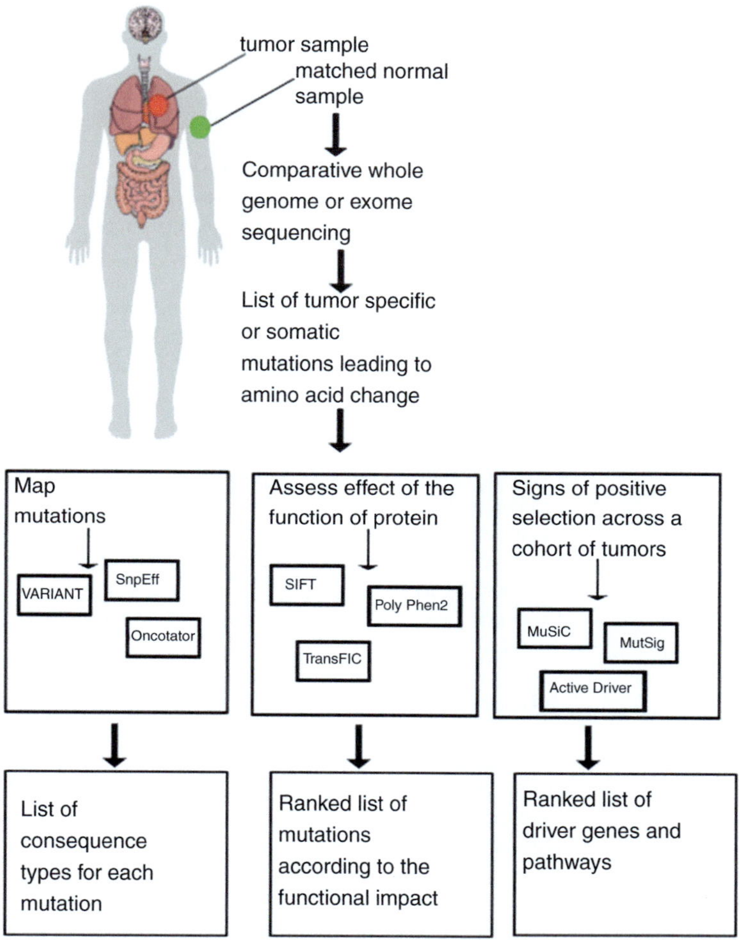

Fig. 13.4 General approaches used in the routine for the analysis of cancer somatic mutation

established MutSigCV that uses the information of replication timing and gene expression to develop a patient-specific mutation model [57].

13.4.2 Functional Impact-Based Approaches

Computational methods offer a fast and an economical way to evaluate the impact of mutations. These methods help the researchers to find the putative mutations that can validate their experimental work. Multiple tools have been developed for the computational approaches. One of the tools is SIFT (The Sorting Intolerant from Tolerant) that finds out the impact of amino acid substitution in protein function. It is based on the extent to which an amino acid is conserved in sequence alignment

Table 13.2 Summary of tools and computational approaches for the identification of driver mutations and SMGs in cancer genome

Mutation frequency-based approaches	
MuSiC	An approach for determination of the mutational significance in cancer
MutSigCV	An integrative approach that corrects for variants using patient-specific mutation frequency and spectrum and gene-specific background mutation model derived from gene expression and replication timing information
OncodriveCLUST	Identifying genes with a significant bias toward mutation clustering in specific regions of proteins using silent mutations as a background mutation model
ContrastRank	A method based on estimating the assumed defective rate of each gene in tumor against normal samples from the 1000 Genomes Project data
Functional impact-based approaches	
MutationTaster	A tool including evolutionary conservation and splice-site change information for the prediction of functional impacts of DNA sequencing modifications
MutationAssessor	Based on evolutionary conservation patterns, it can predict the functional impacts
SIFT	A tool that uses protein sequence homology for the prediction of biological effect of missense variations
PolyPhen-2	A tool for the prediction of the functional impacts of protein sequence variants by using three structure-based and eight sequence-based predictive features to build naive Bayes classifiers
CHASM and SNVbox	Python programs that use the tumorigenic impact of mutations for cancer-related mutations
Condel	A consensus deleteriousness score for evaluating the functional impact of missense mutations
OncodriveFM	An approach based on functional impact bias using three well-known methods
CanDrA	A tool based on a set of 95 structural and evolutionary features
PROVEAN	For the prediction of functional effects of SNV and in-frame insertions and deletions
FATHMM	A tool based on Hidden Markov model-based tool for functional analysis of driver mutations
CRAVAT	A web-based toolkit for arranging missense mutations related to tumorigenesis
Data integration-based approaches	
MAXDRIVER	An approach that uses the data from copy number variant regions of cancer genomes for the prediction of SMGs
CONEXIC	A computational framework that assimilates copy number variants and gene expression changes for prioritizing SMGs
CAERUS	An approach for the prediction of SMGs using structural information of proteins, protein networks, gene expression, and mutation data
Helios	For prediction of SMGs by the integration of functional and genomic RNAi screening data
OncoIMPACT	A framework based on phenotypic impacts for highlighting SMGs

(continued)

Table 13.2 (continued)

Mutation frequency-based approaches	
OncodriverROLE	An approach that classifies SMGs into LoF and GoF
DOTS-Finder	A tool based on functional and frequency for predicting SMGs in cancer
Structural genomics-based approaches	
ActiveDriver	For prediction of SMGs having driver mutations significantly changing phosphorylation sites of proteins
iPAC	For the prediction of SMGs by using protein 3D structure
MSEA	For the prediction of SMGs based on mutation patterns on domains of protein
CanBind	For the prediction of SMGs using the information on the binding site of protein–ligand
Network or pathway-based approaches	
PARADIGM-SHIFT	It uses belief-propagation algorithm for ordering downstream pathways by a mutation in cancer
PARADIGM	By incorporation of patient-specific genetic data, it detects consistent pathways in cancers
DriverNet	By estimating the effect on mRNA expression networks, it identifies driver mutations
Personalized pathway enrichment map	From individual genome, it identifies alleged cancer genes and pathways
NBS	An approach for stratifying tumor mutations
TieDIE	An approach for identification of cancer-mutated subnetworks
DawnRank	On the basis of PageRank algorithm, it prioritizes SMGs in a single patient
HotNet2	For the detection of mutated subnetworks in cancer, an algorithm is used to overcome the limitations of existing single-gene and network approaches
VarWalker	A novel approach for prioritizing SMGs

derived from the closely related sequences [61, 62]. SIFT can characterize impact of missense mutations. Another software named as Polymorphism Phenotyping v2 (PolyPhen-2) is used with SIFT for better results. It predicts the impact of the variants by three structure-based and eight sequence-based features [63]. Another web server, MutationAssessor, uses a novel functional impact score for the characterization of residual mutation. To define the evolutionary conservation patterns, which are taken from aligned families and subfamilies, it uses combinatorial entropy formalism [64]. The three methods mentioned above are useful for nonsynonymous SNVs only. Multiple methods incorporate domain information to predict the functional impact of SNVs. One of them is OncodriveFM. It identifies low recurrent candidate SMGs by utilizing the features of SIFT, MutationAssessor, and PolyPhen-2 [65]. For rapid evaluation of DNA sequence, alteration that is involved in causing the disease can be assessed from MutationTaster. It uses the information from splice-site changes, conservation, and loss of protein features [66]. For somatic missense prediction, CHASM is used. It uses a Random Faster classifier trained with 49 predictive features [67]. Another software based on Hidden Markov model, known as FATHMM, helps in finding the cancer-associated mutations. It differentiates passenger mutations from the amino acid substitutions associated with the cancer. This is achieved by integrating homologous sequence alignment and information of conserved protein domains [68].

CRAVAT toolkit is used to highlight SMGs and mutations using SNVbox and CHASM [69]. Machine learning-based tool CanDrA is based on supporting vector machine (SVM) that incorporates 95 evolutionary and structural features for ranking SMGs [70].

Despite the existence of multiple strategies, there are some limitations of these tools including lack of standard and positive results and selection of nonfunctional mutations.

13.4.3 Data Integration-Based Approach

Cancer data include transcriptome, somatic mutation, proteomics, methylation, and profiles of a tumor and matched normal tissues. It enables the investigators to investigate SMGs and mutations for precision medicine [71]. Data integration-based approaches include Driver Oncogene and Tumor Suppressor (DOTS)-Finder. It categorizes SMGs in cancer by integrating three features of a mutated gene: (1) mutation pattern, (2) mutation frequency, and (3) effect on the gene product's function due to the mutation [72]. It can also predict SMGs specific to oncogenes or tumor suppressor genes. Another unique pipeline SVMerge detects the breakpoints and structural variants by local assembly information and structural variant algorithms [73].

In this regard a favorable direction is to develop an approach that uses the structural variant data like CNVs to rank the SMGs and driver mutations. Driver mutations related to cancer can be identified by CONEXIC. It is done by integrating the CNVs and the genetic expression from tumor-normal samples [74]. They have also developed an algorithm, called Helios, that identifies SMGs within the amplified DNA regions by incorporating cancer genomics data into functional RNA interference (RNAi) data [75]. Helios can assess the potential drivers without a previous genes list.

MAXDRIVER detects alleged SMGs by optimization strategies to build a heterogeneous network by integrating a fused gene functional similarity network with an already existing gene-cancer network [76]. A machine-based learning approach is the OncodriverROLE that categorizes SMGs into activated (Act) and LoF gene [77], although it is a major task for models based on machine learning. A data integration framework OncoIMPACT is based on the phenotypic impacts of patients and forecasts patient-specific SMGs [78].

13.4.4 Structural Genomics-Based Approach

With the advancement in technologies like X-ray crystallography and nuclear magnetic resonance, 3D structures have been generated that are available in different databases like Protein Data Bank (PDB) [79]. In recent years, multiple tools have been developed that require either structure or sequence, because at the structural level, mutations are related with the diseases or drug targets. MSEA (mutation set enrichment analysis) is used to predict alleged SMGs. It is employed using two unique modules (MESA-clust and MESA-domain). MESA-clust is used to screen hotspot regions of mutations by scanning the genomic regions, while MESA-domain is based on the hotspot mutational patterns of protein [80]. Chang et al. developed a network having global kinase-substrate interaction. This network contains 1961 substrates having 36,576 sites for phosphorylation and 7346 pairs connecting 379 kinases [81]. Another approach, ActiveDriver [82], is based on the hypothesis that the cancer-driven mutations may alter the phosphorylation sites of the protein [83]. It analyzes missense point mutations and uses all the phosphorylation sites given in the literature as a mixture training set. A computational pipeline is based on protein pocket to study the functional concerns of somatic mutations in the cancer [84]. Those regions where small molecules and drugs binding occur are known as protein pockets. The mutations lying at these sites may alter the function of protein leading to cancer. SGDriver is based on the relationship among protein 3D structures and somatic mutations to delineate SMG products [85]. SGDriver helps to find out the druggable mutations that can be used in the upcoming field of cancer precision medicine. CanBind is a tool to rank the SMGs that contains the mutations by altering their peptide binding sites or nucleic acids. Identification of Protein Amino acid Clustering iPAC is another algorithm; it prioritizes nonrandom somatic mutations present in the proteins using the 3D structure of a protein [86, 87]. eDriver is another tool to characterize SMGs based on the internal division of somatic missense mutations between protein domains [88]. The development of new tools and approaches will provide exceptional prospects for the clinical applications of cancer genomics data.

13.4.5 Network- or Pathway-Based Approach

Various molecular structures of the cell form a dynamic network. Any genetic change in molecular network frame can cause disturbance in the pathway [89]. Large amount of cancer genomics data obtained from the NGS helps to understand the network-level studies of tumor initiation and progression. As cancer is an intricate disease having changes at the network level, hence there is a dire need to characterize the SMGs and driver mutations. A unique method called PARADIGM detects these pathways by incorporating specific genetic data of the patient. PARADIGM-SHIFT includes downstream pathways which are changed due to mutations by incorporation of gene expression, somatic mutations, and CNVs using a belief-propagation algorithm [90]. It identifies potential functional effects as well such as gain of function (GoF) and loss of function (LoF). TieDIE is based on the network diffusion approach. It is used for the prediction of gene expression changes due to genomic alteration [91]. It identifies a cancer-specific subnetwork by the incorporation of transcriptomic and genomics data into networks originated by

PPIs. The downstream transcriptional alterations due to somatic variations are also recognized. DriverNet is a computational network to recognize the mutations by their effects on mRNA expression network [92]. It identifies rare mutations that mediate oncogenic networks. DawnRank is a computational approach to characterize SMGs on an individual patient using PageRank algorithms [93]. The first personalized tool to rank the SMGs by somatic variation is VarWalker. It uses the somatic variation information from the genome and then adjusts gene length by resampling the mutations. It includes cancer genomics data on a large scale using random walk with restart algorithm [94].

Network-based stratification (NBS) is a unique approach based on network. It stratifies cancer subtypes on the basis of somatic mutation profiles presented in an individual tumor [95]. On the basis of genome-scale interaction network, HotNet identifies mutated pathways in cancer [96]. HotNet2 has been developed by the same group for the detection of subnetworks having mutation. It is done by the insulated heat-diffusing process [96]. They recognized 16 considerably mutated subnetworks that include well-known cancer signaling pathways during pan-cancer analysis to recognize the genes that are occasionally mutated in pan-cancer data sets and in individual cancer data sets. (Pan-cancer analysis revealed that some tumors were more likely to be molecularly and genetically the same due to the types of their rising cells instead of the origin of tissue site.) These approaches are successful, but they have some limitations as well, as the current PPI networks cover only 20–30% pairwise PPIs in humans [97]. This shows that current human interactome may be incomplete [98]. Many structural variants, gene expression and methylation patterns, and noncoding variants are not supposed in the abovementioned approach. Another limitation is that the pathways are sometimes prone to error because they are generated on the computational or experimental data, which are always mixed on the condition specificity. Thus development of an integrative framework to improve human interactome knowledge may offer a complete collection of mutated pathways or networks in the cancer.

In Table 13.2 and in Fig. 13.5, all computational approaches used for the mutational analysis and data resources are shown.

As the technology fastens, tool development for the calculations, measurements, assessment, and integration of data is becoming important [99]. Table 13.2 enlists many online databases that are used for storage of genomic-scale data, regulatory sequence [100], and proteomic analysis [101]. These databases provide the data by which cancer models can be evaluated. As the challenges remain, development of more accurate and biologically powerful in silico tools for representation of human cancer is needed. The general resources and databases used in distributing large amount of data are shown in Table 13.3.

13.5 Precision Medicine

The concept in precision medicine is based on the lifestyle, environment, and genes of a person. With the advancement in the genetics, we have gained the opportunity to make the personalized care of a patient into reality. Precision medicine for breast

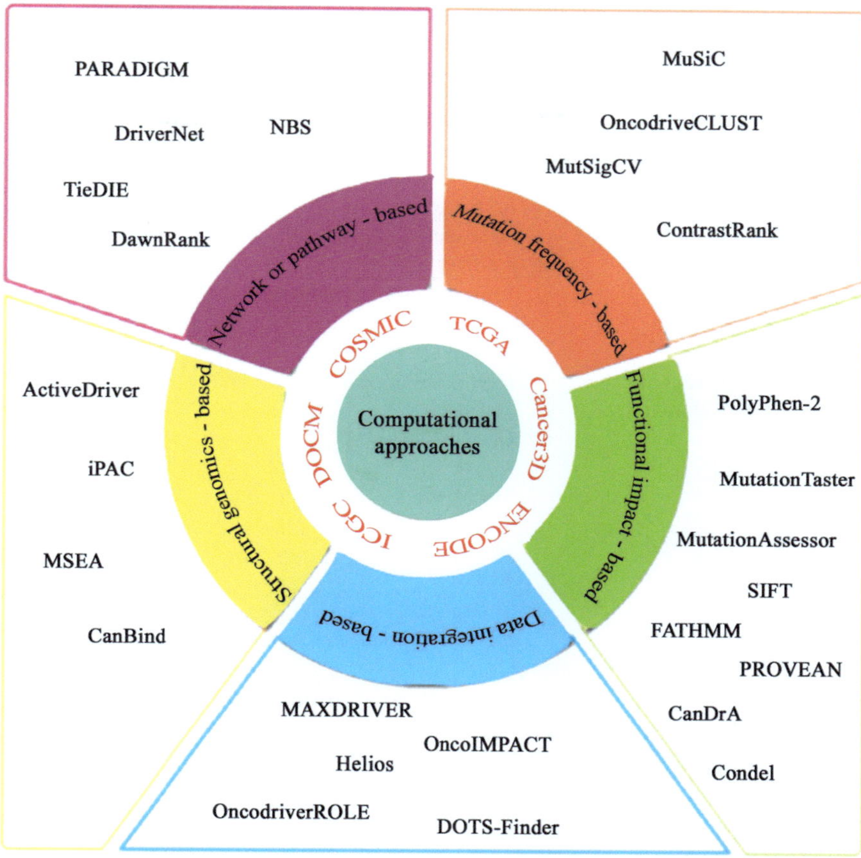

Fig. 13.5 A summarize form of computational approaches used in the cancer mutation analysis

cancer is the most tempting area, but still it is facing a lot of challenges. Other measures may help in early detection of breast cancer like monitoring of circulating tumor DNA and ultradeep sequencing.

13.5.1 Precision Medicine Tools

Identification of genomic changes in patients having the breast cancer helps to adopt the therapy. With the passage of time, different tools are serving for the therapeutic approach; for example, immunohistochemistry was lately used to stratify breast cancer patients with the presence of biomarkers. Now it is used to determine HER2 and ER [125]. To find the copy number, fluorescence in situ hybridization (FISH) is used. DNA array [126], RT PCR [127], or NanoString Technologies [128] is widely used for gene expression quantification. These assays are employed in the early stage detection of breast cancers according to their risk of reversion. NGS is also

Table 13.3 General resources and databases for in silico analysis of cancer

Resource	Database	References
Genome sequence data	Ensemble	Flicek et al. [102]
	UCSC genome browser	Karolchik et al. [103]
Genome annotation data		
Genetic elements	Entrez gene	Maglott et al. [104]
	Gene ontology annotation database	Camon et al. [105]
	Universal protein knowledge base	Apweiler et al. [106]
	Genome reviews	Sterk et al. [107]
Biochemical pathways and functional associations	Kyoto encyclopedia of genes and genomes	Ogata et al. [108]
	Gene ontology	Ashburner et al. [109]
	The SEED	DeJongh et al. [110]
	MetaCyc	Krieger et al. [111]
	BioCyc	Karp et al. [112]
	TransportDB	Ren et al. [113]
Regulatory sequences	Eukaryotic promoter database	Cavin Périer et al. [100]
	Transcriptional regulatory element database	Zhao et al. [114]
Model, model parameter repositories	Kinetic data of biomolecular interactions database	Ji et al. [115]
	BioModels database	Le Novère et al. [116]
	Database of quantitative cellular signaling	Sivakumaran et al. [117]
Protein interaction networks	Database of interacting proteins	Xenarios et al. [118]
	Molecular INTeraction database	Zanzoni et al. [119]
	Mammalian protein-protein interaction database	Pagel et al. [120]
High-throughput genome-scale data		
Transcriptomics	Gene expression omnibus	Edgar et al. [121]
	Stanford microarray database	Sherlock et al. [122]
Proteomics	Proteomics identifications database	Martens et al. [101]
Visualization and data management software packages	Cytoscape	Shannon et al. [123]
	The Gaggle	Shannon et al. [124]

used for the identification of dominant mutations in multigene panel. For the detection of minor sub-clonal alterations, ultradeep sequencing can be used. Nucleic acid detection as well as protein expression pattern is required for the comprehensive molecular profile of the tumors.

13.5.2 Limitations of Precision Medicine

Although there are multiple applications and high-throughput technologies, still many limitations and several challenges are needed to be addressed. A few of them are described below.

13.5.2.1 Logistical and Operational Challenges

- It is very challenging to complete drug testing trials in genomic segments, although these variations are rare and still randomized clinical trials are needed for the approval.
- Genomic results for a certain amount of patients cannot be delivered as biopsy is not achievable for all the patients. Previously known DNA alterations are not enough to explain the progression of cancer in large amount of patients.
- Development of drug and its access is limited due to lesser amount of patients and locations. Genomic tests are very expensive and unaffordable as a private company runs those genomic tests.

13.5.2.2 Scientific Challenges

- Response rates are very low, as multiple pathways are activated resulting in the failure to recognize oncogenic driver.
- Due to the pressure of treatment, additional genomic changes may occur, causing secondary resistance [129].

13.6 Genomic Medicine

Genomic medicine uses the genetic information of an individual as part of his care. It helps to predict disease risk and plots disease course. Genomic medicine makes the plan management according to the need of the patient [130]. The technologies such as high-throughput sequencing and analytical tools help to analyze thousands of molecules simultaneously. Together with computational biology, we can interpret large amount of data sets obtained. The demand for molecular characterization of the disease has been increased to identify the markers for prognosis by the introduction of targeted therapy. This also assists in developing new therapies [131]. Such analyses will also help in early cancer detection and better treatment [132].

13.6.1 Genomic Sequencing for Assessment of Disease

In personalized medicine, NGS has provided us with several promising applications. Genome sequencing may also provide important assistance for reproductive health. This includes prescreening of mothers for mutations related to metabolic and other disorders [133]. Exome sequencing also offers molecular-based diagnosis as it identifies the novel mutation.

The applications of genomic medicine are as follows:

1. Inspection of difference among healthy individuals
2. Disease hindrance
3. Understanding disease risk, susceptibility, and etiology
4. Diagnosis of challenging cases with indecisive results for clinical parameters
5. Classification of accurate disease based on molecular signature
6. Early diagnosis to modify disease course
7. Identification of new mutations related to disease
8. Development of new targeted therapies
9. Personal drug-related profile identification
10. Patients selection for clinical trials
11. Monitoring disease status
12. Evolution of tumor in response to treatment
13. Health management

Furthermore, risk assessment for diseases like diabetes, cancer, and hypertension is economically efficient. It will significantly decrease the treatment problems and may be followed up for prolonged time period [134]. In Fig. 13.6, multistep process is shown.

13.6.2 Genomics Databases

Many genome-wide studies have been applied for the analysis of single nucleotide polymorphisms (SNPs) to examine the genetic variants in different individuals and their effects and its relation with disease risk. In 2005, age-related macular degeneration was investigated [135]. Since then, almost 4000 more associations of SNPs with the disease have been identified [136]. Several international projects have been designed on the oncology frontier to enlist somatic alterations at different levels through exome sequence analysis, mRNA and microRNA (miRNA) production, DNA copy numbers, and promoter methylation. These projects include the Cancer Genome Atlas (http://cancergenome.nih.gov/) [137], the Cancer Genome Project [138], and Hudson et al. [28]. Furthermore, NIH has initiated extensive genomic variation analyses in different diseases by launching various initiatives. Overall, collection of large amount of data at different levels holds a great promise to understand disease management [133]. There are several databases that collect the data to gain a meaningful conclusion.

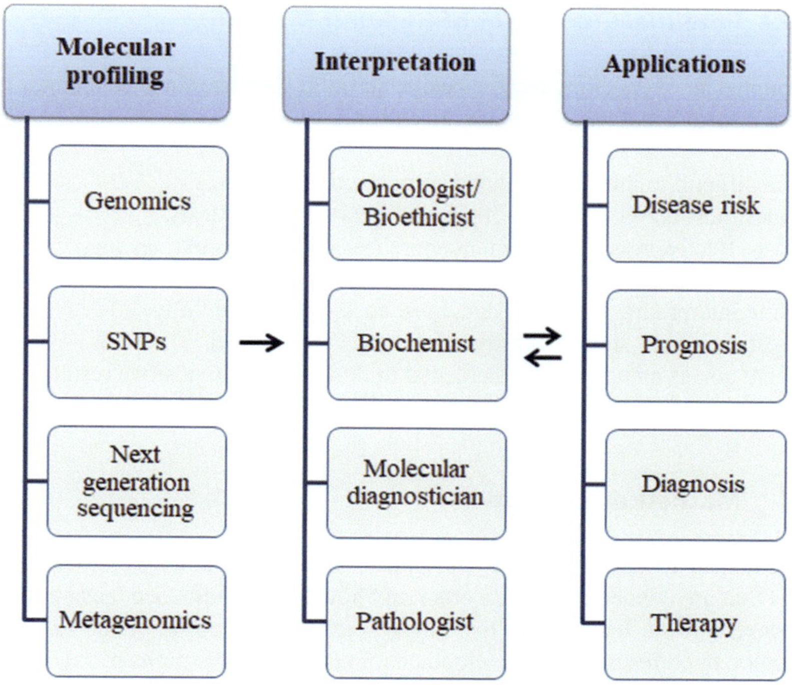

Fig. 13.6 A multistep process for translating genomics to clinical data

Examples of such databases are i2b2 (Informatics for Integrating Biology and the Bedside; https://www.i2b2.org) [139] and locus-specific mutation databases, such as the Human Gene Mutation Database or HGMD (http://www.hgmd.cf.ac.uk/ac/index.php) [140]. Hence data taken from NGS must be inferred in the perspective of environmental conditions and clinical variables for better results.

13.6.3 Monitoring the Personal Genome

Integrative personal omics profiling (iPOP) is a new approach for monitoring personal genome as it combines metabolomics, genomic, proteomic, transcriptomic, and autoantibody profiles of the same person to follow genomic and transcriptomic composition over long periods. By the connection of genetic information with dynamic "omics" activities, it can evaluate disease state and healthy state. These profiles associated with different states are integrated in this approach at multiple time points. An extensive database may be generated with the profiles from more individuals having different kinds of diseases. Such databases might be useful in the monitoring, diagnosis, and disease treatment [141].

13.6.4 Potential Challenges of Genomic Medicine

Although a lot of development has been made, still there are some challenges in the genomic medicine; few of them are given here:

- It is difficult to interpret data and extract actionable items.
- Rules must be set in implementation of new molecular tests.
- Cost-effectiveness. An important apprehension in molecular testing.
- Patient heterogeneity that occurs with the same cancer type and ethnic variation while interpreting genomics data must be addressed carefully.
- "Test accuracy" should improve with time.
- There also is a huge risk of incidental findings and false-positive results.
- Training and teamwork efforts are also needed [142].

13.7 Mathematical Models

Mathematical models allow the researchers and investigators in intricating processes that are connected to each other and how their disturbance leads to the disease development. It also helps to analyze system perturbations systematically and to develop hypothesis for the development of new tests for experiments. Ultimately, new therapeutic targets can be evaluated. Models that describe biological system are very complex to handle manually that is why they are handled numerically. One of the biggest advantages of the mathematical model for the biological systems is computer simulations. These simulations have a lot of benefits. Firstly, a comprehensive molecular scenario can be seen by looking at the discrepancies between the behavior of system projected by mathematical modeling and its actual behavior calculated in experiments. Secondly, with the help of mathematical modeling system, various perturbations can be seen, for example, after drug administration and developmental signals, etc. Thirdly, mathematical simulations are not bound like wet experiments; different experimental conditions can quickly be investigated by computer simulations [143].

13.7.1 Mathematical Equations for Biological Systems Behaviors Modeling

Understanding the biological system is the first step for modeling as different kinds of mathematical frameworks have been developed to model various biological systems. It is important to understand the biological process for selecting the optimal modeling approach because for modeling of different biological systems, diverse mathematical frameworks have been developed. For instance, dynamic processes govern different cellular systems so that the cell adapts its environmental changes. For the description of time-dependent phenomena, it is vital to select mathematical equations that can capture the dynamic effects. Modeling of metabolic processes is essential for a living organism. It provides the energy to the cell by delivering building blocks for the large molecules. Biological research has been dedicated to metabolism for many years, and still full pathways are not known. A main factor is metabolic flux in any metabolic study, that is, conversion rate of metabolites together with a metabolic pathway.

Modeling of signaling and regulatory pathways functions as the central control machinery of a cell. It firmly regulates responses of the cell to the stimuli. These pathways involve the signal transmission from cell membrane into the nucleus of the cell. Pathways are mainly triggered by binding of certain extracellular biomolecules to the receptor as a result; the receptor's 3D structure may be changed. Modeling of comparatively simpler signaling networks revealed that signal transmission from the cell shows unexpected behaviors, such as periodic enhancement patterns of the initial signals [144].

13.8 Conclusion

NGS have assisted researchers to produce large amount of somatic mutations and cancer genomics data in rare and common cancer types. Genetic alterations containing small insertions or deletions, single nucleotide variants, large chromosomal rearrangements; gene fusions are cause of causing cancers. Many computational tools have been developed for pinpointing the cancer genes and driver mutations from millions of somatic cancer mutations. The chapter focused on computational methods for the prediction of mutations based on their structure, analysis of missense mutations in the 3D protein structure, and its effects on stability and interactions. Albeit cancer genomics is still in its beginning, the exceptional production of cancer genomics data assured the better prediction of novel cancer genes. With the increase in number of tumor samples, these computational methods and approaches helped in interpretation of tumor heterogeneity. It facilitated the identification of cancer-driven mutations and delineation of dysregulated pathways which can be targeted by drugs through precision and genomic medicine.

References

1. Breitling R (2010) What is systems biology? Front Physiol 1:9. https://doi.org/10.3389/fphys.2010.00009
2. Palsson BO, Abrams M (2011) Systems biology: simulation of dynamic network states. Cambridge University Press, Cambridge. https://doi.org/10.1017/CBO9780511736179
3. Tavassoly I, Goldfarb J, Iyengar R (2018) Systems biology primer: the basic methods and approaches. Essays Biochem 62:487–500. https://doi.org/10.1042/EBC20180003
4. Chergui M (2009) Physical biology from atoms to medicine edited by Ahmed Zewail. Angew Chem Int Ed 48:3014–3016. https://doi.org/10.1002/anie.200900611
5. Longo G, Montévil M (2014) Perspectives on organisms. Springer, Berlin. https://doi.org/10.1007/978-3-642-35938-5

6. Hood L, Heath JR, Phelps ME, Lin B (2004) Systems biology and new technologies enable predictive and preventative medicine. Science 306:640–643. https://doi.org/10.1126/science.1104635
7. Barillot E (2012) Computational systems biology of cancer. CRC Press, Boca Raton. https://doi.org/10.1201/b12677
8. Werner HMJ, Mills GB, Ram PT (2014) Cancer systems biology: a peek into the future of patient care? Nat Rev Clin Oncol 11:167–176. https://doi.org/10.1038/nrclinonc.2014.6
9. Gentles AJ, Gallahan D (2011) Systems biology: confronting the complexity of cancer. Cancer Res 71:5961–5964. https://doi.org/10.1158/0008-5472.CAN-11-1569
10. Morozova O, Marra MA (2008) Applications of next-generation sequencing technologies in functional genomics. Genomics 92:255–264. https://doi.org/10.1016/j.ygeno.2008.07.001
11. Wang Z, Gerstein M, Snyder M (2009) RNA-Seq: a revolutionary tool for transcriptomics. Nat Rev Genet 10:57–63. https://doi.org/10.1038/nrg2484
12. Rual J-F, Venkatesan K, Hao T et al (2005) Towards a proteome-scale map of the human protein-protein interaction network. Nature 437:1173–1178. https://doi.org/10.1038/nature04209
13. German JB, Hammock BD, Watkins SM (2005) Metabolomics: building on a century of biochemistry to guide human health. Metabolomics 1:3–9. https://doi.org/10.1007/s11306-005-1102-8
14. Tyson JJ, Novák B (2010) Functional motifs in biochemical reaction networks. Annu Rev Phys Chem 61:219–240. https://doi.org/10.1146/annurev.physchem.012809.103457
15. Kafri R, Levy J, Ginzberg MB et al (2013) Dynamics extracted from fixed cells reveal feedback linking cell growth to cell cycle. Nature 494:480–483. https://doi.org/10.1038/nature11897
16. Iyengar R, Zhao S, Chung S-W et al (2012) Merging systems biology with pharmacodynamics. Sci Transl Med 4:126ps7. https://doi.org/10.1126/scitranslmed.3003563
17. Federoff HJ, Gostin LO (2009) Evolving from reductionism to holism: is there a future for systems medicine? JAMA 302:994–996. https://doi.org/10.1001/jama.2009.1264
18. Ayers D, Day PJ (2015) Systems medicine: the application of systems biology approaches for modern medical research and drug development. Mol Biol Int 2015:698169. https://doi.org/10.1155/2015/698169
19. Cardinal-Fernández P, Nin N, Ruíz-Cabello J, Lorente JA (2014) Systems medicine: a new approach to clinical practice. Arch Bronconeumol 50:444–451. https://doi.org/10.1016/j.arbr.2014.09.001
20. Tillmann T, Gibson AR, Scott G et al (2015) Systems medicine 2.0: potential benefits of combining electronic health care records with systems science models. J Med Internet Res 17:e64. https://doi.org/10.2196/jmir.3082
21. Costa J (2008) Systems medicine in oncology. Nat Rev Clin Oncol 5:117–117. https://doi.org/10.1038/ncponc1070
22. Jin G, Wong STC (2014) Toward better drug repositioning: prioritizing and integrating existing methods into efficient pipelines. Drug Discov Today 19:637–644. https://doi.org/10.1016/j.drudis.2013.11.005
23. Jin G, Fu C, Zhao H et al (2012) A novel method of transcriptional response analysis to facilitate drug repositioning for cancer therapy. Cancer Res 72:33–44. https://doi.org/10.1158/0008-5472.CAN-11-2333
24. Mestdagh P, Lefever S, Pattyn F et al (2011) The microRNA body map: dissecting microRNA function through integrative genomics. Nucleic Acids Res 39:e136. https://doi.org/10.1093/nar/gkr646
25. Dimitrakopoulos CM, Beerenwinkel N (2017) Computational approaches for the identification of cancer genes and pathways. Wiley Interdiscip Rev Syst Biol Med 9:e1364. https://doi.org/10.1002/wsbm.1364
26. Forbes SA, Bindal N, Bamford S et al (2011) COSMIC: mining complete cancer genomes in the catalogue of somatic mutations in cancer. Nucleic Acids Res 39:D945–D950. https://doi.org/10.1093/nar/gkq929

27. Weinstein JN, Collisson EA, Cancer Genome Atlas Research Network et al (2013) The Cancer Genome Atlas pan-cancer analysis project. Nat Genet 45:1113–1120. https://doi.org/10.1038/ng.2764
28. Hudson TJ, Anderson W, International Cancer Genome Consortium et al (2010) International network of cancer genome projects. Nature 464:993–998. https://doi.org/10.1038/nature08987
29. Gao J, Aksoy BA, Dogrusoz U et al (2013) Integrative analysis of complex cancer genomics and clinical profiles using the cBioPortal. Sci Signal 6:11. https://doi.org/10.1126/scisignal.2004088
30. Porta-Pardo E, Hrabe T, Godzik A (2015) Cancer3D: understanding cancer mutations through protein structures. Nucleic Acids Res 43:D968–D973. https://doi.org/10.1093/nar/gku1140
31. Venter JC, Adams MD, Myers EW et al (2001) The sequence of the human genome. Science 291:1304–1351. https://doi.org/10.1126/science.1058040
32. ENCODE Project Consortium (2012) An integrated encyclopedia of DNA elements in the human genome. Nature 489:57–74. https://doi.org/10.1038/nature11247
33. Andersson R, Gebhard C, Miguel-Escalada I et al (2014) An atlas of active enhancers across human cell types and tissues. Nature 507:455–461. https://doi.org/10.1038/nature12787
34. Kundaje A, Meuleman W, Roadmap Epigenomics Consortium et al (2015) Integrative analysis of 111 reference human epigenomes. Nature 518:317–330. https://doi.org/10.1038/nature14248
35. GTEx C (2015) The Genotype-Tissue Expression (GTEx) pilot analysis: multitissue gene regulation in humans. Science 348:648–660
36. Ainscough BJ, Griffith M, Coffman AC et al (2016) DoCM: a database of curated mutations in cancer. Nat Methods 13:806–807. https://doi.org/10.1038/nmeth.4000
37. Griffith M, Spies NC, Krysiak K et al (2017) CIViC is a community knowledgebase for expert crowdsourcing the clinical interpretation of variants in cancer. Nat Genet 49:170–174. https://doi.org/10.1038/ng.3774
38. Cheng F, Zhao J, Zhao Z (2016) Advances in computational approaches for prioritizing driver mutations and significantly mutated genes in cancer genomes. Brief Bioinform 17:642–656. https://doi.org/10.1093/bib/bbv068
39. Cheng F, Jia P, Wang Q et al (2014) Studying tumorigenesis through network evolution and somatic mutational perturbations in the cancer interactome. Mol Biol Evol 31:2156–2169. https://doi.org/10.1093/molbev/msu167
40. Croft D, Mundo AF, Haw R et al (2014) The reactome pathway knowledgebase. Nucleic Acids Res 42:D472–D477. https://doi.org/10.1093/nar/gkt1102
41. Kelder T, van Iersel MP, Hanspers K et al (2012) WikiPathways: building research communities on biological pathways. Nucleic Acids Res 40:D1301–D1307. https://doi.org/10.1093/nar/gkr1074
42. Schaefer CF, Anthony K, Krupa S et al (2009) PID: the pathway interaction database. Nucleic Acids Res 37:D674–D679. https://doi.org/10.1093/nar/gkn653
43. Cerami EG, Gross BE, Demir E et al (2011) Pathway Commons, a web resource for biological pathway data. Nucleic Acids Res 39:D685–D690. https://doi.org/10.1093/nar/gkq1039
44. Leiserson MDM, Vandin F, Wu H-T et al (2015) Pan-cancer network analysis identifies combinations of rare somatic mutations across pathways and protein complexes. Nat Genet 47:106–114. https://doi.org/10.1038/ng.3168
45. Chatr-Aryamontri A, Breitkreutz B-J, Heinicke S et al (2013) The BioGRID interaction database: 2013 update. Nucleic Acids Res 41:D816–D823. https://doi.org/10.1093/nar/gks1158
46. Keshava Prasad TS, Goel R, Kandasamy K et al (2009) Human protein reference database--2009 update. Nucleic Acids Res 37:D767–D772. https://doi.org/10.1093/nar/gkn892
47. Ceol A, Chatr Aryamontri A, Licata L et al (2010) MINT, the molecular interaction database: 2009 update. Nucleic Acids Res 38:D532–D539. https://doi.org/10.1093/nar/gkp983
48. Kerrien S, Aranda B, Breuza L et al (2012) The IntAct molecular interaction database in 2012. Nucleic Acids Res 40:D841–D846. https://doi.org/10.1093/nar/gkr1088

49. Franceschini A, Szklarczyk D, Frankild S et al (2013) STRING v9.1: protein-protein interaction networks, with increased coverage and integration. Nucleic Acids Res 41:D808–D815. https://doi.org/10.1093/nar/gks1094
50. Cowley MJ, Pinese M, Kassahn KS et al (2012) PINA v2.0: mining interactome modules. Nucleic Acids Res 40:D862–D865. https://doi.org/10.1093/nar/gkr967
51. Hornbeck PV, Kornhauser JM, Tkachev S et al (2012) PhosphoSitePlus: a comprehensive resource for investigating the structure and function of experimentally determined post-translational modifications in man and mouse. Nucleic Acids Res 40:D261–D270. https://doi.org/10.1093/nar/gkr1122
52. Diella F, Cameron S, Gemünd C et al (2004) Phospho.ELM: a database of experimentally verified phosphorylation sites in eukaryotic proteins. BMC Bioinf 5:79. https://doi.org/10.1186/1471-2105-5-79
53. Minguez P, Letunic I, Parca L, Bork P (2013) PTMcode: a database of known and predicted functional associations between post-translational modifications in proteins. Nucleic Acids Res 41:D306–D311. https://doi.org/10.1093/nar/gks1230
54. Mosca R, Céol A, Aloy P (2013) Interactome3D: adding structural details to protein networks. Nat Methods 10:47–53. https://doi.org/10.1038/nmeth.2289
55. Meyer MJ, Das J, Wang X, Yu H (2013) INstruct: a database of high-quality 3D structurally resolved protein interactome networks. Bioinformatics 29:1577–1579. https://doi.org/10.1093/bioinformatics/btt181
56. Mosca R, Céol A, Stein A et al (2014) 3did: a catalog of domain-based interactions of known three-dimensional structure. Nucleic Acids Res 42:D374–D379. https://doi.org/10.1093/nar/gkt887
57. Lawrence MS, Stojanov P, Polak P et al (2013) Mutational heterogeneity in cancer and the search for new cancer-associated genes. Nature 499:214–218. https://doi.org/10.1038/nature12213
58. Dees ND, Zhang Q, Kandoth C et al (2012) MuSiC: identifying mutational significance in cancer genomes. Genome Res 22:1589–1598. https://doi.org/10.1101/gr.134635.111
59. Tian R, Basu MK, Capriotti E (2014) ContrastRank: a new method for ranking putative cancer driver genes and classification of tumor samples. Bioinformatics 30:i572–i578. https://doi.org/10.1093/bioinformatics/btu466
60. Tamborero D, Gonzalez-Perez A, Lopez-Bigas N (2013) OncodriveCLUST: exploiting the positional clustering of somatic mutations to identify cancer genes. Bioinformatics 29:2238–2244. https://doi.org/10.1093/bioinformatics/btt395
61. Kumar P, Henikoff S, Ng PC (2009) Predicting the effects of coding non-synonymous variants on protein function using the SIFT algorithm. Nat Protoc 4:1073–1081. https://doi.org/10.1038/nprot.2009.86
62. Sim N-L, Kumar P, Hu J et al (2012) SIFT web server: predicting effects of amino acid substitutions on proteins. Nucleic Acids Res 40:W452–W457. https://doi.org/10.1093/nar/gks539
63. Adzhubei IA, Schmidt S, Peshkin L et al (2010) A method and server for predicting damaging missense mutations. Nat Methods 7:248–249. https://doi.org/10.1038/nmeth0410-248
64. Reva B, Antipin Y, Sander C (2011) Predicting the functional impact of protein mutations: application to cancer genomics. Nucleic Acids Res 39:e118. https://doi.org/10.1093/nar/gkr407
65. Gonzalez-Perez A, Lopez-Bigas N (2012) Functional impact bias reveals cancer drivers. Nucleic Acids Res 40:e169. https://doi.org/10.1093/nar/gks743
66. Schwarz JM, Rödelsperger C, Schuelke M, Seelow D (2010) MutationTaster evaluates disease-causing potential of sequence alterations. Nat Methods 7:575–576. https://doi.org/10.1038/nmeth0810-575
67. Wong WC, Kim D, Carter H et al (2011) CHASM and SNVBox: toolkit for detecting biologically important single nucleotide mutations in cancer. Bioinformatics 27:2147–2148. https://doi.org/10.1093/bioinformatics/btr357

68. Shihab HA, Gough J, Cooper DN et al (2013) Predicting the functional consequences of cancer-associated amino acid substitutions. Bioinformatics 29:1504–1510. https://doi.org/10.1093/bioinformatics/btt182
69. Douville C, Carter H, Kim R et al (2013) CRAVAT: cancer-related analysis of variants toolkit. Bioinformatics 29:647–648. https://doi.org/10.1093/bioinformatics/btt017
70. Mao Y, Chen H, Liang H et al (2013) CanDrA: cancer-specific driver missense mutation annotation with optimized features. PLoS One 8:e77945. https://doi.org/10.1371/journal.pone.0077945
71. Brunak S, De La Vega FM, Rätsch G, Stuart JM (2013) Cancer panomics: computational methods and infrastructure for integrative analysis of cancer high-throughput "omics" data-session introduction. In: Biocomputing 2014. World Scientific, Singapore, pp 1–2
72. Melloni GE, Ogier AG, de Pretis S et al (2014) DOTS-Finder: a comprehensive tool for assessing driver genes in cancer genomes. Genome Med 6:44. https://doi.org/10.1186/gm563
73. Wong K, Keane TM, Stalker J, Adams DJ (2010) Enhanced structural variant and breakpoint detection using SVMerge by integration of multiple detection methods and local assembly. Genome Biol 11:R128. https://doi.org/10.1186/gb-2010-11-12-r128
74. Akavia UD, Litvin O, Kim J et al (2010) An integrated approach to uncover drivers of cancer. Cell 143:1005–1017. https://doi.org/10.1016/j.cell.2010.11.013
75. Sanchez-Garcia F, Villagrasa P, Matsui J et al (2014) Integration of genomic data enables selective discovery of breast cancer drivers. Cell 159:1461–1475. https://doi.org/10.1016/j.cell.2014.10.048
76. Chen Y, Hao J, Jiang W et al (2013) Identifying potential cancer driver genes by genomic data integration. Sci Rep 3:3538. https://doi.org/10.1038/srep03538
77. Schroeder MP, Rubio-Perez C, Tamborero D et al (2014) OncodriveROLE classifies cancer driver genes in loss of function and activating mode of action. Bioinformatics 30:i549–i555. https://doi.org/10.1093/bioinformatics/btu467
78. Bertrand D, Chng KR, Sherbaf FG et al (2015) Patient-specific driver gene prediction and risk assessment through integrated network analysis of cancer omics profiles. Nucleic Acids Res 43:e44. https://doi.org/10.1093/nar/gku1393
79. Berman HM, Westbrook J, Feng Z et al (2000) The protein data bank. Nucleic Acids Res 28:235–242. https://doi.org/10.1093/nar/28.1.235
80. Jia P, Wang Q, Chen Q et al (2014) MSEA: detection and quantification of mutation hotspots through mutation set enrichment analysis. Genome Biol 15:489. https://doi.org/10.1186/s13059-014-0489-9
81. Cheng F, Jia P, Wang Q, Zhao Z (2014) Quantitative network mapping of the human kinome interactome reveals new clues for rational kinase inhibitor discovery and individualized cancer therapy. Oncotarget 5:3697–3710. https://doi.org/10.18632/oncotarget.1984
82. Reimand J, Bader GD (2013) Systematic analysis of somatic mutations in phosphorylation signaling predicts novel cancer drivers. Mol Syst Biol 9:637. https://doi.org/10.1038/msb.2012.68
83. Wang Y, Cheng H, Pan Z et al (2015) Reconfiguring phosphorylation signaling by genetic polymorphisms affects cancer susceptibility. J Mol Cell Biol 7:187–202. https://doi.org/10.1093/jmcb/mjv013
84. Vuong H, Cheng F, Lin C-C, Zhao Z (2014) Functional consequences of somatic mutations in cancer using protein pocket-based prioritization approach. Genome Med 6:81. https://doi.org/10.1186/s13073-014-0081-7
85. Zhao J, Cheng F, Wang Y et al (2016) Systematic prioritization of druggable mutations in ~5000 genomes across 16 cancer types using a structural genomics-based approach. Mol Cell Proteomics 15:642–656. https://doi.org/10.1074/mcp.M115.053199
86. Ghersi D, Singh M (2014) Interaction-based discovery of functionally important genes in cancers. Nucleic Acids Res 42:e18. https://doi.org/10.1093/nar/gkt1305
87. Ryslik GA, Cheng Y, Cheung K-H et al (2013) Utilizing protein structure to identify non-random somatic mutations. BMC Bioinf 14:190. https://doi.org/10.1186/1471-2105-14-190

88. Porta-Pardo E, Godzik A (2014) e-Driver: a novel method to identify protein regions driving cancer. Bioinformatics 30:3109–3114. https://doi.org/10.1093/bioinformatics/btu499
89. Pe'er D, Hacohen N (2011) Principles and strategies for developing network models in cancer. Cell 144:864–873. https://doi.org/10.1016/j.cell.2011.03.001
90. Ng S, Collisson EA, Sokolov A et al (2012) Paradigm-shift predicts the function of mutations in multiple cancers using pathway impact analysis. Bioinformatics 28:i640–i646. https://doi.org/10.1093/bioinformatics/bts402
91. Paull EO, Carlin DE, Niepel M et al (2013) Discovering causal pathways linking genomic events to transcriptional states using tied diffusion through interacting events (TieDIE). Bioinformatics 29:2757–2764. https://doi.org/10.1093/bioinformatics/btt471
92. Bashashati A, Haffari G, Ding J et al (2012) DriverNet: uncovering the impact of somatic driver mutations on transcriptional networks in cancer. Genome Biol 13:R124. https://doi.org/10.1186/gb-2012-13-12-r124
93. Hou JP, Ma J (2014) DawnRank: discovering personalized driver genes in cancer. Genome Med 6:56. https://doi.org/10.1186/s13073-014-0056-8
94. Jia P, Zhao Z (2014) VarWalker: personalized mutation network analysis of putative cancer genes from next-generation sequencing data. PLoS Comput Biol 10:e1003460. https://doi.org/10.1371/journal.pcbi.1003460
95. Hofree M, Shen JP, Carter H et al (2013) Network-based stratification of tumor mutations. Nat Methods 10:1108–1115. https://doi.org/10.1038/nmeth.2651
96. Vandin F, Upfal E, Raphael BJ (2011) Algorithms for detecting significantly mutated pathways in cancer. J Comput Biol 18:507–522. https://doi.org/10.1089/cmb.2010.0265
97. Stumpf MPH, Thorne T, de Silva E et al (2008) Estimating the size of the human interactome. Proc Natl Acad Sci U S A 105:6959–6964. https://doi.org/10.1073/pnas.0708078105
98. Menche J, Sharma A, Kitsak M et al (2015) Disease networks. Uncovering disease-disease relationships through the incomplete interactome. Science 347:1257601. https://doi.org/10.1126/science.1257601
99. Perco P, Rapberger R, Siehs C et al (2006) Transforming omics data into context: bioinformatics on genomics and proteomics raw data. Electrophoresis 27:2659–2675. https://doi.org/10.1002/elps.200600064
100. Cavin Périer R, Junier T, Bucher P (1998) The eukaryotic promoter database EPD. Nucleic Acids Res 26:353–357. https://doi.org/10.1093/nar/26.1.353
101. Martens L, Hermjakob H, Jones P et al (2005) PRIDE: the proteomics identifications database. Proteomics 5:3537–3545. https://doi.org/10.1002/pmic.200401303
102. Flicek P, Aken BL, Beal K et al (2008) Ensemble 2008. Nucleic Acids Res 36:D707–D714. https://doi.org/10.1093/nar/gkm988
103. Karolchik D, Kuhn RM, Baertsch R et al (2008) The UCSC genome browser database: 2008 update. Nucleic Acids Res 36:D773–D779. https://doi.org/10.1093/nar/gkm966
104. Maglott D, Ostell J, Pruitt KD, Tatusova T (2005) Entrez gene: gene-centered information at NCBI. Nucleic Acids Res 33:D54–D58. https://doi.org/10.1093/nar/gki031
105. Camon E, Magrane M, Barrell D et al (2004) The Gene Ontology Annotation (GOA) database: sharing knowledge in Uniprot with Gene Ontology. Nucleic Acids Res 32:D262–D266. https://doi.org/10.1093/nar/gkh021
106. Apweiler R, Bairoch A, Wu CH et al (2004) UniProt: the universal protein knowledgebase. Nucleic Acids Res 32:D115–D119. https://doi.org/10.1093/nar/gkh131
107. Sterk P, Kersey PJ, Apweiler R (2006) Genome reviews: standardizing content and representation of information about complete genomes. OMICS 10:114–118. https://doi.org/10.1089/omi.2006.10.114
108. Ogata H, Goto S, Sato K et al (1999) KEGG: kyoto encyclopedia of genes and genomes. Nucleic Acids Res 27:29–34. https://doi.org/10.1093/nar/28.1.27
109. Ashburner M, Ball CA, Blake JA et al (2000) Gene ontology: tool for the unification of biology. The Gene Ontology Consortium. Nat Genet 25:25–29. https://doi.org/10.1038/75556

110. DeJongh M, Formsma K, Boillot P et al (2007) Toward the automated generation of genome-scale metabolic networks in the SEED. BMC Bioinf 8:139. https://doi.org/10.1186/1471-2105-8-139
111. Krieger CJ, Zhang P, Mueller LA et al (2004) MetaCyc: a multiorganism database of metabolic pathways and enzymes. Nucleic Acids Res 32:D438–D442. https://doi.org/10.1093/nar/gkh100
112. Karp PD, Ouzounis CA, Moore-Kochlacs C et al (2005) Expansion of the BioCyc collection of pathway/genome databases to 160 genomes. Nucleic Acids Res 33:6083–6089. https://doi.org/10.1093/nar/gki892
113. Ren Q, Chen K, Paulsen IT (2007) TransportDB: a comprehensive database resource for cytoplasmic membrane transport systems and outer membrane channels. Nucleic Acids Res 35:D274–D279. https://doi.org/10.1093/nar/gkl925
114. Zhao F, Xuan Z, Liu L, Zhang MQ (2005) TRED: a transcriptional regulatory element database and a platform for in silico gene regulation studies. Nucleic Acids Res 33:D103–D107. https://doi.org/10.1093/nar/gki004
115. Ji ZL, Chen X, Zhen CJ et al (2003) KDBI: kinetic data of bio-molecular interactions database. Nucleic Acids Res 31:255–257
116. Le Novère N, Bornstein B, Broicher A et al (2006) BioModels Database: a free, centralized database of curated, published, quantitative kinetic models of biochemical and cellular systems. Nucleic Acids Res 34:D689–D691. https://doi.org/10.1093/nar/gkj092
117. Sivakumaran S, Hariharaputran S, Mishra J, Bhalla US (2003) The database of quantitative cellular signaling: management and analysis of chemical kinetic models of signaling networks. Bioinformatics 19:408–415. https://doi.org/10.1093/bioinformatics/btf860
118. Xenarios I, Salwínski L, Duan XJ et al (2002) DIP, the database of interacting proteins: a research tool for studying cellular networks of protein interactions. Nucleic Acids Res 30:303–305
119. Zanzoni A, Montecchi-Palazzi L, Quondam M et al (2002) MINT: a molecular interaction database. FEBS Lett 513:135–140
120. Pagel P, Kovac S, Oesterheld M et al (2005) The MIPS mammalian protein-protein interaction database. Bioinformatics 21:832–834. https://doi.org/10.1093/bioinformatics/bti115
121. Edgar R, Domrachev M, Lash AE (2002) Gene expression omnibus: NCBI gene expression and hybridization array data repository. Nucleic Acids Res 30:207–210. https://doi.org/10.1093/nar/30.1.207
122. Sherlock G, Hernandez-Boussard T, Kasarskis A et al (2001) The stanford microarray database. Nucleic Acids Res 29:152–155
123. Shannon P, Markiel A, Ozier O et al (2003) Cytoscape: a software environment for integrated models of biomolecular interaction networks. Genome Res 13:2498–2504. https://doi.org/10.1101/gr.1239303
124. Shannon PT, Reiss DJ, Bonneau R, Baliga NS (2006) The Gaggle: an open-source software system for integrating bioinformatics software and data sources. BMC Bioinf 7:176. https://doi.org/10.1186/1471-2105-7-176
125. Wolff AC, Hammond MEH, Hicks DG et al (2013) Recommendations for human epidermal growth factor receptor 2 testing in breast cancer: American Society of Clinical Oncology/College of American Pathologists clinical practice guideline update. J Clin Oncol 31:3997–4013. https://doi.org/10.1200/JCO.2013.50.9984
126. van de Vijver MJ, He YD, van't Veer LJ et al (2002) A gene-expression signature as a predictor of survival in breast cancer. N Engl J Med 347:1999–2009. https://doi.org/10.1056/NEJMoa021967
127. Paik S, Shak S, Tang G et al (2004) A multigene assay to predict recurrence of tamoxifen-treated, node-negative breast cancer. N Engl J Med 351:2817–2826. https://doi.org/10.1056/NEJMoa041588
128. Sorlie T, Tibshirani R, Parker J et al (2003) Repeated observation of breast tumor subtypes in independent gene expression data sets. Proc Natl Acad Sci U S A 100:8418–8423. https://doi.org/10.1073/pnas.0932692100

129. Arnedos M, Vicier C, Loi S et al (2015) Precision medicine for metastatic breast cancer--limitations and solutions. Nat Rev Clin Oncol 12:693–704. https://doi.org/10.1038/nrclinonc.2015.123
130. Ligthart S, Vaez A, Võsa U et al (2018) Genome analyses of >200,000 individuals identify 58 loci for chronic inflammation and highlight pathways that link inflammation and complex disorders. Am J Hum Genet 103:691–706. https://doi.org/10.1016/j.ajhg.2018.09.009
131. Abrahams E (2008) Right drug-right patient-right time: personalized medicine coalition. Clin Transl Sci 1:11–12. https://doi.org/10.1111/j.1752-8062.2008.00003.x
132. Metias SM, Lianidou E, Yousef GM (2009) MicroRNAs in clinical oncology: at the crossroads between promises and problems. J Clin Pathol 62:771–776. https://doi.org/10.1136/jcp.2009.064717
133. Ashley EA, Butte AJ, Wheeler MT et al (2010) Clinical assessment incorporating a personal genome. Lancet 375:1525–1535. https://doi.org/10.1016/S0140-6736(10)60452-7
134. Abelson S, Collord G, Ng SWK et al (2018) Prediction of acute myeloid leukaemia risk in healthy individuals. Nature 559:400–404. https://doi.org/10.1038/s41586-018-0317-6
135. Klein RJ, Zeiss C, Chew EY et al (2005) Complement factor H polymorphism in age-related macular degeneration. Science 308:385–389. https://doi.org/10.1126/science.1109557
136. Johnson AD, O'Donnell CJ (2009) An open access database of genome-wide association results. BMC Med Genet 10:6. https://doi.org/10.1186/1471-2350-10-6
137. Cancer Genome Atlas Network (2012) Comprehensive molecular characterization of human colon and rectal cancer. Nature 487:330–337. https://doi.org/10.1038/nature11252
138. Stephens PJ, Tarpey PS, Davies H et al (2012) The landscape of cancer genes and mutational processes in breast cancer. Nature 486:400–404. https://doi.org/10.1038/nature11017
139. Natter MD, Quan J, Ortiz DM et al (2013) An i2b2-based, generalizable, open source, self-scaling chronic disease registry. J Am Med Inform Assoc 20:172–179. https://doi.org/10.1136/amiajnl-2012-001042
140. Stenson PD, Ball EV, Howells K et al (2009) The human gene mutation database: providing a comprehensive central mutation database for molecular diagnostics and personalised genomics. Hum Genomics 4:69. https://doi.org/10.1186/1479-7364-4-2-69
141. Chen R, Mias GI, Li-Pook-Than J et al (2012) Personal omics profiling reveals dynamic molecular and medical phenotypes. Cell 148:1293–1307. https://doi.org/10.1016/j.cell.2012.02.009
142. Pasic MD, Samaan S, Yousef GM (2013) Genomic medicine: new frontiers and new challenges. Clin Chem 59:158–167. https://doi.org/10.1373/clinchem.2012.184622
143. Fischer HP (2008) Mathematical modeling of complex biological systems: from parts lists to understanding systems behavior. Alcohol Res Health 31:49–59
144. Vera J, Wolkenhauer O (2008) A system biology approach to understand functional activity of cell communication systems. Methods Cell Biol 90:399–415

Part V

Biostatistics in Clinical Oncology

14

Gaurav Roy, Atanu Bhattacharjee, and Iqra Khan

14.1 Introduction

In oncology, precision plays a crucial role. The scientific attributes of biostatistics in clinical oncology encompass a broad spectrum of medical applications ranging from inclusion of patients in clinical trials to the diligent identification of a better treatment regimen as against existing ones to the reasoned selection of the most effective drug dosages to finding genes that cause cancer.

Oncology is the most dynamic research domain towards better treatment outcome. The treatment outcomes can only be compared through proper scientific structured design and analysis. It helps to produce robust scientific outcomes. The scientifically robust outcome can only be obtained through bridging the statistics in oncology research.

Oncology research becomes complex due to the involvement of human over there. There are multidimensional variations. The variation may be due to genetics and social causes. Magnitudes of these factors are indiscernible and thus may have unpredictable interactions with each other, causing massive heterogeneity in data. The unobserved measurement or error due to measurement is defined as an error. It is possible to use error to define the variation in patient outcomes due to unobserved factors. Further, an error can be split into random and bias.

G. Roy (✉)
Molecular Genetics Laboratory, Institute of Medical Genetics and Genomics, Sir Ganga Ram Hospital, New Delhi, India

A. Bhattacharjee
Section of Biostatistics, Centre for Cancer Epidemiology, Tata Memorial Centre & Homi Bhaba National Institute, Mumbai, India

I. Khan
Microbiology and Biotechnology Research Lab, Fatima Jinnah Women University, Old Presidency, Pakistan

N. Masood, S. Shakil Malik (eds.), *'Essentials of Cancer Genomic, Computational Approaches and Precision Medicine*,
https://doi.org/10.1007/978-981-15-1067-0_14

The challenge is to reduce random error vis-a-vis controlling the systematic bias. Merging of clinical research with statistics is currently the need of the hour.

Oncology research is gradually progressing on an increased understanding of biological functions. Therefore, identification and assessment of disease-related biomarkers and exploration of novel methodologies shall open up newer vistas in cancer management. It is much applicable to precision medicine. Precision medicine is standing with exploring the gene expression risk factor for specific cancer. It is also useful for the molecular establishment for enrichment analysis. Studies involved with data exploration shows the relation between explanatory factors and therapeutic outcomes.

The advantage of observational study is that the investigator cannot modify any prognostic factor. However, observation commonly generated from the field or hospital.

Owing to the large number of discovery-based nature of clinical studies, investigators may be overwhelmed by several combinations of potential analyses possible for a data set or may be distracted by false positives. Herein lay the rationale for a clinically and statistically sound study design. A typically robust and in-depth study design formulated with several points like (1) formulated with a specific objective, (2) optimum sample size calculation involved, and (3) formulated to obtain clinical and statistical outcomes. (4) It is easy to control the confounding factors and bias outcome.

Finally, a statistical analysis plan becomes important in creating an executable study. It is useful to calculate the amount of bias in results. Alternatively defining a statistical analysis plan is important towards executable study. It helps to explore and refine the study design. It is important for patient selection criteria as well.

In this chapter, we highlight several critical aspects concerning the application of biostatistics in the realm of clinical oncology and how such representations define the work-flow of a scientifically designed oncology research study.

14.2 Variables and Their Distribution

14.2.1 Common Types of Variables

A variable may be defined as a measured value or characteristic which can vary from one individual to another. Here several common and less common variables are listed out for at a glance understanding. These are:

Categorical Variable: Variables put into categories.

Confounding Variable: Confounding variable describes the association between the dependent (outcome) and independent (predictor) variables in a way that it affects their relationship. Both predictor and outcome variables are associated with confounding variable.

Continuous Variable: It is infinite number and measured only by numerical scale, such as time or weight. These are not countable.

Control Variable: An experimental element which does not change in the whole experiment. It remains constant throughout experiment.

Dependent Variable: It is outcome of an experiment which is tested in experiment. It allows investigators to decide about the success or failure of their experiment.

Discrete Variable: These variables are described in finite number of values as these are countable.

Independent Variable: It is unchanged or unaffected during the experiment by anything that researcher does.

Lurking Variable: It is hidden variable and affects the relationship of predictor and outcome variables.

Measurement Variables: These are also called as numeric or quantitative variables. Such variables are measurable with numerical values, for example, 5 cm.

Nominal Variables: These are actually categorical variables with no numerical values like occupation.

Ordinal Variables: These are also categorical variables, but their values can be set into an order.

Qualitative Variables: These variables have no numerical value that's why they are expressed in frequencies or proportions, and these can be ordinal or categorical.

Quantitative Variables: These variables can be counted that's why they had numerical value and include ratio and discrete variables.

Random Variables: Their values are outcomes of random phenomenon.

Ranked Variables: These are actually ordinal variables in which each data point is set into order. We may not know the exact value but can say which point comes first and which later.

Ratio Variable: It is an interval variable having significant ratio between its any two values.

14.2.2 Less Common Variables

Active Variable: It can be controlled by investigator in the experiment, as it is manipulated by researcher himself.

Antecedent Variable: It cannot explain any apparent association between cause and effect variables and usually comes before independent or dependent variables.

Attribute Variables: It cannot be manipulated or controlled in design of experiment and is also called passive variable.

Binary Variable: This kind of variable has only two values or states usually in form of binary data 0 or 1, male or female, etc.

Collider Variable: It is a variable in statistics and casual graphs represented by node and are influenced by usually two or more than two variables.

Covariate Variable: A covariate may be of direct interest (independent variable) or confounding variable (not variable of interest). It can increase accuracy of results and affects outcome of study.

Criterion Variable: It is dependent variable being predicted in regression analysis.

Dichotomous Variable: It is just like binary variable possessing only two values.

Dummy Variables: These are variables having value one or zero to show presence or absence of categorical variables that were considered to alter outcome of experiment.

Endogenous Variables: These are like dependent variables in statistical model and are determined by other functional variables within model.

Exogenous Variable: Variable which is not affected by any variable in the system but affects other variables in the system is called exogenous variable.

Explanatory Variable: It is manipulated by investigator in study and is type of independent variable used to explain response variable.

Extraneous Variables: These are undesirable variables which are not intentionally studied in system, but they might influence outcome of experiment.

Grouping Variables: Summarize data into groups and discrete values and are a categorical variable. These are also called as coding variables.

Identifier Variables: The singular categorical variables having only one individual per category. No data analysis can be performed on them as they are single, that's why they are used to identify results only.

Indicator Variable: Also known as dummy variable.

Interval Variable: Is a type of continuous variable, and difference between the values of two intervals is measureable and equal.

Intervening Variable: Is a hypothetical variable which cannot be measured in experiment but it describes association between variables.

Latent Variable: Is a hidden variable that is inferred from other variables which can be observed directly in model and is not measured even observed directly.

Manifest Variable: Is a variable which is necessary for latent variable to check whether it is present or not. It can be measured and observed directly.

Manipulated Variable: Is an independent variable that can be changed.

Moderating Variables: Affect or change the strength of relationship between two variables usually dependent and independent and is also called moderator.

Nuisance Variable: Is undesirable variable that elevates variability overall.

Observed Variable: Manifests variable and opposite of latent variable, or we can say measureable variable.

Outcome Variable: Is a dependent variable which is being investigated in experiment by changing independent variables.

Polychotomous Variables: Can be ordered because they possess more than two values.

Predictor Variable: Independent variable.

Responding Variable: Manipulated or independent variable.

Scale Variable: Has numeric value and is measurement variable.

Study Variable: Any variable that is studied during research and has effect on cause and result of study. It is also known as research variable.

Test Variable: Is a dependent variable which is investigated during the course of study.

Treatment Variable: Independent variable manipulated by researcher in study.

14.3 Sample Size Calculations

Sample size calculation evaluates minimum number of subjects that should be included in a study to assess clinically relevant treatment effect. Therefore sample size computation is vital in quantitative research studies. Because of the some constraints of time, cost, and ethics, the number of individuals in a study is usually limited. For example, it is difficult to detect crucial existing effects if sample size is too small. However, too many participants may render resources to be redundant. The optimum sample size calculation is critical. So, interpretation of the expected outcome of study computation of the sample size plays a vital role. Generally, larger sample size is prerequisite for assessing the integrity of an observed effect with greater variability in the outcome variable. Contrarily, tested treatment is more effective with smaller sample size for detection of any effect. Four basic attributes of sample size calculation for clinical trials are discussed here.

1. Type I error (alpha): In clinical oncology, probability of type I error is stated as alpha and is also known as false-positive error. In hypothesis-testing process, type I and type II errors are present. In type I, null hypothesis (H_0) is rejected by fault, and false-positive result is picked up. Simply we can say that false-positive type I is incorrect rejection of null hypothesis (H_0). So, SSC is a prerequisite for defining exact quantity of samples for significant conclusion. Mostly alpha is set at 0.05 allowing only <5% false-positive conclusion. The p value higher than 0.05 is considered clinically insignificant. However, p value less than this specified alpha might not necessarily be clinically significant.
2. Power: Researchers may erroneously accept false positives such as accepting H_0. The null hypothesis must never be accepted. This type of error is referred as type II error or beta. Usually beta is fixed at 0.20 which means that investigator have <20% of chance for false-negative interpretation. One should know power of study for sample size calculation. Power refers to capability of picking up an effect which must exist in that population by applying a sample-based test on that population (true positive). It is also referred as complement of beta, that is, power will be 80% if beta is 0.20 which reflects the probability of rejecting null hypothesis correctly or evading false-negative interpretation.
3. Smallest effect of interest: It is also known as minimal clinically relevant difference, abbreviated as (MCRD). When the researcher wants to detect minimal difference between two studied categories and believes this would be clinically relevant is referred as smallest effect of interest. The MCRD has always a numerical value difference for continuous outcome variables. Minor change in predicted difference in treatment cause huge effect on estimated sample size. This happens because of indirect relation of sample size to square of difference.
4. Variability: The last attribute for sample size calculation is centered on population variance of specified outcome variable. When considering continuous outcome, it is estimated from standard deviation. Variance is not a known entity, that's why researchers generally use information from precedent study or pilot study. Sometimes, the MCRD and variability are united together and expressed

as standardized difference (multiple of standard deviation of observations), also known as effect size. The formula for standardized difference calculation is,

$$\text{Standardized difference} = \frac{\text{difference between the means in the two treatment groups}}{\text{population standard deviation}}$$

The calculation of sample size with full precision is very difficult due to lack of good estimates of the vital parameters that researchers should have. Unluckily sample size must fulfill criterion with respective parameters. Most of the time, alpha with 0.05 and power of 0.80 is sufficient. Anyhow, while considering the area of study, some other assumptions can also be taken into consideration. Sample size will be directly influenced by changing the assumption of power or alpha like larger sample size will be required for lower alpha and higher power leading to higher costs. One should know the impact of any kind of change in these parameters. This can be done by performing sensitivity analysis in which sample size calculation can be done by various values of parameter. Largest sample size should be selected in any kind of uncertainty. The estimate of sample size calculation is one of the significant steps in randomized clinical trials (RCT) design. Generally target difference between treatments of primary outcome is specified before calculation of required sample size. SSC plays an important role in RCT conduct and interpretation. Sample sizes certify about trial high probability and needed statistical power of identifying target difference between treatment strategies that must present. For randomized clinical trials, the DELTA (Difference ELicitation in TriAls) guidance assists in justification of sample size and target difference. Target difference is attaining much attention nowadays regardless their statistical significance. So, target difference specifications along with sample size calculations need to be investigated more and in improved way.

Moreover, various software programs are now also available for assisting in sample size calculations. Advisor, nQuery, PASS, and "Power and Precision" are some authentic and user-friendly programs that can be used for sample size calculation of different data types and study designs. All these programs limitation are paid license requirement. While one can also calculate sample size by some other websites without any license. But the problem is their authenticity and is not sometimes reliable. One of the authentic and freely available websites for sample size calculation is http://www.stat.uiowa.edu/~rlenth/Power/index.html. A multicentric clinicopathological study conducted by Malik et al. calculated sample size calculation of their study with G power software while taking consideration of 80% power and 5% margin of error. Scientific community usually accepts statistical power of 80–90% of any study as it is directly dependent on sample size. Scientific community usually less considers the research studies that lack sample size and power analysis. Sample size formula usage verifies minimum sample size along with pre-specified statistical power.

14.4 Meta-analysis

14.4.1 Overview

The term meta-analysis has been defined as an objective, quantitative mode of summarizing research findings that enable the identification of scientific associations. This statistical methodology integrates results of independent but related studies to synthesize summaries [1]. In conditions where individual studies are too small to offer validated outcomes, meta-analysis increases power, reduces error risk, and promotes exploratory analyses that facilitate the development of future research hypotheses [2].

14.4.2 Methodology

A typical meta-analysis commands a robust and in-depth study design. The strong foundation of a well-structured meta-analysis is built on diligent and a strategic study selection. This is followed by a reasoned inclusion and exclusion criteria, data extraction, pooling of study results, evaluation of publication bias and confounding factors, and a final interpretation of the data that would represent a new paradigm in the already existing knowledge of clinical cancer research. An example of an ideal methodology that ought to be followed while establishing a meta-analysis may be summarized as follows:

Step 1: Literature should be searched in PubMed, Embase, CBM (Chinese Biomedical Literature database), and the Cochrane Database of Systematic Reviews (CDSR).

Step 2: Manuscripts that are eligible should be recouped and their references probed for relevant studies. No inhibition on time period, sample size, population, language, or type of report must be imposed.

Step 3: Justified and well-reasoned inclusion and exclusion criteria are crucial for any meta-analyses. When multiple reports are available for a single unique study population only, the most recent or largest report should be included. Additionally, it is equally important to exclude interim analyses and comparisons of laboratory methods.

Step 4: In order to ascertain accuracy of data extraction and study design, two researchers must unearth information independently, and the difference in interpretation and opinion must be normalized by a unanimous agreement between the investigators. The subgroup analyses ought to be performed by ethnicity and area and ethnic groups should be defined as Caucasian, Asian, and African, while the area must be defined as high-rate, medium-rate, or low-rate areas according to incidence.

Step 5: The significance of the pooled odds ratio (OR) should be determined by Z testing, and a probability level of $p < 0.05$ should be considered to be statistically significant.

Step 6: Next, the random effects and the fixed effects models should be conducted for dichotomous outcomes. The random effects model may be evaluated using the DerSimonian and Laird's method [3], while the fixed effects model might be evaluated through the Mantel-Haenszel method [4].

Step 7: For an accurate assessment of the between-study heterogeneity, both the chi-square-based Cochran's Q statistic [5] and the I2 statistic tests [6] should be deployed for calculation.

Step 8: In order to identify outliers as probable sources of heterogeneity, the Galbraith plot may be a good option [7]. Furthermore, for an improved investigation of the possible sources of between-study heterogeneity, a meta-regression analysis gives us very good results.

Step 9: In order to validate the credibility of outcomes in a meta-analysis, a sensitivity analysis must be computed by sequential omission of individual studies or by omitting studies plotted by the Galbraith plot method as the possible major source of heterogeneity.

Step 10: Finally, publication bias should be investigated by the funnel plot. In context, the funnel plot asymmetry should be assessed by the Egger's linear regression test [8]. In order to ensure reliability and accuracy of results, two investigators should independently enter data into the same statistical software program and should obtain the same output.

14.4.3 Importance of Meta-analysis in Clinical Oncology

The assessment of heterogeneity is probably the most crucial aspect in meta-analysis, and the Cochrane Collaboration is perhaps the most rigorous and innovative leader which has stood the test of time in developing protocols in this regard [9]. These include the development of protocols that provide a structure for literature search and newer and extended analytic and diagnostic methods for evaluation of the output. The judicious use of methods outlined in the handbook should provide a consistent approach to the conduct of meta-analysis. Additionally, the PRISMA (Preferred Reporting Items for Systematic reviews and Meta-Analyses) statement that replaced the QUOROM (Quality of Reporting of Meta-analyses) statement is an extremely useful tool for the improved reporting of systematic reviews and meta-analyses [10–12].

Systematic reviews encompass meta-analyses. A systematic review collates empirical evidence that fits prefixed eligibility criteria in order to address a specific research question. The key characteristics of a systematic review are:

(a) A defined set of objectives with predefined eligibility criteria
(b) A methodology that is explicit and reproducible
(c) Systematic search strategy that attempts to identify all studies qualifying the eligibility criteria
(d) Evaluation of the validity of the findings of the included studies
(e) Last, but not in the least, a systematic presentation and synthesis of the attributes from the studies utilized

Systematic methods, as against traditional review methods, minimize bias and provide reliable results that facilitate the scientific establishment of inferences and decisions [13, 14]. The validity of meta-analytical approaches in observational studies was considerably controversial in the fact that these studies were likely to be subject to unidentified sources of confounding and risk modification [15]. In addition, studies displayed that in meta-analyses, nonrandomized studies showed larger treatment effects than the randomized ones [16].

Meta-analyses are conducted with a view to address the strength of evidence present on a disease and treatment and to obtain a single summary estimate of the effect. The results of a meta-analysis can improve precision of estimates of effect, answer questions not posed by the individual studies, settle controversies arising from apparently conflicting studies, and generate new hypotheses. The examination of heterogeneity is vital to the development of new hypotheses [17].

Meta-analysis on individual patient data (IPD) is the gold standard [18]. This allows standardized analytical techniques across studies, testing of interaction effects with covariates at patient level, and the use of consistent analyses for time-to-event outcomes [19, 20]. In context, in a recent study, a flexible data harmonization platform (DHP) was created to harmonize IPD from multiple studies [21]. The study illustrated the development and use of a flexible DHP that was initially developed for the Predicting OptimaL cAncer RehabIlitation and Supportive care (POLARIS) study [22–24].

14.4.4 Meta-analysis in Cancer Genetics: The Future Is Now

High-throughput genotyping consequentially has produced a large epidemiological data on gene-disease associations. Genetic polymorphisms play a crucial role in susceptibility to cancer through a plethora of functional mechanisms such as DNA repair and cell cycling [25]. Meta-analyses have been computed for key polymorphisms in genes involved in these mechanisms [26, 27]. Results of these endeavors might facilitate the increase of statistical power that is adequate enough for patient counseling on the risk of cancer development. Data on predisposition to cancer may help to induce lifestyle-related changes on the population such as cessation of smoking, reduction of alcohol intake, adherence to healthy diet, and regular exercise in addition to avoidance of occupational exposures [28].

In spite of the low association (OR = 1.1–1.5) of polymorphism and cancer, it is a crucial genetic marker in relation to public health [29]. In this context, reports indicate that a small mathematical change in the association between polymorphisms and cancer may have deleterious consequences on cancer incidence in the general population [30]. Studies have suggested that meta-analyses might facilitate the critical transfer of knowledge from bench to bedside, allowing for re-evaluation and identification of high-risk subjects in accordance with their genetic constitution. Additionally, such studies enable the analyses of crucial patient subgroups and identify high-risk individuals for cancer [31].

Overall, a meta-analysis is a cheaper alternative to the primary study. However, on a higher scale involving larger patient cohorts, meta-analysis is expensive and logistically confusing. A rigorous meta-analysis substantiates the required count of subjects and is detected with improved confidence and statistical precision. Over the years, there has been an accumulating evidence of published data on gene-disease associations [32]. In order to decipher disease-specific risk factors for cancer, it is imperative to logically select out the relevant data. The traditional review article, used to evaluate groups of studies, rarely conjures up the same standards of scientific objectivity as evidenced in original epidemiologic studies. A review article has been crudely visualized as a coarse representation of meta-analysis that does not follow a rigorous pattern in selecting or combining results. On the other hand, however, following a dynamic and in-depth protocol, a meta-analysis succeeds in reducing the potential bias present in review articles. Although a meta-analysis is able to estimate a relative risk with far more precision than the individual studies it contains, it is rarely a validation. A critical challenge for investigators performing meta-analysis is to consider differences in study design and study quality.

A meta-analysis ought to consider the strengths and weaknesses of published data before applying an explicit, objective, and quantitative methodology. Such an exercise of combining studies minimizes biases and provides a scientific output. Conclusively, efforts must be zeroed in on evidences that rigorously minimize bias while diligently and scientifically using all available data [33].

14.5 Statistical Models and Challenges Faced During Analyzing Data on Quality of Life in Cancer Patients

According to the World Health Organization (WHO), quality of life (QoL) has been illustrated as an individual perception of life, values, objectives, standards, and interests in the realm of culture. QoL is being widely used as a primary measure in studies in order to assess treatment effectiveness [34–37]. Patients, instead of measuring lipoprotein levels, glucose, blood pressure, and cardiac functions, take decisions about their health by virtue of the QoL that elucidates the effects on outcomes essential for themselves [38]. A hallmark of oncology nowadays is to evaluate QoL in cancer [39]. QoL associated with cancer is related to all disease stages [40, 41]. Several studies show that the involvement of any cancer patients, general QoL measurement may be useful for assessing the therapeutic effect of treatment and overall health status. However, data display that cancer-specific instruments specifically assess the impact of specific cancer on QoL [39]. In certain malignancies such as glioma, QoL is important and considered the main outcome in a study. In oncology frequently observed measurement is QoL as primary objective [42].

Accumulating lines of evidence have shown to elucidate the impact of cancer disease burden on social and psychological variables. Recent studies have proposed a framework to integrate the biological attributes of cancers and its clinical applications with the behavioral and social influences on patient subjects using a quantitative approach [43]. Data display the assessment of QoL among survivors with breast cancer using nonparametric statistical tools such as Wilcoxon rank sum test, the Fisher's exact test, and Spearman correlation coefficients [44]. In this study, in spite of a good QoL, women subjects were shown to present with significant anxiety, depression, mental anguish, hopelessness, and apprehension about their disease. Studies have also evaluated the psychological impact of cancer survivors with QoL [45]. In this regard, hierarchical linear regression models have been used to analyze the independent effects of cancer perception on distress and QoL. However, there is a paucity of data on the integration of inference-based intelligence tools with multivariate statistical approaches in solving the impact of diseases towards patients.

Health-related quality of life (HRQOL) is another emerging area of cancer research that comprehensively evaluates patients' perception of the impact of therapy and their health status on QoL [46]. The American Society of Clinical Oncology has acknowledged HRQOL as a key treatment outcome [47]. Subsequently, this has been utilized as a primary or secondary end point across all cancer clinical trials [48]. Intent to treat (ITT) enables comparison between studies and therefore is the preferred method to prevent bias. In the AURELIA (Avastin Use in Platinum-Resistant Epithelial Ovarian Cancer) trial, the ITT population had HRQOL data available at baseline for individual patients [49, 50]. The ITT population was also known as patient-reported outcome population. Sensitivity analyses also integrate all ITT patients after multiple imputations.

14.6 Conclusion

Mathematical distributions are the mainstay of statistical computations. Unearthing such distributions may open up newer vistas on easier visualization of data which in turn may expedite statistical model building. However, such experiments are never a substitute to manual data extraction and distribution. Distributions represent the actual percentage of data within a certain range. Reports reveal the same data to elicit different responses if interposed on different distributions. Therefore, for a correct interpretation of statistical analysis, data must be entered onto the correct distribution [51].

The future of research in clinical oncology is exciting. Recent advances in molecular methods and the immune landscape of tumors are bringing complexity to a whole new level. With the advent of next-generation sequencing and its massive output of genomic, transcriptomic, proteomic, and other molecular data in addition to demographic and clinicopathological variables, data obtained from multicentric studies and those data that are accessible for free are a real defiance to the understanding of big data. Such humongous data is merging into a new fascinating frontier in oncology which is known as the molecular-targeted therapy. This when collaborated with newer immunological discoveries caters to a more personal and precise treatment regimen for patients. Newer vistas in bioinformatics have emerged categorically in order to facilitate the quest for improved approaches that will expedite and improve the accuracy of diagnostic and therapeutic interventions. However, present methodologies in vogue cannot entirely answer questions prompted by the myriad of information obtained. Nevertheless, the recent astonishing advances in communication, computation, and artificial intelligence have been both fascinating and intriguing. New approaches in methodology are warranted and should be the way for the future [52].

References

1. Yuan Y, Hunt RH (2009) Systematic reviews: the good, the bad, and the ugly. Am J Gastroenterol 104(5):1086–1092
2. Gotzsche PC (2000) Why we need a broad perspective on meta-analysis. It may be crucially important for patients. BMJ 321(7261):585–586
3. DerSimonian R, Laird N (1986) Meta-analysis in clinical trials. Control Clin Trials 7(3):177–188
4. Mantel N, Haenszel W (1959) Statistical aspects of the analysis of data from retrospective studies of disease. J Natl Cancer Inst 22:719–748
5. Cochran WG (1994) The combination of estimates from different experiments. Biometrics 10:101–129
6. Higgins JP, Thompson SG, Deeks JJ, Altman DG (2003) Measuring inconsistency in meta-analyses. BMJ 327:557–560
7. Galbraith RF (1988) A note on graphical presentation of estimated odds ratios from several clinical trials. Stat Med 7:889–894
8. Egger M, Davey Smith G, Schneider M, Minder C (1997) Bias in meta-analysis detected by a simple, graphical test. BMJ 315:629–634
9. Higgins JPT, Green S (eds) (2009) Cochrane Handbook for Systematic Reviews of Interventions Version 5.0.2. The Cochrane Collaboration, 2009. www.cochrane-handbook.org
10. Liberati A, Altman DG, Tetzlaff J, Mulrow C, Gøtzsche PC, Ioannidis JP, Clarke M, Devereaux PJ, Kleijnen J, Moher D (2009) The PRISMA statement for reporting systematic reviews and meta-analyses of studies that evaluate health care interventions: explanation and elaboration. J Clin Epidemiol 62:e1–e34
11. Moher D, Liberati A, Tetzlaff J, Altman DG (2009) PRISMA group. Preferred reporting items for systematic reviews and meta-analyses: the PRISMA statement. J Clin Epidemiol 62:1006–1012
12. Moher D, Cook DJ, Eastwood S, Olkin I, Rennie D, Stroup DF (1999) Improving the quality of reports of meta-analyses of randomized controlled trials: the QUOROM statement. Quality of reporting of meta-analyses. Lancet 354:1896–1900
13. Antman EM, Lau J, Kupelnick B, Mosteller F, Chalmers TC (1992) A comparison of results of meta-analyses of randomized control trials and recommendations of clinical experts: treatments for myocardial infarction. JAMA 268:240–248
14. Oxman AD, Guyatt GH (1993) The science of reviewing research. Ann N Y Acad Sci 703:125–133
15. Greenland S (1994) Invited commentary: a critical look at some popular meta-analytic methods. Am J Epidemiol 140:290–296
16. Ioannidis JP, Haidich AB, Pappa M, Pantazis N, Kokori SI, Tektonidou MG, Contopoulos-Ioannidis DG, Lau J (2001) Comparison of evidence of treatment effects in randomized and non-randomized studies. JAMA 286:821–830
17. Haidich AB (2010) Meta-analysis in medical research. Hippokratia 14(1):29–37
18. Chalmers I (1993) The Cochrane collaboration: preparing, maintaining, and disseminating systematic reviews of the effects of health care. Ann N Y Acad Sci 703:156–163
19. Riley RD, Lambert PC, Abo-Zaid G (2010) Meta-analysis of individual participant data: rationale, conduct, and reporting. BMJ 340:c221

20. Tierney JF, Vale C, Riley R, Smith CT, Stewart L, Clarke M, Rovers M (2015) Individual participant data (IPD) meta-analyses of randomised controlled trials: guidance on their use. PLoS Med 12(7):e1001855
21. Kalter J, Sweegers MG, Verdonck-de Leeuw IM, Brug J, Buffart LM (2019) Development and use of a flexible data harmonization platform to facilitate the harmonization of individual patient data for meta-analyses. BMC Res Notes 12(1):164
22. Buffart LM, Kalter J, Chinapaw MJ, Heymans MW, Aaronson NK, Courneya KS, Jacobsen PB, Newton RU, Verdonck-de Leeuw IM, Brug J (2013) Predicting Optimal Cancer Rehabilitation and Supportive Care (POLARIS): rationale and design for meta-analyses of individual patient data of randomized controlled trials that evaluate the effect of physical activity and psychosocial interventions on health-related quality of life in cancer survivors. Syst Rev 2(1):75
23. Buffart LM, Kalter J, Sweegers MG, Courneya KS, Newton RU, Aaronson NK, Jacobsen PB, May AM, Galvão DA, Chinapaw MJ, Steindorf K, Irwin ML, Stuiver MM, Hayes S, Griffith KA, Lucia A, Mesters I, van Weert E, Knoop H, Goedendorp MM, Mutrie N, Daley AJ, McConnachie A, Bohus M, Thorsen L, Schulz KH, Short CE, James EL, Plotnikoff RC, Arbane G, Schmidt ME, Potthoff K, van Beurden M, Oldenburg HS, Sonke GS, van Harten WH, Garrod R, Schmitz KH, Winters-Stone KM, Velthuis MJ, Taaffe DR, van Mechelen W, Kersten MJ, Nollet F, Wenzel J, Wiskemann J, Verdonck-de Leeuw IM, Brug J (2017) Effects and moderators of exercise on quality of life and physical function in patients with cancer: an individual patient data meta-analysis of 34 RCTs. Cancer Treat Rev 52:91–104
24. Kalter J, Verdonck-de Leeuw IM, Sweegers MG, Aaronson NK, Jacobsen PB, Newton RU, Courneya KS, Aitken JF, Armes J, Arving C, Boersma LJ, Braamse AMJ, Brandberg Y, Chambers SK, Dekker J, Ell K, Ferguson RJ, Gielissen MFM, Glimelius B, Goedendorp MM, Graves KD, Heiney SP, Horne R, Hunter MS, Johansson B, Kimman ML, Knoop H, Meneses K, Northouse LL, Oldenburg HS, Prins JB, Savard J, van Beurden M, van den Berg SW, Brug J, Buffart LM (2018) Effects and moderators of psychosocial interventions on quality of life, and emotional and social function in patients with cancer: an individual patient data meta-analysis of 22 RCTs. Psychooncology 27(4):1150–1161
25. Gonzalez FJ (1995) Genetic polymorphism and cancer susceptibility: 14th Sapporo Cancer seminar. Cancer Res 55:710–715
26. Pabalan N, Bapat B, Sung L, Jarjanazi H, Francisco-Pabalan O, Ozcelik H (2008) Cyclin D1 Pro241Pro (CCND1-G870A) polymorphism is associated with increased cancer risk in human populations: a meta-analysis. Cancer Epidemiol Biomark Prev 17:2773–2781
27. Pabalan N, Francisco-Pabalan O, Sung L, Jarjanazi H, Ozcelik H (2010) Meta-analysis of two polymorphisms, Lys751Gln and Asp312Asn, in the DNA repair gene, XPD (ERCC2) with breast cancer. Breast Cancer Res Treat 17:27
28. Brennan P (2012) Gene-environment interaction and aetiology of cancer: what does it mean and how can we measure it? Carcinogenesis 23(3):381–387
29. Zintzaras E, Lau J (2008) Trends in meta-analysis of genetic association studies. J Hum Genet 53:1–9
30. Taioli E (2005) Biomarkers of genetic susceptibility to cancer: applications to epidemiological studies. Future Oncol 1:51–56
31. Ioannidis JP (2004) The value of meta-analysis in rheumatology research. Autoimmun Rev 3(Suppl 1):S57–S59
32. Pabalan N (2010) Meta-analysis in cancer genetics. Asian Pacific J Cancer Prev 11:33–38
33. Morris RD (1994) Meta-analysis in cancer epidemiology. Environ Health Perspect 102(Suppl 8):61–66
34. Guyatt GH, Feeny DH, Patrick DL (1993) Measuring health-related quality of life. Ann Intern Med 118(8):622–629
35. Spilker B (ed) (1996) Quality of life and pharmacoeconomics in clinical trials. Lippincott-Raven, Philadelphia, pp 1–1259
36. Testa MA, Simonson DC (1996) Assessment of quality-of-life outcomes. N Engl J Med 334(13):835–840

37. Wilson IB, Cleary PD (1995) Linking clinical variables with health-related quality of life. A conceptual model of patient outcomes. JAMA 273(1):59–65
38. Oldridge N, Gottlieb M, Guyatt G, Jones N, Streiner D, Feeny D (1998) Predictors of health-related quality of life with cardiac rehabilitation after acute myocardial infarction. J Cardpulm Rehabil 18(2):95–103
39. Boscolo-Rizzo P, Maronato F, Marchiori C, Gava A, Da Mosto MC (2008) Long-term quality of life after total laryngectomy and postoperative radiotherapy versus concurrent chemoradiotherapy for laryngeal preservation. Laryngoscope 118(2):300–306
40. Hörnquist JO (1990) Quality of life: concept and assessment. Scand J Soc Med 18(1):69–79
41. Thatcher N, Hopwood P, Anderson H (1997) Improving quality of life in patients with non-small cell lung cancer: research experience with gemcitabine. Eur J Cancer 33(Suppl 1):S8–S13
42. Mauer ME, Bottomley A, Taphoorn MJ (2008) Evaluating health-related quality of life and symptom burden in brain tumour patients: instruments for use in experimental trials and clinical practice. Curr Opin Neurol 21(6):745–753
43. Hiatt RA, Breen N (2008) The social determinants of cancer: a challenge for trans disciplinary science. Am J Prev Med 35:S141–S150
44. Meisel JL, Domchek SM, Vonderheide RH, Giobbie-Hurder A, Lin NU, Winer EP, Partridge AH (2012) Quality of life in long-term survivors of metastatic breast cancer. Clin Breast Cancer 12(2):119–126
45. Zebrack BJ, Landier W (2011) The perceived impact of cancer on quality of life for post-treatment survivors of childhood cancer. Qual Life Res 20(10):1595–1608
46. Osoba D (2011) Health-related quality of life and cancer clinical trials. Ther Adv Med Oncol 3:57–71
47. American Society of Clinical Oncology (1996) Outcomes of cancer treatment for technology assessment and cancer treatment guidelines. J Clin Oncol 14:671–679
48. Efficace F, Fayers P, Pusic A, Cemal Y, Yanagawa J, Jacobs M, la Sala A, Cafaro V, Whale K, Rees J, Blazeby J (2015) European Organization for Research and Treatment of Cancer quality-of-life group (patient-reported outcome measurements over time in oncology registry). Quality of patient-reported outcome reporting across cancer randomized controlled trials according to the CONSORT patient-reported outcome extension: a pooled analysis of 557 trials. Cancer 121:3335–3342
49. Stockler MR, Hilpert F, Friedlander M et al (2014) Patient-reported outcome results from the open-label phase III AURELIA trial evaluating bevacizumab-containing therapy for platinum-resistant ovarian cancer. J Clin Oncol 32:1309–1316
50. Stockler MR, Hilpert F, Friedlander M, King MT, Wenzel L, Lee CK, Joly F, de Gregorio N, Arranz JA, Mirza MR, Sorio R, Freudensprung U, Sneller V, Hales G, Pujade-Lauraine E (2014) Patient-reported outcome results from the open-label phase III AURELIA trial evaluating bevacizumab-containing therapy for platinum-resistant ovarian cancer. J Clin Oncol 32(13):1309–1316
51. Parab S, Bhalerao S (2010) Choosing statistical test. Int J Ayurveda Res 1(3):187–191
52. Roy J, Winter C, Schroeder M (2016) Meta-analysis of Cancer gene profiling data. Methods Mol Biol 1381:211–222

Part VI

History of Drug Reaction in Children Suffering from Cancer

15

Bisma Zafar, Maliha Ghaffar, and Hina Salahuddin

15.1 History of Drug Reaction in Children

People with similar sickness will show inverse respond frequently with identical medication. Some people will have the best response to medication, though some experience slight or no results. Few patients will have contrary drug reactions, while others don't have. Some patients need a high or low dosage related to normal dose demarcated in medical tribunals to get optimal results from the drug. Pharmacogenomics finds the connection between genetic differences and drug responses. Single nucleotide polymorphisms can lead to fluctuation in function and quantity of proteins and so in drug response.

Maximum pharmacogenomic investigations have been done on adults. It is significant to understand that results in the mature population can't be produced in the pediatric population. Processes or systems are under progress in children. Drugs might perform an inverse function in children as compared to adults. Though genetic differences persist, the influence of handling heterogeneity might be diverse at a young age. Pharmacogenomic studies in pediatric cancer focused on forecasting which patients will agonize from adverse ADRs [1].

About 20% of malignant growth in pediatric patients doesn't react to usual treatment [2], and 22% of emergency clinic confirmations in common people are because of antagonistic drug responses [3]. The helpful healing mediators utilized in malignant growth chemotherapy are frequently managed at legal high dosages [4]; this is due to between patient inconstancy and tight remedial extent which ends up in a

B. Zafar
Department of Biotechnology, University of Okara, Okara, Pakistan
e-mail: bismazafar10@gmail.com

M. Ghaffar (✉) · H. Salahuddin
Department of Zoology, University of Okara, Okara, Pakistan
e-mail: malihaghaffar@yahoo.com; hina.salahuddin3@gmail.com

N. Masood, S. Shakil Malik (eds.), *'Essentials of Cancer Genomic, Computational Approaches and Precision Medicine*,
https://doi.org/10.1007/978-981-15-1067-0_15

range of results from extreme toxicities to underexposure. Some portion of this fluctuation can be credited to innate hereditary varieties influencing the medication pharmacodynamics and pharmacokinetics. The investigation of the connection between hereditary qualities and medication work is most normally known as pharmacogenetics or pharmacogenomics. Pharmacogenomics is a valid, recognized, and personalized approach of treatment and has the potential to build up drug safety levels and efficiency [5, 6]. Most of the patients react diversely to a drug because of their constitutive genetic shuffling, yet also because of transformations or epigenetic marks gained among the procedure of neogenesis or treatment. This survey expects to concentrate on germ line varieties that may influence treatment adequacy and toxic quality [7, 8]. By October 2015, in Budapest (Hungary), during 3rd congress under (ESPT) European Society of Pharmaco-genomics and Personalized Therapy, a preface conference was held with an aim of establishing individualized pediatric treatment involved therapy in Hematology and Oncology sections and testing on children's would be the goal. The fundamental reason for existing was to encourage the exchange and coordination of pharmacogenetic analysis from investigational study into applied clinics, to unite essential and translational research, and to teach well-being experts all through Europe as this information is essential to achieve the future goals in pharmacogenomics.

15.2 Ontogeny Role in Pharmacogenomics

Pharmacogenomics in youngsters, in contrast to adults, must be seen concerning body improvement apart from the physiological changes because of the disorder. When an infant becomes an adult, variations happen in physique structure. For example, an untimely newborn of about 1.5 kg has only 3% of physique fat, which prompts 12% with the aid of the 40th week development and farther 25% by the 4th month [9]. Correspondingly, the protein will increase from 25% at the beginning to 50% in a fully grown individual. These progressions need to be observed while examining the distinctions in pharmacokinetic information in connection to the genotypes. An additional issue of significance for the scientific efficacy of pharmacogenetic tests in youngsters is ontogeny of drug-metabolizing enzymes (DMEs), target proteins. One of the best examples is an expansion of drug metabolism capacity linked with expression of cytochrome P450 (CYP) [10]. These enzymes of the CYP3A family can make a change in their activity from fetus to adulthood which includes four types of members in humans that are 3A4, 3A5, 3A7, and 3A43, respectively. CYP3A4 is richly expressed CYP in a small digestive system and liver recovering 35–45% of CYP proteins. CYP3A4 has a very stumpy action during childbirth, coming to around 35–45% of grown-up movement by the principal month and adult action by the 6th month of an adult, surpassing grown-up action of an adult (120%) somewhere in the range of 1 and 4 years old, and diminishing to grown-up levels after adolescence [11]. CYP3A5 and CYP3A4 both are homologous about 83% and represent themselves in kidneys and the liver but at very low levels, whereas CYP3A5 and CYP2B6 are among two CYPs alongside with the phase II of enzyme

N-acetyltransferase showing no change in appearance and the functioning of genetic variants in developmental stages from childhood to adulthood. In contrast, CYPs of family CYP3A7 and CYP3A4 which are mostly expressed in newborns, fetal, and in the embryonic liver, are 90% homologous [12]. Comparable inconstancy in articulation amid improvement is noted for CYP2D6. It was shown that embryos under 30 weeks old express under 5% of the CYP2D6 movement in contrast with the grown-ups. Once after birth, movement bit by bit increases, between days 8 and 28 the action is 30%, and between about a month and 5 years, the action is 70% in adults. Also, CYP articulation and movement can be influenced by basic medical issues, for example, nonalcoholic greasy liver ailment and neonatal diabetes.

Like DMEs, the ontogeny of medication targets is likewise significant in the assessment and performance of pharmacogenetics. For example, multi-drug resistant protein 1 and ATPs binding cassette, whereas G2 is articulated earlier in childhood, though different transporters like Organic anion transporter or multi-drug safe protein 2 (MRP-2) display delayed the development and decreased articulation levels with the main long stretches of adolescence contrasted with the adults [13].

The above-described cases are only a couple of instances of ontogeny commitment to quality control variances. A current publication demonstrates that up to 689 types of genes are otherwise articulated in developmental stages advancement just in lymphoblastic cells. Utilizing genetic articulation profiling of lymphoblast cells, scientists had the option to recognize three specific gatherings: prepubertal which is under 7, pubertal that is from 7 years to 17 years, and early adulthood gathering which is more than 17 [5] proposing a lot of formative genes which may express in a freeway.

The effects of drugs and their responses to children or adults may reveal the importance of ontogeny. More exposure to ototoxicity with cisplatin and its treatment [14, 15], consequences for neurological advancement connected to methotrexate [16], more consent of the tacrolimus or lethargy to codeine in newborn children are nevertheless a couple of cases [17]. Finally, few of related cancer diseases include acute lymphoblastic leukemia (ALL), osteosarcoma (OS), and neuroblastoma (NB) and may appear primarily in younger ones than adults so that's why it is linked to ontogeny giving extra help that pediatric pharmacogenomics ought to be considered as an unmistakable field. The shortage of data and agreement on ontogeny is as yet one of the significant constraints for an unmistakable comprehension of the utility of hereditary variations [18].

The primary step to evaluating gene-drug associations is to highlight individual drugs widely used across European clinics to treat pediatric cancer patients for conditions like brain tumors, leukemia, lymphomas, and solid tumors [19]. Primary drugs were included only to simplify the search, whereas any auxiliary treatments such as prophylactics or co-medications were ruled out. Secondly, it was important to check whether these drugs had gene-drug associations that were enlisted in the Pharmacogenomics Knowledgebase and were integrated into clinical guidelines of the Clinical Pharmacogenetics. PharmGKB is an accessible complete resource that checks and integrates facts on the effect of the genetic differences in drug reactions for clinical application or research. It is programmed to systematically extract gene-drug associations from scientific databases and evaluate evidence. Since CPIC is responsible for the preparation of medical strategies for the gene or drug associations that mollify the utmost criteria of confirmation with special emphasis on clinical importance, PharmGKB beautifully collaborates with it to give stunning gene-drug pairs and evidence for clinicians and researchers worldwide.

The method used to extract data on pediatric oncology pharmacogenomics starts with identifying and defining of drugs used in Europe. CPIC and PharmGKB collectively function to search out drug-gene pairs and the strongest evidence for their application. In terms of strength of evidence, genes are grouped accordingly into four classes. Finally, the research found in the pediatric section in CPIC is reviewed and evaluated.

As previously mentioned, PharmGKB rates gene-drug associations into four comprehensive groups founded on power (with "1" being the resilient and "4" being the feeblest) of indication for the association. The first level contains a gene or drug relations that indicate important *p* values in more than one cohort and rather with a larger magnitude of consequence. The second level consists of suggestions that were reproducible with studies besides them that do not show worth with the association showing the smaller magnitude of the effect. The third level is built on solitary studies presenting substantial association with the indication not reproduced. The fourth level is centered on individualized reports and in vitro, molecular, or functional assays [20]. The PharmGKB approach was tailored for this review with a few amendments in group 3rd and 4th level and both groups were merged in a solo group of a gene-drug linkage having a fairly little possibility of the entering medical trial in a period whereas group 1 and 2 were kept segregated.

15.3 Drugs with Pharmacogenetic Evidence

By the early screening, we were capable to classify the following drug-gene pairs with pharmacogenetic evidence like thiopurines/thiopurine S-methyltransferases (TPMT) pair, and cisplatin, carboplatin, irinotecan, and vincristine have moderate pharmacogenetic evidence.

15.3.1 Thiopurines/Thiopurine S-Methyltransferases (TPMT) Pair

Pharmacogenomic pair of thiopurines with TPMT is perhaps the peak extensively deliberate drug-gene interface in medicine of pediatrics. Thiopurines are functional as prodrugs that transformed into thioguanine nucleotides by hypoxanthine-guanine phosphoribosyltransferase. TGNs are very cytotoxic mixtures that function by integrating into DNA or RNA producing damage to nucleic acids, finally leading to the expiry of cancerous cells. On the downside, TGNs can generate apoptosis in resistant cells producing ADRs mostly neutropenia, thrombocytopenia, as well as hepatotoxicity, commonly manifesting as a veno-occlusive disease [21]. TGNs inactivate through S-methylation by the cytosolic TPMT. TPMT action is affected by polymorphisms occurring in the gene [22, 23]. In medical determinations, the individuals are dispersed into three main groups: ordinary, intermediary, and reduced metabolizers created on the existence of one or two damages of functional alleles. Alleles 2, 3A, 3B, and 3C are by remote the most widely found irregular alleles and are expected to forecast up to 90% of the TPMT function [24]. Apart from the aforementioned, a total of 34 TPMT alleles have been discovered and termed in multiple inhabitants but with minor regularities [25] (Fig. 15.1).

This drug-gene link takes significant medical effects because treatment consequences of childhood ALL with 6MP are very closely linked to maximum tolerable drug dose. The notion is supported by observations of concentration of TGNs and TPMT genotype, which collectively work in an inversely linked relationship to the capability of patients to tolerate full doses of 6MP. Subjects showing poor metabolism of TMPT were able to tolerate not more than 7% of 6MP dose in the children, with those with intermediate and normal metabolism ranging from 65% to 84% tolerance of the treatment in the treatment regime. TPMT metabolizers lost 2% of entire treatment weeks, the indifference of 16–76% of missed weeks for TPMT transitional and TPMT deprived metabolizers, respectively [27]. The normal metabolism of TMPT allowed lag of 2% in total handling weeks, whereas patients with intermediate and poor metabolism demonstrated a lack of response in 16% and 76% of total weeks, respectively. CPIC has developed guidelines that state dosage for patients with normal metabolism traits. A 30–70% decrease is optional

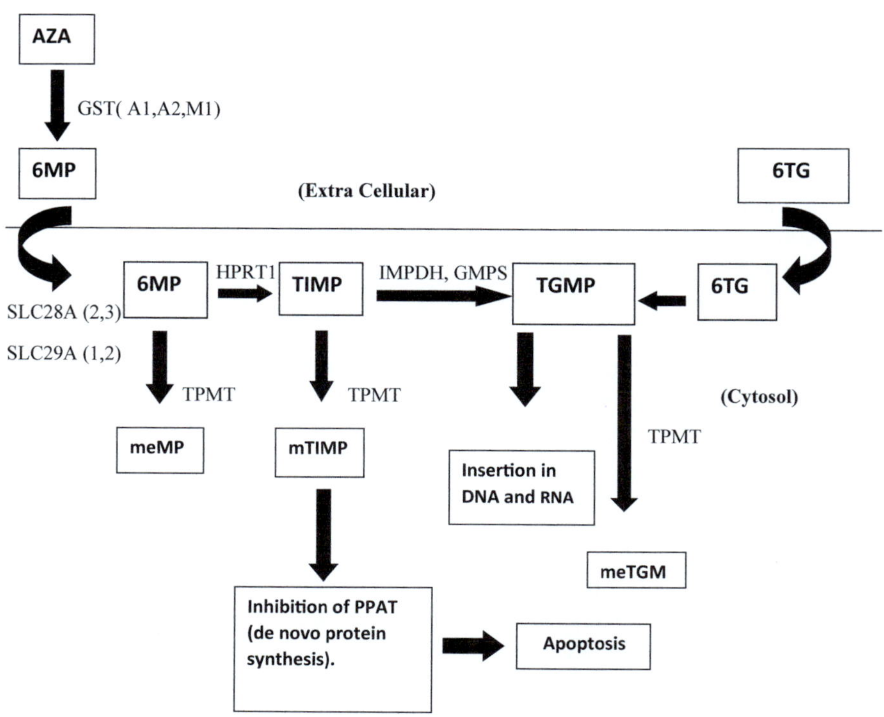

Fig. 15.1 Metabolism of TPMT thiopurine S-methyltransferase [26]

for 6MP and 30–50% reduction for 6TG for the intermediate metabolizer class. Poor metabolism traits demanded to get 6MP or 6TG with a 90% decrease in dosage direction decreased to three times per week to avoid ADRs. Proactive patient testing has been actively called to reduce the chances of contrary drug responses in the situation of cancerous disease or to diminish time wanted for mounting titration of drug dose [28].

Identifying the significance of ontogeny, the indication on thiopurines and TPMT association assembled in pediatric cohorts. Childhood leukemia is flourishing childhood neoplastic disease, and a bulk amount of studies has been directed in the populace of pediatric in this regard [29].

15.3.2 Vincristine

Vincristine is extensively used as a mixture chemotherapeutic negotiator for handling brain tumors, leukemias, lymphomas, neuroblastoma, retinoblastoma, and rhabdomyosarcoma in pediatrics. Vincristine prevents microtubule formation by its toxic properties by ultimately leading to mitotic arrest and apoptosis. Twenty-five percent of both pediatric and adult patients grow medically important vincristine-induced peripheral neuropathy, influencing indirect activities that embrace reduction in dose or termination of cure [30]. CYP3A5 has mostly tangled vincristine metabolism and is articulated only in about 10–20% Caucasians and 80% of Americans [31]. Some contradictory rumors with most of the cases of lesser vincristine clearance in the patients holding deprived CYP3A5 metabolism are more susceptible to the development of VIPN [32]. Also, some populace transformations were detected for this association [33].

Fresh genome extensive suggestion research recognized an irregularity in the centrosomal protein 72 gene link with the VIPN throughout the extension phase of ALL handling with a large number of vincristine dosages [34]. Authors revealed in a similar study that a minor expression of CEP72 produced and enhanced the sensitivity to vincristine. These conclusions elevated confidence for safe vincristine dosage expectancy in ALL usage procedures. However, another reviewing study through the beginning stage of ALL conduct in children of Spanish could not support this link, due to alterations in the study project, populace, and phase of handling protocol [35].

15.4 Conclusion

The baseline recommendations for adults put forward by pediatric pharmacogenomics for thiopurines/TPMT association have shown consistency in results across multiple studies and depicted a profound effect on patients, and the study needs more attention. Thiopurines are one of the few drugs that were supported by strong evidence with its association with TPMT, but further research into the drug-gene relationship is needed before it can be put to practice in hospitals. Sensible indication gene-drug connections were typically formed for pharmacogenetics. Research turns up as either scarce or too complex to allow comparison due to variance created diagonally handling procedures, diseases, populaces, and assessable consequences. On the contrary, vincristine has been found sufficiently quoted in Dutch and French guidelines, suggesting a reduction of the drug dose in some cases of patients exhibiting low metabolism. CYP3A5 is a possible alternative to use lower doses while also implementing a protracted treatment regime. Lack of data available for this gene-drug pair in pediatric pharmacogenetics opens new doors to research on this gene. Pharmacogenetic gene-drug association studies, thereby urging vast study designs to produce reasonable results.

15.5 Future Directions

Before any extra gene-drug interaction-based trials can be initiated in hospitals, rigorous and in-depth analysis yielding strong evidence of gene-drug associations must be performed. PharmGKB provides a valuable platform for clinicians and scientists to analyze and interpret data from pharmacogenomics. Though it facilitates the end user, caution must be taken while interpreting lower-level gene-drug associations as statistics may vary in terms of gene-drug associations. A lacking element in pediatric pharmacogenomics deals with an ontology that requires proper comprehension of the impact of genetic variants. Multiple combinations of drugs used in the treatment of cancer also present a hurdle, which makes it difficult to identify the effect of a single drug component. Future research can be enhanced by creating a standardized treatment regimen spread over different institutions and pinpoint the exact genetic association with the overall treatment cycle.

References

1. McLeod HL, Evans WE (2001) Pharmacogenomics: unlocking the human genome for better drug therapy. Annu Rev Pharmacol Toxicol 41:101–121
2. Pritchard-Jones K, Dixon-Woods M, Naafs-Wilstra M, Valsecchi MG (2008) Improving recruitment to clinical trials for cancer in childhood. Lancet Oncol 9(4):392–399
3. Mitchell AA, Lacouture PG, Sheehan JE, Kauffman RE, Shapiro S (1988) Adverse drug reactions in children leading to hospital admission. Pediatrics 82(1):24–29
4. MacNeil M, Eisenhauer E (1999) High-dose chemotherapy: is it standard management for any common solid tumor? Ann Oncol 10(10):1145–1161
5. Nebert DW (1999) Pharmacogenetics and pharmacogenomics: why is this relevant to the clinical geneticist? Clin Genet 56(4):247–258
6. Stevens A, Hanson D, Whatmore A, Destenaves B, Chatelain P, Clayton P (2013) Human growth is associated with distinct patterns of gene expression in evolutionarily conserved networks. BMC Genomics 14(1):547
7. Holohan C, Van Schaeybroeck S, Longley DB, Johnston PG (2013) Cancer drug resistance: an evolving paradigm. Nat Rev Cancer 13(10):714
8. Longley D, Johnston P (2005) Molecular mechanisms of drug resistance. J Pathol 205(2):275–292
9. Bar-Shalom D, Rose K (2014) Pediatric formulations: a roadmap, vol 11. Springer, New York

10. Kearns GL, Abdel-Rahman SM, Alander SW, Blowey DL, Leeder JS, Kauffman RE (2003) Developmental pharmacology—drug disposition, action, and therapy in infants and children. N Engl J Med 349(12):1157–1167
11. Leeder JS, Kearns GL (1997) Pharmacogenetics in pediatrics: implications for practice. Pediatr Clin N Am 44(1):55–77
12. de Wildt SN, Kearns GL, Leeder JS, van den Anker JN (1999) Cytochrome P450 3A. Clin Pharmacokinet 37(6):485–505
13. Brouwer KL, Aleksunes LM, Brandys B, Giacoia GP, Knipp G, Lukacova V, Meibohm B, Nigam SK, Rieder M, de Wildt SN, Pediatric Transporter Working Group (2015) Human ontogeny of drug transporters: review and recommendations of the pediatric transporter working group. Clin Pharmacol Ther 98(3):266–287
14. Finkielstain GP, Forcinito P, Lui JC, Barnes KM, Marino R, Makaroun S, Nguyen V, Lazarus JE, Nilsson O, Baron J (2008) An extensive genetic program occurring during postnatal growth in multiple tissues. Endocrinology 150(4):1791–1800
15. Knight KRG, Kraemer DF, Neuwelt EA (2005) Ototoxicity in children receiving platinum chemotherapy: underestimating a commonly occurring toxicity that may influence academic and social development. J Clin Oncol 23(34):8588–8596
16. Kushner BH, Budnick A, Kramer K, Modak S, Cheung NKV (2006) Ototoxicity from high-dose use of platinum compounds in patients with neuroblastoma. Cancer 107(2):417–422
17. Bleyer W, Fallavollita J, Robison L, Balsom W, Meadows A, Heyn R, Sitarz A, Ortega J, Miller D, Constine L (1990) Influence of age, sex, and concurrent intrathecal methotrexate therapy on intellectual function after cranial irradiation during childhood: a report from the Children's Cancer Study Group. Pediatr Hematol Oncol 7(4):329–338
18. Lazaryan M, Shasha-Zigelman C, Dagan Z, Berkovitch M (2015) Codeine should not be prescribed for breastfeeding mothers or children under the age of 12. Acta Paediatr 104(6):550–556
19. Uppugunduri RS, Ansari M (2016) Commentary: a myriad aberrations on information of ontogeny of drug metabolizing enzymes in the pediatric population: an obstacle for personalizing drug therapy in the pediatric population. Drug Metab Lett 10(2):72–74
20. Whirl-Carrillo M, McDonagh EM, Hebert J, Gong L, Sangkuhl K, Thorn C, Altman RB, Klein TE (2012) Pharmacogenomics knowledge for personalized medicine. Clin Pharmacol Ther 92(4):414–417
21. Szumlanski C, Otterness D, Her C, Lee D, Brandriff B, Kelsell D, Spurr N, Lennard L, Wieben E, Weinshilboum R (1996) Thiopurine methyltransferase pharmacogenetics: human gene cloning and characterization of a common polymorphism. DNA Cell Biol 15(1):17–30
22. Weinshilboum RM, Sladek SL (1980) Mercaptopurine pharmacogenetics: monogenic inheritance of erythrocyte thiopurine methyltransferase activity. Am J Hum Genet 32(5):651
23. Collie-Duguid E, Pritchard S, Powrie R, Sludden J, Collier D, Li T, McLeod H (1999) The frequency and distribution of thiopurine methyltransferase alleles in Caucasian and Asian populations. Pharmacogenetics 9(1):37–42
24. Appell ML, Berg J, Duley J, Evans WE, Kennedy MA, Lennard L, Marinaki T, McLeod HL, Relling MV, Schaeffeler E, Schwab M, Weinshilboum R, Yeoh AE, McDonagh EM, Hebert JM, Klein TE, Coulthard SA (2013) Nomenclature for alleles of the thiopurine methyltransferase gene. Pharmacogenet Genomics 23(4):242
25. Relling MV, Hancock ML, Rivera GK, Sandlund JT, Ribeiro RC, Krynetski EY, Pui CH, Evans WE (1999) Mercaptopurine therapy intolerance and heterozygosity at the thiopurine S-methyltransferase gene locus. J Natl Cancer Inst 91(23):2001–2008
26. Mlakar V, Huezo-Diaz Curtis P, Satyanarayana Uppugunduri C, Krajinovic M, Ansari M (2016) Pharmacogenomics in pediatric oncology: review of gene—drug associations for clinical use. Int J Mol Sci 17(9):1502
27. Relling M, Gardner E, Sandborn W, Schmiegelow K, Pui CH, Yee S, Stein CM, Carrillo M, Evans WE, Klein TE, Clinical Pharmacogenetics Implementation Consortium (2011) Clinical pharmacogenetics implementation consortium guidelines for thiopurine methyltransferase genotype and thiopurine dosing. Clin Pharmacol Ther 89(3):387–391

28. Swen J, Nijenhuis M, de Boer A, Grandia L, Maitland-van der Zee A-H, Mulder H, Rongen GA, van Schaik RH, Schalekamp T, Touw DJ, van der Weide J, Wilffert B, Deneer VH, Guchelaar HJ (2011) Pharmacogenetics: from bench to byte—an update of guidelines. Clin Pharmacol Ther 89(5):662–673
29. Pui C-H, Evans WE (2006) Treatment of acute lymphoblastic leukemia. N Engl J Med 354(2):166–178
30. Jordan MA, Toso RJ, Thrower D, Wilson L (1993) Mechanism of mitotic block and inhibition of cell proliferation by taxol at low concentrations. Proc Natl Acad Sci 90(20):9552–9556
31. Egbelakin A, Ferguson MJ, MacGill EA, Lehmann AS, Topletz AR, Quinney SK, Li L, McCammack KC, Hall SD, Renbarger JL (2011) Increased risk of vincristine neurotoxicity associated with low CYP3A5 expression genotype in children with acute lymphoblastic leukemia. Pediatr Blood Cancer 56(3):361–367
32. Xie H-G, Wood AJ, Kim RB, Stein CM, Wilkinson GR (2004) Genetic variability in CYP3A5 and its possible consequences. Pharmacogenomics 5(3):243–272
33. Moore AS, Norris R, Price G, Nguyen T, Ni M, George R, van Breda K, Duley J, Charles B, Pinkerton R (2011) Vincristine pharmacodynamics and pharmacogenetics in children with cancer: a limited-sampling, population modelling approach. J Paediatr Child Health 47(12):875–882
34. Sims RP (2016) The effect of race on the CYP3A-mediated metabolism of vincristine in pediatric patients with acute lymphoblastic leukemia. J Oncol Pharm Pract 22(1):76–81
35. Diouf B, Crews KR, Lew G, Pei D, Cheng C, Bao J, Wheeler HE (2015) Association of an inherited genetic variant with vincristine-related peripheral neuropathy in children with acute lymphoblastic leukemia. JAMA 313(8):815–823

Pharmacogenomics of Cisplatin-Induced Toxicity in Children 16

Aadil Rasheed, Maliha Ghaffar, and Hina Salahuddin

16.1 Introduction

Cisplatin belongs to the effective group of chemotherapeutics and has a wide range of action to treat the different types of cancers. In children it can be used to treat different tumors such as hepatoblastoma, neuroblastoma, germ cell tumors, relapsed lymphoma, refractory lymphoma, and osteosarcoma. In adults it has its applications in treating the tumors that include cervical, testicular, ovarian, neck, bladder, head, and lung cancers. Cisplatin has a cure rate of about 85% and is regarded as one of the most effective chemotherapeutic agents. It is an alkylating agent that is used to treat different sorts of cancers. Cisplatin has a platinum atom that has two ammonia groups and two chloride groups attached at the *cis* position. Cisplatin is activated when two water molecules are replaced with two chloride ligands that is a replacement reaction; because of which, platinum cation is formed. The cation then reacts with DNA by covalently binding the purines forming inter- and intrastrand cross-links.

16.2 Discovery

In the 1960s cisplatin for the first time was found to have an anticancer activity, and its clinical success developed the interest of using metal compounds to treat cancers [1].

Barnett Rosenberg at the University of Michigan performed an experiment to study the role of electrical current in cellular division. He grew *Escherichia coli* in NH_4Cl buffer and applied current using inert platinum electrodes 9. After some time, *E. coli* cells were found to be larger than usual [2]. This was found to be due to reason that cell division was inhibited. Later, it was found that this effect was not caused by

A. Rasheed · M. Ghaffar · H. Salahuddin (✉)
Department of Zoology, University of Okara, Okara, Pakistan
e-mail: aadilrasheed96@gmail.com; malihaghaffar@yahoo.com; hina.salahuddin3@gmail.com

N. Masood, S. Shakil Malik (eds.), *'Essentials of Cancer Genomic, Computational Approaches and Precision Medicine,*
https://doi.org/10.1007/978-981-15-1067-0_16

the current; instead the product formed by the hydrolysis of platinum was the reason of inhibition of division [3]. Then different metal compounds of the group 10 transition metals were used in different experiments and resulted in enlargement of *E. coli* cells. It was also discovered that only *cis* form of platinum (IV) complex resulted in enlargement or inhibition of division and *trans* form did have no effect [4].

With these results it was thought that these complexes may prove valuable for having anticancer activity. Mice with sarcoma tumors were subjected to the platinum complexes. Large tumors in mice were reduced in size and they survived. After 24 weeks all the signs of cancer disappeared in the treated mice [5, 6]. The results lead to clinical trials of cisplatin, which now has become one of the most effective anticancer therapeutic agents.

16.3 Synthesis

Michel Peyrone in 1845 was the first to synthesize cisplatin that later was subjected to convicting discussion for its structure [7, 8]. About a half century later, Alfred Werner proposed square planar structure of this molecule, while it helped him in establishing his theory of coordination chemistry. *Cis*- and *trans*-isomers, i.e., cisplatin and transplatin, were also differentiated [8–10], and Werner was awarded Nobel Prize in Chemistry for his work in 1913 [9].

There have been brought many improvements in process of synthesizing cisplatin. Old methods did not tend to be trustworthy as they included some by-products as impurities. So alternative methods with the goal of improved quality of cisplatin and increased yield of reaction were adopted. In 1970 Dhara reported about "A rapid method for synthesis of *cis*-[PtC12(NH3)2]" on which most modern methods of producing cisplatin are based. This procedure included the conversion of the raw material, $K_2[PtCl_4]$, to the tetra-iodo analogue, $K_2[PtI_4]$, and a concentrated solution of KI is added. NH_3 is also added that results in formation of yellowish compound, *cis*-$[PtI_2(NH_3)_2]$, and then an aqueous solution of $AgNO_3$ is also added to purify *cis*-$[PtI_2(NH_3)_2]$ that results in the formation of precipitates of insoluble AgI. The whole solution is filtered and AgI is eliminated. The filtrate that contains *cis*-$[Pt(OH_2)_2(NH_3)_2]^{2+}$ forms final product in the form of precipitates by treating with KCl. The final product is *cis*-$[PtCl_2(NH_3)_2]$ (cisplatin), in the form of yellow powder [11].

16.4 Mode of Action

Cisplatin acts as an anticancer drug when it interacts with DNA and induces apoptosis, i.e., programmed cell death (Fig. 16.1) [1, 12]. The bloodstream contains a high concentration of chloride ions in the plasma of blood, so cisplatin must face this higher concentration, and replacing the chloride ions by water molecules is limited (aquation process is inhibited) [13, 14]. Nevertheless, some proteins present in the plasma find it easier to attack cisplatin [15, 16]. These proteins include especially those having thiol group, which are albumin of human serum and cysteine [17, 18]. It has been found that about 90% cisplatin is found bound by proteins in

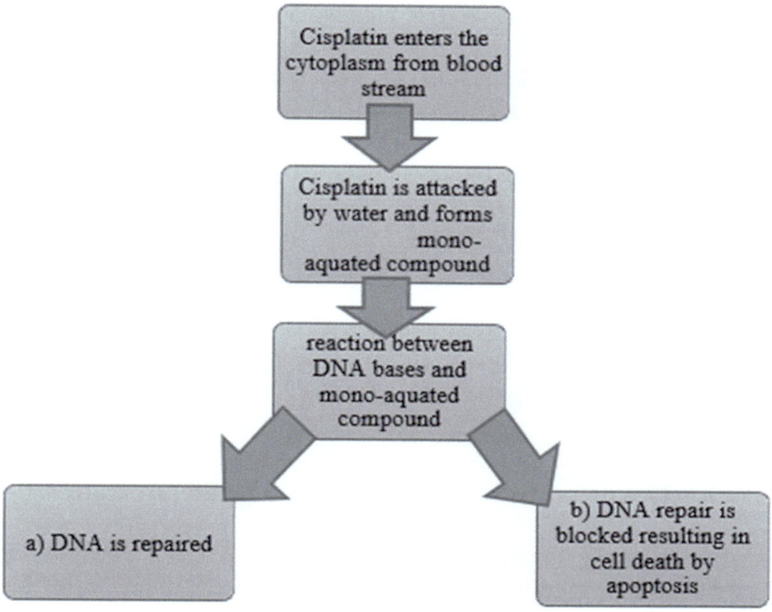

Fig. 16.1 Cisplatin's cytotoxic pathway

plasma after 24 h when the drug has been administered [19–21]. It is believed that cisplatin is deactivated by these proteins [22–26] and results in severe side effects [19, 27–31].

The unreacted cisplatin diffuses through the plasma membrane of the cancer cells and gains entry [32]. It has been also found that cisplatin can also enter tumor cells by active transport across cell membrane by use of Cu-transporting proteins [33]. The concentration of chloride ions is low in intracellular space as compared to blood plasma, and it is easier for cisplatin to be attacked by water molecules and replace one chloride ligand that produces a positive species that is ready to undergo reaction and doesn't diffuse out of the cell. This mono-aquated compound has been found to be responsible for about 98% platinum that binds the DNA in the nucleus of tumor cells by in vitro methods [34].

A monofunctional DNA adduct is formed when reaction occurs between this mono-aquated platinum compound and a base of DNA, mostly guanine [35–37]. The potential sites for binding with platinum with each of DNA bases are nucleophilic nitrogen atoms present in nitrogenous bases. A bifunctional adduct may be formed by the ring closure [38, 39]. Either monofunctional DNA adduct may directly undergo ring closure to form bifunctional adduct, or the second chloride ligand may be aquated after the ring closure. Adenine-guanine and guanine-guanine are included in bifunctional adducts [40]. These bifunctional products distort the DNA significantly. This distorted DNA is recognized by DNA binding proteins. The DNA-binding proteins either start the process of damage repair of DNA or result in signaling the induction of apoptosis. The damage of tumors is caused by induction of apoptosis when different signal transduction pathways are activated to mediate apoptosis [22, 38, 39, 41].

Cisplatin may interact with any of the following [23] leading to activation of transduction pathways:

1. Reactive oxygen species (ROS)
2. DNA
3. Tumor necrosis factors
4. Mitochondria
5. p53
6. Caspases
7. Calcium signaling
8. Multidrug-resistant proteins

16.5 Pharmacogenomics of Cisplatin-Induced Ototoxicity

Cisplatin causes hearing loss in various cancer patients to a great degree in a varied way. Genetic difference can give an illustration of the variations in the disposed patients.

16.5.1 Mechanism of Cisplatin-Induced Ototoxicity

DNA damage and production of acute and chronic reactive oxygen species (ROS) are among the inspections for ototoxicity due to cisplatin. All of the three parts of cochlea, spiral ganglionic cells, lateral wall, and the organ of Corti, have been inspected with elevated production of ROS. The antioxidant enzyme system of cochlea that includes superoxide dismutase, catalase, glutathione peroxidase, glutathione reductase, glutathione S-transferase (GST), etc. is depleted by generation of excess of ROS. This enzyme system scavenges and neutralizes super oxides that are procreated [24]. Consequently, hearing loss results from any polymorphism in these enzymes. An inflammatory cytokine and a superoxide form in the cochlea increasingly by formation of ingrained ROS due to cisplatin. Proapoptotic pathways are activated when ROS are produced unchecked [25].

16.5.2 Megalin, Hearing, and Ototoxicity

Megalin, a multiligand receptor, has multiple functions and seems to be important for hearing. Stria vascularis of the cochlea produces megalin abundantly in its marginal cells. Possibly, cisplatin is ligated by megalin as it has been found to ligate aminoglycoside antibiotics [26, 42]. The association of megalin SNPs with cisplatin-induced ototoxicity was studied. Half of the subjects included in the study lost hearing, while the other half were not affected by cisplatin. An equivalent dose of cisplatin was given to all the subjects. Megalin SNPs were divided into two groups. The group that lost hearing had the SNP rs2075252 of A allele with more frequency. A total of 2 SNPs out of 757 were studied as these were not the same and they were rs2075252 and rs4668123 [43]. Lysine was changed to glutamic acid in rs2075252 SNP as mRNA of megalin at position 12,384 G nucleotide changed to A. Alanine was changed with threonine amino acid in rs4668123 SNP as mRNA of megalin at position 8718 has a transition of A to G nucleotide.

The occurrence of rs2075252 was higher in the subjects with normal hearing impairment, but it was not so in all patients who were affected with cisplatin-induced ototoxicity. In a recent study of a large group of children in Canada, there was no identification that cisplatin ototoxicity is associated with rs2075252 [44]. These findings can neither be refuted nor accepted as more studies of larger samples of cisplatin-induced hearing loss affected patients are required.

16.5.3 Cisplatin-Induced Ototoxicity and GST Polymorphisms

Inner ear expresses two proteins, namely, GSTM and GSTP [45–47]. These two proteins and GSTT1 gene are involved in the induction of cisplatin-induced ototoxicity. GSTP1, GSTT1, and GSTM1 genes control most of GST polymorphisms that are linked with cisplatin ototoxicity. The enzymatic activity of GST is either lowered or lost due to these genes.

Cisplatin ototoxicity-related GST polymorphisms were first studied by Peters et al. [48]. They found that the patients with normal hearing had GSTM∗3B allele oftentimes as compared to those with hearing loss. Thus, the first evidence that the GST polymorphisms are associated with hearing loss due to cisplatin in children was found. Later, Oldenburg et al. communicated the link between the GSTM1 and GSTP1 alleles and protection from hearing loss due to cisplatin [49]. On the other hand, Ross et al. studied about 2000 SNPs to find out variations in 220 genes. He found no link between cisplatin-induced ototoxicity and the alleles GSTP1 or GSTM1.

16.5.4 Thiopurine S-Methyltransferase and Catechol-*O*-methyltransferase and Ototoxicity

Studies have shown variants of catechol-*O*-methyltransferase (COMT) and thiopurine S-methyltransferase (TPMT) linked to ototoxicity caused by cisplatin; these variants are rs12201199 and rs9332377 for TPMT and COMT, respectively. About 90% of patients were diagnosed with COMT risk allele, rs9332377. TPMT is involved in metabolism of exogenous purine compounds, for example, azathioprine metabolites. It is responsible for inactivation of such metabolites. Possibly cisplatin-bound purine inactivity is decreased as the TPMT enzyme synthesis is reduced. So, it results in the formation of greater DNA cross-links with cisplatin, and toxicity is increased. S-adenosylmethionine (SAM) is a methyl donor and required by TPMT and COMT in methionine pathway as they are methyltransferases [44]. Decreased activity of

TPMT and COMT enzymes may result in elevated levels of S-adenosylmethionine that can be the reason of ototoxicity. But studies have shown no proof of SAM ototoxicity. In a study of an enzyme that resembles COMT about 60%, it is revealed that COMT is important for normal hearing in both humans and mice. So, it is suggested that cisplatin-treated patients may loss hearing as COMT level is lowered [50].

16.5.5 Other Genes Related to Cisplatin-Induced Ototoxicity

Mitochondrial DNA was studied for mutations of haplotype by Peters et al. [51]. It was found that more than half of patients administered with cisplatin were characterized with hearing loss. They found that mitochondrial mutations 7472insC, A7445G, and A1555G were not the reason of toxicity but the clustering of haplotype J as they were present in the patients with cisplatin-induced ototoxicity oftentimes.

Eight SNPs were studied by Caronia et al. in patients who were treated with cisplatin [52]. Cisplatin ototoxicity was found to be related to rs2228001 SNP. This SNP in gene XPC had genotypes CC and AA with carrying mutation for hearing loss.

16.6 Cisplatin-Induced Nephrotoxicity

Among different side effects of cisplatin, nephrotoxicity is common and found in the patients with renal cancer who are treated with the drug. Pharmacogenomics of nephrotoxicity has been studied to find out prevention and vulnerability to this adverse drug reaction. Cisplatin nephrotoxicity was found to be due to polymorphisms total eight in number. Out of all these, cisplatin nephrotoxicity was found to be related to only SNP rs316019 of SLCC2A2 gene, OCT2 transporter gene. This SNP resulted in change of serum creatinine (SCr). Transporter function is changed by SNP rs316019 within SLCC2A2 an 808G>T transversion results.

DNA repair mechanism is altered in renal cells and is a notable reason of nephrotoxicity. Nucleotide excision repair genes (ERCC) eliminate lesions due to which helical structure of DNA may be disturbed. If ERCC is varied, proteins for repair are altered and repair function is also altered. ERCC1 is not associated to any SNPs, but ERCC2 is found to have SNP rs13181 where glycine is substituted instead of lysine. DNA repair mechanism is much likely to be affected by SNP rs13181 of ERCC2 [53].

16.7 Limiting Factors

The pharmacogenomics of cisplatin-induced nephrotoxicity has not yet been studied comprehensively due to different limiting factors that include:

1. Different types of cancers
2. Ethnicity

3. Small samples
4. Adjuvant chemotherapies, etc.

16.8 Conclusion

Cisplatin causes toxicity among children in different ways including cisplatin-induced hearing loss or ototoxicity and nephrotoxicity. It reacts with DNA and results in polymorphisms that produce proteins (enzymes and receptors) with altered functions than those vital for body leading to adverse side effects. Despite cisplatin's high cure rate, the adverse side effects of drug cannot be omitted, and it is needed to use some safer chemotherapeutics. Several genetic polymorphisms related to cisplatin-induced toxicity have been reported with conflict in importance of different genes and their variants related to toxicity. Different reports have used several criteria and statistical methods to analyze cisplatin's role in inducing toxicity among children. Naturally different patients having different cancers or tumor types are administrated with varying cumulative dose, so they give varied results. There is a need to carry pharmacogenomic research on larger scale to get robust and relying results for assessing risk related to cisplatin toxicity. As toxicology of cisplatin toxicity is complex, limited works are not much reliable as there may be far more polymorphisms for a single type of toxicity such as ototoxicity. Further there is a need to carry more specific research without adjuvant chemotherapies.

References

1. Lippert B (ed) (1999) Cisplatin: chemistry and biochemistry of a leading anticancer drug. Wiley, Zürich, pp 3–27
2. Rosenberg B, Van Camp L, Krigas T (1965) Inhibition of cell division in Escherichia coli by electrolysis products from a platinum electrode. Nature 205:698–699. https://doi.org/10.1038/205698a0
3. Rosenberg B, Van Camp L, Grimley EB, Thomson AJ (1967) The inhibition of growth or cell division in Escherichia coli by different ionic species of platinum(IV) complexes. J Biol Chem 242:1347–1352
4. Rosenberg B, Renshaw E, Vancamp L et al (1967) Platinum-induced filamentous growth in Escherichia coli. J Bacteriol 93:716–721
5. Rosenberg B, Vancamp L, Trosko JE, Mansour VH (1969) Platinum compounds: a new class of potent antitumour agents. Nature 222:385–386. https://doi.org/10.1038/222385a0
6. Rosenberg B, VanCamp L (1970) The successful regression of large solid sarcoma 180 tumors by platinum compounds. Cancer Res 30:1799–1802
7. Peyrone (1845) Cisplatin. M Ann 51:15
8. Mellor DP (1943) The stereochemistry of square complexes. Chem Rev 33:137–183. https://doi.org/10.1021/cr60105a003
9. Kauffman G (1997) B Plat Met Rev 41:34–40
10. Werner A (1893) Beitrag zur Konstitution anorganischer Verbindungen. Z Anorg Chem 3:267–330. https://doi.org/10.1002/zaac.18930030136
11. Dhara SC (1970) Indian J Chem 8:193–134

12. Basolo F, Pearson RG (1967) Mechanisms of inorganic reactions: a study of metal complexes in solution. Wiley, New York, pp 351–453
13. Natile G, Coluccia M (2001) Coord Chem Rev 216–217:383410
14. Kauffman GB, Cowan DO, Slusarczuk G, Kirschner S (2007) Cis- and trans-Dichlorodiammineplatinum(II). In: Kleinberg J (ed) Inorganic syntheses. Wiley, Hoboken, pp 239–245
15. Sigel A, Sigel H (eds) (2004) Metal ions and their complexes in medication. Marcel Dekker, New York
16. Vollano JF, Al-Baker S, Dabrowiak JC, Schurig JE (1987) J Med Chem 30:716–719
17. Ellis L, Er H, Hambley T (1995) The influence of the axial ligands of a series of platinum(IV) anti-cancer complexes on their reduction to platinum(II) and reaction with DNA. Aust J Chem 48:793–806. https://doi.org/10.1071/CH9950793
18. Galanski M, Keppler BK (1996) Carboxylation of dihydroxoplatinum(IV) complexes via a new synthetic pathway. Inorg Chem 35:1709–1711. https://doi.org/10.1021/ic9509490
19. Ivanov AI, Christodoulou J, Parkinson JA et al (1998) Cisplatin binding sites on human albumin. J Biol Chem 273:14721–14730. https://doi.org/10.1074/jbc.273.24.14721
20. Silvestru C (1994) Metal complexes in cancer chemotherapy. B. K. Keppler (ed) VCH, Weinheim and New York, 1993, 429 pp. DM 196, ISBN 3-527-28425-7 (VCH, Weinheim); ISBN 1-56081-216-8 (VCH, New York). Appl Organomet Chem 8:499–500. https://doi.org/10.1002/aoc.590080511
21. DeConti RC, Toftness BR, Lange RC, Creasey WA (1973) Clinical and pharmacological studies with cis-diamminedichloroplatinum (II). Cancer Res 33:1310–1315
22. Kelland LR (2000) Preclinical perspectives on platinum resistance. Drugs 59(Suppl 4):1–8. https://doi.org/10.2165/00003495-200059004-00001
23. Desoize B (2002) Cancer and metals and metal compounds: part I--carcinogenesis. Crit Rev Oncol Hematol 42:1–3
24. Rybak LP, Mukherjea D, Jajoo S, Ramkumar V (2009) Cisplatin ototoxicity and protection: clinical and experimental studies. Tohoku J Exp Med 219:177–186. https://doi.org/10.1620/tjem.219.177
25. Mukherjea D, Rybak LP, Sheehan KE et al (2011) The design and screening of drugs to prevent acquired sensorineural hearing loss. Expert Opin Drug Discovery 6:491–505. https://doi.org/10.1517/17460441.2011.562887
26. Tauris J, Christensen EI, Nykjaer A et al (2009) Cubilin and megalin co-localize in the neonatal inner ear. Audiol Neurootol 14:267–278. https://doi.org/10.1159/000199446
27. Barnham KJ, Djuran MI, Murdoch P del S et al (1996) Ring-opened adducts of the anticancer drug carboplatin with sulfur amino acids. Inorg Chem 35:1065–1072. https://doi.org/10.1021/ic950973d
28. Lempers ELM, Reedijk J (1991) Adv Inorg Chem 37:175–217
29. Andrews PA, Wung WE, Howell SB (1984) A high-performance liquid chromatographic assay with improved selectivity for cisplatin and active platinum (II) complexes in plasma ultrafiltrate. Anal Biochem 143:46–56. https://doi.org/10.1016/0003-2697(84)90556-6
30. Dolman RC, Deacon GB, Hambley TW (2002) Studies of the binding of a series of platinum(IV) complexes to plasma proteins. J Inorg Biochem 88:260–267. https://doi.org/10.1016/S0162-0134(01)00360-9
31. Borch RF, Pleasants ME (1979) Inhibition of cis-platinum nephrotoxicity by diethyldithiocarbamate rescue in a rat model. Proc Natl Acad Sci 76:6611–6614. https://doi.org/10.1073/pnas.76.12.6611
32. Gately DP, Howell SB (1993) Cellular accumulation of the anticancer agent cisplatin: a review. Br J Cancer 67:1171–1176. https://doi.org/10.1038/bjc.1993.221
33. Ishida S, Lee J, Thiele DJ, Herskowitz I (2002) Uptake of the anticancer drug cisplatin mediated by the copper transporter Ctr1 in yeast and mammals. Proc Natl Acad Sci 99:14298–14302. https://doi.org/10.1073/pnas.162491399
34. Davies MS, Berners-Price SJ, Hambley TW (2000) Slowing of cisplatin aquation in the presence of DNA but not in the presence of phosphate: improved understanding of sequence

selectivity and the roles of monoaquated and diaquated species in the binding of cisplatin to DNA. Inorg Chem 39:5603–5613. https://doi.org/10.1021/ic000847w
35. Lippert B (ed) (1999) Cisplatin: chemistry and biochemistry of a leading anticancer drug. Wiley, Zürich, pp 183–206
36. Lippert B (ed) (1999) Cisplatin: chemistry and biochemistry of a leading anticancer drug. Wiley, Zürich, pp 207–222
37. Lippert B (ed) (1999) Cisplatin: chemistry and biochemistry of a leading anticancer drug. Wiley, Zürich, pp 223–246
38. Jamieson ER, Lippard SJ (1999) Structure, recognition, and processing of cisplatin-DNA adducts. Chem Rev 99:2467–2498
39. Hambley TW (2001) Platinum binding to DNA: structural controls and consequences. J Chem Soc Dalton Trans 2001:2711–2718. https://doi.org/10.1039/B105406F
40. Cohen GL, Ledner JA, Bauer WR, Ushay HM, Caravana C, Lippard SJ (1980) J Am Chem Sot 102:2487–2488
41. Fuertes MA, Castilla J, Alonso C, Pérez JM (2002) Novel concepts in the development of platinum antitumor drugs. Curr Med Chem Anticancer Agents 2:539–551
42. Mizuta K, Saito A, Watanabe T et al (1999) Ultrastructural localization of megalin in the rat cochlear duct. Hear Res 129:83–91. https://doi.org/10.1016/s0378-5955(98)00221-4
43. Riedemann L, Lanvers C, Deuster D et al (2008) Megalin genetic polymorphisms and individual sensitivity to the ototoxic effect of cisplatin. Pharmacogenomics J 8:23–28. https://doi.org/10.1038/sj.tpj.6500455
44. Ross CJD, Katzov-Eckert H, Dubé M-P et al (2009) Genetic variants in TPMT and COMT are associated with hearing loss in children receiving cisplatin chemotherapy. Nat Genet 41:1345–1349. https://doi.org/10.1038/ng.478
45. el Barbary A, Altschuler RA, Schacht J (1993) Glutathione S-transferases in the organ of Corti of the rat: enzymatic activity, subunit composition and immunohistochemical localization. Hear Res 71:80–90. https://doi.org/10.1016/0378-5955(93)90023-t
46. Touliatos JS, Neitzel L, Whitworth C et al (2000) Effect of cisplatin on the expression of glutathione-S-transferase in the cochlea of the rat. Eur Arch Otorhinolaryngol 257:6–9
47. Fujimura T, Suzuki H, Udaka T et al (2008) Immunoreactivities for glutathione S-transferases and glutathione peroxidase in the lateral wall of pigmented and albino guinea pig cochlea. Med Mol Morphol 41:139–144. https://doi.org/10.1007/s00795-008-0405-z
48. Peters U, Preisler-Adams S, Hebeisen A et al (2000) Glutathione S-transferase genetic polymorphisms and individual sensitivity to the ototoxic effect of cisplatin. Anti-Cancer Drugs 11:639–643
49. Oldenburg J, Kraggerud SM, Cvancarova M et al (2007) Cisplatin-induced long-term hearing impairment is associated with specific glutathione s-transferase genotypes in testicular cancer survivors. J Clin Oncol 25:708–714. https://doi.org/10.1200/JCO.2006.08.9599
50. Pussegoda KA (2010) Genetic variants associated with cisplatin-induced hearing loss. Clin Genet 78:33–35. https://doi.org/10.1111/j.1399-0004.2010.01414_2.x
51. Peters U, Preisler-Adams S, Lanvers-Kaminsky C et al (2003) Sequence variations of mitochondrial DNA and individual sensitivity to the ototoxic effect of cisplatin. Anticancer Res 23:1249–1255
52. Caronia D, Patiño-García A, Milne RL et al (2009) Common variations in ERCC2 are associated with response to cisplatin chemotherapy and clinical outcome in osteosarcoma patients. Pharmacogenomics J 9:347–353. https://doi.org/10.1038/tpj.2009.19
53. Zazuli Z, Vijverberg S, Slob E et al (2018) Genetic variations and cisplatin nephrotoxicity: a systematic review. Front Pharmacol 9:1111. https://doi.org/10.3389/fphar.2018.01111

Pharmacogenomics of Methotrexate-Induced Toxicity in Children

17

Amna Riaz, Maliha Ghaffar, and Hina Salahuddin

17.1 Introduction to Methotrexate

Methotrexate (MTX) is an immune system suppressant and a chemotherapy drug. It is also known as amethopterin, methotrexate, mexate, or methyl aminopterin [1]. It is a competitive inhibitor of the enzyme DHFR that helps in the formation of RNA. It also inhibits another enzyme TS used in DNA synthesis [2–4]. It is used in the treatment of various forms of cancer like leukemia, osteosarcoma, lymphoma, and breast cancer [5–9]. Moreover, it is also used in treating other medical conditions such as abortions, ectopic pregnancy, autoimmune diseases like rheumatoid arthritis, psoriasis, and Crohn's disease [10, 11]. MTX efficiently treats various disorders linked with rapid cellular growth. But some patients develop resistance and others experience different toxic side effects. Patients showed sensitivity to MTX, as drug efficacy can be modulated by respective genes that control their activity.

Several studies have reported the potential of MTX as genetically tailored medicine for rheumatoid arthritis and leukemia patients. Methylenetetrahydrofolate reductase and TS genes are the most frequently studied genetic variants that are assumed to have a good predictive role.

A. Riaz · H. Salahuddin (✉)
University of Okara, Okara, Pakistan
e-mail: hina.salahuddin3@gmail.com

M. Ghaffar
Department of Zoology, University of Okara, Okara, Pakistan

N. Masood, S. Shakil Malik (eds.), *'Essentials of Cancer Genomic, Computational Approaches and Precision Medicine*,
https://doi.org/10.1007/978-981-15-1067-0_17

17.2 Discovery

MTX was made in 1947 and recommended for cancer treatment due to less toxicity at that time as compared to other available treatment strategies. In 1947, Sidney Farber with his team of researchers showed that a chemical analog of folic acid aminopterin could be used in the treatment of acute lymphoblastic leukemia (ALL) in children. It was observed that a diet containing folic acid could produce an increase in the effects of disease, whereas the use of folic acid analog worsened leukemia.

In 1950, MTX was proposed as an effectual drug in treating leukemia. In 1951, MTX was used in solid tumors and for temporary recovery from breast cancer. In 1956 some studies showed that MTX had a better therapeutic index than that of aminopterin [12]. Later on, the drug was used for choriocarcinoma and chorioadenoma, metastatic cancer, and mycosis fungoides [13].

17.3 Administration

MTX can be given by mouth or by injection. To limit toxicity the drug is prescribed to be taken weekly and not daily. Routine monitoring of the complete blood count is recommended. Also, after at least every 2 months, creatinine and liver function tests are suggested.

17.4 Structure

MTX has a molecular formula C20H22N8O5 and an average mass of 454.439 Da. Chemical structures of MTX are very similar to folic acid. MTX consists of a pteridine ring and p-aminobenzoic acid plus glutamic acid, whereas the folic acid structure is different due to substitution of a hydroxyl group (OH) for an amine and on the tenth nitrogen of p-aminobenzoic acid by addition of a methyl group in the pteridine ring.

17.5 Mechanism of Action

MTX is an antimetabolite just like other usual cellular materials. They inhibit certain cellular pathways and cell division by competing with normal cellular material. MTX competes with folic acid in cancer cells, which leads to the deficiency of folic acid and hence the death of cells. This is referred to as the chemotherapeutic toxicity of MTX. However, a drawback of MTX is that it causes different side effects by competing with folic acid in other normal cells of the body. These side effects can be diarrhea, liver damage, low blood cell counts, kidney damage, hair loss, nerve damage, and mouth sores.

MTX inhibits the enzymes DHFR and TS, thus limiting DNA and RNA synthesis [2, 3, 14]. It enters cells using an active transport system of folic acid. MTX then undergoes polyglumatation. MTXGlu inhibits the enzymes more effectively. The reduced level of folic acid is maintained by the enzyme DHFR by reducing dihydrofolic acid. DHFR reduces folic acid to an essential cofactor in the purine synthesis, i.e., tetrahydrofolate.

The normal process occurring in a cell is that folic acid (vitamin B9) is converted into dihydrofolate (DHF) by the enzyme DHFR. The same enzyme catalyzes the conversion of dihydrofolate into tetrahydrofolate (THF). Then this THF compound is converted into N5,N10-methylenetetrahydrofolate. N5,N10-methylenetetrahydrofolate helps in the conversion of deoxyuridine monophosphate into thymidine monophosphate by the enzyme TS. In this way, it helps in DNA synthesis, RNA synthesis, and synthesis of purine nucleotides.

MTX inhibits the production of DHFR, so no tetrahydrofolate is produced, and ultimately no N5,N10-methylenetetrahydrofolate is produced. As N5,N10-methylenetetrahydrofolate was required for the action of TS, its absence will affect the cell normal activity mainly cell replication, protein synthesis, DNA and RNA synthesis, and ultimately cell division.

In cancer, it is helpful because it stops the growth and division of cancerous cells, but it also affects the division of non-cancerous or normal body cells.

Cancerous cells and normal cells are different in their cell division. In the case of normal cells contact inhibition, a mechanism is present, i.e., when they encounter similar cells, they will stop dividing. Cancer cells do not possess any inhibition mechanism. Cancer cells divide rapidly and continuously. This uncontrolled proliferation of cancer cells results in the formation of a tumor.

The tumor will shrink if the cancer cells cannot divide. It is achieved through chemotherapy in which the RNA or DNA of cancer cells, that control cell division, is targeted and damaged. Chemotherapy drugs are effective both to dividing cells/cell-cycle specific and to cells that are at rest/cell-cycle non-specific. Type of cancer cells and the rate of their proliferation determine the schedule of chemotherapy.

Chemotherapy drugs cannot differentiate between the cancer cells and the normal cells, so the use of MTX leads to certain side effects like nausea, mouth sores, diarrhea, or hair loss. The normal cells that are usually affected by chemotherapy are cells of hair follicles, mouth, stomach, and blood cells.

Usually, the use of MTX could result in side effects like fever, nausea, increased risk of infection, feeling tired, soreness of mouth and tongue, and low white blood cell counts. Some side effects may be in the form of liver disease, lymphoma, lung disease, and severe form of skin rashes. Patients who are on long-term treatment should be checked regularly for the presence of any side effects. If anyone has kidney problems, lower doses of MTX may be needed. It is also not safe to use this during breastfeeding.

17.6 Introduction to Pharmacogenomics

Pharmacogenetics refers to how variation caused in a single gene will influence the response to a single drug, whereas pharmacogenomics involves the use of genetic information to help the doctor to choose the drug wisely and its dose on an individual basis. So, we can say that pharmacogenomics further includes pharmacogenetics.

17.7 The Foundation of Pharmacogenomics

Certain factors cause a change in the gene, and as a result, every individual responds differently to the drug. This change may be due to mutation or polymorphism. Mutation is due to the difference in the DNA code that occurs in less than 1% of the population. Genetic polymorphism is a difference in DNA sequence among individuals of a population. It occurs in at least 1% of the population but makes up about 90% of all human genetic variation. Polymorphism can result in different stop codons or amino acids. It may also change in the functioning of the protein. By use of pharmacogenomics, we can give patients personalized medicines in which the treatment for a particular disease is chosen based on characteristics of the individual patient rather than the average patient.

17.8 Pharmacogenomics of Methotrexate

MTX is an efficient drug in treating various disorders in which there is rapid cellular growth. But some of the patients develop resistance toward this and others observe toxic side effects [15]. MTX functions by the inhibition of folate-dependent enzymes. The patient show sensitivity to MTX as drug efficacy can be modulated by the genes that control their activity. Several studies that are being conducted mostly in rheumatoid arthritis and leukemia patients have brought into light the potential for tailoring MTX therapy based on the genetics of the patient. MTHFR and TS genes are the most frequently studied genetic variants that are assumed to have a good predictive role.

17.9 Toxicity

We know MTX is a chemotherapeutic agent, and it works by inhibiting the folic acid cycle and an enzyme TS. It is used for the treatment of many diseases like neck cancer, osteosarcoma, ALL, lymphoma, neck and lung cancer, trophoblastic neoplasms, and bladder cancer [16–18]. But sometimes MTX-based chemotherapy can result in many severe toxicities. In such cases, the dose is reduced, or treatment is completely stopped. MTX toxicity can be caused because the patient becomes more sensitive to infections during the treatment. It may also be caused by excessive intrathecal, parenteral administration or intentional oral overdoses of MTX. Therapeutic errors by patients might cause toxicity in some cases, for example, if a patient takes MTX orally daily instead of weekly or in case of self-administration of MTX to induce abortion. This toxicity can cause vomiting, nausea, diarrhea, stomatitis, mucositis, esophagitis, renal failure, an elevated level of hepatic enzymes, acute lung injury, rash, hypotension, tachycardia, stroke-like symptoms neurologic dysfunction like headache, depression, seizures, encephalopathy, and even coma. Toxic effects of MTX might be caused for several hours to days to weeks after normal or excessive use of MTX. Due to variations in pharmacokinetics and pharmacodynamics, from patient to patient, the possible risk for MTX-induced toxicity is not possible at the current time.

It is hypothesized that MTX-induced toxicity is due to mutations in the gene for an enzyme MTHFR that aids in folate metabolism. One of the main assumed factors for causing polymorphism is C to T transition at nucleotide 677 (C677T, rs1801133) as it is involved in increasing homocysteine level and change in folate supply by decreasing the activity of the enzyme [19]. Another factor that affects the activity of enzyme though to less extent is A to C 1298 polymorphism (A1298C, rs1801131).

When the direct investigation for effect of MTX-induced toxicity and the potential for personalized medicine was done on A1298C and MTHFR C677T, the result varied greatly [20]. There is very contradictory evidence about the link between germline variation and MTX-induced toxicity [21]. Also, there is inconsistent evidence about the link between toxicity and MTHFR C677T polymorphisms, whereas it is assumed that both increase and decrease in risk of toxicity are somehow linked with MTHFR A1298C polymorphism.

The risk for carrying a variant allele for different toxicities like hepatic toxicity, gastrointestinal toxicity, oral mucositis, myelosuppression, and hematological toxicity is different [20, 22]. Also, it depends on the type of cancer that MTX is used for because different MTX regimens are used in different types of cancer and patients also respond to these drugs differently.

17.10 Pharmacogenomics of Methotrexate-Induced Toxicity in Children

The genetic determinants of MTX toxicity are discovered by various pharmacogenetic studies. The action of MTX on folate metabolism involves a complex structure that encompasses numerous metabolizing enzymes and several transporters whose expression and/or function have been suggested to be changed by genetic polymorphisms.

Many studies were conducted that showed how chemotherapy toxicity of MTX could have resulted from genetic polymorphisms. According to a study by Moscow in 1995, it was deduced that MTX enters into the cells by the reduced folate carrier 1, whereas it is removed from the cell with the help of numerous ATP-binding cassette (ABC) efflux transporters [23, 24]. According to a study in 1985 by Chabner, it was assumed that in the cell, MTX is metabolized to active polyglutamates, which cause a disturbance in folate metabolic pathway by inhibition of the enzymes required for DNA synthesis [14]. These enzymes are TS and DHFR [2, 3]. In addition to this, MTHFR is also one of the enzymes that aid in the production of 5-methyl-tetrahydrofolate (THF) from 5,10-methylenetetrahydrofolate, an intermediary that is itself synthesized by serine hydroxymethyltransferase (SHMT1) [25]. Also, the production of 5-methyl-tetrahydrofolate is crucial for the biotransformation of homocysteine to methionine. Methionine synthase reductase (MTRR) and methionine synthase (MS) are two of the main enzymes that are included in this conversion.

17.11 Methotrexate and ABC Efflux Transporters

ABC efflux transporters are also associated with MTX-induced toxicity. Polymorphism in ABC efflux transporter leads to neurotoxicity and accumulation of the drug in the brain as they are located in the blood-brain barrier. For example, the presence of the C421A (rs2231142, Gln141Lys) SNP in the ABCG2 gene that codes protein BCRP and the C3435T transition in ABCB1 that codes for the P-glycoprotein are assumed to be involved in causing encephalopathy in children with ALL that is treated with MTX [26]. Also, polymorphism of G-80A, which predicts the intracellular levels of MTX, in the RFC1influx transporter cause toxicity in patients of ALL [27–29].

17.12 Methotrexate Toxicity and 677T Allele

It is assumed that neurotoxicity is caused by 677T allele in young patients of acute lymphocytic leukemia ALL [30–33]. However, this is only seen in clinical case reports. For example, a study was conducted on 53 children suffering from ALL. They were treated with a high-dose of MTX. MTX did not clearly depict the role of 677T allele causing neurotoxicity because only nine of the patients developed it [34]. To overcome this problem, it might be preferable to genotype huge populations of patients who had suffered MTX-induced neurotoxicity. So, we can conclude that some major problems faced in conducting such studies are the low level of people affected, and it also because different SNPs can be associated at a time.

17.13 Methotrexate Toxicity and SLC19A1

ALL and non-Hodgkin malignant lymphoma (NHML) pediatric patients have been studied for mutations in SLC19A1 having MTX-induced adverse drug reactions [35]. In some cases, rs1051266 AA genotype was found to be protected, while in others it showed either no role at all or was associated with an elevated risk of adverse drug reaction due to MTX. Many studies were carried on SNP rs1051266 in SLC19A1 gene and other SNPs. Another SNP rs2832958 with TT genotype was associated with the development of mucositis. Another SNP rs2838951 occurred frequently in patients who did not develop any kind of toxicity due to MTX. About 384 SNPs were investigated by Lopez-Lopez that also included SLC19A1 gene [36]. These SNPs were studied for association with MTX-induced toxicity. The plasma level was not found related to SLC19A1 gene [36]. MTX toxicity was associated with rs11045879 SNP of SLCO1B1 gene [37]. SNPs rs3740065 in ABCC2 and rs9516519 in ABCC4 were related to MTX-induced adverse drug reactions. Another study suggested the ways in which rs1051266 is one of the reasons why MTX toxicity is caused [38]. The SNP rs1051266 along with SNP rs1131956 had a protective role, and rs2838956 had a role in the protection of adverse drug reactions to the skin. The SNPs rs7499, rs2838956, rs3788200, and rs1051266 were also involved in methotrexate-induced gastrointestinal toxicity and rheumatoid arthritis.

17.14 Methotrexate Toxicity and MTHFR

In studying factors related to ALL, MTHFR is studied most. The two most common factors that enhance toxicity caused by MTX are A1298C (rs1801131) and C677T (rs1801133) [39, 40]. But according to the latest and deeper studies of currently available literature, it is assumed that the only important single nucleotide polymorphism (SNP) is caused by C677T, even though some antipodal studies also exist [28, 41, 42].

MTX toxicity has been studied in childhood osteosarcoma patients. Earlier studies suggested the association of MTHFR 677TT gene with methotrexate-induced toxicity such as hepatotoxicity and MTX plasma level, etc. No relation between MTX toxicity and MTHFR 677TT polymorphisms was suggested by Park et al. Alpenc et al. studied ALL patients and did not find a relation between MTHFR 677TT polymorphism and methotrexate-induced toxicity. A study on ALL and osteosarcoma patients showed that MTHFR allele T resulted in hepatotoxicity more as compared to MTHFR C allele. Similarly, hematological toxicity has also been reported to be associated with MTHFR 677TT gene.

17.15 Toxic Effects Caused in Children Using MTX for Treatment of Juvenile Idiopathic Arthritis

Methotrexate (MTX) is the foremost option for the disease-modifying antirheumatic drug (DMARD) for treating juvenile idiopathic arthritis (JIA) [16, 43, 44]. This drug not only reduces arthritis in these children but also has a positive role in both psychosocial and physical quality of life [45]. Despite these advantages, there are some disadvantages of using this drug too. The major drawback is that some children face trouble in taking MTX. The most frequently occurring side effects include vomiting and nausea, and in 10–20% of patients, it causes some abnormalities in liver test [46, 47]. However, folinic acid and folic acid aid in the minimization of the side effects that are resulted from MTX [48, 49]. Sometimes reluctance to MTX and anticipatory nausea may develop if a child kept on experiencing vomiting or nausea after intake of MTX. In some children, it also causes fear of injections or blood monitoring tests that may further give rise to different problems.

The main aim of Sport Aiding Medical Research for Kids (SPARKS) Childhood Arthritis Response to Medication Study (CHARMS) is to study various factors that result in different responses of children with juvenile idiopathic arthritis to MTX [50, 51]. Another study was done to collect data from mothers of children who were suffering from juvenile idiopathic arthritis to know about the factors and extent of methotrexate-related adverse events. One hundred seventy-one mothers took part in the study. The majority of children had vomiting or nausea after taking MTX. Among these, some suffered from anticipatory nausea because they were afraid of injections or giving blood tests. This study concluded that problems in using MTX for treatment of JIA is dominant in an only a notable proportion of children. It also might cause a negative effect on health-related quality of life. We should develop different ways of minimizing these problems [51].

17.16 Folate Metabolic Pathway SNPs as a Pharmacogenetic Marker of Methotrexate

In a study, the pharmacogenetic effect of genetic polymorphisms in folate metabolic pathway genes in Indian rheumatoid arthritis patients taking MTX was evaluated. Twelve polymorphisms in 9 folate pathway genes were studied for the response caused by MTX in 322 patients of Indian rheumatoid arthritis and MTX pharmacokinetics in 94 patients of Indian rheumatoid arthritis. The following results were obtained. Methotrexate-related adverse events were due to polymorphisms in GGH, SHMT1, GGH, and TS, whereas MTX efficacy was associated with SNPs in RFC1/SLC19A1 and MTHFR. The study concluded that polymorphisms in the genes of folate-methotrexate pathway play a significant role in response to MTX [52].

17.17 Current Status and Future Outlook of Pharmacogenomics of Methotrexate

MTX is a folate analog that has a very high therapeutic efficiency in treating cancers and other autoimmune disorders. However, the toxicity and effectiveness of MTX might be changed due to genetic polymorphisms in different genes that are involved in MTX metabolic pathway. To provide a productive, accost effective, and appropriate treatment for patients, we should focus on personalized pharmacotherapy that is based on gene polymorphisms [53].

The effect of SNPs in the genes that are involved in MTX pathway is contradictory. Most of the pharmacogenetic associations are race-specific and disease-specific. The current studies are just limited to a few important diseases and ethnic groups. So, the data from such studies are not helpful enough in clinical practice for the pharmacogenetic application of MTX. In the future, we need to study this on a bigger level and at multiple centers. MTX-PG inhibits folic acid metabolism in three different ways. These three rate-limiting enzymes are TS, MTX hydrofolate reductase, and 5-aminoimidazole-4-carboxamide ribonucleotide. These SNPs have a one-sided function in these genes. Therefore, we need to conduct studies that focus more on the analysis of polymorphism in methotrexate transporters [53].

17.18 Conclusion

Methotrexate (MTX) is an immune system suppressant and a chemotherapy drug that disrupts the folate cycle in the cell by inhibiting the enzymes like DHFR and TS. Proper functioning of these enzymes is important in DNA synthesis, RNA synthesis, protein synthesis, and overall normal cell division. When the activity of these enzymes is inhibited, all these processes are disturbed, and cell division is ceased. This helps limit the growth and proliferation of cancerous cells. However, growth and division of normal cells are also affected which causes various types of toxicities. This part of the study was focused on methotrexate-induced toxicity in children and the variations occurring at the genome level by studying pharmacogenomics of MTX.

The main genes involved in showing important polymorphism are DHFR, MTX-PG, TS, SLC19A1, ATP-binding cassette C1 and two transporters (ABCC1, ABCC2), BCRP, MTHFR, and many others too. A number of studies have demonstrated the relation between MTX and related genes but MTX induced toxicity is not fully understood due to variation in genetic makeup from one individual to another and low level of people affected by the toxic effect of MTX drug.

References

1. Hagner N, Joerger M (2010) Cancer chemotherapy: targeting folic acid synthesis. Cancer Manag Res 2:293–301. https://doi.org/10.2147/CMR.S10043
2. Galivan J (1980) Evidence for the cytotoxic activity of polyglutamate derivatives of methotrexate. Mol Pharmacol 17:105–110
3. Szeto DW, Yung-Chi C, Rosowsky A et al (1979) Human thymidylate synthetase—III: effects of methotrexate and folate analogs. Biochem Pharmacol 28:2633–2637. https://doi.org/10.1016/0006-2952(79)90039-X
4. Visentin M, Zhao R, Goldman ID (2012) The antifolates. Hematol Oncol Clin North Am 26:629–648, ix. https://doi.org/10.1016/j.hoc.2012.02.002
5. Asselin BL, Devidas M, Wang C et al (2011) Effectiveness of high-dose methotrexate in T-cell lymphoblastic leukemia and advanced-stage lymphoblastic lymphoma: a randomized study by the Children's Oncology Group (POG 9404). Blood 118:874–883. https://doi.org/10.1182/blood-2010-06-292615
6. Colleoni M, Cole BF, Viale G et al (2010) Classical cyclophosphamide, methotrexate, and fluorouracil chemotherapy is more effective in triple-negative, node-negative breast cancer: results from two randomized trials of adjuvant chemoendocrine therapy for node-negative breast cancer. J Clin Oncol 28:2966–2973. https://doi.org/10.1200/JCO.2009.25.9549
7. Gennari A, Sormani MP, Pronzato P et al (2008) HER2 status and efficacy of adjuvant anthracyclines in early breast cancer: a pooled analysis of randomized trials. J Natl Cancer Inst 100:14–20. https://doi.org/10.1093/jnci/djm252
8. Jaffe N (2009) Osteosarcoma: review of the past, impact on the future. The American experience. Cancer Treat Res 152:239–262. https://doi.org/10.1007/978-1-4419-0284-9_12
9. Matloub Y, Bostrom BC, Hunger SP et al (2011) Escalating intravenous methotrexate improves event-free survival in children with standard-risk acute lymphoblastic leukemia: a report from the Children's Oncology Group. Blood 118:243–251. https://doi.org/10.1182/blood-2010-12-322909

10. Alghamdi K, Khurrum H (2013) Methotrexate for the treatment of generalized vitiligo. Saudi Pharm J 21:423–424. https://doi.org/10.1016/j.jsps.2012.12.003
11. Dell'anna ML, Picardo M (2006) A review and a new hypothesis for non-immunological pathogenetic mechanisms in vitiligo. Pigment Cell Res 19:406–411. https://doi.org/10.1111/j.1600-0749.2006.00333.x
12. Peiró Cadahía J, Bondebjerg J, Hansen CA et al (2018) Synthesis and evaluation of hydrogen peroxide sensitive prodrugs of methotrexate and aminopterin for the treatment of rheumatoid arthritis. J Med Chem 61:3503–3515. https://doi.org/10.1021/acs.jmedchem.7b01775
13. Mould DR, Hutson PR (2017) Critical considerations in anticancer drug development and dosing strategies: the past, present, and future. J Clin Pharmacol 57(Suppl 10):S116–S128. https://doi.org/10.1002/jcph.983
14. Chabner BA, Allegra CJ, Curt GA et al (1985) Polyglutamation of methotrexate. Is methotrexate a prodrug? J Clin Invest 76:907–912
15. Krajinovic M, Moghrabi A (2004) Pharmacogenetics of methotrexate. Pharmacogenomics 5:819–834. https://doi.org/10.1517/14622416.5.7.819
16. Beresford MW, Baildam EM (2009) New advances in the management of juvenile idiopathic arthritis–1: non-biological therapy. Arch Dis Child Educ Pract Ed 94:144–150. https://doi.org/10.1136/adc.2008.144576
17. Fuchs N, Bielack SS, Epler D et al (1998) Long-term results of the co-operative German-Austrian-Swiss osteosarcoma study group's protocol COSS-86 of intensive multidrug chemotherapy and surgery for osteosarcoma of the limbs. Ann Oncol 9:893–899. https://doi.org/10.1023/a:1008391103132
18. Guardiola E, Peyrade F, Chaigneau L et al (2004) Results of a randomised phase II study comparing docetaxel with methotrexate in patients with recurrent head and neck cancer. Eur J Cancer 40:2071–2076. https://doi.org/10.1016/j.ejca.2004.05.019
19. Hankey GJ, Eikelboom JW (1999) Homocysteine and vascular disease. Lancet 354:407–413. https://doi.org/10.1016/S0140-6736(98)11058-9
20. Yang L, Hu X, Xu L (2012) Impact of methylenetetrahydrofolate reductase (MTHFR) polymorphisms on methotrexate-induced toxicities in acute lymphoblastic leukemia: a meta-analysis. Tumour Biol 33:1445–1454. https://doi.org/10.1007/s13277-012-0395-2
21. Xie L, Guo W, Yang Y et al (2017) More severe toxicity of genetic polymorphisms on MTHFR activity in osteosarcoma patients treated with high-dose methotrexate. Oncotarget 9:11465–11476. https://doi.org/10.18632/oncotarget.23222
22. Umerez M, Gutierrez-Camino Á, Muñoz-Maldonado C et al (2017) MTHFR polymorphisms in childhood acute lymphoblastic leukemia: influence on methotrexate therapy. Pharmgenomics Pers Med 10:69–78. https://doi.org/10.2147/PGPM.S107047
23. Moscow JA, Gong M, He R et al (1995) Isolation of a gene encoding a human reduced folate carrier (RFC1) and analysis of its expression in transport-deficient, methotrexate-resistant human breast cancer cells. Cancer Res 55:3790–3794
24. Strand V, Cohen S, Schiff M, Leflunomide Rheumatoid Arthritis Investigators Group et al (1999) Treatment of active rheumatoid arthritis with leflunomide compared with placebo and methotrexate. Arch Intern Med 159:2542–2550. https://doi.org/10.1001/archinte.159.21.2542
25. Fowler B (2001) The folate cycle and disease in humans. Kidney Int 59:221–229. https://doi.org/10.1046/j.1523-1755.2001.07851.x
26. Erdilyi DJ, Kamory E, Csokay B et al (2008) Synergistic interaction of ABCB1 and ABCG2 polymorphisms predicts the prevalence of toxic encephalopathy during anticancer chemotherapy. Pharmacogenomics J 8:321–327
27. Imanishi H, Okamura N, Yagi M et al (2007) Genetic polymorphisms associated with adverse events and elimination of methotrexate in childhood acute lymphoblastic leukemia and malignant lymphoma. J Hum Genet 52:166–171
28. Kishi S, Cheng C, French D et al (2007) Ancestry and pharmacogenetics of antileukemic drug toxicity. Blood 109:4151–4157. https://doi.org/10.1182/blood-2006-10-054528
29. Shimasaki N, Mori T, Samejima H et al (2006) Effects of methylenetetrahydrofolate reductase and reduced folate carrier 1 polymorphisms on high-dose methotrexate-induced toxicities in

children with acute lymphoblastic leukemia or lymphoma. J Pediatr Hematol Oncol 28:64–68. https://doi.org/10.1097/01.mph.0000198269.61948.90
30. Mahadeo KM, Dhall G, Panigrahy A et al (2010) Subacute methotrexate neurotoxicity and cerebral venous sinus thrombosis in a 12-year-old with acute lymphoblastic leukemia and methylenetetrahydrofolate reductase (MTHFR) C677T polymorphism: homocysteine-mediated methotrexate neurotoxicity via direct endothelial injury. Pediatr Hematol Oncol 27:46–52. https://doi.org/10.3109/08880010903341904
31. Strunk T, Gottschalk S, Goepel W et al (2003) Subacute leukoencephalopathy after low-dose intrathecal methotrexate in an adolescent heterozygous for the MTHFR C677T polymorphism. Med Pediatr Oncol 40:48–50. https://doi.org/10.1002/mpo.10192
32. Vagace JM, Caceres-Marzal C, Jimenez M et al (2011) Methotrexate-induced subacute neurotoxicity in a child with acute lymphoblastic leukemia carrying genetic polymorphisms related to folate homeostasis. Am J Hematol 86:98–101. https://doi.org/10.1002/ajh.21897
33. Vagace JM, de la Maya MD, Caceres-Marzal C et al (2012) Central nervous system chemotoxicity during treatment of pediatric acute lymphoblastic leukemia/lymphoma. Crit Rev Oncol Hematol 84:274–286. https://doi.org/10.1016/j.critrevonc.2012.04.003
34. Kishi S, Griener J, Cheng C, Das S, Cook EH, Pei D et al (2003) Homocysteine, pharmacogenetics, and neurotoxicity in children with leukemia. J Clin Oncol 21:3084–3091
35. Kotnik BF, Jazbec J, Grabar PB et al (2017) Association between SLC19A1 gene polymorphism and high dose methotrexate toxicity in childhood acute lymphoblastic leukaemia and non-Hodgkin malignant lymphoma: introducing a haplotype based approach. Radiol Oncol 51:455–462. https://doi.org/10.1515/raon-2017-0040
36. Lopez-Lopez E, Ballesteros J, Piñan MA et al (2013) Polymorphisms in the methotrexate transport pathway: a new tool for MTX plasma level prediction in pediatric acute lymphoblastic leukemia. Pharmacogenet Genomics 23:53–61. https://doi.org/10.1097/FPC.0b013e32835c3b24
37. Bohanec Grabar P, Leandro-García LJ, Inglada-Pérez L et al (2012) Genetic variation in the SLC19A1 gene and methotrexate toxicity in rheumatoid arthritis patients. Pharmacogenomics 13:1583–1594. https://doi.org/10.2217/pgs.12.150
38. Romão VC, Lima A, Bernardes M et al (2014) Three decades of low-dose methotrexate in rheumatoid arthritis: can we predict toxicity? Immunol Res 60:289–310. https://doi.org/10.1007/s12026-014-8564-6
39. D'Angelo V, Ramaglia M, Iannotta A et al (2011) Methotrexate toxicity and efficacy during the consolidation phase in paediatric acute lymphoblastic leukaemia and MTHFR polymorphisms as pharmacogenetic determinants. Cancer Chemother Pharmacol 68:1339–1346. https://doi.org/10.1007/s00280-011-1665-1
40. Kantar M, Kosova B, Cetingul N et al (2009) Methylenetetrahydrofolate reductase C677T and A1298C gene polymorphisms and therapy-related toxicity in children treated for acute lymphoblastic leukemia and non-Hodgkin lymphoma. Leuk Lymphoma 50:912–917. https://doi.org/10.1080/10428190902893819
41. Chatzidakis K, Goulas A, Athanassiadou-Piperopoulou F et al (2006) Methylenetetrahydrofolate reductase C677T polymorphism: association with risk for childhood acute lymphoblastic leukemia and response during the initial phase of chemotherapy in Greek patients. Pediatr Blood Cancer 47:147–151. https://doi.org/10.1002/pbc.20574
42. Huang L, Tissing WJE, de Jonge R et al (2008) Polymorphisms in folate-related genes: association with side effects of high-dose methotrexate in childhood acute lymphoblastic leukemia. Leukemia 22:1798–1800. https://doi.org/10.1038/leu.2008.66
43. Ferrara G, Mastrangelo G, Barone P et al (2018) Methotrexate in juvenile idiopathic arthritis: advice and recommendations from the MARAJIA expert consensus meeting. Pediatr Rheumatol 16:46. https://doi.org/10.1186/s12969-018-0255-8
44. Giannini EH, Brewer EJ, Kuzmina N et al (1992) Methotrexate in resistant juvenile rheumatoid arthritis. Results of the U.S.A.-U.S.S.R. double-blind, placebo-controlled trial. The Pediatric Rheumatology Collaborative Study Group and The Cooperative Children's Study Group. N Engl J Med 326:1043–1049. https://doi.org/10.1056/NEJM199204163261602

45. Céspedes-Cruz A, Gutiérrez-Suárez R, Pistorio A et al (2008) Methotrexate improves the health-related quality of life of children with juvenile idiopathic arthritis. Ann Rheum Dis 67:309–314. https://doi.org/10.1136/ard.2007.075895
46. Braun J, Rau R (2009) An update on methotrexate. Curr Opin Rheumatol 21:216–223. https://doi.org/10.1097/BOR.0b013e328329c79d
47. Hashkes PJ, Laxer RM (2006) Update on the medical treatment of juvenile idiopathic arthritis. Curr Rheumatol Rep 8:450–458. https://doi.org/10.1007/s11926-006-0041-3
48. Shea B, Swinden MV, Tanjong Ghogomu E, et al. Folic acid and folinic acid for reducing side effects in patients receiving methotrexate for rheumatoid arthritis. Cochrane Database Syst Rev. 2013;CD000951. https://doi.org/10.1002/14651858.CD000951.pub2
49. Van Ede AE, Laan RF, Rood MJ et al (2001) Effect of folic or folinic acid supplementation on the toxicity and efficacy of methotrexate in rheumatoid arthritis: a forty-eight week, multicenter, randomized, double-blind, placebo-controlled study. Arthritis Rheum 44:1515–1524. https://doi.org/10.1002/1529-0131(200107)44:7<1515::AID-ART273>3.0.CO;2-7
50. Moncrieffe H, Hinks A, Ursu S et al (2010) Generation of novel pharmacogenomic candidates in the response to methotrexate in juvenile idiopathic arthritis: correlation between gene expression and genotype. Pharmacogenet Genomics 20:665–676. https://doi.org/10.1097/FPC.0b013e32833f2cd0
51. Mulligan K, Kassoumeri L, Etheridge A et al (2013) Mothers' reports of the difficulties that their children experience in taking methotrexate for Juvenile Idiopathic Arthritis and how these impact on quality of life. Pediatr Rheumatol 11:23. https://doi.org/10.1186/1546-0096-11-23
52. Ghodke-Puranik Y, Puranik AS, Shintre P et al (2015) Folate metabolic pathway single nucleotide polymorphisms: a predictive pharmacogenetic marker of methotrexate response in Indian (Asian) patients with rheumatoid arthritis. Pharmacogenomics 16:2019–2034. https://doi.org/10.2217/pgs.15.145
53. Cao M, Guo M, Wu D-Q, Meng L (2018) Pharmacogenomics of methotrexate: current status and future outlook. Curr Drug Metab 19:1182–1187. https://doi.org/10.2174/1389200219666171227201047

Pharmacogenomics of Thiopurine-Induced Toxicity in Children

18

Hina Salahuddin and Muhammad Junaid Iqbal Tahir

18.1 Introduction

Thiopurines are immunosuppressants, suppress the normal activity of body's immune system [1], and act as purine antimetabolites [2]. Most commonly used thiopurine drugs include azathioprine (AZA), mercaptopurine (6-MP), and thioguanine (6-TG) [3]. Different diseases, like acute lymphoblastic leukemia (ALL) and inflammatory bowel disease (IBD), can be cured by using thiopurine drugs. In the 1950s, Hitchings and Elion synthesize thiopurine drugs including 6-MP and 6-TG that play an important role in ALL (acute lymphoblastic leukemia) treatment [4]. 6-Mercaptopurine (6-MP) is used along with methotrexate (MTX) in ALL therapy. 6-MP and 6-TG act synergistically in inhibiting the synthesis of purine, one of the nucleotides of DNA [5]. These drugs also increase the insertion of thioguanine nucleotide (6-TGN) in nucleic acids (DNA and RNA), thus ultimately inhibiting DNA synthesis [5]. Two-thirds of children suffering from ALL can be cured by using 6-MP. By understanding the pharmacogenetics of thiopurine drugs, we can improve the chances of recovery from disease [2].

18.2 Clinical Use

The following diseases can be treated by using thiopurine drugs:

- Acute lymphoblastic leukemia (ALL) [6]
- Inflammatory bowel disease (IBD) [7]
- Autoimmune disorders (i.e., Crohn's disease, rheumatoid arthritis) [8]
- Organ transplant recipients [8]

H. Salahuddin (✉) · M. J. I. Tahir
University of Okara, Okara, Pakistan
e-mail: hina.salahuddin3@gmail.com; Junaid997981@gmail.com

N. Masood, S. Shakil Malik (eds.), *'Essentials of Cancer Genomic, Computational Approaches and Precision Medicine*,
https://doi.org/10.1007/978-981-15-1067-0_18

18.3 Mode of Action

Thiopurine drugs are basically immunosuppressive drug, inhibiting the production of cells involved in immune response. It is done by blocking various pathways of nucleic acid synthesis, ultimately inhibiting proliferation of cells of immune system [9]. Because of this typical property of these drugs, they are used in cancer treatment, i.e., cancer cells proliferate rapidly and, thus, synthesize their nucleic acid at an extensive rate. Thiopurine drugs inhibit division of cancer cells by blocking synthesis of nucleic acid. Incorporation of 6-TGN (thioguanine nucleotides) into DNA is responsible for anticancer activity of thiopurine drugs [10].

18.4 Metabolism of Thiopurine Drugs

We use thiopurine drugs in their inactive form, and to become active it is necessary to convert them into their metabolites (i.e., 6-MP). First of all, AZA (azathioprine) is converted into 6-MP (6-mercaptopurine) and other imidazole group in a nonenzymatic reaction (Fig. 18.1) [11]. 6-MP and 6-TG (6-thioguanine) undergo a series of metabolic changes to convert into active form and to exhibit their cytotoxic properties. 6-MP and 6-TG inhibit synthesis of purine [3, 12, 13] and replication of DNA (due to incorporation of 6-TGN). 6-TGN, thioguanine nucleotides, is responsible for DNA damage by breakage of single strand or cross linking [14–19].

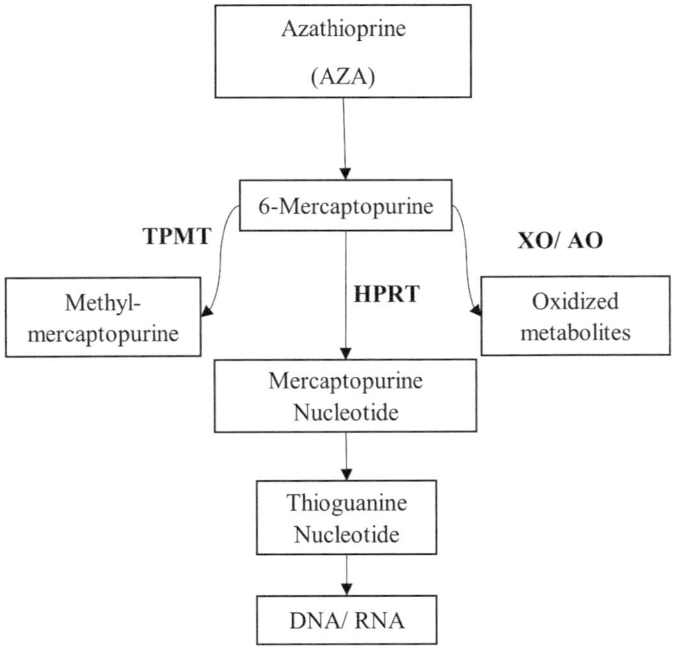

Fig. 18.1 Metabolism of thiopurine drugs

Conversion of 6-MP and 6-TG into 6-TGN is regulated by an enzyme HPRT (hypoxanthine-guanine phosphoribosyltransferase) (Fig. 18.1) [20]. There are many other enzymes like xanthine oxidase (XO), aldehyde oxidase (AO), and thiopurine S-methyltransferase (TPMT) that are used to inactivate thiopurine drugs by converting it into oxidized or methylated metabolites, as shown in Fig. 18.1, thus preventing side effects and accumulation of drug in the body [5, 21]. Metabolites produced by XO and AO pathway have very little cytotoxic effect. That's why mainly TPMT pathway is used for deactivation of thiopurine. TPMT indirectly regulate production of 6-TGN and determine antileukemic effect of thiopurine drugs [22].

18.5 Adverse Drug Reaction (ADR) of Thiopurine

Bone marrow suppression is the most serious side effect of using thiopurine drugs, which is characterized by severe decrease in blood cells (leukocytes, erythrocytes, and platelets), resulting in reduced oxygen carrying capacity and decreased immunity [22]. Other ADR of thiopurine drugs include liver abnormalities, pancreatitis, allergy, increased heart rate, lesions on the lips and in the mouth, and unusual bleeding (from the nose, mouth, or vagina) [23]. Percentage of different adverse drug reactions of thiopurine is shown in Fig. 18.2.

18.6 TPMT Allozymes

TPMT enzyme (thiopurine S-methyltransferase) plays an important role in maintaining thiopurine drug concentration in the body. It inactivates thiopurine drugs by catalyzing S-methylation of heterocyclic aromatic sulfhydryl compounds [24]. TPMT consists of 245 amino acids and its molecular weight is 28.18 kDa. TPMT enzyme is present in nearly all human tissues, but its natural substrate is still unknown [25, 26].

TPMT protein can exist in different protein variants with altered activity. Studies on red blood cells suggest that TPMT activity is trimodal in its distribution. High TPMT activity was observed in 90% of individuals, and they are referred to as high methylators; 10% of individuals show intermediate TPMT activity, and individuals that show low TPMT activity (low methylators) are only 0.3%. Polymorphism of TPMT gene is the reason behind existence of different types of TPMT allozymes [5].

18.7 TPMT Gene

TPMT gene contains coding sequence for TPMT enzyme synthesis. TPMT enzyme is responsible for S-methylation of aromatic or heterocyclic sulfhydryl compounds. This chemical reaction is important for successful regulation of thiopurine drug concentration in our body. TPMT gene inactivates thiopurine drug by metabolizing

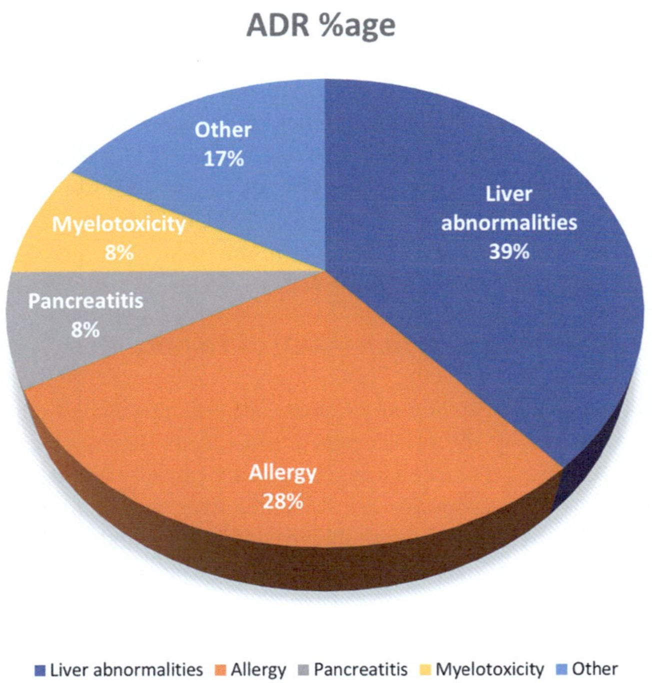

Fig. 18.2 Different ADR percentage of thiopurine drugs

it into nontoxic compounds. The location of TPMT gene is p (short) arm of chromosome number 6 (6p22.3) [26, 27].

18.8 TPMT Genotype

TPMT enzyme exhibits a trimodal distribution pattern. Almost 90% of individuals exhibit wild-type genotype for TPMT and normally metabolize the thiopurine drugs. Three to fourteen percent of individuals have intermediate TPMT activity. In that case, heterozygous mutant genetic variant of TPMT is present (i.e., one of the two alleles of TPMT enzyme contains genetic mutation). In 0.3% of individuals, low TPMT activity (homozygous mutant genetic variant of TPMT) is observed [5] (Table 18.1).

18.9 Clinical Information Related to TPMT

Thiopurine methyltransferase (TPMT) catalyzes the S-methylation of thiopurine drugs. In human thiopurine drugs are metabolized into 6-thioguanine nucleotides (6-TGN) to exhibit their cytotoxic properties [29]; 6-TGN concentration is negatively

Table 18.1 Trimodal distribution pattern of TPMT enzyme

Genotype	Prevalence	Effect	Reference
"Wild type" ($TPMT^H/TPMT^H$)	~90%	Normal metabolism of thiopurine	[5]
"Heterozygous mutant" ($TPMT^H/TPMT^L$)	3–14%	Reduction in thiopurine metabolism	[28]
"Homozygous mutant" ($TPMT^L/TPMT^L$)	0.3%	Drastically reduced or absent thiopurine metabolism	[2, 5, 28]

correlated with RBC TPMT activity [30]. Under normal conditions, TPMT regulate concentration of 6-TGN in blood. Elevated concentration of 6-TGN is because of low activity of TPMT enzyme and results in the development of leukopenia in patients of lymphoblastic leukemia [31]. Risk for development of thiopurine drug toxicity can be predicted by determining TPMT activity level [32–35].

18.10 TPMT Deficiency

Thiopurine methyltransferase deficiency is a condition in which there is significant reduction of enzyme that is responsible for normal metabolism of azathioprine, 6-TG, and 6-MP (thiopurine drugs). Patients with TPMT deficiency may develop life-threatening myelosuppression or severe hematopoietic toxicity if treated with standard doses of thiopurine drugs. TPMT deficiency is an autosomal recessive condition because of mutations in TPMT gene [36].

Therapeutic activity of thiopurine drugs depends upon metabolic conversion of azathioprine, 6-thioguanine, and 6-mercaptopurine to 6-thioguanine nucleotides and the incorporation of these nucleotides (6-TGN) into DNA. TPMT enzyme provides an alternative route to thiopurine drugs and inactivate them by thiomethylation, thus regulating the concentration of 6-TGN in blood, preventing any kind of adverse drug reactions (like myelosuppression and hematopoietic toxicity) [25].

Chances of bone marrow suppression increase in patients with TPMT deficiency. It results in decreased production of erythrocytes, leukocytes, and platelets. Consequently, patients using thiopurine drugs undergo various complications like myelosuppression, anemia, thrombocytopenia, leukopenia, and other life-threatening infections [22].

18.11 TPMT Gene Variants (Haplotype)

Metabolism of thiopurine drugs in our body depends upon the genetic variant of TPMT gene we possess. The number of genetic variants we have along with their special combination (haplotypes) at TPMT gene determines our body's response to thiopurine drugs. There can be many different haplotypes for one gene. Numbering system is used to differentiate among different haplotypes. For instance, one haplotype in the TPMT gene may be called as *3B, while another combination is known as *1. A variety of TPMT allozymes are present because of polymorphism in TPMT

Table 18.2 Some genetic variant in TPMT gene

TPMT variant	Genetic variant	Molecular alterations	Position in TPMT gene	Enzyme activity	Reference
TPMT∗1	Wt (wild type)				
TPMT∗2	c.238G>C	p.Ala80Pro	Exon 5	Low	[36]
TPMT∗3A	c.460G>A and c.719A>G	p.Ala154Thr and p.Tyr240Cys	Exon 7, exon 10	Low	[42]
TPMT∗3B	c.460G>A	p.Ala154Thr	Exon 7	Low	[27, 38]
TPMT∗4	IVS9–1G>A	Exon 10 shortened because of use of cryptic splice site created by G>A substitution	Intron 9/ exon 10	Low	[40]
TPMT∗5	c.146T>C	p.Leu49Ser	Exon 4	Low	[43]
TPMT∗6	c.539A>T	p.Tyr180Phe	Exon 8	Low	[43]
TPMT∗7	c.681T>G	p.His227Glu	Exon 10	Low	[44]
TPMT∗8	c.644G>A	p.Arg215His	Exon 10	Intermediate	[45]

gene. More than 20 genetic variations are identified in TPMT gene (ranging from TPMT∗1 to TPMT∗ 28). Altered TPMT alleles usually consist of one or more single nucleotide polymorphism [37].

Most common TPMT variants include TPMT∗2, TPMT∗3A, TPMT∗3B, and TPMT∗4. TPMT∗2 contain a single nucleotide polymorphism of c.238 G>C, polymorphisms of TPMT∗3A include c.719 A>G and c.460 G>A substitution, TPMT∗3B contain a single c.460 G>A polymorphism, and TPMT∗4 contain a single nucleotide G>A substitution at the 3'end of intron 9. Mostly these SNPs are located within coding sequence of TPMT gene and result in the formation of proteins with altered amino acid sequence [36, 38–40] (Table 18.2).

Despite changes in amino acid sequence, there are haplotypes that result in variable TPMT gene expression by altering transcription and mRNA splicing mechanism. Presence of variable number of tandem repeats in TPMT gene promoter modifies activity level of TPMT because of change in promoter cis-regulatory element [41].

18.12 Clinical Applicability of TPMT Genetic Variants

Patients with reduced TPMT activity can't tolerate standard doses of 6-mercaptopurine. Such cases are also reported in patients of skin diseases and in those suffering from autoimmune disorders [46]. ALL patients with mutant TPMT genotype are unable to metabolize thiopurine drugs properly. Consequently, they accumulate 6-TGN in their body to toxic level resulting in myelosuppression, hematologic toxicity, and hypoplasia of the bone marrow [47–50]. Excessive hematological toxicity can prove fatal, so drug therapy is stopped until the recovery of the bone marrow. But this results in delay of scheduled treatment, resistance against drug, and recurrence of disease. In addition to myelosuppression and hematologic toxicity, ALL patients also become vulnerable to various infections and sepsis [5].

About 2–5% of patients, with reduced TPMT activity level, suffer from mild leukopenia. Cases of severe leukopenia are rare (about 3%). But it can develop suddenly and unpredictably [32]. 6-MP also results in the development of leukopenia in about 2% of patients of IBD. AZA contributes in the induction of myelosuppression and hematologic toxicity in 5% of patients [46].

It is observed that 1–2% of patients experience thiopurine treatment resistance and often don't respond to therapy, even to an elevated level of thiopurine drugs (up to 50%) than standard prescription. These patients develop hepatotoxicity because of elevated level of 6-MP concentration in the therapy. They are referred to as ultra-high methylators [51].

18.13 TPMT Genetic Variants and Thiopurine Drug Intake

TPMT enzyme exhibits a trimodal distribution pattern [5]. Almost 90% of individuals exhibit high activity of TPMT enzyme, and standard dose of thiopurine drugs is used for their treatment [31]. In individuals with low TPMT activity (0.3%), initial dose of thiopurine drugs is reduced by 90%, or an alternate therapy is considered [31, 52]. Three to fourteen percent of individuals possess intermediate TPMT activity. In that case dosage of thiopurine drugs is reduced from 30 to 70% depending upon metabolic activity of TPMT enzyme [52, 53] (Table 18.3).

In addition to genetic variants of TPMT, many nongenetic factors also influence the thiopurine drug metabolism. Only 25% of adverse drug reactions (ADR) are caused by low activity level of TPMT enzyme. Many nongenetic factors like interaction of thiopurine drugs with other drugs, your health conditions, and your lifestyle also contribute in determining the response of your body to thiopurine drugs or any other medication [54–56].

18.14 Conclusion

It is significant to analyze the pharmacogenomics of a drug before its usage on practical basis. Metabolism of thiopurine drugs in our body depends upon the genetic variant of TPMT gene we possess. Because of trimodal distribution pattern of TPMT enzyme, TPMT activity level of the patients, treated with thiopurine drugs, is measured before initiation of therapy. It is necessary to determine TPMT status so that thiopurine drugs dose can be adjusted according to TPMT activity level of the patient. Most common method to determine TPMT status is TPMT genotyping. If TPMT gene is present in homozygous or heterozygous mutant form, then standard dose of thiopurine drugs cannot be used. Because of low activity of TPMT enzyme,

Table 18.3 Thiopurine drug intake based on TPMT activity level

TPMT activity level	Effect	Dosage of thiopurine	References
Normal activity	TPMT enzyme works normally	Standard dose	[31]
Intermediate activity	Increased risk for thiopurine toxicity because of under activity of TPMT enzyme	30–70% of standard dose (depending upon thiopurine metabolism)	[52, 53]
Low/absent activity	Increased risk of adverse drug reactions like myelosuppression, hematologic toxicity, and hypoplasia of the bone marrow	90% reduced dose or consider alternate therapy	[31, 52]

standard doses of thiopurine drug can result in adverse drug reactions like myelosuppression, hematologic toxicity, and hypoplasia of the bone marrow. In that case usually a reduced dose of thiopurine drugs is prescribed, or an alternative treatment is considered to avoid adverse drug reactions.

References

1. O'Connor A, Qasim A, O'Moráin CA (2010) The long-term risk of continuous immunosuppression using thioguanines in inflammatory bowel disease. Ther Adv Chronic Dis 1:7–16
2. Pavlovic S, Zukic B, Nikcevic G (2012) Pharmacogenomics of thiopurine S-methyltransferase: clinical applicability of genetic variants. In: Clinical applications of pharmacogenetics. IntechOpen, Rijeka
3. Coulthard S, Hogarth L (2005) The thiopurines: an update. Investig New Drugs 23:523–532
4. Elion GB (1986) Historical background of 6-mercaptopurine. Toxicol Ind Health 2:1–9
5. Weinshilboum RM, Sladek SL (1980) Mercaptopurine pharmacogenetics: monogenic inheritance of erythrocyte thiopurine methyltransferase activity. Am J Hum Genet 32:651–662
6. Abaji R, Krajinovic M (2017) Thiopurine S-methyltransferase polymorphisms in acute lymphoblastic leukemia, inflammatory bowel disease and autoimmune disorders: influence on treatment response. Pharmgenomics Pers Med 10:143–156
7. Konidari A, Matary WE (2014) Use of thiopurines in inflammatory bowel disease: safety issues. World J Gastrointest Pharmacol Ther 5:63–76
8. Sahasranaman S, Howard D, Roy S (2008) Clinical pharmacology and pharmacogenetics of thiopurines. Eur J Clin Pharmacol 64:753–767
9. Zhou S (2006) Clinical pharmacogenomics of thiopurine S-methyltransferase. Curr Clin Pharmacol 1:119–128
10. Katzung BG (2004) Basic and clinical pharmacology, 9th edn. McGraw-Hill, London
11. Lennard L (1992) The clinical pharmacology of 6-mercaptopurine. Eur J Clin Pharmacol 43:329–339
12. Bertino JR (1991) Improving the curability of acute leukemia: pharmacologic approaches. Semin Hematol 28:9–11
13. Dervieux T, Blanco JG, Krynetski EY et al (2001) Differing contribution of thiopurine methyltransferase to mercaptopurine versus thioguanine effects in human leukemic cells. Cancer Res 61:5810–5816
14. Tay BS, Lilley RM, Murray AW et al (1969) Inhibition of phosphoribosyl pyrophosphate amidotransferase from Ehrlich ascites-tumour cells by thiopurine nucleotides. Biochem Pharmacol 18:936–938

15. Christie NT, Drake S, Meyn RE et al (1984) 6-Thioguanine-induced DNA damage as a determinant of cytotoxicity in cultured Chinese hamster ovary cells. Cancer Res 44:3665–3671
16. Pan BF, Nelson JA (1990) Characterization of the DNA damage in 6-thioguanine-treated cells. Biochem Pharmacol 40:1063–1069
17. Bodell WJ (1991) Molecular dosimetry of sister chromatid exchange induction in 9L cells treated with 6-thioguanine. Mutagenesis 6:175–177
18. Maybaum J, Mandel HG (1983) Unilateral chromatid damage: a new basis for 6-thioguanine cytotoxicity. Cancer Res 43:3852–3856
19. Maybaum J, Mandel HG (1981) Differential chromatid damage induced by 6-thioguanine in CHO cells. Exp Cell Res 135:465–468
20. Karran P, Attard N (2008) Thiopurines in current medical practice: molecular mechanisms and contributions to therapy-related cancer. Nat Rev Cancer 8:24
21. Remy CN (1963) Metabolism of thiopyrimidines and thiopurines. S-Methylation with S-adenosylmethionine transmethylase and catabolism in mammalian tissues. J Biol Chem 238:1078–1084
22. Van Loon J, Weinshilboum RM (1987) Human lymphocyte thiopurine methyltransferase pharmacogenetics: effect of phenotype on 6-mercaptopurine-induced inhibition of mitogen stimulation. J Pharmacol Exp Ther 242:21–26
23. Gearry RB, Barclay ML, Burt MJ et al (2003) Thiopurine S-methyltransferase (TPMT) genotype does not predict adverse drug reactions to thiopurine drugs in patients with inflammatory bowel disease. Aliment Pharmacol Ther 18:395–400
24. Paugh SW, Stocco G, Evans WE (2010) Pharmacogenomics in pediatric leukemia. Curr Opin Pediatr 22:703–710
25. Weinshilboum RM, Raymond FA, Pazmino PA (1978) Human erythrocyte thiopurine methyltransferase: radiochemical microassay and biochemical properties. Clin Chim Acta 85:323–333
26. Zeglam HB, Benhamer A, Aboud A et al (2015) Polymorphisms of the thiopurine S-methyltransferase gene among the Libyan population. Libyan J Med 10:27053
27. Szumlanski C, Otterness D, Her C et al (1996) Thiopurine methyltransferase pharmacogenetics: human gene cloning and characterization of a common polymorphism. DNA Cell Biol 15:17–30
28. Ando M, Ando Y, Hasegawa Y et al (2001) Genetic polymorphisms of thiopurine S-methyltransferase and 6-mercaptopurine toxicity in Japanese children with acute lymphoblastic leukaemia. Pharmacogenetics 11:269–273
29. Elion GB (1989) The purine path to chemotherapy. Science (New York, NY) 244:41–47
30. Lennard L, Van Loon JA, Weinshilboum RM (1989) Pharmacogenetics of acute azathioprine toxicity: relationship to thiopurine methyltransferase genetic polymorphism. Clin Pharmacol Ther 46:149–154
31. McLeod HL, Miller DR, Evans WE (1993) Azathioprine-induced myelosuppression in thiopurine methyltransferase deficient heart transplant recipient. Lancet 341:1151
32. Relling MV, Gardner EE, Sandborn WJ et al (2011) Clinical Pharmacogenetics Implementation Consortium guidelines for thiopurine methyltransferase genotype and thiopurine dosing. Clin Pharmacol Ther 89:387–391
33. Schmiegelow K, Forestier E, Kristinsson J et al (2009) Thiopurine methyltransferase activity is related to the risk of relapse of childhood acute lymphoblastic leukemia: results from the NOPHO ALL-92 study. Leukemia 23:557–564
34. Gurwitz D, Rodríguez-Antona C, Payne K et al (2009) Improving pharmacovigilance in Europe: TPMT genotyping and phenotyping in the UK and Spain. Eur J Hum Genet 17:991–998
35. Relling MV, Altman RB, Goetz MP et al (2010) Clinical implementation of pharmacogenomics: overcoming genetic exceptionalism. Lancet Oncol 11:507–509
36. Krynetski EY, Schuetz JD, Galpin AJ et al (1995) A single point mutation leading to loss of catalytic activity in human thiopurine S-methyltransferase. Proc Natl Acad Sci U S A 92:949–953

37. Feng Q, Vannaprasaht S, Peng Y et al (2010) Thiopurine S-methyltransferase pharmacogenetics: functional characterization of a novel rapidly degraded variant allozyme. Biochem Pharmacol 79:1053–1061
38. Tai HL, Krynetski EY, Yates CR et al (1996) Thiopurine S-methyltransferase deficiency: two nucleotide transitions define the most prevalent mutant allele associated with loss of catalytic activity in Caucasians. Am J Hum Genet 58:694–702
39. Loennechen T, Yates CR, Fessing MY et al (1998) Isolation of a human thiopurine S-methyltransferase (TPMT) complementary DNA with a single nucleotide transition A719G (TPMT*3C) and its association with loss of TPMT protein and catalytic activity in humans. Clin Pharmacol Ther 64:46–51
40. Otterness DM, Szumlanski CL, Wood TC et al (1998) Human thiopurine methyltransferase pharmacogenetics. Kindred with a terminal exon splice junction mutation that results in loss of activity. J Clin Invest 101:1036–1044
41. Wang L, Weinshilboum R (2006) Thiopurine S-methyltransferase pharmacogenetics: insights, challenges and future directions. Oncogene 25:1629–1638
42. Tai HL, Krynetski EY, Schuetz EG et al (1997) Enhanced proteolysis of thiopurine S-methyltransferase (TPMT) encoded by mutant alleles in humans (TPMT*3A, TPMT*2): mechanisms for the genetic polymorphism of TPMT activity. Proc Natl Acad Sci U S A 94:6444–6449
43. Otterness D, Szumlanski C, Lennard L et al (1997) Human thiopurine methyltransferase pharmacogenetics: gene sequence polymorphisms. Clin Pharmacol Ther 62:60–73
44. Spire-Vayron de la Moureyre C, Debuysere H, Sabbagh N et al (1998) Detection of known and new mutations in the thiopurine S-methyltransferase gene by single-strand conformation polymorphism analysis. Hum Mutat 12:177–185
45. Hon YY, Fessing MY, Pui CH et al (1999) Polymorphism of the thiopurine S-methyltransferase gene in African-Americans. Hum Mol Genet 8:371–376
46. Wang L, Sullivan W, Toft D et al (2003) Thiopurine S-methyltransferase pharmacogenetics: chaperone protein association and allozyme degradation. Pharmacogenetics 13:555–564
47. Campbell S, Ghosh S (2001) Is neutropenia required for effective maintenance of remission during azathioprine therapy in inflammatory bowel disease? Eur J Gastroenterol Hepatol 13:1073–1076
48. Posthuma EF, Westendorp RG, van der Sluys Veer A et al (1995) Fatal infectious mononucleosis: a severe complication in the treatment of Crohn's disease with azathioprine. Gut 36:311–313
49. Connell WR, Kamm MA, Ritchie JK et al (1993) Bone marrow toxicity caused by azathioprine in inflammatory bowel disease: 27 years of experience. Gut 34:1081–1085
50. Schutz E, Gummert J, Mohr F et al (1993) Azathioprine-induced myelosuppression in thiopurine methyltransferase deficient heart transplant recipient. Lancet 341:436
51. Schaeffeler E, Fischer C, Brockmeier D et al (2004) Comprehensive analysis of thiopurine S-methyltransferase phenotype-genotype correlation in a large population of German-Caucasians and identification of novel TPMT variants. Pharmacogenetics 14:407–417
52. Swen JJ, Nijenhuis M, de Boer A et al (2011) Pharmacogenetics: from bench to byte—an update of guidelines. Clin Pharmacol Ther 89:662–673
53. Relling MV, Hancock ML, Rivera GK et al (1999) Mercaptopurine therapy intolerance and heterozygosity at the thiopurine S-methyltransferase gene locus. J Natl Cancer Inst 91:2001–2008
54. Raaschou-Nielsen O, Reynolds P (2006) Air pollution and childhood cancer: a review of the epidemiological literature. Int J Cancer 118:2920–2929
55. Belson M, Kingsley B, Holmes A (2007) Risk factors for acute leukemia in children: a review. Environ Health Perspect 115:138–145
56. Linabery AM, Ross JA (2008) Trends in childhood cancer incidence in the U.S. (1992-2004). Cancer 112:416–432

Pharmacogenetics in Cancer Treatment: Challenges and Recent Trends

19

Riffat Batool, Wasim Akhtar, and Ejaz Aziz

19.1 Introduction

Cancer is a genetic disorder of the genome caused by different types of genetic mutations that change the behavior of cells. The research of genomic and post-genomic analysis has provided insight into the molecular level of cancer progression. The sequencing technologies have improved the analysis of cancer genomes in first-time determination. Genome sequence of thousands of patients showed the discrete sets of potential gene alterations among patients with the same cancer tissue type. The single-cell sequencing disclosed the heterogeneity within the subclones of single tumors during evolution. Identification and characterization of these mutations and their assorted variety are crucial for treatments. Next-generation sequencing (NGS) has also been used for study of epigenomes and transcriptomes of cancer providing a comprehensive understanding of cancer pathology. This method gives an inclusive bench-to-bedside overview of cancer genomics, beneficial to researchers and clinicians alike. Available researches show that cancer genomics has improved the cancer prognosis leading toward the potential future therapeutic.

R. Batool (✉)
University Institute of Biochemistry and Biotechnology, PMAS, Arid Agriculture University Rawalpindi, Rawalpindi, Pakistan
e-mail: riffatqau@gmail.com

W. Akhtar
Department of Botany, University of Azad Jammu and Kashmir, Muzaffarabad, Pakistan
e-mail: wasimakhtarqau@gmail.com

E. Aziz
Department of Botany, Government Degree College Khanpur,
Haripur, Khyber Pakhtunkhwa, Pakistan
e-mail: ejaz.aziz.qau@gmail.com

N. Masood, S. Shakil Malik (eds.), *'Essentials of Cancer Genomic, Computational Approaches and Precision Medicine*,
https://doi.org/10.1007/978-981-15-1067-0_19

19.2 Cancer and Genomics

Methodological achievements have revolutionized transcriptome profiling during recent decades. The RNA-sequencing (RNA-seq) made it possible to sequence and quantify the transcriptional profiles of cells. These transcriptomes show a linkage between cellular phenotypes and their molecular groundworks, the mutations. In the context of tumor, this link shows a prospect to reveal the complexity and heterogeneity of cancers and also expose the implications of new diagnostic biomarkers or therapeutic procedures [1].

Tissue morphology and risk assessment through clinical data standards help in the classification and identification of brain tumors. Modernization in genomics and epigenomics recently accompanied an epoch of describing cancers relying on molecular basis. These techniques have developed accuracy for recognizing oncogenic-driving events which eventually increased accuracy in clinical result. Brain cancer spreads through situation of inherited tendency syndromes like Li-Fraumeni or Gorlin syndrome. However, it commonly arises from attainment of somatic mutations and chromosomal variations in tumor cells. From the study of various cancer pathways, certain refrains arise and serve like drivers of cancer. These include DNA harm reparation, genomic variability, mechanical target of rapamycin path, sonic hedgehog way, hypoxia, and epigenetic dysfunction. Consideration of these pathways is vital in developing targeted therapies and recognizing the correct patients with right therapies [2].

The TC-induced macrophages tempted IL-32 translation in TC cells within which TAM- derivative TNFα was the driver of IL-32β expression in TC cells. The overproduction of IL-32β and IL-32γ cannot induce TC cell immigration but amplified the cell death. Higher expression of IL-32β promotes more transcription of the pro-survival cytokine IL-8. TAM-derived TNFα induced IL-32β in TC cells. However, IL-32β is not responsible for TC cell movement, alternate merging of IL-32 to the IL-32β isoform responsible for TC cell existence by inducing pro-survival cytokine IL-8 [2].

Quantitative next-generation sequencing shows increasing buildup of microsatellite variability between paired endometrial and atypical hyperplasia/endometrial intraepithelial neoplasia. Tumor mutations were much greater in endometrial carcinoma than in paired atypical hyperplasia/endometrial intraepithelial neoplasia specimens. This tumor mutational burden was significantly related to percent unstable microsatellite loci. Endometrial carcinoma and paired atypical hyperplasia/endometrial intraepithelial neoplasia specimens showed a progressive accumulation of unstable microsatellite loci after loss of mismatch repair protein expression. Comprehensive next-generation sequencing-based testing of endometrial carcinomas offers new insights into endometrial carcinogenesis and opportunities for improved tumor surveillance, diagnosis, and management [3].

Prominin (PROM1) and PROM2 expression differentially modifies clinical prognosis of cancer. The relationship between mutations and copy number variations in prominin genes and several types of cancers has been reported earlier. The genes that correlated PROM1 and PROM2 in certain cancers were based on their expression levels. Gene ontology and pathway analyses have been utilized to assess the effect of these correlated genes on various cancers. It was found that PROM1 was often overexpressed in esophageal, liver, and ovarian cancers which is negatively associated with prognosis, while PROM2 overexpression was related with poor total survival in lung and ovarian cancers. Owing to characteristics of prominins, it can be concluded that PROM1 and PROM2 expression differentially modulates the clinical outcomes of cancers [4].

19.3 Drug Resistance and Cancer

Cancer possesses the ability to attain resistance against traditional treatments. The growing occurrence of drug-resilient tumor requires more research and therapies. The mechanisms that prompt the drug resistance, namely, drug deactivation, drug target modification, drug efflux, reparation of damaged DNA, reverse of cell death, and epithelial-mesenchymal transition as well as how inherent tumor cell heterogeneity, also promote drug resistance. The epigenetic modifications cause drug resistance that promote the development of cancer progenitor cells which cannot be killed by conventional cancer therapies. The most probable treatment for current drug resistance in cancer is to stop the development of cancer progenitor cells [5].

Anticancer drug resistance is an intricate phenomenon developed by altering drug goals. Developments in DNA microarray, proteomics, and targeted treatments offer novel plans to avoid the drug resistance. The resistance of cancer cell toward anticancerous agents could be made by several aspects like personal individual's genetic variances particularly in cancer somatic cells. Such resistance might be acquired by different processes such as cell death inhibition, multidrug resistance, difference in the drug digestion, epigenetic and drug goals, increasing maintenance of DNA, and gene multiplication [6].

The anticancer agents were involved significantly in the development of sterile existence and excellence of life in tumor patients. But, in several cases, after promising initial response to treatment, cancer reappearance happens. This acquired resistance to therapy is a problem for the efficiency of cancer therapy. It is a type of inherent resistance in which proteins of membrane-linking transports are involved in fundamental drug fight by varying drug carriage and its propelling out from cancer cells. Further, the steady attainment of specific genetic and epigenetic mutations in tumor cells can enhance the acquired drug resistance. The clinical data shows that the problematic nature of anti-drug property appears with an undesirable effect on molecularly targeted anticancer drugs. The medical experts suggest the recognition of such resistance mechanisms and designing the new drugs which can remove this complicacy [7].

Several features and limits must be considered as real tumor treatment using antineoplastic drugs. The way of drug management and the greatest tolerated dose can finish cancer cells while minimizing it can result in adverse effects [8, 9]. The "maximum tolerable dose" or "maximum tolerated dose" (MTD) is good known as the maximum sole dose of an agent or therapy that does not cause significant or intolerable/opposing effects. For several drugs, the optimum dose does not essentially overlap with the MTD revealing a potency of the optimal dose stances a great challenge [10].

19.4 Cancer Genomics and Personalized Medicines

Personalized medicine practices traditional and is developing ideas of the hereditary and external foundation of ailment to modify anticipation, analysis, and action. Adapted genomics has a dynamic part without limitation, in up-to-date model of personalized medicine. The differences between genomics and genetic medicine are extra quantitative than qualitative. Ideologies developed by genomics and genetics features of medicine comprise the practice of variations as indicators for diagnosis, forecast, anticipation, targets for treatment, and clinically authenticated alternatives which are not functionally categorized. The separation of these alternatives in Mendelian and non-Mendelian factors, epigenitic charcters and the dependency on sign for medical helpfulness have serious impacts on social science. In this present change from examination to exercise, customers should be saved from problems of early version investigation outputs and encourage the advanced and profitable application of these genomic findings that raise the adapted medicinal repair [11].

High-throughput, data-intensive biomedical research assays and technologies have created a need for researchers to develop strategies for analyzing, integrating, and interpreting the massive amounts of data they generate. Although a variety of statistical methods have been designed to accommodate "big data," experiences with the use of artificial intelligence (AI) techniques suggest that they might be particularly appropriate. In addition, the results of the application of these assays reveal a great heterogeneity in the pathophysiologic factors and processes that contribute to disease, suggesting that there is a need to tailor, or "personalize," medicines to the nuanced and often unique features possessed by each patient. Given how important data-intensive assays are to show proper intervention targets and strategies for treating an individual with a disease, AI can show a significant role for personalized medicines development. We describe many areas where AI can play such a role and argue that AI's ability to advance personalized medicine will depend critically not only on the refinement of relevant assays but also on ways of storing, aggregating, accessing, and ultimately integrating the data they produce. We also point out the limitations of many AI techniques in developing personalized medicines as well as consider areas for further research [12].

Variable quantity of drug can be generated by 3D printing skill with instant release tablets, pulsatile release pills, and transdermal dose types. The 3D printing skill would be discovered positively to make modified medicines that can show a dynamic part for deadly illnesses treatment. The 3D printing-based personalized drug delivery scheme can also be examined in chemotherapy of cancer patients with value of the reduction in side effects [13].

A single human physique is a place of above 1 trillion microorganisms with a diversity of commensal microbes which carry out vital roles for health. These microorganisms exist in various places including oral cavity, skin, gut, etc. These microbes vary in types and abundance in different organs; also these can vary among people. The genetic makeup of these microbes and their bionetwork establish a microbiome. Different features such as diet, environment, host genetics, etc. determine this wide microbial biodiversity. Experiments on human microbiome revealed a diverse microbiota between fit and unhealthy ones. This change in microbiome is due to the increased expression of genes that bring about composite ailments like cancer. Changes in microbiome may be caused by probiotics or synbiotics, diet or prebiotics. Modern sequence of genome and analysis of metagenomic deliver us the wider understanding of these probiotics with their distinctive features of microbiome in healthy and disease conditions. Molecular pathological epidemiology is helpful in providing understandings of pathological phenomena of ailment arousal and movement by defining the specific etiological features. Novel strategies target the microbial genome for therapeutic drives by which adapted medicines can be generated for curing numerous types of cancers. Screening programs can support in identifying patients about to gain cancer and in delivering appropriate approaches according to individual risk modes so that disease could be ceased [14].

19.5 Future of Pharmacogenomics in Cancer

The present pharmacogenetic methodologies face many hindrances. Candidate gene-based methodologies don't give a solid analysis of typical tissue danger and effects of drugs on tumor due to incomplete understanding of each risk factor involved in carcinogenesis. Genome-wide association study gives a progressively vigorous stage to pharmacogenetic examination as has been reported by Watters et al. [15]. These practices have different issues in clinical settings, for example, quality control which is expected due to phenotypic heterogeneity; lengthy duration involved in validation of pharmacogenetic markers; choice of the most suitable board of SNPs; investigation of the connection between genotypes, enzyme action, and gene expression; criteria for hazard appraisal and limits; and thought of ethnic varieties as the circulation and recurrence of SNPs change among various ethnic groups which makes it hard to extrapolate the discoveries of one group on another [16]. More up-to-date targeted treatments are likewise picking up fame. Trastuzumab (Herceptin), a refined recombinant monoclonal immunizer (IgG), targets HER2 (human epidermal growth factor receptor 2); Avastin (bevacizumab) represses the tyrosine kinase activity of the epidermal growth factor receptor, the expansion of which to standard chemotherapy regimens has demonstrated improved survival rates and response reaction in the treatment of metastatic colorectal malignant growth [17]. In similar manner, Erbitux (cetuximab), a monoclonal antibody, focusing on EGFR has likewise indicated promising outcomes in neck and head cancers and colorectal malignancy.

Future advancements in some key territories will assume a basic job in choosing the general impact of pharmacogenetic information on therapeutic decisions. More research is required in genome-based technologies, such as high-throughput innovations and improvement of gene expression arrays and genome-wide outputs which could distinguish already unidentified SNPs and SNP chips and functionally significant candidate genes. Mouse models could be used for genome-wide scans in progeny from phenotypically particular mice from vulnerable and resistant strains. Transgenic and knockout approaches could likewise be utilized for setting up the key components that helps in drug response.

Candidate gene methods could be improved by consolidating a metabolic pathway approach and by information picked up from genome-wide procedures. The expense of genomic innovation (SNP) should be less expensive. For incorporation of a genetic test into clinical practice, it must give dependable, prescient, and significant data that would have generally been obscure [18]. Prior to clinical usage, solid proof from randomized controlled clinical trials is required.

During shifting toward clinical practice, validation and replication of pharmacogenomic characteristics raise difficulties. It is often hard to portray, consistently treat, and efficiently assess patients to impartially measure the medication reaction phenotype. The standard of consideration ought to be to get genomic DNA from all patients went into clinical medication preliminaries, alongside proper consent to allow pharmacogenetic studies. This is currently practiced in most huge preliminaries being led by pharmaceutical organizations and is normal for a portion of the NCI clinical trials gatherings [19–21], yet has not turned out to be standard for foundation supported or academic trials.

The main challenge for future application is the proper use of new data and the need to guarantee that following up on a pharmacogenomic marker is to the greatest advantage of the patient. The dependence on forthcoming, randomized, controlled trials as the best way to legitimize clinical implementation isn't useful and ensures that new data will have a 5- to 10-year lag, while studies are developed, led, and translated. There is likewise a separation between the funding bodies and the prioritization of this kind of study, regarding budgetary duty, clinical trial framework, and capacity to quickly sanction new techniques. There have been a few endeavors to create approaches to pick up trust in early appropriation of pharmacogenomic information, based on agreement working among establishments around the use of genetic data to medicate treatment. One such exertion is the Clinical Pharmacogenetics Implementation Consortium (CPIC), which incorporates members from >80 institutions crosswise over 4 continents [22]. There is a need to devise a structure whereby any source of variation in a clinically credentialed pathway can be advanced toward clinical execution.

The time has come to be increasingly practical as we move ahead. Although significant advancement has been made in recognizing and describing pharmacogenomic phenomena, interpretation of this information into viable clinical application remains moderate. A variety of components add to this issue, including an absence of clearness on the measure of information expected to demonstrate clinical utility, the scarcity of interventional pharmacogenetic ponders, and uncertain practical consideration, for example, how to build up and execute clear rules in departments that oversee malignancy. There are additionally societal components having an effect on everything, including acknowledgment of across-the-board genetic testing just as suggestions for protection inclusion and risk. These issues should be investigated and tended to before the promise of genetically tweaked medication can turn into a reality.

Meanwhile we risk that crucial inventions of anticancer pharmacogenomic might not arise from growing the sample size of medical pharmacogenomic data. This is based upon insight information and revolutions of other disciplines such as medicine discoveries or designing of novel anticancerous drugs and guidelines of drug mixtures [23, 24]. Response of cancer patients follows a very heterogeneous pattern. Inherited differences of interindividual drug deposition and their effects can determine the goal of choosing the optimal drug for each patient. Cancer therapies are very significant in terms of pharmacogenetics as it shows severe toxicity and efficiency. Genetic polymorphism of genes accounts for metabolic enzymes and cellular targets for cancer chemotherapeutic agents from which the consequence chemotherapy is not possible. This particular genetic determination of drug response can transform the utility of medications. Determination of severe toxicity can help treatment leading to individualized cancer therapy for cancer patients. Guessing the cancer treatment outcome from gene polymorphism is now possible for many types of chemotherapy agents. But further research is needed from larger cancer populations along with validated pharmacogenetic markers prior to application in diagnostics [25].

19.6 Conclusion

Cancer is a heterogeneous ailment with distinctive phenotypic and genomic features that differ between individual patients and even among individual tumor regions. It is concluded that for efficient cancer therapies, characterization and identification of genomic mutations and their diversity are vital. So, linking cancer genomics with pharmacological factors is the only way to develop potent cancer therapies. For this modern technologies including next-generation sequencing, candidate gene-based analysis, etc. can play an important role in cancer therapeutics. Novel strategies target the microbial genome for therapeutic drives by which adapted medicines can be generated for curing numerous types of cancers. Future advancements in some key territories will assume a basic job in choosing the general impact of pharmacogenetic information on therapeutic decisions. The main challenge for future application is proper utilization of new data and the need to guarantee that there is strong information supporting that following up on a pharmacogenomic marker is to the greatest advantage of the patient.

References

1. Cieślik M, Chinnaiyan AM (2018) Cancer transcriptome profiling at the juncture of clinical translation. Nat Rev Genet 19:93

2. Archer TC, Ehrenberger T, Mundt F et al (2018) Proteomics, post-translational modifications, and integrative analyses reveal molecular heterogeneity within medulloblastoma subgroups. Cancer Cell 34:396–410
3. Chapel DB et al (2019) Quantitative next-generation sequencing-based analysis indicates progressive accumulation of microsatellite instability between atypical hyperplasia/endometrial intraepithelial neoplasia and paired endometrioid endometrial carcinoma. Mod Pathol 32:1508
4. Saha SK, Islam SR, Kwak KS et al (2019) PROM1 and PROM2 expression differentially modulates clinical prognosis of cancer: a multiomics analysis. Cancer Gene Ther. https://doi.org/10.1038/s41417-019-0109-7
5. Housman G et al (2014) Drug resistance in cancer: an overview. Cancers 6:1769–1792
6. Mansoori B, Mohammadi A, Davudian S et al (2017) The different mechanisms of cancer drug resistance: a brief review. Adv Pharm Bull 7:339
7. Nikolaou M, Pavlopoulou A, Georgakilas AG et al (2018) The challenge of drug resistance in cancer treatment: a current overview. Clin Exp Metastasis 35:309–318
8. Carlson RW, Sikic BI (1983) Continuous infusion or bolus injection in cancer chemotherapy. Ann Intern Med 99:823–833
9. Steuart C, Burke P (1971) Cytidine deaminase and the development of resistance to arabinosyl cytosine. Nat New Biol 233:109
10. Marangolo M et al (2006) Dose and outcome: the hurdle of neutropenia. Oncol Rep 16:233–248
11. Offit K (2011) Personalized medicine: new genomics, old lessons. Hum Genet 130:3–14
12. Schork NJ (2019) Artificial intelligence and personalized medicine. In: Precision medicine in cancer therapy, Springer, Cham, pp 265–283
13. Afsana, Jain V, Haider N, Jain K (2018) 3D printing in personalized drug delivery. Curr Pharm Des 24:5062–5071
14. Rajpoot M, Sharma AK, Sharma A et al (2018) Understanding the microbiome: emerging biomarkers for exploiting the microbiota for personalized medicine against cancer. In: Seminars in cancer biology, vol 52. Elsevier, New York, pp 1–8
15. Watters JW, Kraja A, Meucci MA et al (2004) Genome-wide discovery of loci influencing chemotherapy cytotoxicity. Proc Natl Acad Sci U S A 101:11809–11814
16. Oscarson M (2003) Pharmacogenetics of drug metabolising enzymes: importance for personalised medicine. Clin Chem Lab Med 41:573–580
17. Hurwitz H, Fehrenbacher L, Novotny W et al (2004) Bevacizumab plus irinotecan, fluorouracil, and leucovorin for metastatic colorectal cancer. N Engl J Med 350:2335–2342
18. McLeod HL (2013) Cancer pharmacogenomics: early promise, but concerted effort needed. Science 339:1563–1566
19. Baldwin RM, Owzar K, Zembutsu H et al (2012) A genome-wide association study identifies novel loci for paclitaxel-induced sensory peripheral neuropathy in CALGB 40101. Clin Cancer Res 18:5099–5109
20. Innocenti F, Owzar K, Cox NL et al (2012) A genome-wide association study of overall survival in pancreatic cancer patients treated with gemcitabine in CALGB 80303. Clin Cancer Res 18:577–584
21. Ratain MJ, Miller AA, McLeod HL et al (2006) The cancer and leukemia group B pharmacology and experimental therapeutics committee: a historical perspective. Clin Cancer Res 12:3612s–3616s
22. Relling MV, Klein TE (2011) CPIC: clinical pharmacogenetics implementation consortium of the pharmacogenomics research network. Clin Pharmacol Ther 89(3):464–467
23. Lu D-Y, Lu T-R (2010) Antimetastatic activities and mechanisms of bisdioxopiperazine compounds. Anticancer Agents Med Chem 10:564–570
24. Lu D-Y, Lu T-R, Wu H-Y (2012) Development of antimetastatic drugs by targeting tumor sialic acids. Sci Pharm 80(3):497–508
25. Ruwali M (2019) Pharmacogenetics and cancer treatment: progress and prospects. In: Molecular medicine. IntechOpen, Rijeka

Precision Nutraceutical Approaches for the Prevention and Management of Cancer

20

Ali Asghar, Muhammad Shafqat Rasool, Talha Younas, Muhammad Basit, Ouswa Amjad, and Lillah

20.1 Nutraceuticals, Apoptosis, and Disease Prevention

The way of life has improved with financial advancement of the general population. But with this advancement, lifestyle diseases have increased due to poor living habits. An increase in the consumption pattern of junk food has been observed in recent era which also has triggered several health related issues especially prevalence of lack of important essential nutritional constituents in diet. For the healthy and active lifestyle, deficiency of important constituent of diet can be fulfilled by the use of nutraceuticals. There are tremendous nutritional improvements that help to prevent or treat disease generated using crude herbals. Nutraceuticals are already in use since ages in the form of traditional herbs and plants and their health benefits are also well acclaimed. Modifications in our eating habits and patterns can reduce the risk of several diseases by including important nutracdeuticals as the part of our daily diet [1].

20.2 Nutraceuticals and Apoptosis

Plants like garlic, ginger, soybean, and tea can be a good source of nutraceuticals which are basically phytochemicals. They have preventive activity against malignant growth occurrence which is likely identified with apoptosis [2].

A. Asghar (✉) · M. S. Rasool · T. Younas · M. Basit · O. Amjad · Lillah
National Institute of Food Science and Technology, University of Agriculture, Faisalabad, Pakistan
e-mail: Ali.asghar@uaf.edu.pk

N. Masood, S. Shakil Malik (eds.), *'Essentials of Cancer Genomic, Computational Approaches and Precision Medicine*,
https://doi.org/10.1007/978-981-15-1067-0_20

20.3 Apoptosis

Apoptosis which is a programmed cell death includes morphological changes like chromatin condensation, fragmentation of the nucleus, and cell shrinkage. Apoptosis includes complex molecular processes with more than 100 separate enzymes participating efficiently in signal transduction, zymogen-type course, precise implementation of important cytoskeletal structures, and signalized DNA within the selected cell. These opportunities contribute to discontinuity of DNA, blebbing, growth of apoptotic bodies, and ultimately destruction of cells. In addition, phagocytes overwhelm the withering of cells due to phosphatidylserine introduction and changes in surface sugars. This mechanism of apoptosis can without much of a stretch be actuated by nutraceuticals. Apoptosis by nutraceuticals can be a tremendous approach for disease prevention especially cancer [2].

20.4 Disease Prevention

The term "nutraceutical" derived from the terms "food" and "pharmaceutical" was established in 1989 to describe substances that can be used as a source of nutrition that can improve health [3].

By utilizing nutraceuticals, it might be conceivable to diminish or dispose the requirement for traditional prescriptions, lessening the odds of any unfriendly impact. Nutraceuticals frequently have interesting synthetic activities that are inaccessible in pharmaceuticals. The whole world is battling maladies normal for the cutting-edge age, for example, stoutness, osteoporosis, diabetes, hypersensitivities, and dental issues. Supplements, herbals, and nutritional intensifications are major components of nutraceuticals that make them innovative in well-being, acting against various diseases and thus advancing individual satisfaction. It is prestigious to use sustenance products to promote well-being and treat illness [4].

20.5 Nutraceutical Prevention of Disease Through Apoptosis

The following are the structural classes of nutraceuticals: carotenoids, flavonoids, stilbenes, sulfur-containing compounds, or other phenolic compounds [2].

20.6 Carotenoids

Various epidemiological studies have shown that tomato consumption is associated with lower risk of malignant tumor growth and cardiovascular disorders. Tomatoes are a rich source of many types of carotenoids. In tomatoes lycopene is a precursor of beta-carotene that resembles the lycopene cyclase gene and linked with regulation of gene associated with aging. Lycopene and β-carotene have the ability to initiate the process of apoptosis in prostate's mutated cells and dangerous lymphoblast cells at a 3–30 μM concentration and time duration of 24 h. Apoptosis that is initiated by carotenoids includes the disruption of DNA, cleavage of poly-ADP-ribose polymerase (PARP), and caspase-3 enactment [2].

20.7 Flavonoids

Flavonoids comprise of more than 4000 polyphenolic compounds that are present normally in food that are obtained from plants. These plant components have a typical structure of phenyl benzopyrone (C6–C3C6) and are ordered by the level of immersion and opening of the focal pyran ring, mainly in flavones, flavonols, isoflavones, flavanone, and flavanonols. Compounds present in tea like polyphenols, quercetin, and genistein have a therapeutic role and chemopreventive potential. The link between the consumption of tea and reduced chances of having a malignant tumor is not clearly demonstrated. According to animal trials, there is no visible effect of concentrations of tea or its polyphenols on cancer treatments. In other studies, it has an effect on prevention of malignant tumor growth, and it can fight inflammations, infections, and cardiovascular diseases. In some studies, epigallocatechin gallate (EGCG) and catechin effects on human lymphoid leukemic cells and human carcinoma cells have been investigated. It is capable of decreasing the likelihood of pulmonary tumor cell lines, colon malignant cells, breast cancer cells and virally altered human fibroblasts, prostate malignant cells, stomach cancer cells, cerebral tumor cells, head and neck squamous carcinoma, and cervical malignant growth cells. The apoptotic ability of EGCG is in the scope of 20–100 μM in mutated cells, and the time duration ranges between 10 and 30 h [2].

20.8 Stilbenes

Resveratrol (3,5,4′-trihydroxy-trans-stilbene), a phytoalexin with natural sources such as grapes, peanuts and pines, has cancer prevention effects against inflammation and helps in quick fixing of Leguminosae that hinders cell association with tumor inception. Resveratrol can trigger cell death in laboratory studies and stop the development of various human tumor cells, particularly oral squamous carcinoma, human breast malignant growth cells, prostate cancer cells, esophageal carcinoma cells, pancreatic malignant cells, and monocytic leukemia cells. The concentration of resveratrol consumed in different investigations has changed somewhere in the range of 10 and 300 μM, with apoptosis showing up somewhere in the range of 24 and 96 h. Acceptance of p53 at the mRNA and protein levels is the most normally observed impact of resveratrol and is viewed as the significant reason for cancer cell death. Resveratrol does not express any significant inhibitory impact toward changed human fibroblasts. Strangely, a resveratrol simple, 3,4,5,4′-tetrahydroxystilbene, is stronger than resveratrol in enhances death of changed cells, however has no impact on ordinary partners at increased concentrations [2].

20.9 Sulfur-Containing Compounds

The consumption of garlic in diet as a cancer-preventing agent has been studied. The compound allyl sulfur present in garlic has a positive effect in the prevention of further spread of malignant tumors in humans. Diallyl sulfide and diallyl disulfide can initiate programmed cell death in diseased lung cells, in prostate malignant cell growth, and in malignant cancers of the breast. Z-ajonene, an active ingredient in garlic, can also cause cell death of HL-60 cells. Treatment of cancer with these active compounds has shown changes in ratio of Bax gene to Bcl-2. *Brassica* plants (e.g., broccoli and cauliflower) have an active compound named glucosinolates, which further changed into isothiocyanates, for example, sulforaphane. According to various studies, isothiocyanates can prevent malignancy and have chemopreventive properties. In various studies, sulforaphane can enhance the chances of programmed cell death in colon disease cells, prostate malignant growth cells, and leukemia cells. These studies revealed the expansion of Bax in the treated cells is due to the positive effect of sulforaphane on programmed cell death [2].

20.10 Other Phenolic Compounds

Caffeic corrosive phenethyl ester, a functioning phenolic segment removed from bumble bee propolis, can prevent tumor formation in two steps in animals with malignant growth in the skin that showed significant effect with 12-O-tetradecanoylphorbol-13-acetic acid derivation. Caffeic acid phenethyl ester increased the programmed cell death in HL-60 leukemic cells and epidermal JB6 Cl 41 cells. Various other studies can also clearly depict the activity of caffeic acid phenethyl ester in mechanism of anticancer activity in various frameworks. Curcumin, which is a diferuloylmethane, sustain the strong flavor of turmeric and contains polyphenols, is a major biologically active ingredient which can prevent the fabrication of cancer causing agent in skin of mice. Use of curcumin on surface can suppress the artificially initiated skin cancer formation. Curcumin can cause programmed cell death in colon carcinoma cells, leukemic cells, prostate malignancy cells, melanoma cells, and breast cancer cells. By initiation of a p53-subordinate pathway, curcumin also initiates programmed cell death [2].

20.11 Prevention of Various Diseases by Nutraceuticals

20.11.1 Obesity-Related Colorectal and Liver Carcinogenesis

Obesity and its related complications are insulin-resistant and changes in the insulin-like development factor-1 (IGF-1)/IGF-1 receptor (IGF-1R) and its aggravation conditions can increase chances of having colorectal disease (CRC) and hepatocellular carcinoma (HCC). These findings additionaly demonstrate that metabolic issues of stoutness may be compelling factors to counteract the improvement of colorectal cancer and hepatocellular carcinoma in large people. Green tea catechins (GTCs) have cancer-preventive and chemopreventive properties against malignancy in different organs, including the colorectum and liver. GTCs have also a leading role in managing obesity, diabetes management and palliative impacts, which revealed that the GTCs interfere with the weightrelated colorectal and liver cancer formation. Branched-chain amino acids (BCAA) can improve the protein status of individuals and also prevent liver failure in patients with already prevailing hepatic illness; furthermore their supplementation can prevent the chances of having hepatocellular carcinoma in patients who are obese and have cirrhosis. Branched-chain amino acids revealed these health-promoting properties since their role in the improvement of insulin resistance. These properties make a link between the metabolic issues and improvement in colorectal cancers and hepatocellular carcinoma. Additionally treatment of colorectal cancer and hepatocellular carcinoma with the utilization of GTC and BCAA according to clinically proven research has the ability to correct metabolic irregularities and by different pathways can improve colorectal cancer and hepatocellular carcinoma in obese individuals [5].

20.11.2 Lung Cancer

Tea, obtained from the plant *Camellia sinensis*, has worldwide importance because of its refreshing properties. Different studies have revealed that tea has a therapeutic potential and consumption of tea is linked with reduced chances of developing cancer. An important part in anticancer properties of green tea is the presence of epigallocatechin gallate (EGCG), which is a bioactive compound. The pathways by which it can regulate the cancer causing elements is by the use of various chemicals and receptors, cell cycle capture and programmed cell death, cell flagging pathways balance and hiding the initiation factors and inhibits the further proliferation of malignant tumor. These are the anticancer and restorative properties of green tea and its bioactive ingredients particularly EGCG [6].

20.11.3 Bladder Cancer

Epithelial-mesenchymal transition (EMT) is an important step in the proliferation of malignant cells. Butein is an active polyphenolic compound which can prevent the proliferation of malignant tumor cells. Butein can stop the relocation and attack through the ERK1/2 and NF-kappa B flagging pathways in human bladder malignant growth cells and inversion of EMT which is an inhibitory impact. These outcomes were asserted by RNAi-interceded concealment of NF-kappa B, which incompletely turns around EMT and represses cell obtrusive capacity in vitro. These results have shown that butein has a tendency to inhibit bladder malignant cell growth [6].

20.11.4 Miscellaneous

Curcumin can prevent leukemia, lymphomas, multiple myeloma, brain cancer, melanoma, and skin, lung, prostate, breast, ovarian, liver, gastrointestinal, pancreatic, and colorectal epithelial cancers (Mimeault & Batra, 2011). Dietary monoterpenes can prevent skin, liver, lung, and stomach cancers. These compounds have nonnutritive components, and essential oils of citrus are its natural source (Crowell, 1999). Skin, prostate, lung, and liver cancers can be prevented by consuming foods rich in genistein, resveratrol, lycopene, ellagitannins e.g., pomegranate and lupeol [7].

20.11.5 Future of Nutraceuticals

The modern nutraceutical market focuses on products which have additional dietary advantages and provide nourishments as well as target the preventable properties. The comprehensive approaches can propel the development of nutraceuticals. Many researchers described that many natural ingredients can increase the demands in nutraceuticals. "Catalysts have been underemployed. They will be a hot region later on." Utilization of microorganism and the process of fermentation to make innovative products also have therapeutic potential. This is the multidisciplinary approaches that are needed in the production of innovative products. It includes the interlink of science, innovative products promotion, and customers feedbacks that cannot be neglected. Some nutraceuticals have medical advantages because of good bioavailability, and it can be provided through oral or transdermal pathways. With the advancement of "Smart Nutraceuticals," a Futuristic *Doctor's Desk Reference* would contain data on individual hereditary profiles to be coordinated with explicit nourishing intercessions also. This would be an immense improvement over current dietary proposals which being too summed up are accounted for to profit just 60% of the population [8].

20.12 Novel Nutraceuticals in Cancer Prevention

20.12.1 Carotenoids and Cancer Prevention

Carotenoids naturally occur as orange, red, and yellow pigments that are widely distributed. These lipid-soluble pigments are present in different fruits, vegetables, and flowers and some kinds of animals and fungi. Carotenoids are present in human as well as animal cells such as zeaxanthin and lutein in the eyes, and astaxanthin is present in salmon which is obtained from diet [9].

During metabolism and respiration, reactive oxygen species (ROS), singlet oxygen, and free radicals are produced naturally in the human body. Other free radicals from the exogenous sources such as smoking, air pollution, and pesticides lead to the exceeding levels of ROS in the body. The higher level of ROS causes the development of oxidative stress. Carotenoids have natural antioxidant potential which protects the cells from damage and deterioration. ROS would react with lipids of plasma membranes, proteins, enzymes, and endothelial cell that result in cellular damage, deterioration, mutation, and inflammation, which are related to aging and incidence of chronic, degenerative disorders and cancer. Carotenoid-rich diet consumption has been stated to reduce the risks of different disorders caused by oxidative damage. The antioxidant action of carotenoids depends upon their physical scavenging activity [10].

Various studies demonstrated the relationship between the carotenoid intake and cancer risks. Lycopene is found in tomatoes and tomato-based food products. More intake of lycopene-rich food sources such as tomatoes exhibited significant decreased cancer risk in subjects afflected with cancer of the gastrointestinal tract [11].

It has been hypothesized that carotenoid intake reduces head and neck cancer risk due to its antioxidant properties. A systematic review and meta-analysis of the epidemiological studies determined the association between consumption of specific dietary carotenoid and combined carotenoids, with the risk of head and neck cancer. From literature, a review of 15 case-control studies and one prospective cohort study showed significant reduction in cancer risk associated with consumption of β-carotene equivalent intakes that were 45% for oral cavity cancer and 56% for laryngeal cancer. β-Cryptoxanthin and lycopene also minimized the risk for laryngeal cancer. β-Cryptoxanthin, lycopene, and α-carotene showed association with at least 25% reduction in the oral and pharyngeal cancer rate. Systematic review and meta-analysis on dietary carotenoid consumption and head and neck cancer showed that carotenoids have protective role against HNC, in comparison to most of single-nutrient intakes [12].

Another meta-analysis of epidemiological studies, including 6 cohort and 11 case-control studies, exhibited that the consumption of tomatoes and tomato-containing foods and gastric cancer risk is inversely related. A comparison between groups with highest and lowest intake of tomato-based foods showed 28% reduction in the risk of gastric cancer (lycopene caused 11% reduction in cancer risk, while the decrease was not significant statistically) [12].

Another case-control study showed similar results. Over the course of 20 years, plasma levels of carotenoids have been determined in 18,744 women. Women with high carotenoid levels in plasma demonstrated significant reduction of 18–27% in breast cancer risk. Furthermore, carotenoid concentrations and recurrence of breast cancer showed strong inverse relationship. Beta-carotene reduced the risk of breast cancer recurrence by 67% when the highest and lowest level quantiles were compared [13].

Consumption of carotenoids such as lycopene, alpha and beta-carotene, lead to reduction in the risk of prostate tumor and breast cancer. Beta-carotene also reduces the risk of breast cancer recurrence [14].

20.12.2 Polyphenols and Cancer Prevention

Polyphenols are plants' secondary metabolites which show protective effects against various disorders. Polyphenols are classified into five distinct groups such as flavonoids, phenolic acids, curcuminoids, stilbenes, and lignans. Depending upon their structure and functions, flavonoids are further classified into different groups such as flavanols, flavonols, flavones, isoflavones, and anthocyanins.

Polyphenols in pinecone are bioactive dietary components that exhibit antioxidant and immunoregulatory properties and play important role in health promotion, cancer prevention, and treatment. A study was conducted to examine the antioxidant, antitumor, and immunoregulatory actions of the 40% ethanol eluent of polyphenols from pinecone on rat models. The results demonstrated that pinecone polyphenols exhibit antitumor activity by stimulating the mitochondrial apoptotic pathway and by its immunoregulatory and antioxidant properties [15].

Plant polyphenols have anti-oxidative, anti-inflammatory, anti-angiogenic, and pro-apoptotic properties. They can modify the roles of some important functional proteins and receptors, such as IGF, IGF-1R, and IGBPs proteins in insulin-like growth factor system. The IGF system plays an important role in carcinogenesis, cell proliferation, differentiation and apoptosis. They modulate different signal transduction pathways and perform a significant role in cancer prevention. Different mechanisms of action show that polyphenols also have potential in the prevention and inhibition of tumors and cancers.

In old age, the leading cause of death is cancer. Consumption of fruits and vegetables decreases the risk of cancer incidence and mortality. Because of their chemopreventive and chemotherapeutic capacity, a number of fruits rich in polyphenols are researched. Pomegranate helps boost anticancer activity because its high polyphenol content. Pomegranate has antiproliferative and antimetastatic effect that induces apoptosis through modulation, upregulation, and downregulation processes. Pomegranate helps to block the activation of inflammatory pathways including the NF-κB pathway. Before suggesting the use of pomegranate or its polyphenols for cancer-related therapeutic purposes, certain parameters like an accurate risk or safety assessment should be made [16].

Studies investigating the relationship between the consumption of dietary polyphenol and the risk of cancer have shown diverse outcomes. The inconsistency of results is because of the difficulty in the assessment of polyphenol intake and polyphenol diversity. However various studies have shown that intake of natural polyphenols, such as anthocyanins, curcumin, epigallocatechin-3-gallate (EGCG), and resveratrol, exhibit anticancer activities. The mechanisms of action chiefly involve modulation of different molecular events and cell signaling pathways linked with its survival, propagation, differentiation, migration, angiogenesis, detoxification enzymes, and immunity. In addition, the effects of polyphenol against cancer vary according to the type of cancer and dose of polyphenols. It must be noted that genistein and daidzein are polyphenols that have antagonistic effects on hormone-related cancer. Therefore, these polyphenols should be utilized with caution in any type of cancer. Moreover, there are less clinical trials about the anticancer activity of polyphenols. To assess the impact of dietary polyphenols on cancer risks, further epidemiological studies are needed. Further studies are required for the assessment and comparison of mechanisms of action of different polyphenols. Larger randomized clinical trials should be carried out to provide more clear evidence about safety and bioavailability of polyphenols [16].

Multiple studies after the discovery of noncoding RNAs (ncRNAs) have investigated that polyphenols, such as EGCG, resveratrol, and curcumin, can regulate different tumor suppressor and oncogenic ncRNAs which regulate progression of different cancer types [17].

Polyphenols are present in green tea in the form of epigallocatechin-3-gallate (EGCG) and have a role in inhibition of tumors. There is need to investigate antitumor action of EGCG. A study was conducted for EGCG antitumor effect on the human esophageal squamous cell carcinoma cell lines, in vivo and in vitro. The results demonstrated that EGCG induced apoptosis and inhibited proliferation through production of ROS, caspase-3 activation, and a decrease in VEGF expression in vitro and in vivo. In the future EGCG may have clinical applications to prevent or treat cancer of the esophagus [18].

20.12.3 Phytosterols and Cancer

Plant sterols that are present in plants cell membrane are called phytosterols. They play their role in plants as cholesterol performs its functions in the human body.

It has been reported that plant sterols and stanols have various other functions except their role in cardiovascular diseases. Current studies showed that phytosterols have inhibitory actions in different types of cancers such as stomach, lung, breast, and ovarian cancers. Different mechanisms of actions are involved including inhibition of carcinogens synthesis, growth of cancerous cell, angiogenesis, metastasis and apoptosis. Phytosterol intake may help in the reduction of oxidative stress by increasing the antioxidant activity. Phytosterols are thought to encourage apoptosis by reducing blood cholesterol levels. Studies revealed that daily consumption of 2 g phytosterols does not pose any health issues [19].

Phytochemicals show preventative effects against chronic disorders such as obesity, CVD, diabetes, and cancer. It was estimated that diets rich in phytochemicals can decrease the risk of disease as much as 20%. Phytosterols are structurally similar to cholesterol but are present solely in plants. It is revealed by epidemiological studies that phytosterol content in the diet helps to reduce common cancers including colon, breast, and prostate cancers.

Phytosterols enable vigorous anticancer response in host system by boosting immune function for the recognition of cancerous cells and by influencing hormonal-dependent propagation of endocrine tumors. It directly slows down the tumor growth by altering cell cycle, inducting apoptosis, and inhibiting metastasis of tumors [20].

A case-control study for investigating phytosterols' role in cancer prevention included 1363 control and colorectal cancer patients, and they were given five subclasses of phytosterols (stigmasterol, campesterol, B-sitosterol, campestanol, and B-sitostanol) over a period of 5 years. Results revealed that consumption of different subclasses of phytosterols showed inverse relationship with risk of colorectal cancer. However, stigmasterol showed nonsignificant association with colorectal cancer [20].

A side effect linked with phytosterols' intake is that they reduce carotenoid levels in blood. However, it has been proposed that this impact can be compensated by increasing consumption of carotenoid-containing foods and through supplementation of carotenoids [21].

Phytosterols have shown decreased development in multiple cancer cells in the liver, lungs and breast, although exact mechanisms involved in inhibition of cancerous cell growth are not well explained. Different mechanisms involved are angiogenesis reduction, invasion of cancerous cell, and ROS production. Phytosterols have acquired more insight for their protective impact against numerous types of cancer; however, additional information is needed to fully comprehend their functions and processes as less data is available on human subjects [22].

20.13 Mechanism of Antioxidant Action

20.13.1 Oxidative Stress

Oxygen exhibits both positive and potentially harmful effects for living systems. Due to its reactive properties, it helps in high-energy electron transfer reactions and production of ATP via oxidative phosphorylation. It therefore enables the growth of complicated multicellular organisms but also assumes responsibility for attacking any biological molecule, be it a protein, lipid, or DNA. As a consequence, reactive oxygen species (ROS) are constantly attacking our body. This attack by reactive oxygen species (ROS) is maintained in equilibrium by an advanced complicated antioxidant defense mechanism. This equilibrium can sometimes be unsettled, resulting in oxidative stress. Oxidative stress plays a major part in the pathophysiology of many distinct illnesses including problems during pregnancy [22].

This subject focuses on studies in the clinical and fundamental sciences. When the inherent antioxidant defenses are submerged by the manufacturing of reactive oxygen organisms, then oxidative stress occurs. Reactive oxygen species play a main position in cell retention with their adjacent setting in homeostasis situation. Reactive oxygen species generate undiscriminating harm to biological molecules at an intense rate, resulting in cell failure to operate correctly and cell death eventually. In this section, we will come to understand critically how oxygen reactive species are produced, how they are detoxified in human placenta, and their function in homeostatic levels [23].

20.13.2 Action of Nutraceuticals Against Oxidative Stress

Because of their chemical reactivity in combination with hunting and decreasing of free radicals produced during cell metabolism, plant nutraceuticals have been noted to have a distinctive immediate antioxidant activity. The quenching or diminishing of free radicals relates to the reduction of electrophilic species, such as radicals of peroxyl and hydroperoxide, while the scavenging or hunting exercise depicts the development of a more stable phenoxyl radical item by the response of phenol loop hydroxyl group (OH) with a reactive oxygen species. This demonstrates that the bioactivity of nutraceuticals relies on a direct and undeviating response with oxidized species and also on their location, adsorption, dispersal, absorption, and excretion. These nutraceuticals can meet with organisms at cellular and molecular levels by regulating gene expression, protein and DNA repair, and epigenetic controls. Several trials have evaluated the cellular and molecular function of nutraceuticals in livestock, taking benefit of high-throughput screening. Nutraceuticals can modify gene expression and signaling processes. Nutrigenomic studies have revealed that nutraceuticals can also be useful in the processes of cell apoptosis, drug metabolism, immune modulation and metabolism.

20.13.3 Precision Nutrition

Precision Nutrition is a medical model that suggests nutritional customization with nutritional choices, items, or processes available to the individual. Analytical testing is often used in this model to select appropriate and optimal biomarker-based dietary elements, including the inheritances of the individual, or the results of other cellular or molecular tests.

Examples are:

- Precise selection of omega-3 fatty acids for individuals with low omega-3 indexes (von Schacky, 2014)
- Accurate selection of immune-stimulating supplements [24]
- Suitable recommendations for zinc or phytochemicals to avoid molecular degeneration based on heritable information

Precision Nutrition study thus provides a number of easy to implement measures to avoid disease and compress disease:

- Many dietary interventions are tested over time, and positive results are supported by observational trials.
- Different dietary interventions are affordable and easy to use [25].

20.13.4 Precision Nutraceutical Approaches

Nutraceuticals are food or portion of food that provides medical advantages including disease prevention and treatment. Adding nutraceuticals to diet in adequate quantities may prevent the occurrence of chronic diseases such as hypertension, cancer, coronary heart disease, and obesity. Nutraceuticals captured the attention and fantasy of customers seeking the convenience of food that contains nutraceuticals which are beneficial for health. Nutraceutical-added foods can substitute dietary supplements [26].

It is possible to add nutraceuticals in different foods in liquid, semiliquid, powder, or semisolid form. Scientists consider various distinct factors while developing the product containing nutraceuticals. These factors affect the physical, chemical, and natural properties of nutraceuticals which result in change in taste, strength, and sustainability of the product. Furthermore, enriched and fortified foods with nutraceuticals include enriched dairy products, fortified cereal and grain products, functional drinks, high-energy beverages, snack bars, candy parlors, etc.

20.13.5 Nutraceutical Incorporation Approaches

Nutraceuticals can be incorporated in the food for appropriate health benefits, optimal medical benefit and due to visual attraction [27].

20.13.5.1 Encapsulation

Encapsulation is a process in which an active ingredient (nutraceutical) is captured in another material (matrix or encapsulant). Encapsulated active substance is shielded from external conditions for a certain time period until it is transported in the field. The design of an encapsulated element with the anticipated features and composition must be done carefully.

- Natural physicochemical characteristics of matrix and active components
- Active ingredient and matrix stability in various media
- Mutual interactions of matrix and active ingredient
- The technology used to prepare the encapsulated ingredient

The encapsulation generally involves the reinforcement of the binding component, consideration of the conditions under which the encapsulated component is available and it requires protection from external harsh conditions. When the encapsulation is in the constituent state, during food processing, food storage, or food consumption, there is a trigger such as the activity of the enzyme or the pH that releases it into the digestive tract until it hits the required body location [26] (Table 20.1).

Table 20.1 Different types of encapsulated nutraceuticals

Class	Examples
Proteins	Milk proteins (e.g., whey protein isolates, caseinates, individual caseins, micellar casein, bovine serum albumin, plant proteins (e.g., soy protein isolate, wheat protein, oat protein, zein)
Gelatins (e.g., fish gelatin, collagen)	Carbohydrates, sugars (e.g., glucose, sucrose, lactose, trehalose, glucose syrups, honey, oligosaccharides)
Starch and starch derivatives	For example, native starches, modified starches, resistant starches, maltodextrins Nonstarch polysaccharides (e.g., alginate, pectin, carrageenan, chitosan, plant fibers, gum acacia, gum Arabic
Lipids and waxes	Vegetable fats and oils (e.g., canola oil, palm oil, sunflower oil, and fractions of these) Milk fat and milk fat fractions (e.g., olein and stearin)
Surfactants	Natural surfactants (e.g., milk phospholipids) Synthetic surfactants (e.g., tweens, spans, polyglycerol polyricinoleate, sucrose esters), $\omega - 3$ fatty acids, and probiotics
Phenolic compounds, phytochemicals	Vitamins and minerals, bioactive peptide, carotenoids, and tocopherols

20.13.6 Product Trends and Emerging Nutraceuticals

Nutraceuticals are generally directed to diverse demographic and market requirements. Food can be delivered on the basis of health advantages, age groups, and religious or cultural nutritional needs. In the future older people will make significant use of the development of functional and nutraceutical food products. Sensory preferences of old consumers (e.g., taste, texture) are very different from those of young consumers. Therefore, in manufacturing functional foods for old consumers, it is important to remodel existing products with different tastes and textures.

It is well recognized that the nutritional requirements of individuals differ depending on their age and medical condition, and the nutraceutical and functional food industry can deliver products developed for specific age group. The main products of concern to elderly clients are functional foods that influence lung health (omega-3 fatty acids), cardiovascular health (probiotics), aging (resveratrol and antioxidants), and GIT health (probiotics). Likewise, for healthy eyes (lutein, zeaxanthin) and for healthy bone and skeleton (calcium, vitamin D3) are important. Products that encourage brain development (such as omega-3 fatty acids) and immunological health (such as probiotics, oligosaccharides) are of biggest concern to infants and young kids.

The exclusive functional foods and drink products are the most fast-growing functional foods in the globe after recipes for neonates, energy drinks and probiotic yogurts. Nondairy options were identified as the fastest-growing functional beverage classification, for example, rice, oats, hemp, and walnut milk, given increased weight of food intolerance and welfare concerns associated with milk and soybeans.

Foods carrying a combination of nutraceutical components are increasing quickly in the market due to their probable synergistic health effects. This contributes an extra amount of difficulty to the encapsulation systems technological growth in potential functional foods. Advances and efficiency in nutrigenomics will provide a better knowledge of collaboration and a driving force to gradually increase the effect of diet and lifestyle on well-being and prosperity. The distribution of nutraceuticals offers a variety of products to assist customers to satisfy their health and wellness needs for more useful dietary choices.

Research based on evidence will assist customers achieve trust in acquiring functional food products along with nutraceuticals and improving nutraceuticals and functional food laws. These laws are the contradictions between countries, and they must be considered when producing functional foods for global markets. In food industry generally, encapsulation is used to add nutraceutical component in food. It is used to overcome the challenges of adding nutraceuticals in an effective dose without affecting the sensory properties and storage strength of the food.

There are various encapsulation methods, and the selection of method relies on the nutraceutical element characteristics and the target application. When using food as a means of delivering nutraceuticals, new formulated strategies and food structures are also created.

Regardless of the strategy implemented, it is necessary to understand the interaction during processing between the nutraceuticals and the different components of the food matrix. These relationships can influence the added nutraceutical content's bioavailability and bioactivity. Additional studies are needed to understand the relationship between nutraceuticals and complex dietary matrices, to demonstrate the health advantages of nutraceuticals added to foods, and to understand the composition of the intestinal tract and how the encapsulant may impact this process.

20.13.7 Role of Precision Nutraceuticals in Preventive and Curative Approaches Against Cancer Novel Trends

Sensitive foods contribute to the protection and promotion of health as plant foods. It has been found to be useful in the control of diseases such as cancer and diabetes. Some research has shown that daily consumption of 21–31% of multivitamins as a public benefit for plant nutrients serves to prevent and cancer. Studies have shown that some selected plants have nutraceuticals that can manage cancer cell growth. Plants with nutraceutical nutrients have proven to be a low-cost nutritional supplement. Partially, medicinal plants must be washed thoroughly from the microbial load and heavy metals to obtain a properly reinforced product [28].

As indicated by epidemiological studies and animal models, nutraceuticals can have chemopreventive actions, primarily phytochemicals obtained from medicinal plants such as tea, ginger, garlic, soy, tea, honey, propolis, and others. Various studies found that their ability to reduce the occurrence of disease is linked to apoptosis. Use of nutraceuticals as potential chemo-protective reagents has led to an increase in in vitro studies on cultured human cells. Chemoprevention involves the use of small molecules that contain dietary or herbal chemicals to prevent cancer, unlike chemotherapeutics where mostly synthetic chemicals are used to relieve or alleviate signs of cancer. While the notion of chemoprevention has been common in the East for thousands of years, lately in the West, it attained scientific acceptance.

Large-scale clinical trials have shown that tamoxifen, raloxifene, estrogen receptor antagonists, and synthetic retinoids such as fenretinide are effective in protecting women against breast diseases. The American Cancer Research Association's Chemoprevention Working Group study was a watershed suggesting that chemoprevention was considered a feasible option for cancer therapy. It is therefore important to investigate the possibility of using phytochemicals or other nutritional substances as an inhibitor of cancer agents. In addition, examining the biological effects of these phytochemicals at the cellular level provides the molecular basis for antitumor functions and helps to develop a platform for producing stronger chemopreventive agents and chemotherapy agents.

Apoptosis performs a role in multiple normal physiological mechanisms such as immunity, homeostasis, development of tissues, or any other process that may increase or decrease the balance between organism's life and death. Therefore, in some functional deficit and degenerative disorders such as Alzheimer's, Parkinson's, and Huntington's disease, multiple sclerosis, myocardial infarction, and arteriosclerosis, the loss of essential cells from postmitotic tissues due to increased cell death may play a significant part. Garlic utilization as an antitumor process has been due to compounds extracted from garlic such as allyl sulfur compounds which has an important anticarcinogenic property against human cancers. Our increased research and understanding of the biology and chemistry of nutraceuticals have brought us to chemopreventive area. The following preventive activities should be taken into consideration during the use of nutraceuticals in the future:

1. Synergistic effect: Each nutraceutical molecular understanding elaborates that testing of synergistic effect can be done by using two or more nutraceuticals or their derivatives on the chemoprevention.
2. Defining molecular objectives: The molecular objectives of nutraceuticals have been identified; it is now feasible to create finer and target-specific nutraceuticals that select shared locations usually.
3. Synthesis of analogues: Efficacy of nutraceuticals has been increasing; this could be used as chemical template for combinational synthesis [29].

One nutraceutical that has been linked to soy, named as genistein, is gaining much popularity to fight tumors. Epidemiological evidence indicates that there are positive relationships between the main cause of genistein, chemoprevention, and soy consumption. Soy can inhibit tumor angiogenesis in mice and the growth of transplantable human carcinomas.

Apples are widely consumed in the human diet, which is the main supplier of phytochemicals. Apples are rich source of dihydrochalcones, flavonols, anthocyanins, hydroxycinnamic acids, flavam-3-procyanidins, chlorogenic acids, catechins, quercetin 3-glycosides (Q3G), phlorizin, and cyanidin-3-glycosides; these are the major phenolics. Consumption of apples can lower the risk of cancer, asthma, pulmonary disorders, and type 2 diabetes.

Tea belongs to *Theaceae* family and *Camellia sinensis* species. Tea is the most ancient, after water; it is the most largely consumed hot drink worldwide. Tea is high in polyphenols that have strong anticancer, anti-inflammatory, antioxidant, and antimutagenic properties. Tea polyphenols also inhibit proliferation and increase apoptosis in carcinogenic cells. Black tea, green tea, and soy essence have expressively reduced the tumor rate, growth, and proliferation, serum androgen level, and prostate tumor in mice in single or more diets.

Pomegranate is highly consumed as fresh and in the form of beverage juice or wines. The peel and juice of pomegranate have high content of polyphenols, antioxidants, tannins, anthocyanins, and ellagitannins. These compounds show chemopreventive, anti-inflammatory, and chemotherapeutic effects.

Organosulfur component of garlic demonstrates chemopreventive property for human cancers, just like colon and lung cancers. Combination therapy treatments for skin cancer are more helpful than individual treatments [30].

20.13.8 Constraints

Functional foods provide energy and basic nutrition to health that have advantages beyond basic nutrition. Nutraceuticals are the compounds that could be in the form of food or any food element that offer health advantages such as disease prevention and treatment. The expansion of nutraceutical elements to food in adequate values may suppress the beginning of enduring sicknesses, for example, coronary illness, tumor, hypertension, and heftiness. There are in any event two noteworthy classes of useful sustenance and nutraceuticals. First incorporates food that are normally rich in nutraceutical, and the other incorporates sustenance detailed with added nutraceutical fixings in adequate amounts, regularly with a medical advantage or ailment counteractive action focus at the top of the priority list.

The second group of functional foods that are added to nutraceuticals and gained the attention of consumers are those which are concerned about eating the supplemented diets for the betterment of health. This has been a motivation for the food industry in the presence of functional foods. There is an alternative to the dietary supplements which are available in tablet and capsule forms. The alternative is functional foods with the addition of nutraceuticals.

The normal diet parts including beverages and foods are food source of nutraceuticals. Consumers are increasingly demanding for healthier food and their derived products. Food manufacturing and processing industries produce food that is cost-effective, safe, and consumer-friendly. Many marketing, technological, and regularity encounters still need to address functional foods to be thrived in the market places.

20.13.9 Complexities of Nutraceutical Incorporation

The process of incorporating, fortifying, and adding nutraceuticals to food is complicated. Adding and fortifying new components to an existing item impact the physicochemical and sensory characteristics and structures of the original food or drink. The structure and its flavor, shelf life, and texture are enhanced. The solubility and format of nutraceutical elements increase the formulation processing of the product.

With the help of added nutraceuticals, anticipated characteristics are attained. The direct addition of nutraceuticals is not possible.

This impacts the food characteristics in which nutraceuticals are added. Direct inclusion of nutraceuticals in products is often not feasible because many nutraceuticals are prone to degradation and can interfere with other elements in the food, leading to the loss of nutraceutical element's bioactivity and a decrease in nutritional quality of the food item. Therefore, the effective introduction of nutraceuticals into products needs to be secured by a well-designed delivery system specifically developed for the delivery of specific products [31].

20.13.10 Challenges for Incorporation of Nutraceuticals in Foods

The need to manage an efficient dose of nutraceutical agent for a specific health advantage is a significant task as it impacts the finished product's flavor and aftertaste. Some difficulties are the following:

- Race prevents the unwanted effects of nutraceuticals from interacting with the other components of food and environment.
- Balance the nutraceutical components of food during the shelf life of the finished product.
- Make sure that foods containing nutraceuticals provide the expected health benefit after consumption.

Nutraceuticals are less stable after being isolated from many sources of bioactive and natural foods. In addition, encapsulation of nutraceutical is necessary so it might not interact with food component making it bio-unavailable.

Finish the application of food and the desired health result. Sensitive nutrition is difficult for several reasons. There are still no systematic intervention studies, and some of the few studies that are currently being carried out are uncertain.

- The effects of nutrition on health biomarkers tend to be small, which requires further studies to confirm the significant findings.
- The final visualization of long-term positive results requires long follow-up periods, and research on the interaction of nutritional interventions based on biomarkers (synergistic) is at an early stage [32].

20.14 Conclusion

However, sensible nutrition should be part of the concepts of medical therapy, protection, and normal health and concepts of healthy aging. More than 400 million people worldwide suffer from diabetes, with a high impact on metabolic diseases. It is estimated that more than 600 million people in 2040 will have diabetes. Sensitive nutrition can have a sustainable effect to reduce this growing number.

Providers of hospitals that offer sensitive medicine must also offer sensitive nutrition as part of the concepts of sustainable medical treatment oriented to results. Subsequently, sensible nutrition should be part of normal daily life to prevent and reduce the morbidity that we normally observe in metabolic diseases.

There will be an emerging trend of complete value chain of medicine-sensitive prevention-sensitive nutrition, that will incorporate new food logistics services, combining the concepts of new direct food delivery services for patients to the surrounding restaurants and cooking courses precisely all integrating into the food supply chain.

- The first sensitive nutrition success stories are introduced.
- The first well-approved health biomarkers (biological age) are available.
- Now we should carry out systematic studies of precision of nutrition on a large scale.

References

1. Dang R (2017) Nutraceuticals for healthy life. Indian J Pharm Educ Res 51(3):S148–S151
2. Gosslau A, Chen KY (2004) Nutraceuticals, apoptosis, and disease prevention. Nutrition 20(1):95
3. Estevinho L (2018) Special issue "Nutraceuticals in human health and disease". Int J Mol Sci 19:1213
4. Chintale Ashwini G, Kadam Vaishali S, Sakhare Ram S, Birajdar Ganesh O, Nalwad Digambar N (2013) Role of nutraceuticals in various diseases: a comprehensive review. Int J Res Pharm Chem 3:290–299
5. Shimizu M, Kubota M, Tanaka T, Moriwaki H (2012) Nutraceutical approach for preventing obesity-related colorectal and liver carcinogenesis. Int J Mol Sci 13(1):579–595
6. Khan N, Mukhtar H (2015) Dietary agents for prevention and treatment of lung cancer. Cancer Lett 359(2):155–164
7. Khan N, Adhami VM, Mukhtar H (2010) Apoptosis by dietary agents for prevention and treatment of prostate cancer. Endocr Relat Cancer 17(1):R39–R52
8. Kumar K, Kumar S (2015) Role of nutraceuticals in health and disease prevention: a review. South Asian J Food Technol Environ 1:116–121
9. Kaczor A, Barańska M, Czamara K (2016) Carotenoids: overview of nomenclature, structures, occurrence and functions. Carotenoids: nutrition, analysis and technology, 1st edn. Wiley, London, pp 1–13
10. Lerfall J (2016) Carotenoids: occurrence, properties and determination. In: Encyclopedia of food and health. Elsevier, Amsterdam, pp 663–669

11. Burton-Freeman B, Reimers K (2011) Tomato consumption and health: emerging benefits. Am J Lifestyle Med 5(2):182–191
12. Leoncini E, Nedovic D, Panic N, Pastorino R, Edefonti V, Boccia S (2015) Carotenoid intake from natural sources and head and neck cancer: a systematic review and meta-analysis of epidemiological studies. Cancer Epidemiol Prev Biomarkers 24(7):1003–1011
13. Eliassen AH, Liao X, Rosner B, Tamimi RM, Tworoger SS, Hankinson SE (2015) Plasma carotenoids and risk of breast cancer over 20 y of follow-up. Am J Clin Nutr 101(6):1197–1205
14. Ruiz RB, Hernández PS (2016) Cancer chemoprevention by dietary phytochemicals: epidemiological evidence. Maturitas 94:13–19
15. Yi J, Qu H, Wu Y, Wang Z, Wang L (2017) Study on antitumor, antioxidant and immunoregulatory activities of the purified polyphenols from pinecone of Pinus koraiensis on tumor-bearing S180 mice in vivo. Int J Biol Macromol 94:735–744
16. Turrini E, Ferruzzi L, Fimognari C (2015) Potential effects of pomegranate polyphenols in cancer prevention and therapy. Oxidative Med Cell Longev 2015:938475
17. Huarte M (2015) The emerging role of lncRNAs in cancer. Nat Med 21(11):1253
18. Liu L, Hou L, Gu S, Zuo X, Meng D, Luo M, Zhang X, Huang S, Zhao X (2015) Molecular mechanism of epigallocatechin-3-gallate in human esophageal squamous cell carcinoma in vitro and in vivo. Oncol Rep 33(1):297–303
19. Woyengo T, Ramprasath V, Jones P (2009) Anticancer effects of phytosterols. Eur J Clin Nutr 63(7):813
20. Bradford PG, Awad AB (2007) Phytosterols as anticancer compounds. Mol Nutr Food Res 51(2):161–170
21. Jones PJ, AbuMweis SS (2009) Phytosterols as functional food ingredients: linkages to cardiovascular disease and cancer. Curr Opin Clin Nutr Metab Care 12(2):147–151
22. Ramprasath VR, Awad AB (2015) Role of phytosterols in cancer prevention and treatment. J AOAC Int 98(3):735–738
23. Burton GJ, Jauniaux E (2011) Oxidative stress. Best Pract Res Clin Obstet Gynaecol 25(3): 287–299
24. Kwak JH, Baek SH, Woo Y, Han JK, Kim BG, Kim OY, Lee JH (2012) Beneficial immunostimulatory effect of short-term Chlorella supplementation: enhancement of natural killer cell activity and early inflammatory response (randomized, double-blinded, placebo-controlled trial). Nutr J 11(1):53
25. Fuellen G, Schofield P, Flatt T, Schulz R-J, Boege F, Kraft K, Rimbach G, Ibrahim S, Tietz A, Schmidt C (2016) Living long and well: prospects for a personalized approach to the medicine of ageing. Gerontology 62(4):409–416
26. Augustin MA, Sanguansri L (2015) Challenges and solutions to incorporation of nutraceuticals in foods. Annu Rev Food Sci Technol 6:463–477
27. Yao Z, Liu X-C, Gu Y-E (2014) Schisandra chinensis Baill, a Chinese medicinal herb, alleviates high-fat-diet-inducing non-alcoholic steatohepatitis in rats. Afr J Tradit Complement Altern Med 11(1):222–227
28. Nithya DM, Brindha P (2014) Herbal nutraceuticals in the management of cancer and chronic diseases-a select study. Int J Pharm Pharm Sci 6(1):21–34
29. Salami A, Seydi E, Pourahmad J (2013) Use of nutraceuticals for prevention and treatment of cancer. Iran J Pharm Res 12(3):219
30. Shukla Y, George J (2011) Combinatorial strategies employing nutraceuticals for cancer development. Ann N Y Acad Sci 1229(1):162–175
31. Özdemir V, Kolker E (2016) Precision nutrition 4.0: a big data and ethics foresight analysis—convergence of agrigenomics, nutrigenomics, nutriproteomics, and nutrimetabolomics. OMICS 20(2):69–75
32. Celis-Morales C, Livingstone KM, Marsaux CF, Macready AL, Fallaize R, O'Donovan CB, Woolhead C, Forster H, Walsh MC, Navas-Carretero S (2016) Effect of personalized nutrition on health-related behaviour change: evidence from the Food4me European randomized controlled trial. Int J Epidemiol 46(2):578–588

Part VII

Cancer Genomics in Precision Oncology: Applications, Challenges, and Prospects

21

Michele Araújo Pereira, Marianna Kunrath Lima, Patrícia Gonçalves Pereira Couto, Michele Groenner Penna, Luige Biciati Alvim, Thaís Furtado Nani, Maíra Cristina Menezes Freire, and Luiz Henrique Araújo

21.1 Introduction

The completion of the Human Genome Project (HGP) in 2001 led to a better understanding of human biology, its particularities, and variabilities. Since then, considerable time and effort have been dedicated to decoding the patterns of human and cancer genomes. In 2015, the President of the United States, Barack Obama, launched the Precision Medicine Initiative (PMI), a new effort to revolutionize medicine and improve health and disease treatment, as opposed to a "one-size-fits-all" medicine approach [1]. Precision medicine aims to deliver the right treatment to the right patient, at the right dose, and at the right time. In this context, precision medicine offered new strategies and opportunities for surveying cancer genomes. Many molecular genetic tests have been developed and used for several different purposes in cancer research (e.g., differential diagnosis, prognosis, pharmacogenomics, treatment, disease monitoring, and risk assessment (Fig. 21.1).

DNA sequencing has become the main molecular tool for cancer research [2, 3]. Sequencing has been possible since 1977 when Frederick Sanger developed the "chain-termination" method which became the most commonly used (first-generation) DNA sequencing method [4]. However, the arrival of next-generation sequencing (NGS) in 2005 changed the landscape of precision medicine. NGS has overtaken Sanger sequencing due to its high throughput, parallel operation, and

M. A. Pereira (✉) · M. K. Lima · P. G. P. Couto · M. G. Penna · L. B. Alvim · T. F. Nani · M. C. M. Freire
Instituto Hermes Pardini, Vespasiano, Brazil
e-mail: mi.araujop@hotmail.com; kunrathlimam@gmail.com; patriciagpcouto@gmail.com; michelepenna@gmail.com; luigebiciati@yahooo.com.br; thaisfnani@gmail.com; freiremcm@hotmail.com

L. H. Araújo
Instituto COI & Instituto Nacional de Câncer, Rio de Janeiro, Brazil
e-mail: luizaraujo.md@gmail.com

N. Masood, S. Shakil Malik (eds.), *'Essentials of Cancer Genomic, Computational Approaches and Precision Medicine*,
https://doi.org/10.1007/978-981-15-1067-0_21

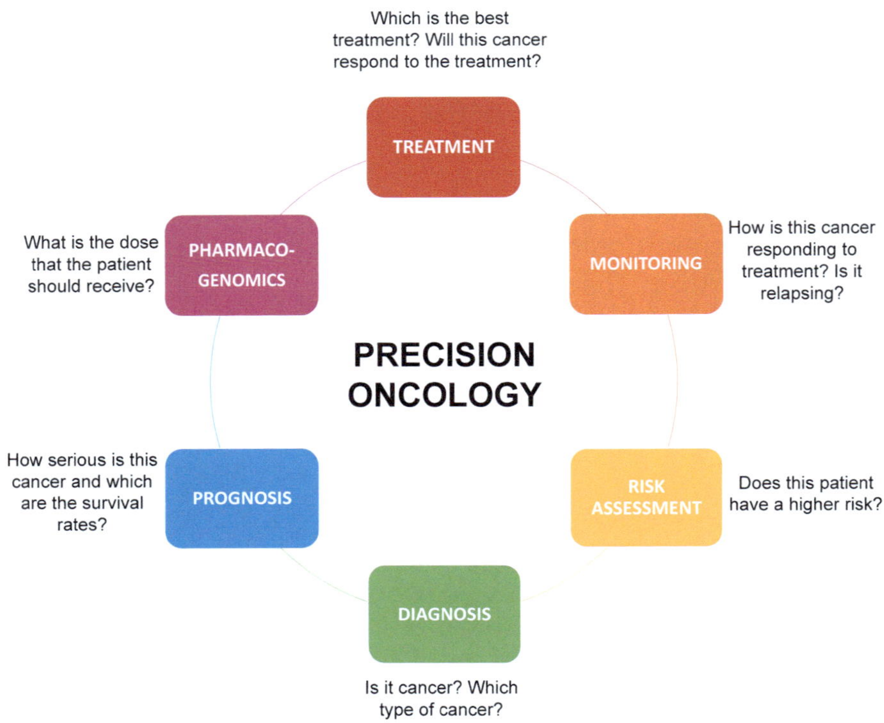

Fig. 21.1 Clinical uses of molecular diagnostics test in precision oncology

lower cost per base pair. The analysis of multiple genomic fragments simultaneously has allowed the identification of the full catalogue of germline and somatic mutations, epigenetic alterations, the characterization of cancer cell transcriptomes, and the discovery of new biomarkers [3, 5].

A variety of molecular diagnostic tests use NGS (e.g., single- and multigene sequencing panels, whole-exome sequencing (WES), whole-genome sequencing (WGS)) and other polymerase chain reaction (PCR)-based approaches (e.g., quantitative PCR (qPCR) and digital PCR (dPCR)). Therefore, understanding the application and limitations of these different approaches is of utmost importance in clinical practice. The following topics will detail current applications and challenges on genomic research, clinical case studies on the role of precision oncology, and future perspectives of cancer genomics.

21.2 Applications and Challenges on Cancer Genomics

A diagnostic test encompasses three main different phases: pre-analytical (i.e., test design and specimen handling issues), analytical (i.e., sample analysis), and post-analytical (i.e., results interpretation and report). This section aims to provide further contributions for the applications, challenges, and solutions found in all phases of genetic testing in oncology.

21.2.1 Pre-analytical Phase

The pre-analytical phase comprises the first stages involved in a diagnostic assay, from test design to patient sample collection and processing. This is one of the most important steps during genetic test development because it ensures reliable delivery and quality results and is now increasingly being appreciated not only by laboratory researchers but also by doctors and patients [6]. Several factors that influence the pre-analytical phase have already been described and include (1) correct indication for the test, (2) correct preparation for sampling, (3) sample type, (4) sampling time, (5) sample handling, (6) patient preparation, (7) standardized and validated collection, (8) analyte transport, and (9) pretest laboratory steps, among others [7].

Currently, the definition of what tests and treatments should be used does not occur only from the physician's decision. Doctor-patient communication plays a central role in building a doctor-patient test/therapeutic relationship. This is important in providing excellent healthcare, which is the objective of precision medicine. Good communication can ensure the sharing of pertinent information for proper diagnosis of patient health issues, adherence to guidelines, and prescribed treatment [8]. A very relevant point in this communication is the physician's role in explaining all the peculiarities of an exam and the possible results. Clinical labs and research centers should provide manuals with clear and objective information to healthcare professionals (doctors, nurses, and others) on all requirements necessary for the pre-analytical phase. This care is fundamental, since most diagnostic errors occur during this phase [9]. These errors are usually related to a lack of standardized protocols, from test design to sampling acquisition. This is also the case in precision medicine. Therefore, careful design of a test and its execution must be well-planned in order to have reliable results. This section will review some pre-analytical challenges in precision oncology and discuss approaches for overcoming them.

21.2.1.1 Test Design

Designing a good assay is the first task when a test is being developed. There are many experimental options available, and understanding each step and the possible limitations is essential but challenging [10]. The design depends on intrinsic (e.g., sample type, disease's characteristics, number of targets, sequencing platform) and extrinsic (e.g., samples availability, cost, time, transport conditions) factors.

When choosing a genetic test, there are doubts regarding which mutations to assess. Should the entire gene-coding sequence be analyzed? Or only point mutations? One gene, or several genes? Single-nucleotide variants (SNVs; point mutations), for example, are the most frequent mutation type in solid tumors and hematological malignant diseases [11]. In somatic oncology, attention should be directed to mutations or variants that have clinical importance, having an impact on treatment choice, or acting as agnostic/prognostic markers. For non-small-cell lung cancer (NSCLC), for example, mutations in the *EGFR* gene that confer sensitivity or resistance to tyrosine kinase inhibitors (TKIs) are well-described [12]. The three most relevant are deletion at exon 19 (Del19) and L858R, both making tumors sensitive to EGFR TKIs, and T790M, which confers resistance to first- and second-generation TKIs but is sensitive to third-generation TKIs [12]. Given the importance of these mutations to NSCLC treatment, molecular tests for patients affected by this cancer type should cover, at least, the codons affected by such mutations.

A major issue involving cancer genomics is the types of gene panels. Certain types of cancer have landmark-mutated genes, whereas other cancer types do not possess signature mutated genes. In any of the cases, the number of genes, which genes, and the mutation types that should be tested are questions with answers that are not so simple. Germline or sporadic cancer applications, as somatic testing for solid tumors or hematological malignancies, may require the use of different genes/panels. Commercially available NGS panels (e.g., Illumina's TruSight™ Oncology 500, Thermo Fisher's Oncomine™ Focus Assay, or Agilent's ClearSeq Comprehensive Cancer Panel) may be attractive for multiple indications. However, custom gene panels should be necessary for cost saving. Designing a custom panel became relatively straightforward due to sophisticated and easy-to-use bioinformatics tools. The Association for Molecular Pathology (AMP) and College of American Pathologists (CAP) recommend understanding the panel's intended use prior to making a panel choice (e.g., search for therapeutic targets or diagnosis and patient prognostication) and to include solely genes that have sufficient scientific grounds for the disease diagnosis, prognostication, or treatment [11].

Once the genes or mutations to be tested are defined, another question emerges: should the assay be qualitative or quantitative? Most qualitative tests are for diagnostic purposes, while quantitative tests are for disease follow-up or response monitoring. A renowned case is BCR-ABL fusion (Philadelphia chromosome (Ph)) in chronic myeloid leukemia (CML) [13]. The National Comprehensive Cancer Network (NCCN) and LeukemiaNet guidelines strongly suggest that qualitative search of Ph, by molecular methods or by cytogenetics, should be employed for diagnostic testing, whereas Ph quantitative search is indicated for monitoring drug response and minimal residual disease (MRD) [14, 15]. For allele ratio (in the case of rare alleles search), quantification can be used for prognostic risk stratification, as for *FLT3* in acute myeloid leukemia (AML), where *FLT3-ITD* (internal tandem duplication) mutation allele ratio is considered for stratifying patients [16]. Tumor mutational burden (TMB) is a different case, where the total amount of mutations present within a tumor is quantified to help direct immunotherapy and patient stratification [17].

Choosing the best methodology involves careful analysis of specificity, sensibility, costs, and benefits of each technique available. For example, quantification of rare alleles can be assessed by qPCR, dPCR or sequencing (Sanger or NGS) [18–20]. With qPCR, probes are preferred instead of intercalating dyes, such as SYBR Green, because even though probes are more expensive than intercalating dyes, they are more specific for a gene region. However, when compared to dPCR, qPCR is less sensitive and also demands a standard curve, as it is not an absolute quantification method. Sequencing, especially NGS, could be the most sensitive method for rare allele quantification [18], but its costs, when analyzing a small number of mutations, could be prohibitive for some laboratories and patients.

Beyond the aforementioned points, test design should consider logistical aspects (transport and sample conservation time), technical and analytical team (properly trained for sample acquisition, sample processing, results analysis), and assay cost (Fig. 21.2). Taken together, complications regarding lack of design standardization could be reduced.

21.2.1.2 Sampling

Establishing the sample type is also an important step. Several primary materials may be used, depending on the type of nucleic acid modification to be evaluated and the assay methodology to be employed (e.g., whole blood, saliva, bone marrow, liquor, formalin-fixed paraffin-embedded (FFPE) tissues, etc.). Liquid biopsies, as it is indicated by its name, use nonsolid biological tissue samples, with whole blood being the most extensively used. There are many studies involving other body fluids ([21]; for more information, see, Sect. 21.2.2.5). Leukemia tests are based on whole blood and bone marrow samples, as this area comprises liquid tumors originated in blood cells [14, 15]. Solid tumors are usually molecularly studied by nucleic acid extracted from slides derived from FFPE [22]. Furthermore, DNA and/or RNA can be used. For example, for MRD in chromosome fusions in oncohematology, the nucleic acid studied is RNA, since most fusions occur at intronic regions [23].

Sample collection tubes are a major concern. Most molecular assays are inhibited by the presence of heparin, which makes ethylenediaminetetraacetic acid (EDTA) the main choice anticoagulant on molecular genetics [24]. There are some patented tubes available, such as Qiagen's PAXgene® and Streck's BCT® tubes, which contain special preservative products that stabilize cells and/or nucleic acids for longer than normal tubes [25]. This brings more quality for the assays and enables safer transport between distant locations. For liquid biopsies, it is well-described that blood storage and processing methods have a strong influence on ctDNA (circulating tumor DNA) concentration [26].

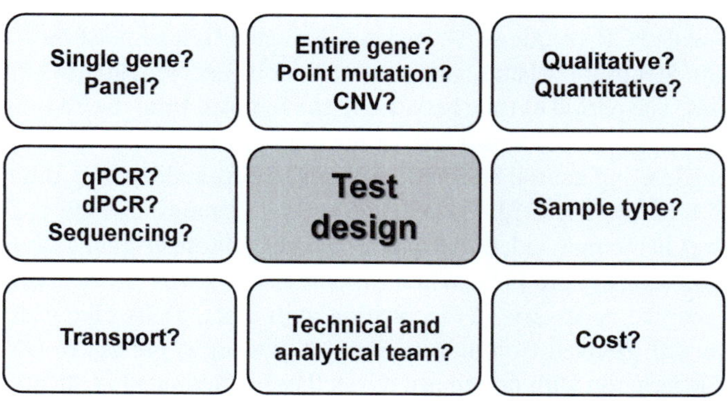

Fig. 21.2 Points that should be considered when designing a test for molecular precision oncology. This scheme summarizes some of the aspects that must be evaluated during the test design phase: number of genes analyzed, target(s) definition, methodology (including qualitative or quantitative methods), sample type, logistics, qualified working team, and costs, among others

Sample volume is also thought to interfere with an assay final result [27]. In the case of liquid specimens, like samples for RNA-based MRD evaluation in oncohematology and plasma for liquid biopsy, where the targeted mutation/variant may be present in extremely low quantities, initial sample volumes are directly involved in the test quality and sensibility [27, 28]. Regarding FFPE samples, small-sized tumors (e.g., alveolar lung cancers) and small tumoral areas provide reduced amounts of material for nucleic acid extraction, which can be very challenging for later applications [27].

When RNA is used, it is important to remember that it is less stable than DNA, so sample conservation times are reduced and extraction conditions must be carefully controlled [29]. Malentacchi et al. [30] have also described that tubes containing cellular RNA stabilizers (e.g., PAXgene® Blood RNA Tube) significantly affect the transcript levels of *FOS*, *IL8*, *FOSB*, and *TNFRSF10c* genes, maintaining these transcript levels close to the ones observed at time zero (T_0). RNA should be extracted from samples as soon as possible, 48–72 h is the maximum time allowed for RNA extraction from fresh blood samples, which can be challenging for long distance transportation. These samples must be kept refrigerated until RNA is extracted. New technologies that permit dry storage at room temperature are promising. Dried RNA has been shown to have comparable results to cryopreserved RNA in downstream applications, even after 1 year of storage [31]. RNA can be degraded by naturally occurring enzymes (RNases), which makes ambient RNase removal important when handling this type of nucleic acid. After extraction, samples need to be kept at −80 °C, and repeated freeze-thaw cycles may decrease RNA quality, so the use of multiple aliquots is recommended [32].

FFPE samples have particular issues regarding their preparation and analysis. At the pre-analytical phase, sample quality can be affected by fixative solution pH, duration of tissue fixation, storage conditions and age of tissue blocks, and extraction method [33]. Small tissue samples can provide smaller nucleic acid yields, as previously described. Different tissue types may need additional treatments due to their specific characteristics. For example, melanin binds to Taq DNA polymerase, interfering with PCR reactions, so melanin-enriched tissues must be treated with bovine serum albumin [34] and bone tissues must be decalcified using EDTA [35], among others. The period of time between tissue removal from the body and its fixation may interfere with methods used for nucleic acid analysis [35]. Tissue fixation should be made using neutral buffered formalin (4% formaldehyde), diluted no longer than 24 h before use [33]. Fixing time and temperature can affect DNA/RNA integrity, so it is recommended that this step takes no longer than 72 h and should occur at room temperature [35]. When extracting DNA from FFPE samples, other treatments may be necessary: (1) incubation with uracil-DNA glycosylase (UDG) to remove uracil (derived from deamination of cytosines) present in DNA and (2) prolonging incubation with proteinase K and thermal treatment at 90 °C, to remove possible cross-links (protein-protein, DNA-protein, formaldehyde-DNA, or even DNA interstrand cross-links) caused by the formaldehyde present in formalin [36]. The age of the blocks could interfere with the quality of DNA that is degraded over the years. Storage time is also a limiting factor to DNA quality in FFPE tissues, irrespectively of the extraction method [37]. Slides derived from FFPE samples should be accurately manufactured, so they represent the genuine tumoral milieu. Good quality paraffin blocks and tissue slides are essential for an effective pathological review, in which the pathologist identifies tumor-rich and necrotic-rich areas, in order to enhance analytic sensitivity [36].

As it is invasive and, in some cases, difficult to make a tissue biopsy every time a new exam is needed, the characterization of several genetic biomarkers in plasma samples by liquid biopsy is an emerging approach in precision medicine. Levels of these biomarkers are increased in certain types of malignant cancer, such as lung, colorectal, and breast tumors, and in late-stage cancers [38]. Prior cancer treatments can also change the quantity of ctDNA in patient plasma [39]. Thus, the analysis of liquid biopsy results must consider these variables.

Tumor heterogeneity is another challenge for genetic analysis. This phenomenon is generated due to genomic instability and, in certain types of cancer, polyclonality of cancer cells. The patient with intratumoral heterogeneity could have a poor prognosis because therapeutic selection pressure may promote an expansion of a resistant subclonal population, promoting the evolution of drug-resistant cells, which changes the profile of possible target-directed therapies against the tumor. Multiregional tissue sampling, single-cell sequencing, and research autopsies are all methodological approaches that have the capacity to enable high-resolution identification of complex clonal changes [40]. Liquid biopsies are also recommended, as they may be able to detect ctDNA from all tumor clones, reflecting the tumor genome heterogeneity [41].

Regarding nucleic acid extraction, there are good automated and manual (solution-based or column-based) methods available [42]. Automated extraction can decrease variability and reduce hands-on time for the execution of a test, whereas manual extraction can generate higher nucleic acid yields and is usually less expensive [43, 44]. For RNA, despite the demanding hands-on time, phenol-chloroform manual extraction is still the main choice for liquid samples, as it is less expensive than automated methods and very effective [45, 46]. For FFPE, semiautomated methods are the main choice [47]. Care must be taken concerning magnetic bead extraction when using droplet digital PCR (ddPCR), once these beads impair droplet generation, and deparaffinization of tissue blocks need to be efficient, because formalin and paraffin may cause cross-links between nucleic acids and proteins, jeopardizing downstream sample applications. Table 21.1 summarizes the points related to sampling.

21.2.2 Analytical and Post-analytical Phases

21.2.2.1 Sanger Sequencing

To date, Sanger sequencing is the gold standard in diagnostic tests. Although NGS has a much higher processing capacity, confirmation of genetic findings is still made by the Sanger method in many clinical laboratories [48]. Sanger sequencing workflow has very easy-to-use and familiar protocols. However, it is important to

Table 21.1 Main attention points for sampling in precision oncology

Sample type or methodology	Attention points
FFPE	Tumor size, additional treatments for particular cancer types, time between biopsy and fixation, fixative solution pH, duration of tissue fixation, cross-links removal, age and storage conditions of tissue blocks, determination of tumor-rich and necrotic-rich areas, tumor heterogeneity, nucleic acid extraction method
Liquid biopsy	Sample volume, cancer type, available biomarkers, sampling time (cancer stage and previous treatments), special conservative tubes, nucleic acid extraction method
Oncohematology	EDTA as anticoagulant for sample collection, sample volume, RNA stability and conservation time, nucleic acid extraction method

highlight some challenges and limitations including (1) primer design, (2) inability to perform parallel investigation of multiple targets, (3) lower scalability due to increasing sample input requirements, (4) less cost-effective for high numbers of targets, (5) worse sequence quality in the first 15–40 bases and after 600–1000 bases, (6) lower mutation resolution (size of the mutation identified), and (7) lower sensitivity (limit of detection ~15–20%). Although Sanger sequencing and PCR are routinely used to identify clinically relevant mutations, these techniques are insensitive to changes occurring at an allele frequency lower than 20%, apart from qPCR, dPCR and NGS techniques, which could reach higher sensitivity [49–51]. Therefore, somatic cancer mutations can be difficult to detect with the Sanger method especially without performing microdissections since tumors are heterogeneous and often mixed with normal tissue [52]. Another challenge in Sanger sequencing analysis is the difficulty in dealing with normal/polymorphic genomic variations in the patient sample that may interfere with variant detection. A variant present at the primer annealing site can generate sequencing of only one of the DNA strands, generating misleading results. Other challenges include primer design, primer self-looping, and primer dimers. These problems are also present in NGS amplicon-based assays, which will be covered later in this section.

While Sanger sequencing has a lower sample throughput, NGS sequences millions of fragments simultaneously per run, offering greater discovery power to detect novel or rare variants with deep sequencing [53–55]. Sanger sequencing can be a good choice when (1) sequencing specific mutations, (2) sequencing amplicon targets up to 1 Kb, (3) identifying microbes, and (4) analyzing fragments and analyzing short tandem repeats (STRs). Otherwise, NGS is preferred because it allows for (1) simultaneous sequencing of many genes, (2) expansion of the number of targets for finding novel variants, (3) samples with low input amounts of starting material, and (4) somatic mutations at low allele frequency (above 20%) [56].

21.2.2.2 Pyrosequencing

The era of parallel massive sequencing became known as the second generation of DNA sequencing. Pyrosequencing developed by Nyrén et al. in 1996 [57] was the first method of this generation and the first alternative to the conventional Sanger method [58–60]. In this method, 454 pyrophosphate-based sequencing (thus the name pyrosequencing) builds on a sequencing by synthesis (SBS) approach and can be defined as a method capable of defining the DNA sequence by capturing visible light through a series of enzymatic reactions from the release of a pyrophosphate during the synthesis [54, 57, 61].

The pyrosequencing technique is recommended for sequencing up to 100 bases and is generally used for analysis of single nucleotide polymorphisms (SNPs) and for identification of short DNA sequences [62–65]. Pyrosequencing technology performance proved to also be applicable in several types of analysis including mutation detection, DNA methylation, tag sequencing of a selected cDNA library, clone checking, etc. [66–71]. This method is simple, robust, fast, sensitive, and cost-effective [72]. There are a number of studies that have applied the pyrosequencing technique in somatic cancer analysis – especially for *KRAS*, *NRAS*, *BRAF*, and *EGFR* genes – allowing detection of genetic variants in an allele frequency around 12.5%, using low amounts of DNA, with robust and fast results in an extremely simple protocol [73].

The major challenge of this technology is to enhance read lengths while maintaining reliability and accuracy. There are important reasons that inhibit the system from performing longer reads accurately, like uncertainties in homopolymeric regions and loss of synchronism. In long homopolymeric regions, it is difficult to interpret the light signal when many identical nucleotides are incorporated into a single cycle [63]. Other challenges include an inability to detect complex mutations, primer design, enzyme and nucleotide dispensation, primer self-looping, primer dimers, cross-hybridizations, and de novo sequencing of polymorphic regions in heterozygous DNA material [58].

21.2.2.3 NGS Sequencing

Currently the NGS technique has been used for a wide variety of clinical and research applications due to the proven cost reduction of reagents, equipment, related products, and improved data analysis solutions [74]. Defining the library method and sequencing platform is an important choice to consider when choosing NGS technology for clinical and research applications [75]. There are two main forms of library methods, hybridization-based and amplicon-based methods, that differ in the way they amplify and sequence target regions as well as detect genetic variants. For sequencing platforms, there are two major chemistry choices: SBS and semiconductor technology [75]. For each chemistry choice, there is a balance of advantages and disadvantages [76].

SBS platforms usually generate higher throughput per run and utilize single base extension and competitive nucleotide addition, resulting in highly accurate sequencing [76], but sequencing by synthesis technology has well-known base substitution errors [77, 78]. Semiconductor technologies run shorter reads, and the most relevant limitation is the error rate in homopolymer regions (repetitive regions), which requires robust bioinformatics pipeline and analytical expertise to reduce error rate [79]. However, it delivers the fastest throughput and shortest run time [76, 80].

When comparing different platforms, simplified workflows, runtime, time processing, and analysis are taken into account when defining which option is the best to work with [76]. Hybridization and amplicon approaches have different flows that should be evaluated, being amplicon method the simplified workflow, for example [75]. Additionally, amplicon-based methods have short preparation time compared to other methods [80] and also offer an advantage in being able to work with smaller quantities of DNA than hybridization assays [76]. On the other hand, amplicon assays, although ideal for small numbers of well-defined regions, are challenging to multiplex. Another important challenge of amplicon assays, as well as in Sanger sequencing, is the presence of variants at the primer annealing site, resulting in erroneous results. Hybridization capture method, in turn, performed better in complex regions and also in uniformity quality measures than amplicon-based methods [75], is less restricted by variant position, and can still enrich all strands and alleles equally, even in the presence of multiple novel variants. It has been demonstrated, however, that regions with high or low GC content may affect probe hybridization and PCR bias [81, 82].

Finally, cost is always an important factor. Sequencing cost is generally comparable but may also be affected by the target region size, on-target rate, and depth coverage [75]. The hybridization method is the most economical for large target regions. On the other hand, for smaller panels, the amplicon method turns out to be the most cost-effective. The final cost should be calculated taking into account the desired quality parameters as well as any additional experiments that may be required [76].

NGS assay is composed of three main distinct and interdependent parts: library construction, sequencing, and data analysis [74]. Regardless of the method chosen (hybridization or amplicon-based), the massive number of sequence data produced by NGS is computationally intensive, reinforcing the need of robust pipelines [54, 83, 84].

A bioinformatics pipeline involves numerous file transformations interacting with information from different databases, software components, and operational environments (i.e., the environment in which users run application software). They are typically specific to each sequencing platform and can be customized [85]. A bioinformatics pipeline consists of the following major steps: (1) a first analysis, where the sequence is generated by base calling and quality score generation; (2) a second analysis, where alignment occurs to the reference sequence; and (3) a tertiary analysis, where the variant is called, annotated, filtered, and interpreted as to its clinical relevance [85, 86].

Although bioinformatics tools continue to improve, important challenges still remain concerning variant-calling process. There are somatic and germline genetic variants, depending on their origin. Germinal variants are inherited or occur at a very early time during embryogenesis [87]. Somatic genetic variants are acquired as a result of internal or external events. Cumulative somatic mutations are an intrinsic characteristic of cancer and tumors throughout its development shows new changes from small point changes to large genomic rearrangements [88]. Germline and somatic NGS data differ at several points that need to be considered during analysis [89], including the following:

1. Expected allele frequency: as stated earlier, somatic variants may have very-low-frequency values (NGS sensitivity ~5%), and germline variant frequency remains 50% (heterozygous) or 100% (homozygous).
2. Mean coverage depth: must be greater in somatic (~1500x) than in germline (~200x).
3. Sample quantity and quality: tumor is usually scarce and of poor quality, being variable according to pre-analytical care and biological factors (e.g., the extensive tissue necrosis found in many cancers).

SNV and small indels are the most frequent variations in genome; however, large DNA rearrangements are a fundamental part of the development of many diseases and particularly in cancer. Copy number variation (CNV) was earlier described as DNA regions with at least 1 kb in size, involving gains or losses of base pairs in genomic DNA that presented different copy number in comparison with a reference genome [90, 91]. However, we know that CNVs can range considerably in size, and smaller sizes (e.g., 50 bp) may also be considered as CNVs. As the detection technologies and the knowledge about CNVs advanced, the increased available data could provide accurate information on CNVs related to cancer diagnosis and management. CNV detection is usually performed by multiplex ligation-dependent probe amplification (MLPA), array-based comparative genomic hybridization (aCGH), fluorescence in situ hybridization (FISH), and qPCR. Most of these techniques are low-throughput assays (with the exception of aCGH, which is a genome-wide array), but it is possible to make CNV analysis by high-throughput techniques (e.g., NGS). The hybridization-based method presents a better coverage and uniformity than the amplicon-based method allowing large genetic rearrangement computational analysis [75]. There are many software available to identify and call CNVs [92], but all quality parameters should be verified and validated to call CNVs correctly, reducing false-positive (FP) or false-negative (FN) results. The most critical point is the sequencing depth; when it does not reach the minimum established for the test, CNV cannot be detected. This is a real challenge to CNV analysis on NGS platforms. It has been shown that CNV can be found in a gene or gene region when it is overgrown by at least five amplicons in well-validated protocols [93]. Sequencing systematic noise and array data still stands as significant challenge to CNV determination in cancer genome analysis, but there are some initiatives trying to reduce this kind of issue [94, 95].

Both germline (CNV) and somatic copy number alterations (SCNAs) are present in cancer and can affect oncogenes or tumor suppressor genes. The identification of these alterations allows better cancer categorization and a better characterization of cancer pathways. Comparison of CNV and SCNA signatures showed that SCNAs are larger than the germline CNVs, due to high rates of somatic events [96].

Concerning NGS variant annotation, bioinformatics tools collect data from several databases to characterize and provide auxiliary data for each called variant, such as variant location (chromosome, gene, exon/intron), predicted cDNA and amino acid sequence changes (c. and p., respectively), allele frequencies, and in silico prediction of pathogenicity (e.g., SIFT, PolyPhen, Human Splicing Finder (HSF)) [85]. Databases include ClinVar, Single-Nucleotide Polymorphism Database (dbSNP), Online Mendelian Inheritance in Man (OMIM), the Genome Aggregation Database (gnomAD), Catalogue of Somatic Mutations in Cancer (COSMIC), and The Cancer Genome Atlas (TCGA), among others. All this data is used to further filter, classify, and interpret variants.

Sequence variant nomenclature needs to be precise, unequivocal, stable, but flexible enough for all known sequence variation classes (substitution, deletion, duplication, insertion, conversion, inversion, deletion-insertion, and repeated sequence) [97]. The Human Genome Variation Society (HGVS) nomenclature is the standard recommendation for the description of DNA, RNA, or protein sequence variants in molecular diagnostics [98], and different algorithms can be used to check HGVS nomenclature, as Mutalyzer [99]. Indels and complex variants represent one of the main challenges of an accurate sequence variant nomenclature, and NGS analysis

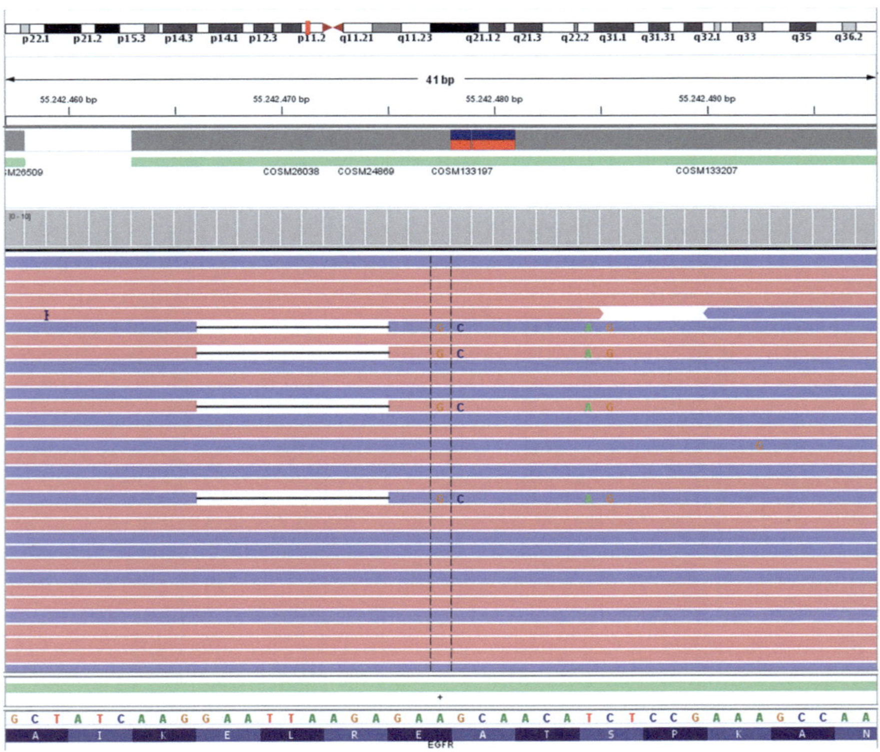

Fig. 21.3 Complex *EGFR* variant detection (deletion followed by four base substitutions). This alteration could be interpreted as three different mutational events (LRG_304t1:c.2236_2244del(;)2247_2248delinsGC(;)2254_2255delinsAG), two different mutational events (LRG_304t1:c.2238_2248delinsGC(;)2254_2255delinsAG) or as a unique event (LRG_304t1:c.2238_2255delinsGCCAACAAG). It is the consensus of the scientific community to consider all mutations in the same event

sometimes may be limited to provide the correct nomenclature. Figure 21.3 illustrates the detection of a complex variant (one deletion followed by four base substitutions) in the *EGFR* gene. There are distinct ways to interpret this alteration: one, two, or three mutational events. In evolutionary terms, three different mutational events are unlikely to occur at once. Furthermore, it is the consensus of the scientific community to consider all mutations in the same event, being this variant description as LRG_304t1:c.2238_2255delinsGCCAACAAG.

A key step is to achieve robust and reliable results by defining well-validated bioinformatics pipeline quality parameters. A team of experienced professionals should validate analytical parameters that deal with various challenges in NGS analysis. It is important, for example, to exclude FP artifacts through analysis of mapping quality, base-calling quality, and strand bias [85]. One example is the comparison of libraries from fresh frozen tissue and from FFPE libraries, with the former having significantly lower quality, thereby increasing the number of artifacts in the final data [100]. In this context, the use of orthogonal assays (e.g., Sanger sequencing) to confirm pathogenic variants detected by NGS is a standard practice in many clinical laboratories.

Orthogonal methods should be also used in various complex occasions like homologous pseudogenes sequences, homopolymer regions, GC-rich regions, or regions with low coverage [101]. However, the adoption of different applications is necessary to overcome the limitations presented. Three kinds of multigene panel tests are useful for this purpose: (A) >99% of the interest region is covered, and all the gaps are filled with Sanger sequencing; (B) regions sequenced are reported and some specific gaps (only in important genes) are filled with Sanger; and (C) no additional Sanger sequencing is performed [102]. It is recommended to define the horizontal coverage report as well as the limitations of each test [103].

Other techniques might be useful to confirm variants when technical bias (e.g., directional artifacts) is detected. Figure 21.4 illustrates the different detection of the *EGFR* Del19 variant on the positive (forward) and on the negative (reverse) strands. According to Barnell et al. [104], artifacts in sequencing may be affected by DNA polymerase acting more in one direction than in the other (complement strand) and can also be caused during alignment or during post-sequencing base/read processing, when a small molecule is preferentially amplified and is not removed through analysis programs. Another problem could be the occurrence of polymorphisms at prime annealing sites in one of the strands for amplicon-based methods. When such an event is detected, it is recommended to perform a second test in order to confirm the real presence of the variant, such as qPCR (e.g., cobas® *EGFR* Mutation Test v2) and/or MLPA. It is of utmost importance to understand the limitations of all molecular techniques for defining the best option to confirm NGS findings (e.g., cobas® kit uses specific mutation probes, which limits the identification of variants, such as the complex *EGFR* Del19 variants, which are not detected by this assay). For the case described in Fig. 21.4, it would be interesting to apply another orthogonal technique on samples (**b**) and (**c**) to understand the real reason for the limitation of the *EGFR* Del19 variants to negative strands.

Another interesting case is the occurrence of two different start and end positions at *EGFR* Del19: LRG_304t1(*EGFR*):c.2236_2250del; p.(Glu746_Ala750del) and LRG_304t1(*EGFR*):c.2238_2252del; p.(Glu746_Ala751del) in lung cancer (Fig. 21.5).

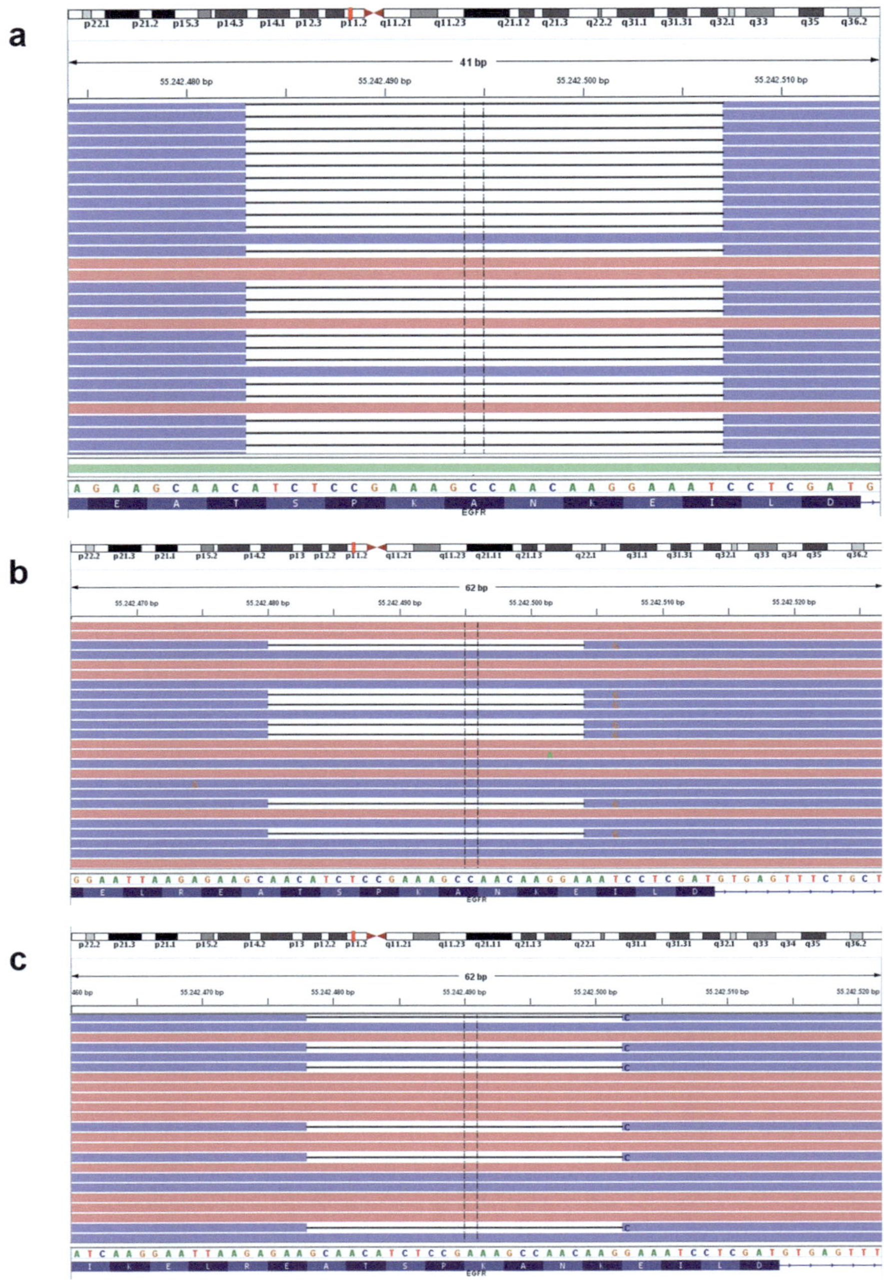

Fig. 21.4 *EGFR* Del19 variants detection limited to negative strands. (**a**) LRG_304t1(*EGFR*):c.2253_2276del. (**b**) LRG_304t1(*EGFR*):c.2252_2276delinsG. (**c**) LRG_304t1(*EGFR*):c.2248_2272delinsC. Samples were also tested by cobas® EGFR Mutation Test v2 (data not shown), but only variant (**a**) was confirmed. These *EGFR* Del19 had uncommon start and end positions, which could not be detected by cobas® assay

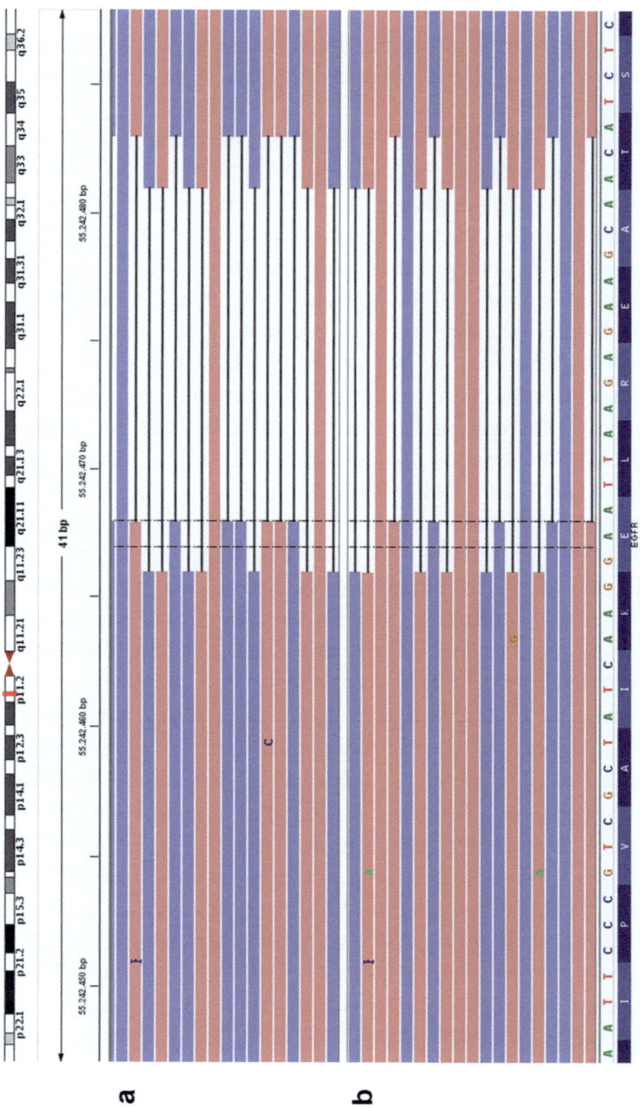

Fig. 21.5 NGS data from two different experiments (**a**) and (**b**). Both presented two different start and end positions of *EGFR* Del19 for the same sample

Variants were detected in both directions (no strand bias), and the result was confirmed by a second NGS experiment using a new DNA extraction. To our knowledge, this is the first case showing this phenomenon for *EGFR* Del19 that may be explained by tumor heterogeneity. Melanoma and lung cancers are tumor types that harbor a relevant mutational burden, because of the high possibility of involvement of exogenous mutagens (e.g., ultraviolet light and tobacco carcinogens) [105]. According to Barnell et al. [106], it is recommended to perform an orthogonal confirmation of the variant. Unlike the case mentioned previously, cobas® is not recommended for this case, since both mutations will not be differentiated by this assay.

International guidelines for NGS validation do not present a consensus recommendation regarding the necessity of NGS confirmation [98]. It is commonly accepted that quality thresholds for high-confidence calls and orthogonal confirmation for low-quality variants should ensure the highest sensitivity and sensibility of the assay [48, 98]. However, some studies suggest that confirmation may not always be necessary [107, 108] or has limited utility [109]. Some criteria need to be established in order to identify which NGS-derived variants do not require validation [110].

Difficult-to-call variants may be interpreted as a FP result when the reviewer is not confident about variants called features and corresponding reads. As mentioned previously, homopolymer regions represent a big challenge for amplicon-based NGS sequencing. Figure 21.6 illustrates an error affecting the homopolymer region. The pathogenic variant LRG_293t1(*BRCA2*):c.956dupA (Fig. 21.6a) is a commonly detected technical artifact for amplicon-based NGS sequencing. Sanger sequencing orthogonal confirmation for two patients showed the variant as TP for Patient 1 (Fig. 21.6b) and FP for Patient 2 (Fig. 21.6c). This example reinforces the importance of secondary confirmation as this relevant clinical variant would easily pass automatic high-quality control filters and could be considered as a technical artifact for all samples.

NGS sequencing are also contributing to reveal somatic mosaicism. Somatic mosaicism refers to the co-existence of two or more genetically distinct cell lines in the same individual as a result of a genetic event after zygote formation [111]. Mutant cells may appear with different mosaic ratio in patient's tissues, usually in an allele frequency below 30%, being the majority below 20% [112], and NGS provides opportunities to assess medium- and low-grade mosaicism through reading depth information [113, 114]. Figure 21.7 illustrates a genetic testing for hereditary cancer screening that identified a *TP53* mutation at an unexpected heterozygous/homozygous ratio for a germline variant. A pathogenic LRG_321t1(*TP53*):c.659A>G variant was detected in an 80-year-old woman (Fig. 21.7a). Two other variants (LRG_293t1(*BRCA2*):c.280C>T LRG_321t1(*TP53*):c.1010G>A) were also detected, at ~50% frequency (data not shown). NGS analysis showed the presence of LRG_321t1(*TP53*):c.659A>G at a medium variant allele frequency (VAF = 18%). A careful examination of Sanger sequencing electropherograms revealed a weak signal corresponding to the mutant peak in this DNA position (Fig. 21.7b). This case could be a mosaicism event; however, other tissue testing is necessary to confirm this. It is important to highlight that low-grade mosaicism is often missed by Sanger sequencing as the mutant peak may not be distinguished from the

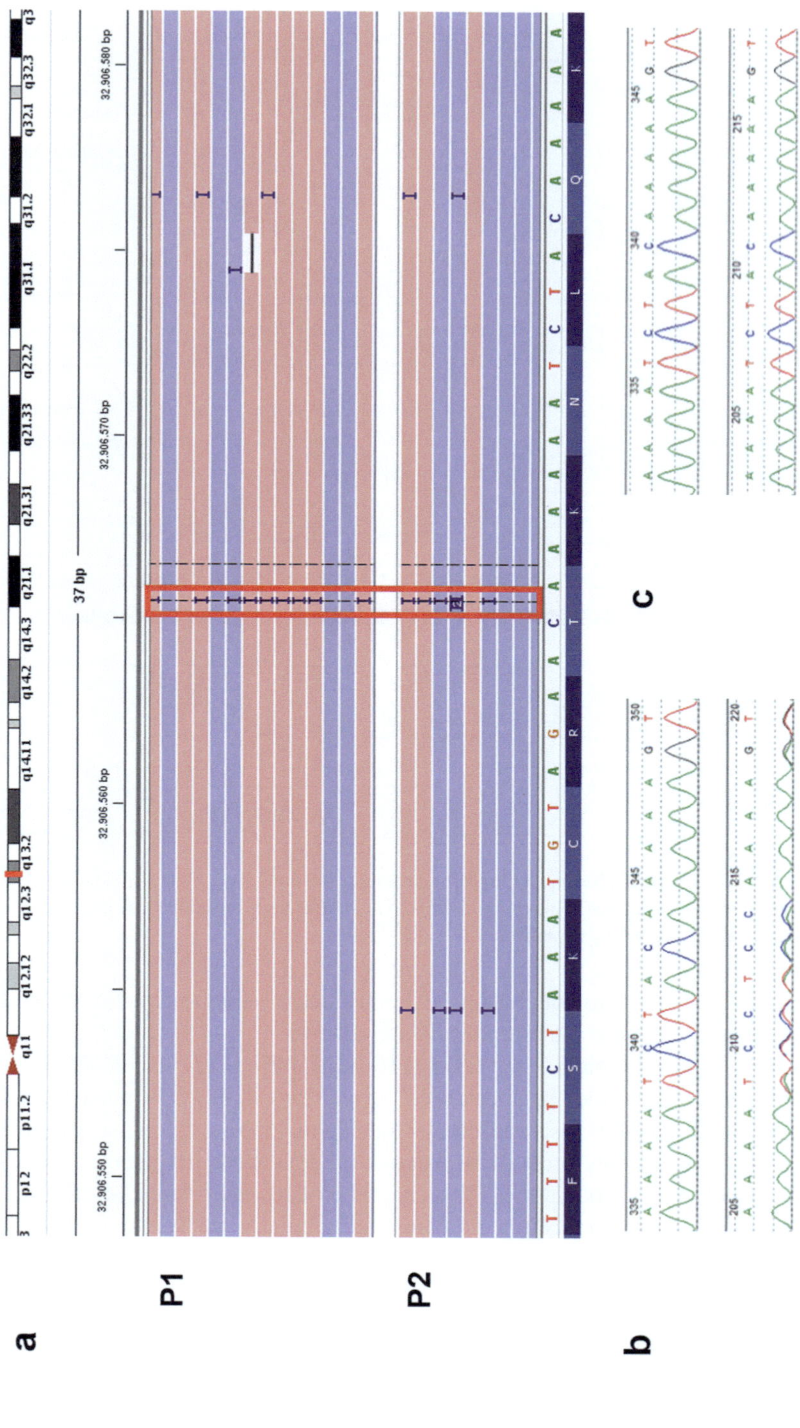

Fig. 21.6 (**a**) Pathogenic variant LRG_293t1(*BRCA2*):c.956dupA in homopolymer region identified for two patients (P1 and P2) by NGS. (**b**) Sanger sequencing orthogonal confirmation for P1. (**c**) Sanger sequencing revealing the commonly detected technical artifact

a

b

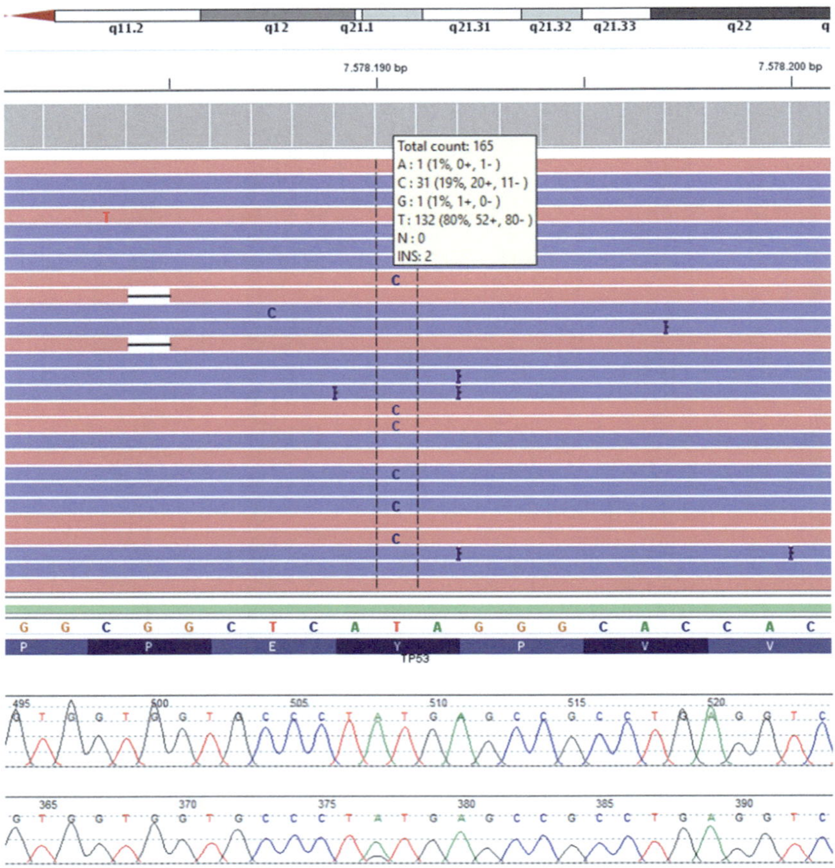

Fig. 21.7 (**a**) NGS and (**b**) Sanger sequencing of the germline mutation LRG_321t1(*TP53*):c.659A>G at an unexpected heterozygous/homozygous ratios. This could be a mosaicism event; however, other tissue testing is necessary to confirm this

background noise [115]. In conclusion, VAF verification is important for an accurate zygosity and germline/somatic variant assessment.

Similar cases can be found, e.g., *TP53* [116–121], *NF1* [122], and *PTEN* [123] genes. Studies demonstrated that aberrant cell expansions were a common phenomenon on NGS multipaneled tests caused by clonal hematopoiesis, and somatic variants guiding to clonal outgrowth of hematopoietic cells were frequent in persons above the age of 70 years old [116]. These factors produce important clinical implications because of the application of unjustified clinical interventions. Another point of observation that comes from mosaicism reports is that they may indicate an adverse clinical outcome, a hematologic neoplasia, or an increased non-hematologic mortality. The challenge is to analyze and report these variants, as there are currently no guidelines for NGS standard quality control measures. A good practice for laboratories is to be transparent about their policies regarding the detection, reporting, and follow-up of cases with germline variants at lower VAF [121].

21.2.2.4 Variant Classification Challenge

Once NGS become routinely used in research and clinical practice, the number of genetic variants identified has increased significantly. Added to this, deciphering which of the observed variants are pathogenic is challenging since the majority of human variants is part of normal human variation [124]. Clinical diagnostic laboratories need to be able to classify variants accurately, since the promise of personalized medicine relies on consistent variant interpretation, which can define diagnosis, treatment, prognosis, and genetic counseling [125]. Therefore, the interpretation of NGS data requires qualified professionals with in-depth knowledge in molecular genetics and sequence technologies, especially NGS [85].

The process of variant classification, which aims to determine whether a DNA variant causes a disease, is complex and requires checking a set of evidence mainly based on patient and disease characteristics and literature reports. These include verifying the disease mechanism, which type of variant (e.g., frameshift, nonsense, missense, silent, splice site), and its effect on DNA, RNA, or protein, whether the variant has been previously described in a patient with similar clinical features and also has not been reported in controls individuals, etc. Even after all the analysis, a considerable amount of variants can still remain unclassified due to conflict or lack of evidence. These cases are reported as variants of uncertain significance (VUS) [126].

An example that highlights the complexities of variant interpretation was a lawsuit filed in 2016, in the United States [127]. A mother of a child with epilepsy alleges that a genetic laboratory failed to accurately classify her son's *SCN1A* variant as a VUS. In 2007, the child's blood sample was sent to a laboratory to gauge if it had mutations in the *SCN1A* gene, which causes Dravet syndrome, a rare inherited form of epileptic encephalopathy. The genetic test detected a VUS variant, meaning that there was not sufficient evidence at that moment to link the mutation to epilepsy or to determine it as benign. The child continued to receive contraindicated treatment, his condition worsened, and he died following a severe seizure. Based on the child's medical records, the opinions of experts and the scientific literature, the complaint is convinced that there was enough evidence at the time to assert the variant as disease-causing. The lawsuit cites two papers published [128, 129] that mention the same specific mutation in another patient with epileptic encephalopathy. The case is complex, and a legal resolution is likely to take some time.

To improve the standardization of variant interpretation by clinical testing laboratories, the American College of Medical Genetics and Genomics (ACMG) and AMP issued the standards and guidelines for variant interpretation for Mendelian disorders which established six categories of variant classification: benign, likely benign, VUS, likely pathogenic, and pathogenic [98]. Later, the Clinical Genome Resource (ClinGen) established the SVI working group to support the refinement and evolution of the ACMG/AMP criteria, increasing the uniformity and consistency of sequence variant interpretation [104, 130–138]. In addition, AMP/CAP developed a guideline for interpreting somatic cancer variants which categorize them into four categories based on their clinical impact (tier I, variants with strong clinical significance; tier II, variants with potential clinical significance; tier III, variants with unknown clinical significance; and tier IV, variants that are benign or likely benign) [139].

These guidelines define different evidence codes capturing different types of information for or against variant pathogenicity/actionability; they aid in reducing the subjectivity of classification and increase the consistency in results in laboratories [125, 140]. Standardization, however, has its limitations. Even when the same classification program is used on identical datasets, different groups may come up with different interpretations due to the use of professional judgment and non-standardized criteria [140]. Currently, a considerable number of studies have identified discrepancies in variant classification between and within laboratories, between disease-specific databases, and even within individual databases [141–143]. These classification approaches are usually more stringent than laboratories have applied in their routine, resulting in a larger proportion of VUS.

There are many intriguing findings in NGS analysis concerning variant classification. The co-occurrence of relevant variants could be challenging for genetic counselors and patients. Patient A was found to carry two variants: a pathogenic LRG_321t1(*TP53*):c.1010G>A and a VUS LRG_292t1(*BRCA1*):c.4410A>T. Wh en two heterozygous variants are identified in a patient for a dominant disease and one variant is known to be pathogenic, finding the variants in *trans* provide evidence for a benign impact [98]. In this case, VUS variant could be reclassified through *cis/trans* testing and variant segregation analysis with the disease [98, 144, 145]. Patient B was found to carry three variants: LRG_292t1(*BRCA1*):c.3331_3334del(;) c.3454G>A NM_016081.3(*PALLD*):c.1273A>T, a pathogenic, and two VUS, respectively. As mentioned before, VUS reclassification should be performed as co-occurrence in *trans* with a pathogenic variant decreases the clinical relevance of these variant. Patient C was found to carry two pathogenic variants in *BRCA1* and *TP53* genes: LRG_292t1(*BRCA1*):c.1961del LRG_321t1(*TP53*):c.537T>G, and Patient D was found to carry two likely pathogenic variants in *TP53* gene: LRG_321t1(*TP53*):c.641A>G(;)c.713G>A. For genetic counseling, it is of utmost importance to test proband parents or other family members with cancer from both sides (i.e., maternal and paternal) [144, 145]. Without knowing phase information and which side of the family each variant is being inherited, misdiagnosis can occur, leading to late detection of the disease.

Reclassification of VUS to (likely) pathogenic, (likely) benign, or actionability (in the case of somatic variants) is strongly recommended as more scientific information becomes available [98, 140, 146]. However, several policy and ethical questions should be highlighted, such as the duty to recontact patients, informed consent process, data sharing, and further research to improve VUS interpretation [147]. Challenges involving variants of unknown significance also include possible misperceptions of VUS as deleterious variants by patients or health professionals, due to lack of formal training in genetics [148, 149]. Moreover, VUS carriers are sometimes counseled to undergo prophylactic risk reduction surgeries [150].

Besides that, VUS carriers cannot take the same benefit of therapeutic measures and genetic counseling that is available to carriers of known pathogenic variants [147, 151].

The variant reclassification process requires good public database practices. It is essential to promote the curation of scientific data available in databases as well as to keep them up-to-date [152]. In addition, for a reclassification it is important to have critical judgment and expertise knowledge of the available scientific evidence. Large research centers and clinical laboratories hold a huge volume of data that needs to be shared with the scientific community in a responsible and ethical manner to ensure the responsible dissemination of knowledge [141, 142, 153].

Even for popular genes (e.g., *BRCA1/2*), new VUS continue to occur [147], often causing patient frustration due to an unclear and ambiguous clinical meaning of the result [154]. In the United States, for example, VUS results are reported in about 5% of *BRCA1/2* tests [155]. In an effort to reclassify all VUS variants in *BRCA1* and *BRCA2* genes detected by Instituto Hermes Pardini (Brazil) between June 2014 and July 2017, our group reviewed 294 variants in 2018, following the criteria of the ACMG/AMP guideline [98] (unpublished work). As previous findings for variant reclassification on hereditary cancer syndromes [145, 156–158], the majority (28.3%) of VUS were downgraded to (likely) benign, with a substantially smaller fraction (1.7%) being upgraded to (likely) pathogenic (Fig. 21.8).

VUS will continue to challenge both patients and healthcare providers with an uncertain measure of disease risk, thereby complicating decisions regarding cancer surveillance and prevention. In women with an increased risk of breast and/or ovarian cancer, for example, identifying a VUS in *BRCA1* or *BRCA2* increases the complexity of genetic counseling and medical decision-making. As mentioned before, this is a critical task as the risk of misunderstanding is high among uneducated genetic counselors [159]. Irreversible treatment decisions may be made without knowing whether or when the VUS will be reclassified. Certainly, several other

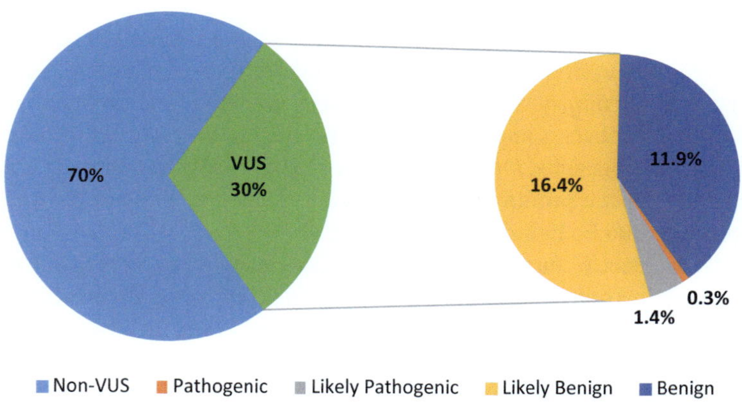

Fig. 21.8 VUS reclassification in *BRCA1/2* genes following the criteria of the ACMG/AMP guideline [98]. Thirty percent for VUS received new classification, being 1.7% (likely) pathogenic and 28.3% (likely) benign

factors may impact a patient's clinical decision-making process [159–161]. Personal and family experience of cancer is likely to influence surgical decisions [162, 163]. Also, the variant available data (e.g., characteristics of the genetic variant, results of functional assays, or observed co-segregation of VUS with disease) may give clues about the direction the variant may be reclassified (pathogenic or benign), what may influence patient's perception of a VUS. With this, a multidisciplinary work is essential: genetic counselors, physicians, patients, laboratories, and all the scientific community must become engaged in international initiatives to develop VUS-related guidelines for standard classification, disclosure, management, and follow-up.

In conclusion, it is clear that the interpretation of genetic variation represents one of the most complex and challenging fields of clinical genetics [141], but this can be easier through standardization, transparent documentation, and knowledge sharing. It is expected that this process will have an effective impact on both consistency and accuracy of variant classification and will decrease the number of variants being reported as VUS or disease-causing without having enough evidence for that classification [140].

21.2.2.5 Liquid Biopsy

The cancer genome sequencing projects allowed us to know the variety of genetic alterations that are present in different types of cancer and that can be applied for detection, monitoring, and determining the appropriate treatment protocols for patients. However, biopsies of primary tumors and metastases are typically not practical because the tissue is often inaccessible or reachable only by invasive procedures. Due to these limitations, new ways to observe tumor genetics and dynamics have evolved [164, 165].

Liquid biopsy refers to noninvasive techniques that detect fragments of DNA or cells. Blood samples are often used as the source for tumor DNA detection. However, other research groups have detected tumor DNA in non-blood body fluids [166], including urine [167–170], saliva [171, 172], sputum [173–175], stool [176–178], cerebrospinal [179–181], ovarian cysts [182], and gastric washes [183]. Apart from the invasiveness of conventional biopsy, liquid biopsy also offers several advantages compared to tissue biopsy. The amount of tissue sampled is one limitation of traditional biopsy. Moreover, sample may not reflect the tumor molecular profile due to intratumoral heterogeneity. On the other hand, liquid biopsy can provide a real and representative genetic profile of cancerous cells, since any parts of the tumor can shed molecules into body fluids [164, 184, 185].

The first evidence of tumor cells in the bloodstream was provided by the pathologist Thomas Ashworth 50 years ago, through microscopic observation of circulating tumor cells (CTCs) of a man with metastatic cancer [186]. In 1948, Mandel and Metais [187] reported the presence of cell-free DNA in human plasma of healthy and sick individuals. Over time it became clear that, in addition to normal cells, tumors also shed DNA fragments into the circulation and that these fragments mirror the genetic landscape of the tumor [188].

A range of analytes can be isolated from the blood samples including CTCs, cell-free DNA (cfDNA, especially ctDNA), and eventually other tumor-derived material (e.g., exosomes) [165, 189]. Molecular analysis of these different components can provide distinct and complementary information.

Primary and metastatic lesions release CTCs in the bloodstream from all cancer types studied so far. Also, the more aggressive the disease, the more CTCs are found. However, they are highly diluted, no matter how advanced is the metastatic disease (on average 1 CTCs per 1×10^9 normal blood cells) [190, 191]. CTCs are isolated from total blood cells by size-based selection methods (they are usually larger than normal blood cells) or using markers (cocktails of antibodies) commonly expressed on the surface of these cells [21, 165]. In terms of output, CTCs allow the analysis of SNV, genetic rearrangements, loss of heterozygosity (LOF), changes in gene and protein expression, alternative splicing, and drug sensitivity [191].

In contrast, ctDNA is released via tumor cells apoptosis, necrosis, phagocytosis, and active cellular secretion [192, 193], representing a small portion of cfDNA levels in the blood plasma (<0.1–10%) [165, 193]. The quantity of ctDNA may vary substantially depending on tumor type and even among patients with the same tumor. This variation is a consequence of, e.g., TMB, inflammation levels, and cellular turnover [165, 191]. It is possible to capture cfDNA from plasma as a mixture of DNA fragments released from nonmalignant cells and from ctDNA by several centrifugation and filtration steps [165]. A typical output for ctDNA analysis is the assessment of SNV, CNV, and rearrangements in well-established cancer-associated genes [191, 194].

Liquid biopsy specimens are challenging analytes because they are present in a relatively small fraction in a complex background of germline DNA that originates from normal cells. Additionally, circulating material is highly fragmented, which further reduces the concentration of intact target sequence [21, 188]. As such, technologies with high analytical sensitivity and specificity have been developed, since traditional DNA analyses (e.g., Sanger sequencing) are insufficient for the detection of somatic mutations in plasma. In general, methods can be separated into two broad approaches depending on the genomic coverage and analytical sensitivity: single-gene platform or panel-based platform (Fig. 21.9 and Table 21.2).

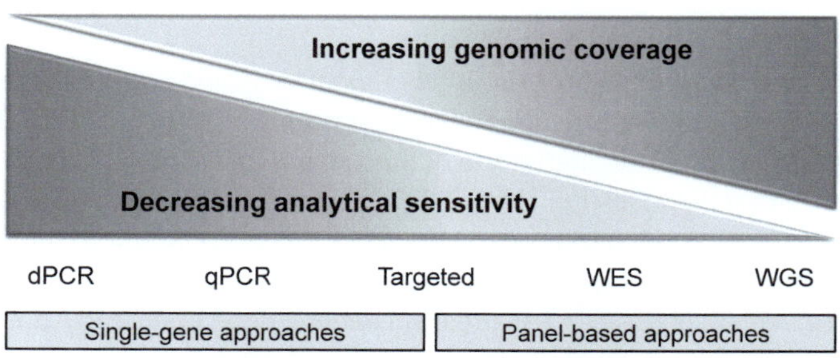

Fig. 21.9 Comparison of methods for analysis in liquid biopsy, according to the genomic coverage and analytical sensitivity. Droplet digital PCR (ddPCR), quantitative PCR (qPCR), whole-exome sequencing (WES), and whole-genome sequencing (WGS)

Table 21.2 Main detection platforms applied in liquid biopsy

Approach	Method	LoD (%)	Advantages	Disadvantages
Single-gene platform	Digital PCR	0.001–0.01	– Rapid – High sensitivity – Low running cost – Streamlined workflow on validated platform	– Only detect limited targets per assay
	qPCR	0.05–0.1		
Panel-based platform	Targeted	0.01–>2	– Does not require any prior knowledge of the molecular alteration – Cost-effective. Screen of mutations in a panel of genes in a single assay	– Long turnaround time due to complex procedure – Bioinformatics expertise required – High running cost
	WES	1–3		
	WGS	0.001		

LoD limit of detection, *qPCR* quantitative PCR, *WES* whole-exome sequencing, *WGS* whole-genome sequencing

With the current interest and advances of cancer targeting therapy, the major techniques applied in molecular laboratories target only critical gene mutations (e.g., driver mutations or actionable mutations) [185]. Such technologies can reach a high resolution besides being mostly PCR-based (e.g., dPCR, qPCR, and amplification refractory mutation system (ARMS)) [164, 188]. In contrast, the panel-based platform can be used for the discovery of new actionable targets in cancer patients, since such techniques allow the analysis of multiple variants/genes without prior knowledge of tumor profile [21, 195]. Moreover, NGS-based approaches can detect not only SNV, indels, or rearrangements but also CNV and gene fusions [196, 197]. However, these methods usually require a larger tumor fraction to achieve informative results [188].

Overall, the liquid biopsy is an important tool for the precision medicine approach, as it provides personalized information about the genomic tumor profile and the patient's eligibility for targeted therapy or clinical trials. Furthermore, the ability to detect a disease prior to the appearance of symptoms and starting treatment at an early stage can reduce or slow patients' potential damages and improve life quality.

21.2.2.6 Regulation of Genetic Tests

Genetic tests are becoming part of routine clinical care, and so far, only a few tests have received regulatory approvals (for some examples, see Sect. 21.4). In general, the government develops regulations to define quality and safety standards for commercialization of genetic testing [198–200]. In the United States, two federal agencies are in charge of regulating genetic tests: the Centers for Medicare and Medicaid Services (CMS) which regulates clinical laboratories through its Clinical Laboratory Improvement Amendments (CLIA) program and the Food and Drug Administration (FDA) which regulates most medical and biological products.

It is of utmost importance to verify the validity and clinical utility of a genetic test. Therefore, regulation involves a three-step evaluation process: (1) analytical validity (i.e., test's ability to predict the presence/absence of genetic variant(s)), (2)

clinical validity (i.e., test's ability to predict the presence/absence/risk of a specific disorder), and (3) clinical utility (i.e., test's ability to provide helpful information about diagnosis, management, treatment, or prevention of a specific disorder, evaluating its risks and benefits). Analytical validity includes technical test performance (e.g., analytic sensitivity and specificity, within- and between-laboratory precision, assay robustness). Clinical validity includes two different and independent aspects: establishment of gene-disease association and clinical test performance measurement (e.g., sensitivity, specificity, positive and negative predictive values (PPV and NPV, respectively)). On the other hand, clinical utility includes test purpose (legitimacy, efficacy, effectiveness, appropriateness) and feasibility (acceptability, efficiency, optimality, equity) of test delivery [198, 200–204]. A review of the different methods proposed for genetic methods evaluation can be found at National Academies of Sciences, Engineering, and Medicine et al. [201]. An expanded framework proposed by the United Kingdom Genetic Testing Network (UKGTN) and the PHG Foundation can be found at PHG Foundation [203].

The CMS regulates analytical validity by controlling the quality of laboratory practices, while the FDA regulates diagnostic test kits. Since not all genetic tests are marketed as in vitro diagnostic (IVD) tests, laboratory developed tests (LDTs) are generally not regulated by the FDA. Due to the advancements in the field of NGS and the progressive use of genetic testing, in 2018, the FDA finished a guidance providing recommendations for using NGS-based tests for clinical diagnostic [205]. Neither agency regulates the clinical utility of a genetic test; instead, consumers, healthcare providers, and healthcare insurance companies are usually responsible for determining this [198, 199, 202]. However, disagreements are common due to different expectations and evidence about genetic test purpose [203]. Time and experience are essential for regulators to define the clinical utility of genetic testing.

21.2.2.7 Genomic Education

The rapid advances in genomic technologies are transforming healthcare by enabling targeted screening, diagnosis, and treatment for disease management. There are now several emerging challenges for genomic knowledge application in patient care and management [206]. This new medicine is fundamentally dependent on a team approach. The use of the right genetic test, the correct interpretation of complex results, the delivery of confidential results, and proper patient follow-up require highly specialized and multidisciplinary professionals (e.g., bioinformaticians, computational biologists, IT technicians, statisticians, molecular biologists, geneticists, genetic counselors, and clinicians) [85]. Due to the constant updates of genetic test approaches, an ongoing and continuing education of this multidisciplinary team regarding emerging technologies, software, databases, and data analysis pipelines that reflect current practice is necessary. Genomic education also needs to be incorporated into medical school curriculums [207, 208].

In the near future, genomic testing will be integrated into a wide range of medical and other healthcare specialties. Genetic counseling is required to apply the benefits from this type of testing, which requires a team of well-trained and well-oriented healthcare professionals that allows the genetic information generated to be appropriately relayed and to provide information and support to individuals and families attempting to comprehend and adjust to a genetic condition [209].

Other relevant issue regarding genomic education concerns ethical, legal, and psychosocial implications related to cancer genetic screening, including the competency of the laboratories and medical professionals performing the testing, the debate of individual rights versus collective rights, discrimination, and stigma. If all these issues are addressed in the implementation of cancer genetic screening in populations, everyone could benefit from cancer prevention and treatment in the era of precision oncology [210].

21.3 Precision Oncology Clinical Case Studies

As precision oncology grows, genetic tests are routinely ordered by healthcare providers. Genetic screening of mutations for breast cancer genes (e.g., *BRCA1/2*, *BRIP1*, *CDH1*, *CHEK2*, *PALB2*, *PTEN*, *STK11*, *TP53*), mismatch repair (MMR) genes (e.g., *MLH1*, *MSH2*, *MSH3*, *MSH6*, *PMS1*, *PMS2*) in colon cancers, and *EGFR* in lung cancers are, nowadays, widely used in clinical practice to determine the susceptibility and the correct treatment for these common types of cancers [211–213]. Clinical case presentations offer new insights into cancer diagnosis, susceptibility, and treatment methods. This section presents two clinical case studies where the multidisciplinary application and deep understanding of precision medicine knowledge were fundamental in patient management.

21.3.1 An Immunotherapy Case Report

A 58-year-old male, white, former smoker, presented with a right hemiparesia in November 2016. After clinical evaluation, a brain magnetic resonance imaging scan was performed and showed a cerebral nodule of 0.9 cm in the right frontoparietal transition, surrounded by edema. Because metastasis was suspected to have occurred, computed tomography of the thorax and abdomen was recommended and demonstrated a large, upper left lobe, parahilar lung mass encasing bronchovascular structures. In addition, several metastatic lung nodules were described, as well as enlarged mediastinal lymph nodes. A transthoracic lung biopsy was conducted and confirmed the diagnosis of poorly differentiated lung adenocarcinoma. Immunohistochemistry analysis was positive for TTF1, CK7, p63, and napsin and negative for CK5/6 and calretinin. NGS detected a *KRAS* G13D (LRG_344t1(*KRAS*):c.38G>A) mutation and wild-type *EGFR*, *NRAS*, and *BRAF*. The patient was initially treated with brain radiosurgery to single brain lesion and was screened for an immunotherapy clinical trial. However, the biopsy tissue was not sufficient for further testing to screen in the protocol. In 2016, immunotherapy was not a standard in the first-line therapy of lung cancer, and PD-L1 was a biomarker to enrich for clinical response in clinical trials. After a long discussion with the patient, the possibility of starting standard treatment with chemotherapy was explained, while he could

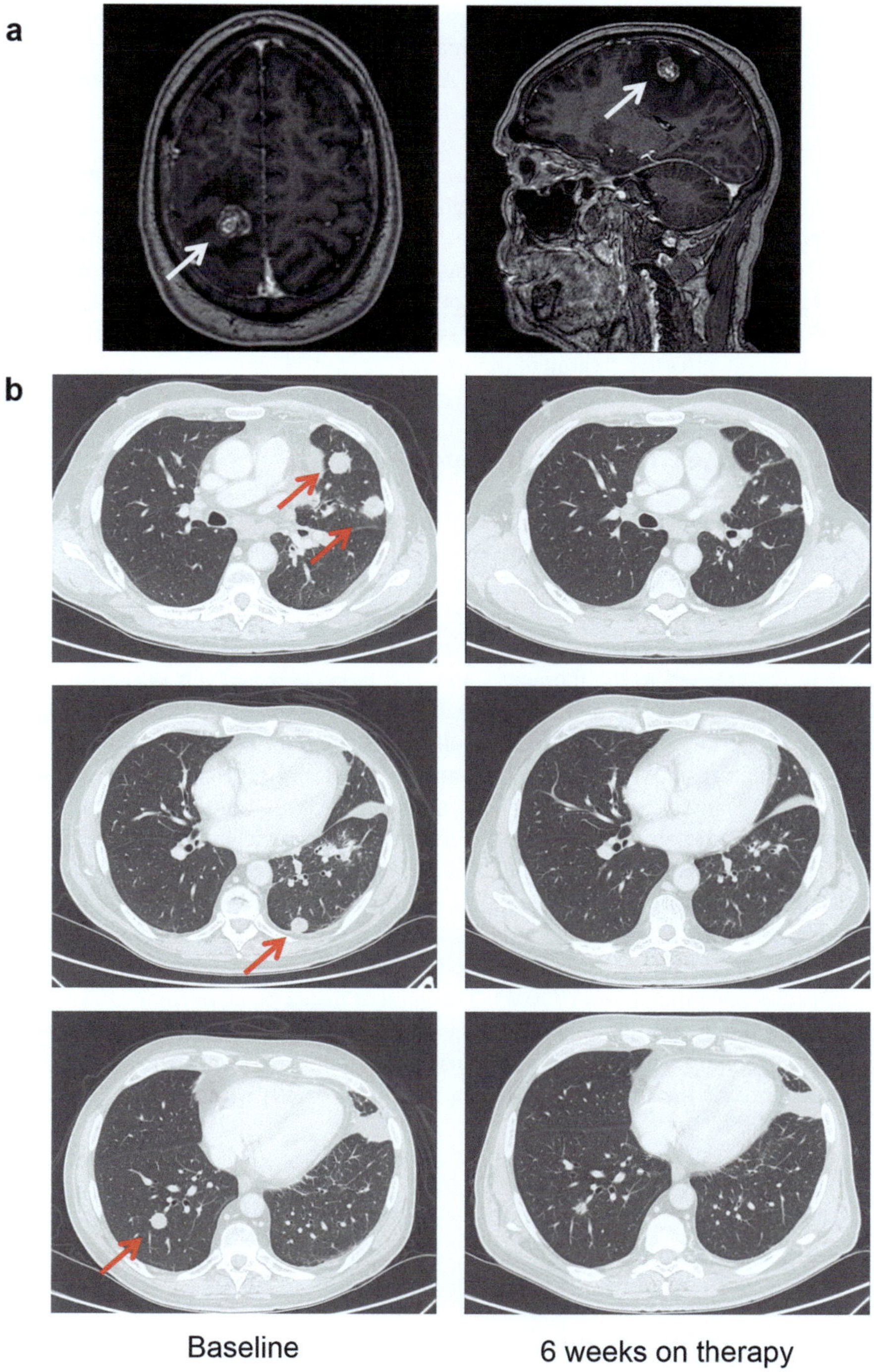

Fig. 21.10 (**a**) Axial and sagittal magnetic resonance sequences with contrast. A small nodule of about 1 cm in the convexity of the right parietal lobe of the brain with significant contrast

also decide to pursue a new biopsy to assess PD-L1 on the trial. The patient decided to go through a new lung biopsy, which confirmed a strong staining for PD-L1 (SP142 antibody; +3) and absence of ALK staining. He was randomized to the immunotherapy arm to receive an anti-PD-L1 antibody (atezolizumab 1200 mg, intravenous, every 3 weeks). After only 6 weeks, new computed tomography scans (CTs) confirmed an exceptional response, with shrinkage of the primary mass and all lung nodules (Fig. 21.10). After roughly 3 years of immunotherapy, this patient presents with almost complete response, asymptomatic, with a great quality of life and absence of adverse events. This case highlights the relevance of pursuing a complete biomarker assessment in the era of precision oncology. Thanks to patient's confidence and understanding, a rebiopsy to run full biomarker analysis led to the use of a highly effective treatment in this case.

21.3.2 A Target Therapy Case Report

A 65-year-old female was diagnosed with a locally advanced, stage III, lung adenocarcinoma in 2013, which manifested with a lung mass and mediastinal lymph node enlargement. She was initially treated with combined chemoradiation until September 2013. In November 2015, she started feeling a back pain again, and disease progression was observed in the bones and pleura. Hypofractionated radiation therapy was applied to the thoracic spine, and biomarker analysis was conducted. *EGFR* sequencing confirmed an exon 19 deletion, while ALK staining was negative. She was started on a first-generation EGFR inhibitor (erlotinib 150 mg daily, orally), which resulted in pain improvement and partial response on the imaging scans. After roughly a year on therapy, a disease progression was detected in the lungs and pleuropericardial space. Treatment was changed to chemotherapy (carboplatin-pemetrexed) in June 2016 and then to immunotherapy (nivolumab, an anti-PD1 antibody) in December 2016. In April 2017, disease progression was noted in the bones, liver, and pleural effusion. At this time, a third-generation inhibitor was available through expanded access program in cases that developed an *EGFR* resistance mutation (T790M). This patient tested positive for T790M in the blood with dPCR (liquid biopsy) and was started on the novel therapy (osimertinib 80 mg daily, orally) with excellent response and symptom improvement (Fig. 21.11). She remained on therapy for over a year, with great quality of life.

Fig. 21.10 (continued) enhancement and marked perilesional edema apparently without midline deviations (white arrow). (**b**) Thorax tomography with lung window in the axial plane. Left images: multiple, tumoral lung nodules spread in both lungs (red arrows). Right images: regression of lung nodules after commencement of anti-PD-L1 antibody

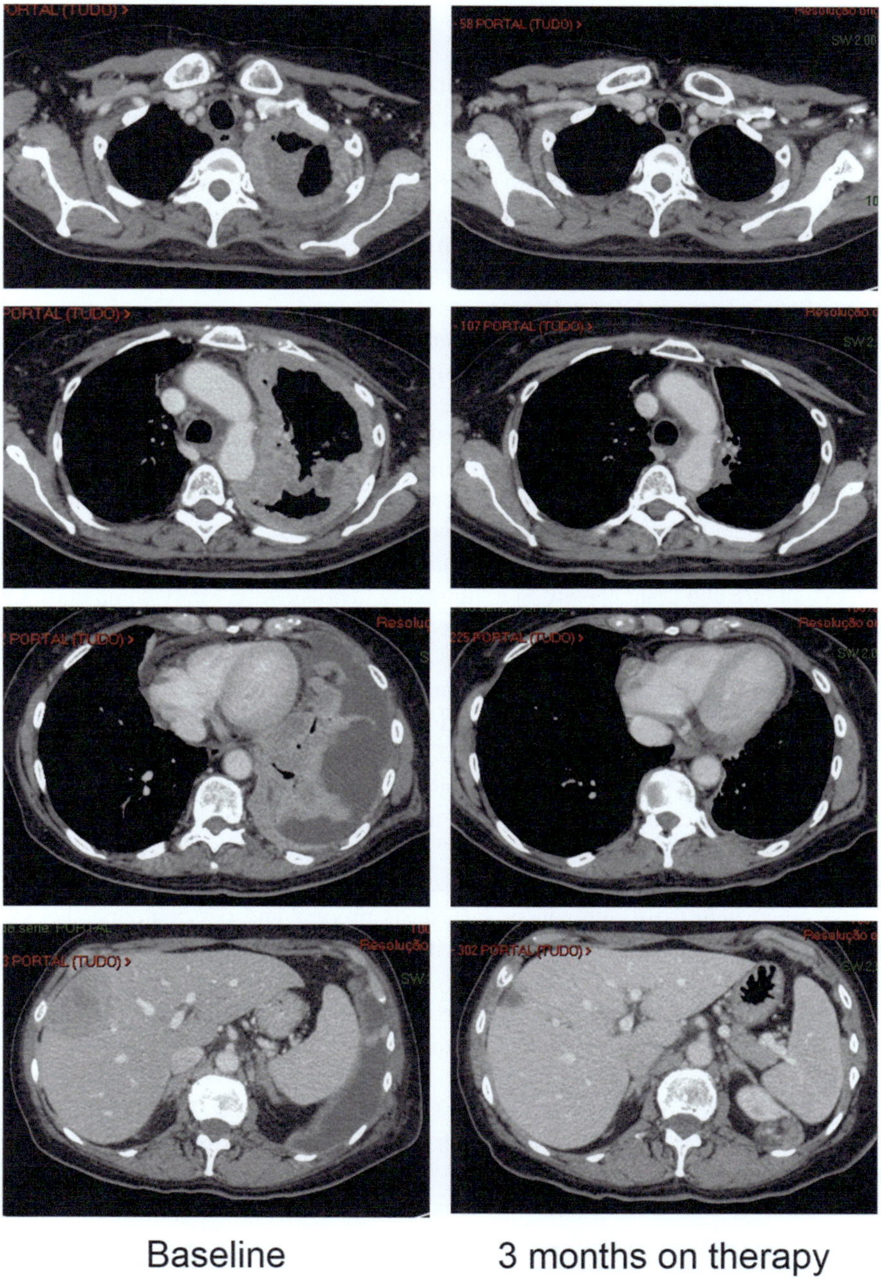

Fig. 21.11 Computed tomography (CT) of the chest and abdomen with mediastinal window. Left side: significant irregular pleural thickening with intense, neoplastic enhancement, associated with a moderate pleural effusion on the same side, leading to parenchymal atelectasis in the left lower lobe. Below a large liver metastasis shown as subcapsular mass in the right lobe of the liver. Right side: complete regression of neoplastic pleural thickening and pleural effusion and significant volume reduction of the liver metastatic mass after osimertinib (bottom image)

21.4 Future Perspectives

As precision oncology expands, the utilization of targeted therapies continues to increase. FDA-approved treatments (e.g., EGFR TKIs for *EGFR* sensitizing mutations; larotrectinib for *NTRK* gene fusions; erdafitinib for *FGFR3* mutations; gilteritinib for *FLT3* mutation; alpelisib for *PIK3CA* mutations; ivosidenib for *IDH1* mutation; enasidenib for *IDH2* mutation) also expand the use of genomic approaches and reinforce their importance in precision oncology. The FDA has already approved some NGS tests (Oncomine™ Dx Target Test, MSK-IMPACT™, FoundationOne® CDx, Praxis Extended RAS Panel, clonoSEQ®) as companion diagnostics, and other companies are seeking FDA marketing authorization. On January 2019, the FDA granted Breakthrough Device Designation for Illumina's pan-cancer assay (TruSight™ Oncology Comprehensive), and on May 2019, Resolution HRD™ Liquid Biopsy Assay also received Breakthrough Device Designation. If approved, Resolution HRD™ could be the first company to detect gene deletions from cell-free DNA (cfDNA) and differentiate between single copy and biallelic (homozygous) gene deletions through a simple blood draw.

Although it is still a nascent field, liquid biopsy holds great promise for cancer understanding and management in a minimally invasive way. Many companies are developing new methods for analyzing biomarkers in fluid samples (e.g., Resolution HRD™ Liquid Biopsy Assay; Guardant Health's LUNAR; CancerSEEK [214]; Predicine's Gene RADAR; Singlera's PanSeer and ColonES assays). Meanwhile, Roche's Cobas® EGFR Mutation Test v2 is currently the only FDA-approved liquid biopsy in patients with metastatic NSCLC. Foundation Medicine is also racing to get FDA approval for the first liquid biopsy test (FoundationOne® Liquid) that includes multiple companion diagnostics and genomic biomarkers, such as TMB.

As mentioned before (see Sect. 21.2.2.5), liquid biopsy can also be performed through isolation of CTCs and extracellular vesicles (EVs). Capturing and studying CTCs could help clarifying cancer metastasis process and personalizing therapy [215]. CTCs are frequently associated with the epithelial mesenchymal transition (EMT) phenomenon, and EMT is directly related to a metastatic phenotype [216]. However, isolation of highly pure CTCs is still challenging. Limitations include (1) low sensitivity, (2) the inefficacy in capturing all types of CTCs, (3) the inability to capture CTCs clusters, (4) contamination of captured CTCs by white blood cells, (5) difficulty in recovering captured cells from the devices, and (6) high production costs [215]. The only FDA-approved platform for CTC capture is the CELLSEARCH® based on immunomagnetic enrichment; however, its sensitivity remains poor. A new method for CTC capture based on microarrays of carbon nanotube (CNT) surfaces was developed by Loeian et al. [215]. The nanotube-CTC-chip technology presented better performance than other reported CTC technologies and has none of the limitations presented by these other technologies [215]. Clinical trials and also point-of-care testing (POCT) diagnostic devices using nanotube-CTC-chip are starting to be globally performed.

Regarding EVs, emerging evidence suggests that they have crucial roles in cancer development, being potential blood or urine biomarkers for cancer diagnosis, prognostication, and management. EVs are membrane-encapsulated particles (exosomes and microvesicles) produced by cancer cells that contain regulatory molecules (functional proteins and nucleic acids) necessary for cell-cell communication within the tumor microenvironment. Due to their biocompatibility, low toxicity, and low immunogenicity, EVs hold great promise as potential vehicles for the delivery of therapeutic agents. A review of EV-associated drug delivery vehicles and exosomal miRNAs can be found at Xu et al. [217] and Rahbarghazi et al. [218]. Since the knowledge of EVs in biological samples is still limited, clinical application of EV technologies remains a challenge [217–219]. On June 2019, the FDA granted Breakthrough Device Designation for Bio-techne's ExoDx® *Prostate(IntelliScore)* (EPI), the first exosome-based liquid biopsy test. EPI is a noninvasive urine exosome gene expression assay that analyzes three exosomal RNA biomarkers (PCA3, prostate cancer antigen 3; ERG, V-ets erythroblastosis virus E26 oncogene homologs; SPDEF, SAM pointed domain-containing Ets transcription factor). The test stratifies men for risk of aggressive prostate cancer, assisting physicians in determining whether a prostate biopsy is necessary in patients with an ambiguous PSA test result [220] (clinical trial information: NCT03031418 and NCT03235687).

Another genomic potential biomarker is TMB, which has been identified as an important quantitative biomarker for predicting the response for cancer immunotherapy. TMB is defined as the number of somatic mutations normalized by a coding area in a cancer genome (Mut/Mb). Tumors harbor mutations that can change amino acids and generate neoantigens, which can be recognized as nonself by the major histocompatibility complex (MHC) system, leading to an antitumor immune response. The first evidence of TMB as a biomarker was in 2014 in melanoma [221], and a large effort has been made to characterize TMB across tumor types over the last years [222–224]. TMB and mutation types vary widely within and across cancer types, and evidence suggests that high TMB is associated with increased neoantigens and better response to immune checkpoint inhibitors in multiple cancers [223, 225, 226]. TMB is not an approved biomarker and requires standardization for clinical use; however, its implementation into clinical routine is still a challenge given the variety of approaches available and several pre-analytical, analytical, and post-analytical caveats. Challenges include standardization, cancer type, intratumoral heterogeneity, sample preparation (e.g., fixation methodology), TMB panel size, library preparation (e.g., amplicon- or capture-based), depth of sequencing, bioinformatics algorithms (e.g., variant calling, filters used, cutoffs), and TMB definition and reporting [223, 225]. It is important to highlight that not all neoantigens presented on the cell surface are immunogenic and other factors also influence the ability of the immune system to recognize the tumor, or may contribute to neoantigenic load [223], such as HLA genotype [227], inactivating mutations in immunologically genes (e.g., *JAK1*, *JAK2*, *B2M* [228]), some immune evasion mechanisms (e.g., TGF-β signaling [229], indoleamine 2,3-dioxygenase (IDO) activity [230]), fusion proteins, and posttranslational modifications of non-mutated proteins [223]. Table 21.3 summarizes different NGS gene panels in development or currently available for TMB measurement.

Table 21.3 NGS gene panels in development or currently available for TMB measurement

Sample type	Test Name	Manufacturer	Size (genes, Mb)
FFPE	CANCERPLEX	KEW	435 genes, 2.8 Mb
FFPE	FoundationOne CDx	FoundationOne	324 genes, 1.8 Mb
FFPE	IBM Watson Genomics	Quest Diagnostic	50 genes, unspecified
FFPE	MI Tumor Seek	Caris Life Sciences	592 genes, 1.4 Mb
FFPE	MSK-IMPACT	Memorial Sloan Kettering Cancer Center	468 genes, 1.5 Mb
FFPE	NEOplus v2 RUO	NEO New Oncology	>340 genes, >1.1 Mb
FFPE	NeoTYPE Discovery Profile	NeoGenomics	326 genes, unspecified
FFPE	Oncomine Tumor Mutation Load Assay	Thermo Fisher	409 genes, 1.7 Mb
FFPE	PGDx Elio tissue complete	PGDx	507 genes, 1.3 Mb
FFPE	Tempus xT	Tempus	596 genes, unspecified
FFPE	TruSight Oncology 500	Illumina	523 genes, 1.94 Mb
FFPE	TruSight Tumor 170	Illumina	170 genes, 0.5 Mb
FFPE/ blood	QIAseq TMB panel	QIAGEN	486 genes, 1.3 Mb
Blood	Guardant OMNI	Guardant Health	500 genes, 2.1 Mb
Blood	FoundationOne Liquid	FoundationOne	394 genes, 1.14 Mb
Blood	PredicineATLAS	Predicine	600 genes, 2.2 Mb

Precision immuno-oncology has also expanded opportunities for personalized cancer vaccines (PCV). The objective of PCV is to induce an immune response specific to each individual patient's tumor by exposing the organism to tumor-associated antigens (TAAs) [231, 232]. These neoantigens have been deployed as messenger RNA (mRNA) vaccine targets in humans, most of these vaccines being therapeutic, rather than prophylactic [231]. The mRNA PCV technology involves the identification and selection of unique mutations on the patient's cancer cells by NGS sequencing. A vaccine that encodes for each of these patient-specific epitopes is created and loaded onto a single mRNA molecule. Once injected into the patient, the mRNA directs cells to produce and express neoantigens (i.e., TAAs), helping the patient's immune system fight cancer. Diverse preclinical and clinical studies have demonstrated the viability of PCV to combat cancer (reviewed in [231, 233]). In

2016, for example, Moderna, a biotechnology company pioneering mRNA therapeutics and vaccines, formed a strategic alliance with Merck to develop mRNA-4157 in combination with Merck's anti-PD-1 therapy, KEYTRUDA (pembrolizumab), for the treatment of multiple types of cancer. In June 2019, a phase I dose escalation study showed that mRNA-4157 is safe and well tolerated at all dose levels tested, supporting the advancement to phase 2 [234] (clinical trial information: NCT03313778). The National Cancer Institute (NCI) also showed safety, tolerability, and immunogenicity data from its phase 1 study of PCV NCI-4650 as monotherapy for patients with advanced metastatic cancers [235] (clinical trial information: NCT03480152). The NCI program uses Moderna's mRNA technology but uses a different neoantigen selection process and study design.

In addition to mRNA-based immunotherapy, RNA interference (RNAi) and RNA-based genome editing technologies holds great potential as a tool for cancer therapy. Noncoding RNA (ncRNA) can inhibit therapeutically relevant genes through at transcriptional or posttranscriptional gene silencing (e.g., mRNA degradation) [236]. Major considerations include (1) toxicity (e.g., off-target effects, immunological effects, or toxic effects due to delivery method), (2) efficacy (e.g., poor annealing of guide strand to target mRNA), and (3) delivery (immune system activation by delivery agents) (reviewed in [237]). Four RNAi classes commonly used in clinical trials are microRNA (miRNA) mimics, short-interfering RNAs (siRNAs), short hairpin RNAs (shRNAs), and Dicer substrate RNAs (dsiRNAs) [237]. Gradalis, another biotechnology company focused on cancer therapeutics, is developing Vigil for the treatment of different types of cancer (e.g., Ewing's sarcoma (clinical trial information: NCT03495921 and NCT02511132), advanced melanoma (clinical trial information: NCT02574533), ovarian cancer (clinical trial information: NCT02346747), and advanced women's cancers (clinical trial information: NCT03073525 and NCT02725489)). The Vigil vaccine is a shRNA-based cancer immunotherapy approach. It expresses granulocyte-macrophage colony-stimulating factor (GMCSF) and two shRNAs targeted to furin mRNA, designed to decrease immunosuppression and to promote tumor antigen presentation, increasing immune system response against cancer cells. Information about other RNAi-based cancer therapy can be found at Bobbin and Rossi [237], Sullenger and Nair [236], and Xin et al. [238].

Gene editing is another promising mRNA-based therapeutic approach. Genome-engineering tools based on programmable nucleases (e.g., zinc-finger nucleases (ZFNs), transcription activator-like effector nucleases (TALENs), RNA-guided engineered nucleases (RGENs), or clustered regularly interspaced short palindromic repeat (CRISPR)-Cas) has the potential to directly correct deleterious mutation or to introduce protective mutations [239, 240]. Comparison of the different programmable nuclease platforms can be found at Cox, Platt, and Zhang [239]. Clinical development of gene-editing technology faces major challenges regarding treatment safety and efficacy, such as specificity of genome editing tools, efficiency of gene correction, and delivery approaches (ex vivo and in vivo) to target cell types [239, 241]. Current therapeutic strategies are primarily focused on ex vivo applications [233, 242, 243]. To date, the CRISPR-Cas9 system is the most robust and commonly used genome editing technique [233, 239, 243, 244]. It has recently emerged as a powerful tool for cancer research and therapy by providing an efficient technology to discover novel targets for drug development and to provide insight about tumorigenesis mechanisms [243, 244]. Applications of CRISPR-Cas9 in oncology include generation of cancer models, synergistic gene interactions studies, functional gene screening, drug target validation, and sensitive gene identification [244]. For example, CRISPR-Cas9 has been used for breast cancer (1) diagnosis by validation of putative cancer drivers in vivo, (2) treatment by inhibition of breast cancer cell proliferation, and (3) drug resistance research by removal of damaging germline *BRCA1* variants [242].

Growing evidence show that human microbiota – the collection of microorganisms that populate the human bodies – has great influence on human health and disease processes [245–248]. For precision oncology it is known that microbiota can affect disease prevention, diagnosis, and, especially, treatment. Microbes present at tumor microenvironment and intratumoral microbes can affect tumor growth and metastasis by three main mechanisms: (1) modifying host cell death and proliferation homeostasis, (2) shaping host immune system responses, and (3) altering host metabolism concerning molecule production, food digestion, and drug metabolization [246]. As there is a connection between microorganisms and host immune system, it is conceivable that these organisms can impact on how the host is going to respond to immunotherapy. A study developed by Iida et al. [249] showed that mice carrying subcutaneous tumors when treated with antibiotics had reduced responsiveness to CpG oligonucleotide immunotherapy. After this study, many research groups started to analyze microbiota influence on human immunotherapy effectiveness, most on inhibitors of immune checkpoints (negative regulators of immune response; [250]). Gopalakrishnan et al. [251] produced one of these works. It was observed that melanoma patients that responded to anti-PD1 therapy had an increased diversity of their intestinal microbiome, when compared to non-responder patients. Moreover, there was a predominance of certain bacteria types in responders and other bacteria types in non-responders. This suggests that intestinal microbiota can modulate antitumor immunity. To overcome possible adverse effects of microbiome on immunotherapy, it has been suggested that patient stool samples should be sequenced, to trace the microorganisms present in the samples, and, in some cases, fecal microbial transplantation could be used, with non-responders receiving material from responder patients [252]. Microbiome could also be targeted for drug usage, to increase immunotherapy effectiveness. Other usual cancer therapies, as chemotherapy and radiotherapy, can be affected by microbiota, as reviewed by Roy and Trinchieri [253].

21.5 Conclusions

Precision medicine is an emerging approach in clinical oncology practice, and its applications in the near future are exciting. With the rapid advancement in molecular knowledge and techniques, a personalized understanding of each patient's behavior will enable new targets for therapies and genetic counseling with maximum efficiency. The success of this proposal depends on conscious application by medical and scientific community based on pre-analytical, analytical, and post-analytical validations, aggregation of data in reliable databases, and robust clinical trials. The multidisciplinary team involved in patient support must understand the limitations and potential benefits of these new technologies in order to help patients make better informed decisions [254].

Despite the great advances, personalized medicine for cancer treatment is not yet part of routine care for most patients. The high therapy costs make it inaccessible to a large part of the population and can become a major challenge for the sustainability of health services, especially for underdeveloped countries [255]. Thus, precision oncology needs to overcome a long list of problems, such as few assays approved by regulatory agencies, scarcity of trained professionals and financial resources, and the complexities of health systems to have an equal implementation for all. Finally, the major questions are if and when will precision medicine be a reality for everyone, once no health innovation comes true without cooperation between all hierarchical levels and education, transparency, leadership, and political will.

References

1. Jaffe S (2015) Planning for US precision medicine initiative underway. Lancet 385(9986):2448–2449. https://doi.org/10.1016/S0140-6736(15)61124-2
2. Carrasco-Ramiro F, Peiró-Pastor R, Aguado B (2017) Human genomics projects and precision medicine. Gene Ther 24(9):551–561. https://doi.org/10.1038/gt.2017.77
3. Rabbani B et al (2016) Next generation sequencing: implications in personalized medicine and pharmacogenomics. Mol BioSyst 12(6):1818–1830. https://doi.org/10.1039/C6MB00115G
4. Sanger F, Nicklen S (1977) DNA sequencing with chain-terminating. Proc Natl Acad Sci U S A 74(12):5463–5467
5. Paolillo C, Londin E, Fortina P (2016) Next generation sequencing in cancer: opportunities and challenges for precision cancer medicine. Scand J Clin Lab Invest 76(sup245):S84–S91. https://doi.org/10.1080/00365513.2016.1210331
6. Domingo G et al (2013) Diagnostic applications of biomaterials. In: Biomaterials science. Elsevier, Saint Louis, pp 1087–1106. https://doi.org/10.1016/B978-0-08-087780-8.00106-6
7. Benson ES (1977) Managing the patient-focused laboratory. JAMA 237(1):69. https://doi.org/10.1001/jama.1977.03270280071032
8. Ha JF, Longnecker N (2010) Doctor-patient communication: a review. Ochsner J 10(1):38–43
9. Lippi G et al (2006) Preanalytical variability: the dark side of the moon in laboratory testing. Clin Chem Lab Med 44(4):358–365. https://doi.org/10.1515/CCLM.2006.073
10. Cree IA et al (2014) Guidance for laboratories performing molecular pathology for cancer patients. J Clin Pathol 67(11):923–931. https://doi.org/10.1136/jclinpath-2014-202404
11. Jennings LJ et al (2017) Guidelines for validation of next-generation sequencing–based oncology panels. J Mol Diagn 19(3):341–365. https://doi.org/10.1016/j.jmoldx.2017.01.011
12. Rolfo C et al (2018) Liquid biopsy for advanced non-small cell lung Cancer (NSCLC): a statement paper from the IASLC. J Thorac Oncol 13(9):1248–1268. https://doi.org/10.1016/j.jtho.2018.05.030
13. Knight TG, Grunwald MR, Copelan EA (2019) Chronic myeloid leukemia (CML). In: Concise Guide to Hematology. Springer, Cham, pp 313–322. https://doi.org/10.1007/978-3-319-97873-4_25

14. Baccarani M et al (2015) A review of the European LeukemiaNet recommendations for the management of CML. Ann Hematol 94(S2):141–147. https://doi.org/10.1007/s00277-015-2322-2
15. Radich JP et al (2018) Chronic myeloid leukemia, version 1.2019, NCCN clinical practice guidelines in oncology. J Natl Compr Cancer Netw 16(9):1108–1135. https://doi.org/10.6004/jnccn.2018.0071
16. Boddu PC et al (2019) Validation of the 2017 European LeukemiaNet classification for acute myeloid leukemia with NPM1 and FLT3 -internal tandem duplication genotypes. Cancer 125(7):1091–1100. https://doi.org/10.1002/cncr.31885
17. Goodman AM et al (2017) Tumor mutational burden as an independent predictor of response to immunotherapy in diverse cancers. Mol Cancer Ther 16(11):2598–2608. https://doi.org/10.1158/1535-7163.MCT-17-0386
18. Druley TE et al (2009) Quantification of rare allelic variants from pooled genomic DNA. Nat Methods 6(4):263–265. https://doi.org/10.1038/nmeth.1307
19. Karlin-Neumann G, Bizouarn F (2018) Entering the pantheon of 21st century molecular biology tools: a perspective on digital PCR. Methods Mol Biol 1768:3–10. https://doi.org/10.1007/978-1-4939-7778-9_1
20. Vargas DY et al (2016) Multiplex real-time PCR assays that measure the abundance of extremely rare mutations associated with Cancer. PLoS One 11(5):e0156546. https://doi.org/10.1371/journal.pone.0156546
21. Siravegna G et al (2017) Integrating liquid biopsies into the management of cancer. Nat Rev Clin Oncol 14(9):531–548. https://doi.org/10.1038/nrclinonc.2017.14
22. Schweiger MR et al (2009) Genome-wide massively parallel sequencing of formaldehyde fixed-paraffin embedded (FFPE) tumor tissues for copy-number- and mutation-analysis. PLoS One 4(5):e5548. https://doi.org/10.1371/journal.pone.0005548
23. Annala MJ et al (2013) Fusion genes and their discovery using high throughput sequencing. Cancer Lett 340(2):192–200. https://doi.org/10.1016/j.canlet.2013.01.011
24. Beutler E, Gelbart T, Kuhl W (1990) Interference of heparin with the polymerase chain reaction. BioTechniques 9(2):166
25. Warton K et al (2017) Evaluation of Streck BCT and PAXgene stabilised blood collection tubes for cell-free circulating DNA studies in plasma. Mol Diagn Ther 21(5):563–570. https://doi.org/10.1007/s40291-017-0284-x
26. Parpart-Li S et al (2017) The effect of preservative and temperature on the analysis of circulating tumor DNA. Clin Cancer Res 23(10):2471–2477. https://doi.org/10.1158/1078-0432.CCR-16-1691
27. Hofman P (2019) The challenges of evaluating predictive biomarkers using small biopsy tissue samples and liquid biopsies from non-small cell lung cancer patients. J Thorac Dis 11(S1):S57–S64. https://doi.org/10.21037/jtd.2018.11.85
28. Müller MC et al (2004) Standardization of Preanalytical factors for minimal residual disease analysis in chronic Myelogenous leukemia. Acta Haematol 112(1–2):30–33. https://doi.org/10.1159/000077557
29. Breit S et al (2004) Impact of pre-analytical handling on bone marrow mRNA gene expression. Br J Haematol 126(2):231–243. https://doi.org/10.1111/j.1365-2141.2004.05017.x
30. Malentacchi F et al (2014) SPIDIA-RNA: second external quality assessment for the pre-analytical phase of blood samples used for RNA based analyses. PLoS One 9(11):e112293. https://doi.org/10.1371/journal.pone.0112293
31. Seelenfreund E et al (2014) Long term storage of dry versus frozen RNA for next generation molecular studies. PLoS One 9(11):e111827. https://doi.org/10.1371/journal.pone.0111827
32. Ellervik C, Vaught J (2015) Preanalytical variables affecting the integrity of human biospecimens in biobanking. Clin Chem 61(7):914–934. https://doi.org/10.1373/clinchem.2014.228783
33. Kresse SH et al (2018) Evaluation of commercial DNA and RNA extraction methods for high-throughput sequencing of FFPE samples. PLoS One 13(5):e0197456. https://doi.org/10.1371/journal.pone.0197456

34. Eckhart L et al (2000) Melanin binds reversibly to thermostable DNA polymerase and inhibits its activity. Biochem Biophys Res Commun 271(3):726–730. https://doi.org/10.1006/bbrc.2000.2716
35. Bass BP et al (2014) A review of Preanalytical factors affecting molecular, protein, and morphological analysis of formalin-fixed, paraffin-embedded (FFPE) tissue: how well Do you know your FFPE specimen? Arch Pathol Lab Med 138(11):1520–1530. https://doi.org/10.5858/arpa.2013-0691-RA
36. Do H, Dobrovic A (2015) Sequence artifacts in DNA from formalin-fixed tissues: causes and strategies for minimization. Clin Chem 61(1):64–71. https://doi.org/10.1373/clinchem.2014.223040
37. Watanabe M et al (2017) Estimation of age-related DNA degradation from formalin-fixed and paraffin-embedded tissue according to the extraction methods. Exp Ther Med 14(3):2683–2688. https://doi.org/10.3892/etm.2017.4797
38. Marrugo-Ramírez J, Mir M, Samitier J (2018) Blood-based Cancer biomarkers in liquid biopsy: a promising non-invasive alternative to tissue biopsy. Int J Mol Sci 19(10):2877. https://doi.org/10.3390/ijms19102877
39. Jia N et al (2019) Serial monitoring of circulating tumor DNA in patients with metastatic colorectal Cancer to predict the therapeutic response. Front Genet 10:470. https://doi.org/10.3389/fgene.2019.00470
40. Dagogo-Jack I, Shaw AT (2018) Tumour heterogeneity and resistance to cancer therapies. Nat Rev Clin Oncol 15(2):81–94. https://doi.org/10.1038/nrclinonc.2017.166
41. Grölz D et al (2018) Liquid biopsy preservation solutions for standardized pre-analytical workflows—venous whole blood and plasma. Curr Pathobiol Rep 6(4):275–286. https://doi.org/10.1007/s40139-018-0180-z
42. Thatcher SA (2015) DNA/RNA preparation for molecular detection. Clin Chem 61(1):89–99. https://doi.org/10.1373/clinchem.2014.221374
43. Dundas N et al (2008) Comparison of automated nucleic acid extraction methods with manual extraction. J Mol Diagn 10(4):311–316. https://doi.org/10.2353/jmoldx.2008.070149
44. Riemann K et al (2007) Comparison of manual and automated nucleic acid extraction from whole-blood samples. J Clin Lab Anal 21(4):244–248. https://doi.org/10.1002/jcla.20174
45. Chomczynski P, Sacchi N (2006) The single-step method of RNA isolation by acid guanidinium thiocyanate–phenol–chloroform extraction: twenty-something years on. Nat Protoc 1(2):581–585. https://doi.org/10.1038/nprot.2006.83
46. Tan SC, Yiap BC (2009) DNA, RNA, and protein extraction: the past and the present. J Biomed Biotechnol 2009:1–10. https://doi.org/10.1155/2009/574398
47. Bohmann K et al (2009) RNA extraction from archival formalin-fixed paraffin-embedded tissue: a comparison of manual, Semiautomated, and fully automated purification methods. Clin Chem 55(9):1719–1727. https://doi.org/10.1373/clinchem.2008.122572
48. Mu W et al (2016) Sanger confirmation is required to achieve optimal sensitivity and specificity in next-generation sequencing panel testing. J Mol Diagn 18(6):923–932. https://doi.org/10.1016/j.jmoldx.2016.07.006
49. Bustin S (2000) Absolute quantification of mRNA using real-time reverse transcription polymerase chain reaction assays. J Mol Endocrinol 25(2):169–193. https://doi.org/10.1677/jme.0.0250169
50. Kohlmann A et al (2011) The Interlaboratory RObustness of next-generation sequencing (IRON) study: a deep sequencing investigation of TET2, CBL and KRAS mutations by an international consortium involving 10 laboratories. Leukemia 25(12):1840–1848. https://doi.org/10.1038/leu.2011.155
51. MacConaill LE (2013) Existing and emerging technologies for tumor genomic profiling. J Clin Oncol 31(15):1815–1824. https://doi.org/10.1200/JCO.2012.46.5948
52. Arsenic R et al (2015) Comparison of targeted next-generation sequencing and Sanger sequencing for the detection of PIK3CA mutations in breast cancer. BMC Clin Pathol 15(1):20. https://doi.org/10.1186/s12907-015-0020-6

53. Mardis ER (2011) A decade's perspective on DNA sequencing technology. Nature 470(7333):198–203. https://doi.org/10.1038/nature09796
54. Metzker ML (2010) Sequencing technologies — the next generation. Nat Rev Genet 11(1):31–46. https://doi.org/10.1038/nrg2626
55. Tucker T, Marra M, Friedman JM (2009) Massively parallel sequencing: the next big thing in genetic medicine. Am J Hum Genet 85(2):142–154. https://doi.org/10.1016/j.ajhg.2009.06.022
56. Hagemann IS (2015) Chapter 1 – overview of technical aspects and chemistries of next-generation sequencing. Clin Genom 3–19. https://doi.org/10.1016/B978-0-12-404748-8.00001-0
57. Nyrén P (2007) The history of pyrosequencing®. Methods Mol Biol 373:1–14. https://doi.org/10.1385/1-59745-377-3:1
58. Fakruddin M et al (2012) Pyrosequencing- principles and applications. Int J Life Sci Pharma Res 2(1):L–65–L–76
59. Margulies M et al (2005) Genome sequencing in microfabricated high-density picolitre reactors. Nature 437(7057):376–380. https://doi.org/10.1038/nature03959
60. Ronaghi M (1998) A sequencing method based on real-time pyrophosphate. Science 281(5375):363–365. https://doi.org/10.1126/science.281.5375.363
61. Gharizadeh B et al (2006) Large-scale pyrosequencing of synthetic DNA: a comparison with results from Sanger dideoxy sequencing. Electrophoresis 27(15):3042–3047. https://doi.org/10.1002/elps.200500834
62. Ahmadian A et al (2000a) Analysis of the p53 tumor suppressor Gene by pyrosequencing. BioTechniques 28(1):140–147. https://doi.org/10.2144/00281rr02
63. Gharizadeh B et al (2002) Long-read pyrosequencing using pure 2′-Deoxyadenosine-5′-O′-(1-thiotriphosphate) Sp-isomer. Anal Biochem 301(1):82–90. https://doi.org/10.1006/abio.2001.5494
64. Milan D (2000) A mutation in PRKAG3 associated with excess glycogen content in pig skeletal muscle. Science 288(5469):1248–1251. https://doi.org/10.1126/science.288.5469.1248
65. Nordström T et al (2000) Direct analysis of single-nucleotide polymorphism on double-stranded DNA by pyrosequencing. Biotechnol Appl Biochem 31(Pt 2):107–112
66. Ahmadian A et al (2000b) Single-nucleotide polymorphism analysis by pyrosequencing. Anal Biochem 280(1):103–110. https://doi.org/10.1006/abio.2000.4493
67. Garcia CA et al (2000) Mutation detection by pyrosequencing: sequencing of exons 5–8 of the p53 tumor suppressor gene. Gene 253(2):249–257. https://doi.org/10.1016/S0378-1119(00)00257-2
68. Nordström T et al (2001) Method enabling fast partial sequencing of cDNA clones. Anal Biochem 292(2):266–271. https://doi.org/10.1006/abio.2001.5094
69. Nourizad N, Gharizadeh B, Nyrén P (2003) Method for clone checking. Electrophoresis 24(11):1712–1715. https://doi.org/10.1002/elps.200305434
70. Uhlmann K et al (2002) Evaluation of a potential epigenetic biomarker by quantitative methyl-single nucleotide polymorphism analysis. Electrophoresis 23(24):4072–4079. https://doi.org/10.1002/elps.200290023
71. Yang AS (2004) A simple method for estimating global DNA methylation using bisulfite PCR of repetitive DNA elements. Nucleic Acids Res 32(3):e38. https://doi.org/10.1093/nar/gnh032
72. Kim HJ et al (2013) Clinical investigation of EGFR mutation detection by pyrosequencing in lung cancer patients. Oncol Lett 5(1):271–276. https://doi.org/10.3892/ol.2012.950
73. Mack E et al (2016) A rational two-step approach to KRAS mutation testing in colorectal cancer using high resolution melting analysis and pyrosequencing. BMC Cancer 16(1):585. https://doi.org/10.1186/s12885-016-2589-2
74. Daber R, Sukhadia S, Morrissette JJD (2013) Understanding the limitations of next generation sequencing informatics, an approach to clinical pipeline validation using artificial data sets. Cancer Genet 206(12):441–448. https://doi.org/10.1016/j.cancergen.2013.11.005

75. Samorodnitsky E et al (2015) Evaluation of hybridization capture versus amplicon-based methods for whole-exome sequencing. Hum Mutat 36(9):903–914. https://doi.org/10.1002/humu.22825
76. Loman NJ et al (2012) Performance comparison of benchtop high-throughput sequencing platforms. Nat Biotechnol 30(5):434–439. https://doi.org/10.1038/nbt.2198
77. Meacham F et al (2011) Identification and correction of systematic error in high-throughput sequence data. BMC Bioinformatics 12(1):451. https://doi.org/10.1186/1471-2105-12-451
78. Nakamura K et al (2011) Sequence-specific error profile of Illumina sequencers. Nucleic Acids Res 39(13):e90–e90. https://doi.org/10.1093/nar/gkr344
79. Bragg LM et al (2013) Shining a light on dark sequencing: characterising errors in ion torrent PGM data. PLoS Comput Biol 9(4):e1003031. https://doi.org/10.1371/journal.pcbi.1003031
80. Simon R, Roychowdhury S (2013) Implementing personalized cancer genomics in clinical trials. Nat Rev Drug Discov 12(5):358–369. https://doi.org/10.1038/nrd3979
81. Asan et al (2011) Comprehensive comparison of three commercial human whole-exome capture platforms. Genome Biol 12(9):R95. https://doi.org/10.1186/gb-2011-12-9-r95
82. Clark MJ et al (2011) Performance comparison of exome DNA sequencing technologies. Nat Biotechnol 29(10):908–914. https://doi.org/10.1038/nbt.1975
83. Leipzig J (2016) A review of bioinformatic pipeline frameworks. Brief Bioinform 18(3):530–536. https://doi.org/10.1093/bib/bbw020
84. Roy S et al (2016) Next-generation sequencing informatics: challenges and strategies for implementation in a clinical environment. Arch Pathol Lab Med 140(9):958–975. https://doi.org/10.5858/arpa.2015-0507-RA
85. Roy S et al (2018) Standards and guidelines for validating next-generation sequencing bioinformatics pipelines. J Mol Diagn 20(1):4–27. https://doi.org/10.1016/j.jmoldx.2017.11.003
86. Chang F, Li MM (2013) Clinical application of amplicon-based next-generation sequencing in cancer. Cancer Genet 206(12):413–419. https://doi.org/10.1016/j.cancergen.2013.10.003
87. Agarwal D et al (2017) Functional germline variants as potential co-oncogenes. NPJ Breast Cancer 3(1):46. https://doi.org/10.1038/s41523-017-0051-5
88. Iourov IY, Vorsanova SG, Yurov YB (2010) Somatic genome variations in health and disease. Curr Genomics 11(6):387–396. https://doi.org/10.2174/138920210793176065
89. Meyerson M, Gabriel S, Getz G (2010) Advances in understanding cancer genomes through second-generation sequencing. Nat Rev Genet 11(10):685–696. https://doi.org/10.1038/nrg2841
90. Redon R et al (2006) Global variation in copy number in the human genome. Nature 444(7118):444–454. https://doi.org/10.1038/nature05329
91. Shlien A, Malkin D (2009) Copy number variations and cancer. Genome Med 1(6):62. https://doi.org/10.1186/gm62
92. Povysil G et al (2017) Panelcn.MOPS: copy-number detection in targeted NGS panel data for clinical diagnostics. Hum Mutat 38(7):889–897. https://doi.org/10.1002/humu.23237
93. Hoogstraat M et al (2015) Simultaneous detection of clinically relevant mutations and amplifications for routine Cancer pathology. J Mol Diagn 17(1):10–18. https://doi.org/10.1016/j.jmoldx.2014.09.004
94. Tabak B et al (2019) The tangent copy-number inference pipeline for cancer genome analyses. bioRxiv:566505. https://doi.org/10.1101/566505
95. Zare F et al (2017) An evaluation of copy number variation detection tools for cancer using whole exome sequencing data. BMC Bioinformatics 18(1):286. https://doi.org/10.1186/s12859-017-1705-x
96. Heng HH (2017) The genomic landscape of cancers. In: Ecology and evolution of cancer. Elsevier, London, pp 69–86. https://doi.org/10.1016/B978-0-12-804310-3.00005-3
97. den Dunnen JT et al (2016) HGVS recommendations for the description of sequence variants: 2016 update. Hum Mutat 37(6):564–569. https://doi.org/10.1002/humu.22981
98. Richards S et al (2015) Standards and guidelines for the interpretation of sequence variants: a joint consensus recommendation of the American College of Medical Genetics and

Genomics and the Association for Molecular Pathology. Genet Med 17(5):405–423. https://doi.org/10.1038/gim.2015.30
99. Wildeman M et al (2008) Improving sequence variant descriptions in mutation databases and literature using the Mutalyzer sequence variation nomenclature checker. Hum Mutat 29(1):6–13. https://doi.org/10.1002/humu.20654
100. Haile S et al (2019) Sources of erroneous sequences and artifact chimeric reads in next generation sequencing of genomic DNA from formalin-fixed paraffin-embedded samples. Nucleic Acids Res 47(2):e12–e12. https://doi.org/10.1093/nar/gky1142
101. Xue Y et al (2015) Solving the molecular diagnostic testing conundrum for Mendelian disorders in the era of next-generation sequencing: single-gene, gene panel, or exome/genome sequencing. Genet Med 17(6):444–451. https://doi.org/10.1038/gim.2014.122
102. Matthijs G et al (2016) Guidelines for diagnostic next-generation sequencing. Eur J Hum Genet 24(10):1515. https://doi.org/10.1038/ejhg.2016.63
103. Weiss MM et al (2013) Best practice guidelines for the use of next-generation sequencing applications in genome diagnostics: a National Collaborative Study of Dutch genome diagnostic laboratories. Hum Mutat 34(10):1313–1321. https://doi.org/10.1002/humu.22368
104. Tavtigian SV et al (2018) Modeling the ACMG/AMP variant classification guidelines as a Bayesian classification framework. Genet Med 20(9):1054–1060. https://doi.org/10.1038/gim.2017.210
105. Alexandrov LB et al (2013) Signatures of mutational processes in human cancer. Nature 500(7463):415–421. https://doi.org/10.1038/nature12477
106. Barnell EK et al (2019) Standard operating procedure for somatic variant refinement of sequencing data with paired tumor and normal samples. Genet Med 21(4):972–981. https://doi.org/10.1038/s41436-018-0278-z
107. Baudhuin LM et al (2015) Confirming variants in next-generation sequencing panel testing by sanger sequencing. J Mol Diagn 17(4):456–461. https://doi.org/10.1016/j.jmoldx.2015.03.004
108. Strom SP et al (2014) Assessing the necessity of confirmatory testing for exome-sequencing results in a clinical molecular diagnostic laboratory. Genet Med 16(7):510–515. https://doi.org/10.1038/gim.2013.183
109. Beck TF, Mullikin JC, Biesecker LG (2016) Systematic evaluation of sanger validation of next-generation sequencing variants. Clin Chem 62(4):647–654. https://doi.org/10.1373/clinchem.2015.249623
110. Lincoln SE et al (2019) A rigorous Interlaboratory examination of the need to confirm next-generation sequencing–detected variants with an orthogonal method in clinical genetic testing. J Mol Diagn 21(2):318–329. https://doi.org/10.1016/j.jmoldx.2018.10.009
111. Freed D, Stevens EL, Pevsner J (2014) Somatic mosaicism in the human genome. Genes 5(4):1064–1094. https://doi.org/10.3390/genes5041064
112. Vázquez-Osorio I et al (2017) Cutaneous and systemic findings in mosaic Neurofibromatosis type 1. Pediatr Dermatol 34(3):271–276. https://doi.org/10.1111/pde.13094
113. Cohen ASA et al (2015) Detecting somatic mosaicism: considerations and clinical implications. Clin Genet 87(6):554–562. https://doi.org/10.1111/cge.12502
114. Gajecka M (2016) Unrevealed mosaicism in the next-generation sequencing era. Mol Gen Genomics 291(2):513–530. https://doi.org/10.1007/s00438-015-1130-7
115. Rohlin A et al (2009) Parallel sequencing used in detection of mosaic mutations: comparison with four diagnostic DNA screening techniques. Hum Mutat 30(6):1012–1020. https://doi.org/10.1002/humu.20980
116. Jaiswal S et al (2014) Age-related clonal hematopoiesis associated with adverse outcomes. N Engl J Med 371(26):2488–2498. https://doi.org/10.1056/NEJMoa1408617
117. Norquist BM et al (2016) Inherited mutations in women with ovarian carcinoma. JAMA Oncol 2(4):482–490. https://doi.org/10.1001/jamaoncol.2015.5495
118. Renaux-Petel M et al (2017) Contribution of de novo and mosaic TP53 mutations to Li-Fraumeni syndrome. J Med Genet 55(3):173–180. https://doi.org/10.1136/jmedgenet-2017-104976

119. Steensma DP et al (2015) Clonal hematopoiesis of indeterminate potential and its distinction from myelodysplastic syndromes. Blood 126(1):9–16. https://doi.org/10.1182/blood-2015-03-631747
120. Swisher EM et al (2016) Somatic mosaic mutations in PPM1D and TP53 in the blood of women with ovarian carcinoma. JAMA Oncol 2(3):370–372. https://doi.org/10.1001/jamaoncol.2015.6053
121. Weitzel JN et al (2018) Somatic TP53 variants frequently confound germ-line testing results. Genet Med 20(8):809–816. https://doi.org/10.1038/gim.2017.196
122. Messiaen L et al (2011) Mosaic type-1 NF1 microdeletions as a cause of both generalized and segmental neurofibromatosis type-1 (NF1). Hum Mutat 32(2):213–219. https://doi.org/10.1002/humu.21418
123. Salo-Mullen EE et al (2014) Mosaic partial deletion of the PTEN gene in a patient with Cowden syndrome. Familial Cancer 13(3):459–467. https://doi.org/10.1007/s10689-014-9709-4
124. Ellard S et al (2017) ACGS best practice guidelines for variant classification 2017. Available at: https://www.acgs.uk.com/media/10792/uk_practice_guidelines_for_variant_classification_2017.pdf. Accessed 2 July 2019.
125. Hoskinson DC, Dubuc AM, Mason-Suares H (2017) The current state of clinical interpretation of sequence variants. Curr Opin Genet Dev 42:33–39. https://doi.org/10.1016/j.gde.2017.01.001
126. Hoffman-Andrews L (2017) The known unknown: the challenges of genetic variants of uncertain significance in clinical practice. J Law Biosci 4(3):648–657. https://doi.org/10.1093/jlb/lsx038
127. Ray T (2016) Mother's negligence suit against quest's athena could broadly impact genetic testing lab. Available at: https://www.genomeweb.com/molecular-diagnostics/mothers-negligence-suitagainst-quests-athena-could-broadly-impact-genetic. Accessed 5 July 2019.
128. Berkovic SF et al (2006) De-novo mutations of the sodium channel gene SCN1A in alleged vaccine encephalopathy: a retrospective study. Lancet Neurol 5(6):488–492. https://doi.org/10.1016/S1474-4422(06)70446-X
129. Harkin LA et al (2007) The spectrum of SCN1A-related infantile epileptic encephalopathies. Brain 130(3):843–852. https://doi.org/10.1093/brain/awm002
130. Abou Tayoun AN et al (2018) Recommendations for interpreting the loss of function PVS1 ACMG/AMP variant criterion. Hum Mutat 39(11):1517–1524. https://doi.org/10.1002/humu.23626
131. Biesecker LG, Harrison SM (2018) The ACMG/AMP reputable source criteria for the interpretation of sequence variants. Genet Med 20(12):1687–1688. https://doi.org/10.1038/gim.2018.42
132. Gelb BD et al (2018) ClinGen's RASopathy expert panel consensus methods for variant interpretation. Genet Med 20(11):1334–1345. https://doi.org/10.1038/gim.2018.3
133. Ghosh R et al (2018) Updated recommendation for the benign stand-alone ACMG/AMP criterion. Hum Mutat 39(11):1525–1530. https://doi.org/10.1002/humu.23642
134. Kelly MA et al (2018) Adaptation and validation of the ACMG/AMP variant classification framework for MYH7-associated inherited cardiomyopathies: recommendations by ClinGen's inherited cardiomyopathy expert panel. Genet Med 20(3):351–359. https://doi.org/10.1038/gim.2017.218
135. Lee K et al (2018b) Specifications of the ACMG/AMP variant curation guidelines for the analysis of germline CDH1 sequence variants. Hum Mutat 39(11):1553–1568. https://doi.org/10.1002/humu.23650
136. Mester JL et al (2018) Gene-specific criteria for PTEN variant curation: recommendations from the ClinGen PTEN expert panel. Hum Mutat 39(11):1581–1592. https://doi.org/10.1002/humu.23636
137. Oza AM et al (2018) Expert specification of the ACMG/AMP variant interpretation guidelines for genetic hearing loss. Hum Mutat 39(11):1593–1613. https://doi.org/10.1002/humu.23630

138. Zastrow DB et al (2018) Unique aspects of sequence variant interpretation for inborn errors of metabolism (IEM): the ClinGen IEM working group and the phenylalanine hydroxylase gene. Hum Mutat 39(11):1569–1580. https://doi.org/10.1002/humu.23649
139. Li MM et al (2017) Standards and guidelines for the interpretation and reporting of sequence variants in Cancer. J Mol Diagn 19(1):4–23. https://doi.org/10.1016/j.jmoldx.2016.10.002
140. Patel RY et al (2017) ClinGen pathogenicity calculator: a configurable system for assessing pathogenicity of genetic variants. Genome Med 9(1):3. https://doi.org/10.1186/s13073-016-0391-z
141. Amendola LM et al (2016) Performance of ACMG-AMP variant-interpretation guidelines among nine Laboratories in the Clinical Sequencing Exploratory Research Consortium. Am J Hum Genet 98(6):1067–1076. https://doi.org/10.1016/j.ajhg.2016.03.024
142. Harrison SM et al (2016) Using ClinVar as a resource to support variant interpretation. Curr Protoc Hum Genet 8(16):1–8.16.23. https://doi.org/10.1002/0471142905.hg0816s89. Hoboken, NJ, USA: John Wiley & Sons, Inc.
143. Pepin MG et al (2016) The challenge of comprehensive and consistent sequence variant interpretation between clinical laboratories. Genet Med 18(1):20–24. https://doi.org/10.1038/gim.2015.31
144. Claustres M et al (2014) Recommendations for reporting results of diagnostic genetic testing (biochemical, cytogenetic and molecular genetic). Eur J Hum Genet. 22(2):160–170. https://doi.org/10.1038/ejhg.2013.125
145. Slavin TP et al (2019) The effects of genomic germline variant reclassification on clinical cancer care. Oncotarget 10(4):417–423. https://doi.org/10.18632/oncotarget.26501
146. Ellard S et al (2019) ACGS best practice guidelines for variant classification 2019. Available at: https://www.leedsth.nhs.uk/assets/Genetics-Laboratory/86fa75f316/ACGS-variant-classification-guidelines-2019.pdf. Accessed 2 July 2019.
147. Cheon JY, Mozersky J, Cook-Deegan R (2014) Variants of uncertain significance in BRCA: a harbinger of ethical and policy issues to come? Genome Med 6(12):121. https://doi.org/10.1186/s13073-014-0121-3
148. Brierley KL et al (2010) Errors in delivery of cancer genetics services: implications for practice. Conn Med 74(7):413–423
149. Brierley KL et al (2012) Adverse events in Cancer genetic testing. Cancer J 18(4):303–309. https://doi.org/10.1097/PPO.0b013e3182609490
150. Easton DF et al (2007) A systematic genetic assessment of 1,433 sequence variants of unknown clinical significance in the BRCA1 and BRCA2 breast Cancer–predisposition genes. Am J Hum Genet 81(5):873–883. https://doi.org/10.1086/521032
151. Burke W et al (1997) Recommendations for follow-up care of individuals with an inherited predisposition to cancer. II. BRCA1 and BRCA2. Cancer genetics studies consortium. JAMA 277(12):997–1003
152. Lincoln SE et al (2017) Consistency of BRCA1 and BRCA2 variant classifications among clinical diagnostic laboratories. JCO Precis Oncol 1:1–10. https://doi.org/10.1200/PO.16.00020
153. Vail PJ et al (2015) Comparison of locus-specific databases for BRCA1 and BRCA2 variants reveals disparity in variant classification within and among databases. J Community Genet 6(4):351–359. https://doi.org/10.1007/s12687-015-0220-x
154. Ardern-Jones A et al (2010) Is no news good news? Inconclusive genetic test results in BRCA1 and BRCA2 from patients and professionals' perspectives. Hered Cancer Clin Pract. 8(1):1. https://doi.org/10.1186/1897-4287-8-1
155. Culver J et al (2013) Variants of uncertain significance in BRCA testing: evaluation of surgical decisions, risk perception, and cancer distress. Clin Genet 84(5):464–472. https://doi.org/10.1111/cge.12097
156. Macklin S et al (2018) Observed frequency and challenges of variant reclassification in a hereditary cancer clinic. Genet Med 20(3):346–350. https://doi.org/10.1038/gim.2017.207
157. Mersch J et al (2018) Prevalence of variant reclassification following hereditary Cancer genetic testing. JAMA 320(12):1266. https://doi.org/10.1001/jama.2018.13152

158. Turner SA et al (2019) The impact of variant classification on the clinical management of hereditary cancer syndromes. Genet Med 21(2):426–430. https://doi.org/10.1038/s41436-018-0063-z
159. Wallace AJ (2016) New challenges for BRCA testing: a view from the diagnostic laboratory. Eur J Hum Genet. 24(Suppl 1):S10–S18. https://doi.org/10.1038/ejhg.2016.94
160. De Leeuw JRJ, van Vliet MJ, Ausems MGEM (2008) Predictors of choosing life-long screening or prophylactic surgery in women at high and moderate risk for breast and ovarian cancer. Familial Cancer 7(4):347–359. https://doi.org/10.1007/s10689-008-9189-5
161. Ray JA, Loescher LJ, Brewer M (2005) Risk-reduction surgery decisions in high-risk women seen for genetic counseling. J Genet Couns 14(6):473–484. https://doi.org/10.1007/s10897-005-5833-5
162. McCullum M et al (2007) Time to decide about risk-reducing mastectomy: a case series of BRCA1/2 gene mutation carriers. BMC Women's. Health 7(1):3. https://doi.org/10.1186/1472-6874-7-3
163. Uyei A et al (2006) Association between clinical characteristics and risk-reduction interventions in women who underwent BRCA1 and BRCA2 testing. Cancer 107(12):2745–2751. https://doi.org/10.1002/cncr.22352
164. Crowley E et al (2013) Liquid biopsy: monitoring cancer-genetics in the blood. Nat Rev Clin Oncol 10(8):472–484. https://doi.org/10.1038/nrclinonc.2013.110
165. Speicher MR, Pantel K (2014) Tumor signatures in the blood. Nat Biotechnol 32(5):441–443. https://doi.org/10.1038/nbt.2897
166. Peng M et al (2017) Non-blood circulating tumor DNA detection in cancer. Oncotarget 8(40):69162–69173. https://doi.org/10.18632/oncotarget.19942
167. Lee DH et al (2018a) Urinary Exosomal and cell-free DNA detects somatic mutation and copy number alteration in Urothelial carcinoma of bladder. Sci Rep 8(1):14707. https://doi.org/10.1038/s41598-018-32900-6
168. Lu T, Li J (2017) Clinical applications of urinary cell-free DNA in cancer: current insights and promising future. Am J Cancer Res 7(11):2318–2332
169. Salvi S, Casadio V (2019) Urinary cell-free DNA: potential and applications. Methods Mol Biol 1909:201–209. https://doi.org/10.1007/978-1-4939-8973-7_15
170. Wang X-S et al (2018) Cell-free DNA in blood and urine as a diagnostic tool for bladder cancer: a meta-analysis. Am J Transl Res 10(7):1935–1948
171. Hyun KA et al (2018) Salivary exosome and cell-free DNA for Cancer detection. Micromachines 9(7):340. https://doi.org/10.3390/mi9070340
172. Wang Y et al (2015) Detection of somatic mutations and HPV in the saliva and plasma of patients with head and neck squamous cell carcinomas. Sci Transl Med 7(293):293ra104. https://doi.org/10.1126/scitranslmed.aaa8507
173. Hubers AJ et al (2013) Molecular sputum analysis for the diagnosis of lung cancer. Br J Cancer 109(3):530–537. https://doi.org/10.1038/bjc.2013.393
174. Hulbert A et al (2017) Early detection of lung Cancer using DNA promoter Hypermethylation in plasma and sputum. Clin Cancer Res 23(8):1998–2005. https://doi.org/10.1158/1078-0432.CCR-16-1371
175. Thunnissen FBJM (2003) Sputum examination for early detection of lung cancer. J Clin Pathol 56(11):805–810. https://doi.org/10.1136/jcp.56.11.805
176. Bailey JR, Aggarwal A, Imperiale TF (2016) Colorectal Cancer screening: stool DNA and other noninvasive modalities. Gut Liver. 10(2):204. https://doi.org/10.5009/gnl15420
177. Dhaliwal A et al (2015) Fecal DNA testing for colorectal cancer screening: molecular targets and perspectives. World journal of gastrointestinal. Oncology 7(10):178. https://doi.org/10.4251/wjgo.v7.i10.178
178. Olmedillas-López S et al (2017) Detection of KRAS G12D in colorectal cancer stool by droplet digital PCR. World J Gastroenterol 23(39):7087–7097. https://doi.org/10.3748/wjg.v23.i39.7087

179. Li Y et al (2016) Tumor DNA in cerebral spinal fluid reflects clinical course in a patient with melanoma leptomeningeal brain metastases. J Neuro-Oncol 128(1):93–100. https://doi.org/10.1007/s11060-016-2081-5
180. Miller AM et al (2019) Tracking tumour evolution in glioma through liquid biopsies of cerebrospinal fluid. Nature 565(7741):654–658. https://doi.org/10.1038/s41586-019-0882-3
181. Pan W et al (2015) Brain tumor mutations detected in cerebral spinal fluid. Clin Chem 61(3):514–522. https://doi.org/10.1373/clinchem.2014.235457
182. Wang Y et al (2016) Diagnostic potential of tumor DNA from ovarian cyst fluid. elife 5:e15175. https://doi.org/10.7554/eLife.15175
183. Pizzi MP et al (2019) Identification of DNA mutations in gastric washes from gastric adenocarcinoma patients: possible implications for liquid biopsies and patient follow-up. Int J Cancer 145(4):1090–1098. https://doi.org/10.1002/ijc.32217
184. Bedard PL et al (2013) Tumour heterogeneity in the clinic. Nature 501(7467):355–364. https://doi.org/10.1038/nature12627
185. Cheung AH-K, Chow C, To K-F (2018) Latest development of liquid biopsy. J Thorac Dis 10(S14):S1645. https://doi.org/10.21037/jtd.2018.04.68
186. Ashworth TR (1869) A case of Cancer in which cells similar to those in the Tumours were seen in the blood after death. Med J Aust 14:146–147
187. Mandel P, Metais P (1948) Les acides nucléiques du plasma sanguin chez l'homme. Comptes rendus des seances de la Societe de biologie et de ses filiales 142(3–4):241–243
188. El-Heliebi A, Heitzer E (2019) State of the art and future direction for the analysis of cell-free circulating DNA. In: Nucleic acid nanotheranostics. Elsevier, Amsterdam, pp 133–188. https://doi.org/10.1016/B978-0-12-814470-1.00005-8
189. Neumann MHD et al (2018) ctDNA and CTCs in liquid biopsy – current status and where we need to Progress. Comput Struct Biotechnol J 16:190–195. https://doi.org/10.1016/j.csbj.2018.05.002
190. Aceto N et al (2015) En route to metastasis: circulating tumor cell clusters and epithelial-to-Mesenchymal transition. Trends Cancer 1(1):44–52. https://doi.org/10.1016/j.trecan.2015.07.006
191. Castro-Giner F et al (2018) Cancer diagnosis using a liquid biopsy: challenges and expectations. Diagnostics 8(2):31. https://doi.org/10.3390/diagnostics8020031
192. Bronkhorst AJ, Ungerer V, Holdenrieder S (2019) The emerging role of cell-free DNA as a molecular marker for cancer management. Biomol Detect quantif 17:100087. https://doi.org/10.1016/j.bdq.2019.100087
193. Chin RI et al (2019) Detection of solid tumor molecular residual disease (MRD) using circulating tumor DNA (ctDNA). Mol Diagn Ther 23(3):311–331. https://doi.org/10.1007/s40291-019-00390-5
194. Goodwin S, McPherson JD, McCombie WR (2016) Coming of age: ten years of next-generation sequencing technologies. Nat Rev Genet 17(6):333–351. https://doi.org/10.1038/nrg.2016.49
195. Heitzer E, Ulz P, Geigl JB (2015) Circulating tumor DNA as a liquid biopsy for Cancer. Clin Chem 61(1):112–123. https://doi.org/10.1373/clinchem.2014.222679
196. Forshew T et al (2012) Noninvasive identification and monitoring of Cancer mutations by targeted deep sequencing of plasma DNA. Sci Transl Med 4(136):136ra68. https://doi.org/10.1126/scitranslmed.3003726
197. Kinde I et al (2011) Detection and quantification of rare mutations with massively parallel sequencing. Proc Natl Acad Sci 108(23):9530–9535. https://doi.org/10.1073/pnas.1105422108
198. Genetic Alliance (2019) Genetic testing: understanding your genes and what they mean for your health. Available at: http://www.geneticalliance.org/advocacy/policyissues/genetictesting. Accessed 2 Aug 2019.
199. NIH (National Institutes of Health) (2019) Help me understand genetics. How can consumers be sure a genetic test is valid and useful? Available at: https://ghr.nlm.nih.gov/primer/testing/validtest. Accessed 2 Aug 2019

200. WHO (World Health Organization) (2019) Quality & safety in genetic testing: an emerging concern. Available at: https://www.who.int/genomics/policy/quality_safety. Accessed 2 Aug 2019
201. National Academies of Sciences, Engineering, and Medicine et al (2017) An evidence framework for genetic testing - 3, genetic test assessment. Available at: https://www.ncbi.nlm.nih.gov/books/NBK425803. Accessed 2 Aug 2019
202. NHGRI (National Human Genome Research Institute) (2018) Regulation of genetic tests. Available at: https://www.genome.gov/about-genomics/policy-issues/Regulation-of-Genetic-Tests. Accessed 2 Aug 2019
203. PHG Foundation (2007) Moving beyond ACCE: an expanded framework for genetic test evaluation. Available at: http://www.phgfoundation.org/documents/369_1409657043.pdf. Accessed 2 Aug 2019
204. Zimmern RL, Kroese M (2007) The evaluation of genetic tests. J Public Health 29(3):246–225. https://doi.org/10.1093/pubmed/fdm028
205. Luh F, Yen Y (2018) FDA guidance for next generation sequencing-based testing: balancing regulation and innovation in precision medicine. NPJ Genom Med 3:28. https://doi.org/10.1038/s41525-018-0067-2
206. Gaff CL et al (2017) Preparing for genomic medicine: a real world demonstration of health system change. NPJ Genom Med 2(1):16. https://doi.org/10.1038/s41525-017-0017-4
207. Rizzo JM, Buck MJ (2012) Key principles and clinical applications of 'next-generation' DNA sequencing. Cancer Prev Res 5(7):887–900. https://doi.org/10.1158/1940-6207.CAPR-11-0432
208. Schrijver I et al (2012) Opportunities and challenges associated with clinical diagnostic genome sequencing: a report of the Association for Molecular Pathology. J Mol Diagn 14(6):525–540. https://doi.org/10.1016/j.jmoldx.2012.04.006
209. Middleton A et al (2017) The role of genetic counsellors in genomic healthcare in the United Kingdom: a statement by the Association of Genetic Nurses and Counsellors. Eur J Hum Genet 25(6):659–661. https://doi.org/10.1038/ejhg.2017.28
210. Olopade OI, Pichert G (2001) Cancer genetics in oncology practice. Ann Oncol 12(7):895–908. https://doi.org/10.1023/A:1011176107455
211. Hall MJ et al (2014) Gene panel testing for inherited cancer risk. J Natl Compr Cancer Netw 12(9):1339–1346
212. John T, Liu G, Tsao M-S (2009) Overview of molecular testing in non-small-cell lung cancer: mutational analysis, gene copy number, protein expression and other biomarkers of EGFR for the prediction of response to tyrosine kinase inhibitors. Oncogene 28(S1):S14–S23. https://doi.org/10.1038/onc.2009.197
213. Stoffel EM (2010) Lynch syndrome/hereditary non-polyposis colorectal Cancer (HNPCC). Minerva Gastroenterol Dietol 56(1):45–53
214. Cohen JD et al (2018) Detection and localization of surgically resectable cancers with a multi-analyte blood test. Science 359(6378):926–930. https://doi.org/10.1126/science.aar3247
215. Loeian MS et al (2019) Liquid biopsy using the nanotube-CTC-chip: capture of invasive CTCs with high purity using preferential adherence in breast cancer patients. Lab Chip 19(11):1899–1915. https://doi.org/10.1039/C9LC00274J
216. Serrano MJ et al (2014) EMT and EGFR in CTCs cytokeratin negative non-metastatic breast cancer. Oncotarget 5(17):7486–7497. https://doi.org/10.18632/oncotarget.2217
217. Xu R et al (2018) Extracellular vesicles in cancer — implications for future improvements in cancer care. Nat Rev Clin Oncol 15(10):617–638. https://doi.org/10.1038/s41571-018-0036-9
218. Rahbarghazi R et al (2019) Tumor-derived extracellular vesicles: reliable tools for Cancer diagnosis and clinical applications. Cell Commun Signal 17(1):73. https://doi.org/10.1186/s12964-019-0390-y
219. Gao D, Jiang L (2018) Exosomes in cancer therapy: a novel experimental strategy. Am J Cancer Res 8(11):2165–2175

220. McKiernan J et al (2016) A novel urine exosome gene expression assay to predict high-grade prostate Cancer at initial biopsy. JAMA Oncology 2(7):882. https://doi.org/10.1001/jamaoncol.2016.0097
221. Snyder A et al (2014) Genetic basis for clinical response to CTLA-4 blockade in melanoma. N Engl J Med 371(23):2189–2199. https://doi.org/10.1056/NEJMoa1406498
222. Chalmers ZR et al (2017) Analysis of 100,000 human cancer genomes reveals the landscape of tumor mutational burden. Genome Med 9(1):34. https://doi.org/10.1186/s13073-017-0424-2
223. Chan TA et al (2019) Development of tumor mutation burden as an immunotherapy biomarker: utility for the oncology clinic. Ann Oncol 30(1):44–56. https://doi.org/10.1093/annonc/mdy495
224. Zehir A et al (2017) Mutational landscape of metastatic cancer revealed from prospective clinical sequencing of 10,000 patients. Nat Med 23(6):703–713. https://doi.org/10.1038/nm.4333
225. Büttner R et al (2019) Implementing TMB measurement in clinical practice: considerations on assay requirements. ESMO Open 4(1):e000442. https://doi.org/10.1136/esmoopen-2018-000442
226. Samstein RM et al (2019) Tumor mutational load predicts survival after immunotherapy across multiple cancer types. Nat Genet 51(2):202–206. https://doi.org/10.1038/s41588-018-0312-8
227. Chowell D et al (2018) Patient HLA class I genotype influences cancer response to checkpoint blockade immunotherapy. Science 359(6375):582–587. https://doi.org/10.1126/science.aao4572
228. Zaretsky JM et al (2016) Mutations associated with acquired resistance to PD-1 blockade in melanoma. N Engl J Med 375(9):819–829. https://doi.org/10.1056/NEJMoa1604958
229. Mariathasan S et al (2018) TGFβ attenuates tumour response to PD-L1 blockade by contributing to exclusion of T cells. Nature 554(7693):544–548. https://doi.org/10.1038/nature25501
230. Banerjee T et al (2008) A key in vivo antitumor mechanism of action of natural product-based brassinins is inhibition of indoleamine 2,3-dioxygenase. Oncogene 27(20):2851–2857. https://doi.org/10.1038/sj.onc.1210939
231. Pardi N et al (2018) mRNA vaccines — a new era in vaccinology. Nat Rev Drug Discov 17(4):261–279. https://doi.org/10.1038/nrd.2017.243
232. Pastor F et al (2018) An RNA toolbox for cancer immunotherapy. Nat Rev Drug Discov 17(10):751–767. https://doi.org/10.1038/nrd.2018.132
233. Kowalski PS et al (2019) Delivering the messenger: advances in technologies for therapeutic mRNA delivery. Mol Ther 27(4):710–728. https://doi.org/10.1016/j.ymthe.2019.02.012
234. Burris HA et al (2019) A phase I multicenter study to assess the safety, tolerability, and immunogenicity of mRNA-4157 alone in patients with resected solid tumors and in combination with pembrolizumab in patients with unresectable solid tumors. J Clin Oncol 37(15_suppl):2523–2523. https://doi.org/10.1200/JCO.2019.37.15_suppl.2523
235. Cafri G et al (2019) Immunogenicity and tolerability of personalized mRNA vaccine mRNA-4650 encoding defined neoantigens expressed by the autologous cancer. J Clin Oncol 37(15_suppl):2643. https://doi.org/10.1200/JCO.2019.37.15_suppl.2643
236. Sullenger BA, Nair S (2016) From the RNA world to the clinic. Science 352(6292):1417–1420. https://doi.org/10.1126/science.aad8709
237. Bobbin ML, Rossi JJ (2016) RNA interference (RNAi)-based therapeutics: delivering on the promise? Annu Rev Pharmacol Toxicol 56(1):103–122. https://doi.org/10.1146/annurev-pharmtox-010715-103633
238. Xin Y et al (2017) Nano-based delivery of RNAi in cancer therapy. Mol Cancer 16(1):134. https://doi.org/10.1186/s12943-017-0683-y
239. Cox DBT, Platt RJ, Zhang F (2015) Therapeutic genome editing: prospects and challenges. Nat Med 21(2):121–131. https://doi.org/10.1038/nm.3793
240. Kim H, Kim J (2014) A guide to genome engineering with programmable nucleases. Nat Rev Genet 15(5):321–334. https://doi.org/10.1038/nrg3686

241. Gori JL et al (2015) Delivery and specificity of CRISPR/Cas9 genome editing Technologies for Human Gene Therapy. Hum Gene Ther 26(7):443–451. https://doi.org/10.1089/hum.2015.074
242. Yang H et al (2018) Break breast Cancer addiction by CRISPR/Cas9 genome editing. J Cancer 9(2):219–231. https://doi.org/10.7150/jca.22554
243. Zhan T et al (2019) CRISPR/Cas9 for cancer research and therapy. Semin Cancer Biol 55:106–119. https://doi.org/10.1016/j.semcancer.2018.04.001
244. Tian X et al (2019) CRISPR/Cas9 – an evolving biological tool kit for cancer biology and oncology. NPJ Precis Oncol 3(1):8. https://doi.org/10.1038/s41698-019-0080-7
245. Alexander JL, Kohoutova D, Powell N (2019) Science in focus: the microbiome and Cancer therapy. Clin Oncol 31(1):1–4. https://doi.org/10.1016/j.clon.2018.09.004
246. Garrett WS (2015) Cancer and the microbiota. Science 348(6230):80–86. https://doi.org/10.1126/science.aaa4972
247. Garrett WS (2019) The gut microbiota and colon cancer. Science 364(6446):1133–1135. https://doi.org/10.1126/science.aaw2367
248. Kroemer G, Zitvogel L (2018) Cancer immunotherapy in 2017: the breakthrough of the microbiota. Nature reviews. Immunology 18(2):87–88. https://doi.org/10.1038/nri.2018.4
249. Iida N et al (2013) Commensal bacteria control cancer response to therapy by modulating the tumor microenvironment. Science 342(6161):967–970. https://doi.org/10.1126/science.1240527
250. York A (2018) Microbiome: gut microbiota sways response to cancer immunotherapy. Nature reviews. Microbiology 16(3):121. https://doi.org/10.1038/nrmicro.2018.12
251. Gopalakrishnan V et al (2018) Gut microbiome modulates response to anti-PD-1 immunotherapy in melanoma patients. Science 359(6371):97–103. https://doi.org/10.1126/science.aan4236
252. Zitvogel L et al (2018) The microbiome in cancer immunotherapy: diagnostic tools and therapeutic strategies. Science 359(6382):1366–1370. https://doi.org/10.1126/science.aar6918
253. Roy S, Trinchieri G (2017) Microbiota: a key orchestrator of cancer therapy. Nature reviews. Cancer 17(5):271–285. https://doi.org/10.1038/nrc.2017.13
254. Schwartzberg L et al (2017) Precision oncology: who, how, what, when, and when not? Am Soc Clin Oncol Educ Book 37:160–169. https://doi.org/10.1200/EDBK_174176
255. Iriart JAB (2019) Medicina de precisão/medicina personalizada: análise crítica dos movimentos de transformação da biomedicina no início do século XXI. Cad Saude Publica 35(3):e00153118. https://doi.org/10.1590/0102-311x00153118

MIX
Papier aus verantwortungsvollen Quellen
Paper from responsible sources
FSC® C105338

If you have any concerns about our products,
you can contact us on
ProductSafety@springernature.com

In case Publisher is established outside the EU,
the EU authorized representative is:
Springer Nature Customer Service Center GmbH
Europaplatz 3, 69115 Heidelberg, Germany

Printed by Libri Plureos GmbH
in Hamburg, Germany